# Biological Activities of Steroids
## in Relation to Cancer

# Biological Activities of Steroids
# in Relation to Cancer

Proceedings of a Conference Sponsored by the
Cancer Chemotherapy National Service Center,
National Cancer Institute, National Institutes of
Health, U. S. Department of Health, Education
and Welfare

*EDITED BY*
Gregory Pincus and Erwin P. Vollmer

COMMITTEE ON ARRANGEMENTS

D. M. BERGENSTAL          E. JENSEN
M. GRAFF                  G. PINCUS
A. HILGAR                 D. J. TAYLOR
D. INGLE                  E. P. VOLLMER
              G. WOOLLEY

1960

ACADEMIC PRESS • New York and London

ACADEMIC PRESS INC.
111 FIFTH AVENUE
NEW YORK 3, N. Y.

*United Kingdom Edition*
Published by
ACADEMIC PRESS INC. (LONDON) LTD.
17 OLD QUEEN STREET, LONDON S.W. 1

*Library of Congress Catalog Card Number 60-14263*

PRINTED IN THE UNITED STATES OF AMERICA

*This volume is dedicated to the memory of*

DELBERT M. BERGENSTAL

*a devoted colleague and leader*

*in the fight against cancer*

# Contributors

FRED J. ANSFIELD, *University of Wisconsin Medical School, Madison, Wisconsin*

WILLIAM H. BAKER, *The John Collins Warren Laboratories of the Huntington Memorial Hospital of Harvard University at the Tumor Clinic of the Massachusetts General Hospital, Boston, Massachusetts*

D. M. BERGENSTAL, *Endocrinology Branch, National Cancer Institute, National Institutes of Health, Bethesda, Maryland*

BARBARA J. BOWMAN, *Department of Endocrinology, The Upjohn Company, Kalamazoo, Michigan*

HERBERT BRENDLER, *New York University School of Medicine, Bellevue Medical Center, New York, New York*

M. J. BRENNAN, *Oncology Division, Henry Ford Hospital, and Detroit Institute of Cancer Research, Detroit, Michigan*

ANNE C. CARTER, *The State University of New York, College of Medicine at New York City, and the Medical Service (Division II) Kings County Hospital, Brooklyn, New York*

WILLIAM H. DAUGHADAY, *Metabolism Division, Department of Medicine, Washington University School of Medicine, St. Louis, Missouri*

MARGARIDA M. DEDERICK, *Division of Oncology, Medical Services, Lemuel Shattuck Hospital, and Department of Medicine, Harvard Medical School, Boston, Massachusetts*

RALPH I. DORFMAN, *Worcester Foundation for Experimental Biology, Shrewsbury, Massachusetts*

VICTOR A. DRILL, *Research Laboratories, G. D. Searle and Company, Chicago, Illinois*

W. F. DUNNING, *Cancer Research Laboratory, University of Miami, Coral Gables, Florida*

EUGENE EISENBERG, *Department of Medicine, University of California School of Medicine, San Francisco, California*

LEWIS L. ENGEL, *The John Collins Warren Laboratories of the Collis P. Huntington Memorial Hospital of Harvard University at the Massachusetts General Hospital, and the Department of Biological Chemistry, Harvard Medical School, Boston, Massachusetts*

GEORGE C. ESCHER, *The State University of New York, College of Medicine at New York City, and The Medical Service (Division II) Kings County Hospital, Brooklyn, New York*

ELAINE BOSSAK FELDMAN, *The State University of New York, College of Medicine at New York City, and the Medical Service (Division II) Kings County Hospital, Brooklyn, New York*

JOSEF FRIED, *The Squibb Institute for Medical Research, New Brunswick, New Jersey*

E. MYLES GLENN, *Department of Endocrinology, The Upjohn Company, Kalamazoo, Michigan*

IRA S. GOLDENBERG, *Department of Surgery, Yale University School of Medicine, New Haven, Connecticut*

THOMAS C. HALL, *Division of Oncology, Medical Services, Lemuel Shattuck Hospital, Boston, Massachusetts*

JOHN J. HARRIS, *Division of Human Tumor Experimental Chemotherapy, Sloan-Kettering Institute for Cancer Research, and Sloan-Kettering Division Cornell University Medical College, New York, New York*

MARK A. HAYES, *Department of Surgery, Yale University School of Medicine, New Haven, Connecticut*

ROY HERTZ, *Endocrinology Branch, National Cancer Institute, National Institutes of Health, Bethesda, Maryland*

CHARLES HUGGINS, *The Ben May Laboratory for Cancer Research, The University of Chicago, Chicago, Illinois*

ROBERT A. HUSEBY, *Department of Surgery, University of Colorado Medical Center, Denver, Colorado*[1]

HERBERT I. JACOBSON, *The Ben May Laboratory for Cancer Research, The University of Chicago, Chicago, Illinois*

ELWOOD V. JENSEN, *The Ben May Laboratory for Cancer Research, The University of Chicago, Chicago, Illinois*

RITA M. KELLEY, *Department of Medicine, Massachusetts General Hospital, Boston, Massachusetts, and Department of Medicine, Pondville Hospital, Walpole, Massachusetts*

SYDNEY KOFMAN, *University of Illinois College of Medicine and Department of Medicine, Presbyterian-St. Luke's Hospital, Chicago, Illinois*

SHUTSUNG LIAO, *The Ben May Laboratory for Cancer Research, and Department of Biochemistry, The University of Chicago, Chicago, Illinois*

S. LIEBERMAN, *Departments of Obstetrics and Gynecology and of Biochemistry, College of Physicians and Surgeons, Columbia University, New York, New York*

---

[1] *Present address:* Eleanor Roosevelt Institute for Cancer Research, American Medical Center, Denver, Colorado.

M. B. Lipsett, *Endocrinology Branch, National Cancer Institute, National Institutes of Health, Bethesda, Maryland*

Stanley C. Lyster, *Department of Endocrinology, The Upjohn Company, Kalamazoo, Michigan*

Ida Kozak Mariz, *Metabolism Division, Department of Medicine, Washington University School of Medicine, St. Louis, Missouri*

Philip C. Merker, *Division of Human Tumor Experimental Chemotherapy, Sloan-Kettering Institute for Cancer Research, and Sloan-Kettering Division Cornell University Medical College, New York, New York*

R. H. Moy, *Endocrinology Branch, National Cancer Institute, National Institutes of Health, Bethesda, Maryland*

O. Mühlbock, *The Netherlands Cancer Institute, Amsterdam, The Netherlands*

Gerald C. Mueller, *The McArdle Memorial Laboratory, The University of Wisconsin Medical School, Madison, Wisconsin*

P. J. Murison, *Alton Ochsner Medical Foundation, and Tulane University School of Medicine, New Orleans, Louisiana*

Hans B. Nevinny, *Division of Oncology, Medical Services, Lemuel Shattuck Hospital, and Harvard Medical School, Boston, Massachusetts*

Kenneth B. Olson, *Albany Medical College, Albany, New York*

Joy E. Palm, *Division of Human Tumor Experimental Chemotherapy, Sloan-Kettering Institute for Cancer Research, and Sloan-Kettering Division Cornell University Medical College, New York, New York[2]*

Mary Ellen Patno, *Department of Statistics, University of Michigan, Ann Arbor, Michigan*

Charles P. Perlia, *Department of Medical Oncology of Presbyterian-St. Luke's Hospital and the Department of Medicine, University of Illinois, College of Medicine, Chicago, Illinois*

S. Lee Richardson, *Department of Endocrinology, The Upjohn Company, Kalamazoo, Michigan*

E. L. Rongone, *Alton Ochsner Medical Foundation, and Tulane University School of Medicine, New Orleans, Louisiana*

Chester B. Rosoff, *Department of Surgery, Beth Israel Hospital, and Harvard Medical School, Boston, Massachusetts*

William Wallace Scott, *The James Buchanan Brady Urological Institute, The Johns Hopkins Hospital, Baltimore, Maryland*

---

[2] *Present address:* Wistar Institute of Anatomy and Biology, Philadelphia, Pennsylvania.

ALBERT SEGALOFF, *Alton Ochsner Medical Foundation, and Tulane University School of Medicine, New Orleans, Louisiana*

W. L. SIMPSON, *Detroit Institute of Cancer Research, and Department of Pathology, Wayne State University College of Medicine, Detroit, Michigan*

HOWARD H. SKY-PECK, *Department of Biochemistry, University of Illinois College of Medicine and Department of Medicine, Presbyterian-St. Luke's Hospital, Chicago, Illinois*

PAUL SPEAR, *Veterans Administration Hospital, Brooklyn, New York*

P. TALALAY, *The Ben May Laboratory for Cancer Research, and Department of Biochemistry, The University of Chicago, Chicago, Illinois*

SAMUEL G. TAYLOR, III, *Department of Medical Oncology of Presbyterian-St. Luke's Hospital, and Department of Medicine, University of Illinois College of Medicine, Chicago, Illinois*

MORRIS N. TELLER, *Division of Human Tumor Experimental Chemotherapy, Sloan-Kettering Institute for Cancer Research, and Sloan-Kettering Division Cornell University Medical College, New York, New York*

R. VANDEWIELE, *Departments of Obstetrics and Gynecology and of Biochemistry, College of Physicians and Surgeons, Columbia University, New York, New York*

ELEANOR Z. WALLACE, *The State University of New York, College of Medicine at New York City, and the Medical Service (Division II) Kings County Hospital, Brooklyn, New York*

J. B. WEETH, *Alton Ochsner Medical Foundation, and Tulane University School of Medicine, New Orleans, Louisiana*

H. G. WILLIAMS-ASHMAN, *The Ben May Laboratory for Cancer Research, and Department of Biochemistry, The University of Chicago, Chicago, Illinois*

RICHARD J. WINZLER, *Department of Biological Chemistry, The University of Illinois College of Medicine, Chicago, Illinois*

JULIUS WOLF, *Medical Service, Veterans Administration Hospital, Bronx, New York*

GEORGE W. WOOLLEY, *Division of Human Tumor Experimental Chemotherapy, Sloan-Kettering Institute for Cancer Research, and Sloan-Kettering Division Cornell University Medical College, New York, New York*

RAYMOND YESNER, *Laboratory Service, Veterans Administration Hospital, West Haven, Connecticut*

# Preface

More than a half century has passed since Beatson showed that excision of the ovaries might be followed by substantial improvement in the condition of patients with breast cancer. Since then much clinical and experimental evidence has implicated the endocrine system in the development, and inferentially in the cure, of this and other types of cancer; but progress in therapy has been disappointingly slow. Perhaps it was because of this promise and this disappointment that the endocrine field was designated to receive special attention in the cancer chemotherapy program set up by the National Cancer Institute in 1955. By the middle of 1956 an endocrinological research program was under way in the Cancer Chemotherapy National Service Center.

Since its beginning, this program has centered about the study of steroids. This apparent preoccupation did not arise from conviction on the part of the advisors—the Endocrinology Panel—that steroids alone were important in the endocrine aspects of the cancer problem. Rather, it was the result of practical considerations, in particular the burgeoning availability of new synthetic steroids, and the parallel accumulation of rich veins of biological information about these compounds. Moreover, the implication of steroids in carcinogenesis and the treatment of tumors, clinical as well as experimental, seemed more clear-cut than that of other endocrine factors. This was the outstanding field of challenge, and the one which seemed to offer the most proximate rewards.

By 1958 a considerable enterprise of steroid procurement and testing was under way. The compounds procured were being assayed for hormonal properties and screened against animal tumors. A number of clinicians, who warmly supported the program from the beginning, formed cooperative groups to subject steroids to careful trials against cancer of the breast and prostate. Also by 1958, the Endocrinology Panel foresaw the need for extensive review and evaluation of such a program. Scientists from diverse fields had become party to the effort, and almost the only word common to their vocabularies was "steroid." There was a need to know not only whether the program was on a promising course, but also, of what the promise of its course consisted. This could be answered best by showing that the program, in its various parts, would ring true in forum with those parts of contemporary science that were relevant. For this reason the Panel recommended evaluation of the first phase of its program in the form of a conference rather than a committee report. The result was the "Conference on the Biological Activities of Steroids in Relation to Cancer," attended by more than 200 scientists at Vergennes, Vermont, September 27 to October 2, 1959. This book is the record of that conference.

These meetings did not lead directly to solutions, and had not been expected to do so. If there was any consensus, it was more a postulate than a conclusion: that the role of steroids in tumor genesis, growth, and regression involves more than a simple drug—target tissue relationship. The phenomena involved range from cell—steroid interaction to steroid metabolic events and repercussing systemic effects. These must be taken into account in the interpretation of clinical results. This postulate on the role of hormones in cancer does not make clinical trial any easier than before, but it does, we believe, bring clinical trial closer to grips with the deceptive natural history of endocrine-conditioned neoplasms.

Conferences of this sort are not conceived and carried through to term without labor. The planning committee—five panel members and four members of the staff—met to draw up the program and set the rules for procedure. This stage was exciting, more pleasure than work. The day-to-day work came later, and in this connection more acknowledgments are due than can be made here. First, we must thank the speakers and other participants, whose contributions made up the substance of the conference. Secondly, we have many to thank in connection with the mechanics of the meeting and the subsequent documentation. Mr. Robert Beach was ubiquitously helpful at the meeting site, and Mr. Werner Ferch produced remarkably complete recordings of discussions. We are particularly indebted to Mrs. Doyn R. Scruggs, Mrs. Georgia Becker, Mrs. Mary Jiuliano, and Mrs. Mabel Jacobson for their able rendering of sound transcriptions into typed manuscript, and a variety of similar tasks. Finally, we wish to thank Miss Gladys Kauffmann for her truly exceptional assistance in editing the manuscripts and galleys, and in preparing the glossary of terms and the index.

*August 1960*

Gregory Pincus
Erwin P. Vollmer

# Contents

# I. INTRODUCTION

## Steroids, Growth, and Cancer[1]

CHARLES HUGGINS

*The Ben May Laboratory for Cancer Research, University of Chicago, Chicago, Illinois*

Just thirty years ago, E. A. Doisy (3) isolated the first crystalline steroid hormone and in so doing initiated an epoch of steroid endocrinology. Since this discovery of estrone in 1929, many hundreds of steroids with biological activity have been isolated as natural products or have been synthesized. Much has been learned about the physiological activity of these compounds and the pathological effects which they evoke. The administration, or the withdrawal, of steroids is now commonly used in medical practice, often with great benefit to patients. Lagging somewhat behind the great developments of steroid chemistry, physiology, and medicine, a significant beginning has recently been made in the biochemistry of modes of action of steroids (19–22). Without doubt, the ensemble represents one of the most brilliant chapters of science and medicine.

In the last three decades it has been established that the hormones which influence growth occupy a place near the center of the cancer problem—in the neoplasms of man and the animals and of plants as well and in the cause or prevention or the treatment of cancer. Tumors of many organs have been induced in susceptible rodents following the administration of steroids (reviewed in 4); only phenolic estrogens have been firmly established in this cancerogenic role in animals. The incidence of hormone-induced cancer of animals is always reduced by appropriate modifications of their endocrine status, and many of these cancers can be absolutely prevented by endocrine means (4).

Moreover, in certain patients it is possible to induce a profound regression of widely disseminated cancer, even in the terminal stages of the disease, by modification of the hormonal status of the host (11). These witherings of extensive cancer, which can last more than a decade in favorable cases, are accompanied by clinical improvement with return to health. Here, alteration of the tumor-host relationship has content and meaning to cancerous man. It is now certain that hormones can be of great significance in the maintenance of four neoplasms those of the breast (7), the prostate, the thyroid gland (17), and also the lymphomas (16).

---

[1] This study was aided by grants from The Jane Coffin Childs Memorial Fund for Medical Research, the American Cancer Society, and the Public Health Service.

1

The control of cancer by hormonal means rests on two principles (5). (*a*) Cancer is not necessarily autonomous. Cancer cells do not differ from normal cells as black differs from white. When the cells of origin of a cancer are dependent on hormones for metabolic activity at a high rate, the cancers derived therefrom can be similarly dependent and both cancer and normal cells undergo atrophy when hormonal support is withdrawn, and this can be accomplished by a number of means; such tumors are by definition *hormone-dependent* tumors. (*b*) The second principle is that cancer can be sustained by hormonal function that is not exaggerated in rate or abnormal in kind, but which is operating at normal or even subnormal levels. It is now appreciated that trace amounts of hormones can lead to such exuberant neoplastic growth that they cause death of the host.

The concept of hormone dependence of cancer arose from a study of prostatic tumors, first of the dog (9) and then of man (11). These common neoplasms of elderly males of these species were found to be dependent on steroids of the androstane series, since in most cases the tumors regress after antiandrogenic measures. Aside from some practical clinical by-products, the significance of this work was the concept that cancer in living creatures could no longer be regarded as a lawless growth; cancer has its laws and these it is forced to obey. Historically, diethylstilbestrol used in the treatment of prostatic cancer (11) happened to be the beginning of chemotherapy of cancer.

The influence of the administration or the withdrawal of steroids on prostatic neoplasms was found out by orderly development in the laboratory, and the hormonal treatment of human prostatic cancer merely represented a transposition of the findings in the experimental animal to man. The discovery of the relation of the endocrine system to human mammary cancer was far different. Many of the most significant facts known about human mammary cancer emerged first in the clinic without the support of preliminary basic experimental observations.

Mammary cancer is one of the most lofty problems of medicine. Cancer of the breast has the highest rate of prevalence of any form of neoplastic disease, in either sex, in three species—man, dog, and mouse. In man and mouse, mammary cancer commonly progresses with relatively great speed and ferocity; in the dog, it grows indolently.

Two difficulties hindered the development in the laboratory of methods for the control of human mammary cancer. First, the biological characteristics of human mammary carcinoma differ significantly from those of canine and murine cancer of the breast. Unfortunately, in contrast to some types of human mammary cancer, carcinoma of the breast of the dog or mouse is not hormone dependent. Removal of the pituitary or the steroid-producing glands induced no remission after mammary cancers of the mouse had reached palpable size (15). Similarly, removal of the ovaries or the adrenals did not effect a diminution in size of canine mammary cancer (12). Until recently (6), there has been no experimental counterpart of human mammary cancer which could be forced to regress by endocrine means, a spectacular phenomenon often observed in the clinic.

A second difficulty in mammary cancer research is that the induction of cancer of the breast in the mouse is very slow; frequently many months or as long as two years elapsed after the inception of an experiment in murine mammary cancer before cancer of the breast developed in this species. For most purposes, two years is an inordinately long time for an experiment in biology. It was necessary to find a species of animal other than dog or mouse whose mammary cancers would be hormone dependent and to devise rapid methods for their induction. These tasks were not difficult.

The rapid and simple method to achieve these goals consisted of the administration of maximal amounts, compatible with life, of 3-methylcholanthrene (3-MC) to young, adult female rats of a *special strain* by way of the gastrointestinal tract. The method is an outgrowth of the Maisin effect.

Research methods for the investigation of mammary cancer have been developed in a discontinuous series of events, often with long intervals between significant discoveries.

Three years after the discovery of estrone, Lacassagne (13) injected this hormone into three male mice of special strain and mammary cancer developed in each of them after 5 months. Lacassagne raised but left unanswered two interpretations of this important experiment: (1) Estrone in provoking the maintenance of the mammary gland of the male mice has only permitted a latent hereditary characteristic (the predisposition to cancer of the breast) to manifest itself in furnishing an anatomical substrate. (2) The excitation produced by the hormone in the mammary region has been the determining cause of mammary cancer.

Soon it was learned that mammary cancer can be evoked by aromatic compounds devoid of hormonal activity. Wieland and Dane (23) prepared 3-methylcholanthrene by degradation of deoxycholic acid in 1933. Maisin and Coolen (14) painted the skin of mice with 3-methylcholanthrene and found that, in addition to skin cancer, carcinoma of the mammary gland developed in high incidence. Bielschowsky (2) induced mammary cancer in the rat by incorporating in the diet another carcinogen, 2-acetylaminofluorene (2 AAF). Armstrong and Bonser (1) were among the first to employ gastric intubation for the administration of a carcinogen (2-AAF). Shay et al. (18) fed 3-methylcholanthrene, 2 mg. daily, to rats by stomach tube. In Shay's experiments mammary tumors developed in 100% of the females in 129–383 days. The incidence of mammary cancer was invariable, but a long time was required to induce the tumors.

## Rapid Development of Mammary Cancer

This technique arose from a systematic quantitative investigation of the relative effectiveness of carcinogenic hydrocarbons in evoking mammary cancer when administered via the gastrointestinal tract. All the experiments were conducted on *female albino rats of the Sprague-Dawley strain* and the administration of the carcinogens by gastric intubation was started at age 50 days; *dosage refers to the amount of carcinogen administered daily 6 days each week for 50 days*. The most effective carcinogen was 3-methyl-cholanthrene and the optimal dose was 10 mg.

After the administration of 3-MC, 2 mg., the first mammary cancer was detected at 69 days, and some rats were free from mammary cancer after 9 months; this finding confirmed an observation of Shay *et al.* (18). Doses of 5 mg. or 10 mg. elicited mammary cancer in all rats, the rate of their development being faster with a dosage level of 10 mg. Severe toxicity was evident when the dosage of 3-MC was increased to 15 mg.; at a dosage of 20 mg., all rats died before any mammary cancer developed.

There were 314 animals in 30 consecutive series of adult Sprague-Dawley females fed 3-MC, 10 mg., 6 days each week for 50 days beginning at age 50 days. Everyone of these rats developed mammary cancer and all within 92 days: range 29–92 days, mean $53.1 \pm 9.4$ days. In this series of 314 rats, there were 14 animals (4.46 %) which developed mammary cancer in 70–92 days. Significantly, no rat developed a tumor of the liver. Mammary cancer was always the first tumor to be observed, and often it was the only neoplasm to develop. Why does fed 3-MC have an overwhelming and highly selective tumor-producing effect in the mammary gland of susceptible rats?

The hormonal status of the rats receiving 3-MC is highly conducive to the development of mammary cancer. This neoplasm did not develop in hypo-physectomized rats. The incidence of cancer was profoundly reduced in the highly hyperplastic mammary glands of rats treated with equine gonado-tropin or estradiol-17β (10). The speed of development of mammary cancer in intact female rats is accelerated by the administration of pro-gesterone or 9α-bromo-11-ketoprogesterone: such enhancement is abolished by the concurrent administration of moderate or large amounts of estradiol-17β.

### Hormone Dependence of Induced Mammary Cancer of the Rat

Many of the established mammary cancers which had been induced in the Sprague-Dawley rats by 3-MC are hormone dependent. This was a novel observation (8) since experimental mammary tumors with these functional characteristics had not been recognized previously.

The hormone-dependent mammary carcinomas undergo a considerable diminution in size after (a) hypophysectomy or (b) ovariectomy or (c) the injection of dihydrotestosterone (8), and the regression is accompanied by atrophic changes, which are often profound, in the malignant epithelial cells. The most effective regressive agency was hypophysectomy; 2 rats with established mammary cancer in a series of 10 animals subjected to hypophysectomy were alive and free from mammary cancer one year after removal of the pituitary. Less commonly, the same hormonal treatments failed to cause regression of the mammary carcinoma and the characteristic atrophy was absent.

It has been observed in some tumors that only a proportion of the epithelial cells underwent profound hormone-withdrawal atrophy in response to ovariectomy while in adjacent areas the cells were hormone independent in character, consisting of actively growing epithelial cells. Clearly, the cell population of these tumors was not uniform in its functional response to ovariectomy; since hormone-independent cells were abundant, these tumors continued to grow despite the presence of a hormone-dependent component. It is certain from this observation that hormone dependence or independence, respectively, is a function of the tumor, and not of the host.

### Summary

When maximal amounts of 3-methylcholanthrene compatible with survival are fed in repeated doses to young normal adult female rats of a special strain, mammary cancer develops selectively, often exclusively, invariably, and in a short time. The functional state of the mammary substratum, determined by the hormonal status of the animals exposed to a carcinogen, is of critical significance in determining whether or not mammary cancer will develop.

Many of the induced mammary carcinomas are hormone dependent. Hormone dependence or independence, respectively, is a function of the tumor and not a quality of the host.

### References

1. Armstrong, E. C., and Bonser, G. M. *J. Pathol. Bacteriol.* **59**, 19 (1947).
2. Bielschowsky, F. *Brit. J. Exptl. Pathol.* **25**, 1 (1944).
3. Doisy, E. A., Veler, C. D., and Thayer, S. *Am. J. Physiol.* **90**, 329 (1929).

4. Huggins, C. *J. Urol.* **68**, 875 (1952).
5. Huggins, C. *Cancer Research* **16**, 825 (1956).
6. Huggins, C. *Klin. Wochschr.* **36**, 1102 (1958).
7. Huggins, C. *J. Roy. Coll. Surgeons Edinburgh* **4**, 1 (1959).
8. Huggins, C., Briziarelli, G., and Sutton, H., Jr. *J. Exptl. Med.* **109**, 25 (1959).
9. Huggins, C., and Clark, P. J. *J. Exptl. Med.* **72**, 747 (1940).
10. Huggins, C., Grand, L. C., and Brillantes, F. P. *Proc. Natl. Acad. Sci. U.S.* **45**, 1294 (1959).
11. Huggins, C., and Hodges, C. V. *Cancer Research* **1**, 293 (1941).
12. Huggins, C., and Moulder, P. V. *J. Exptl. Med.* **80**, 441 (1944).
13. Lacassagne, A. *Compt. rend. acad. sci.* **195**, 630 (1932).
14. Maisin, J., and Coolen, M-L. *Compt. rend. soc. biol.* **123**, 159 (1936).
15. Mühlbock, O. *In* "Endocrine Aspects of Breast Cancer" (A. R. Currie, ed.), p. 291. Livingstone, Edinburgh, 1958.
16. Pearson, O. H., Eliel, L. P. Rawson, R. W., Dobriner, K., and Rhoads, C. P. *Cancer* **2**, 943 (1949).
17. Seidlin, S. M., Marinelli, L. D., and Oshry, E. *J. Am. Med. Assoc.* **132**, 838 (1946).
18. Shay, H., Aegerter, E. A., Gruenstein, M., and Komarov, S. A. *J. Natl. Cancer Inst.* **10**, 255 (1949).
19. Talalay, P., and Williams-Ashman, H. G. *Proc. Natl. Acad. Sci. U.S.* **44**, 15 (1958).
20. Talalay, P., and Williams-Ashman, H. G. *Proc. Natl. Acad. Sci. U.S.* **44**, 862 (1958).
21. Villee, C. A. *J. Biol. Chem.* **215**, 171 (1955).
22. Villee, C. A., and Gordon, E. E. *J. Biol. Chem.* **216**, 203 (1955).
23. Wieland, H., and Dane, E. *Z. physiol. Chem.* **219**, 240 (1933).

## DISCUSSION

**Charles Harris:** I want to congratulate Dr. Huggins for the direct and forceful experimentation which has brought to light certain interrelationships, some of which have not been observed with smaller doses of carcinogen. There are several comments I would like to make relating only to our own experience with smaller doses. First, give 2 mg. of methylcholanthrene daily to an animal for even as short a time as 1 month, and it becomes a much worse insurance risk than an animal that has never received it at all, and it will develop tumors even as long as 11 months after cessation of the drug. Secondly, we analyze our tumors slightly differently, by excising all tumors when they reach 2 cm. in diameter, and this gives us an opportunity in a group of about 20 animals to observe 240 breasts and add to the statistical power so that in any two given groups, where 100% of the animals do develop tumors, we can derive differences in the numbers of tumors and the speed with which they occur, and thus often separate the two groups statistically.

As far as progesterone is concerned, ten years ago we implanted progesterone tablets in female animals that received 2 mg. of methylcholanthrene daily for a 12-month period, and there was no effect.

As far as estrogen is concerned we agree that it exerts a blocking action on tumor induction by methylcholanthrene. Estrogen itself is carcinogenic. About 30% of our animals develop at least one tumor in the course of estrogen implantation, and that this is related to the pituitary is suggested by the work of Dr. Furth. Secondly, when we slow the rapid tumorification of the pituitary and chromophobe adenoma formation induced by estrogen by giving TACE, which inhibits the rate at which estrogen tends to cause this gland to grow, the breast-tumor rate increases even though TACE itself would suppress methylcholanthrene-induced carcinogenesis. Also, estrogen in male animals has an opposite effect from that in females. In males it implements decidedly the amount of breast cancer that develops. You can take a male animal, give it methylcholanthrene, and give it enough estrogen so that the animal will approximate, in incidence and speed with which tumors develop, the incidence of tumors in female rats given methylcholanthrene alone.

Last, I think not least, this question of basket cells. The myoepithelial elements under the influence of estrogen partake in gland formation, but under the influence of androgens they tend to form stroma; I think that this is truly a multipotential cell.

**A. Mittleman:** Dr. Huggins did not mention whether these methylcholanthrene-induced tumors metastasize.

**C. Huggins:** At times, they metastasize to regional lymph nodes and they metastasize to the lungs. For metastases to develop, the animals require special treatment because breast cancers are superficial and one has to be very careful that ulceration of the tumor doesn't set in and kill the animal before metastasis has developed. No question about it, they metastasize—these are real cancers.

**S. Solomon:** Dr. Huggins mentioned that all dogs having mammary tumors had adrenal tumors. Can he please tell us something about the nature of these adrenal tumors?

**C. Huggins:** I think what I said was that all the dogs that we have seen with mammary tumors have adrenal tumors. I wouldn't like to say that every dog everywhere with mammary cancer has an adrenal tumor, but the incidence certainly must be quite high; these are adrenal-corticoid tumors.

**R. L. Noble:** Dr. Huggins, your main thesis of speed really pertains to induction of breast cancer or carcinogenesis. If one is looking for a test method to screen substances for carcinostatic action, presumably one would have to induce the tumor and then treat the animal with the growing tumors. Now do these tumors grow rapidly once they are induced or are they relatively slow growing? In relation to this question do you feel that a compound which inhibits the development of these tumors would also inhibit their growth once they have started to grow? Finally have you had any experience with first-generation transplants of these tumors, and do they retain their hormone dependency?

**C. Huggins:** In an untreated female given methylcholanthrene the tumors grow rapidly. If one gives an enhancing agent like progesterone plus methylcholanthrene the tumor will grow to large size, but sometimes when you stop progesterone the cancers regress temporarily but always come back at a subsequent time. These are rapidly growing tumors. I haven't tried to transplant these tumors. I worked for several years on the transplantable fibroadenoma, with which Professor Noble has done so much. With steroids you can block growth of this benign tumor very effectively and you could learn useful things, but once the tumor had arisen you couldn't make it disappear. It was like a fire, perhaps gutting the interior of the building, but the tumor remained of large size. It is an advantage that this other tumor is not a benign tumor and one can make it disappear in untreated females if one is interested, in that methylcholanthrene induces a rapid-growing tumor, which never regresses spontaneously, and it is possible to make it disappear. If you are interested in prevention of carcinogenesis this cancer can be prevented absolutely. There are a half dozen techniques for doing that.

**U. Kim:** I think I could give an answer to Dr. Noble's question. We also confirmed Dr. Huggins' mammary tumor induction data in highly inbred Wistar and Fischer rats. The mammary tumors induced by 3-methylcholanthrene are almost all adenocarcinomas and they do metastasize when they become very large. We grafted many methylcholanthrene-induced mammary carcinomas into an isologous strain of rats and did parallel studies comparing their hormone responsiveness with the primary tumors from which the grafts derived. We have observed that there was a perfect parallelism between the primary tumors and the first-generation grafts in their magnitude of hormone responsiveness. However, from the second generation on, the results were irregular. Some tumors were parallel as long as third or fourth subpassage generations, and some changed or became autonomous from the second generation on.

**M. J. Brennan:** Dr. Huggins made the statement that methylcholanthrene goes straight to the mammary gland and thereupon produces the tumor. I would like to know whether or not there is direct evidence that methylcholanthrene concentrates in the breast tissue which subsequently becomes carcinomatous.

**C. Huggins:** I don't think the quantitative aspects have been studied yet, but it is quite easy qualitatively to detect this fluorescence by examination with a quartz lamp. I have the impression that 3-methylcholanthrene does not concentrate in mammary gland but that it goes there and induces the carcinogenic process almost immediately.

## II. STEROID STRUCTURE AND FUNCTION

# Some Recent Advances in Steroid Chemistry

JOSEF FRIED

*The Squibb Institute for Medical Research, New Brunswick, New Jersey*

It is quite obvious that in a review paper of this type it is impossible to do justice to all that has been accomplished in recent years, to outline all the trends and currents in the field of steroid chemistry that are discernible from the many publications in this field. Some selection had to be made, and I wish to apologize in advance in case you should notice a certain bias in favor of the author's laboratory.

There is little question that the ever-increasing activities in the field of cancer biology and medicine are stimulating the chemist to compose new variations on a well-known theme, the steroid nucleus. Selected by the evolutionary process to perform some of the most fundamental biological functions, this relatively simple chemical ring system not only has served to inspire several generations of endocrinologists, but also has become the basis for some of the most phenomenal accomplishments in organic chemistry. The establishment of the chemical architecture of cholesterol and of the bile acids, the isolation and elucidation of structure of the steroid hormones, the development of conformational analysis, and the various total syntheses of the steroid hormones exemplify the caliber of the responses to the challenge presented by this molecule.

It has been, and probably will remain, the fate of steroid chemistry periodically to be pronounced dead and incapable of yielding another finding of chemical or biological significance, only to be revived shortly thereafter and raised to new heights by some new discovery. During the last decade steroid chemistry has been thriving on the stimulus provided by the discovery of the anti-inflammatory properties of the cortical hormones. The chemical problems that arose from this far-reaching discovery were largely concerned with the efficient introduction of hydroxyl groups in the $11\beta,17\alpha$- and 21-positions of the steroid nucleus. It is fortunate that the answers to these questions have enabled us to advance a great deal beyond the original goal. I am thinking here particularly of the microbiological hydroxylation reaction first reported by Murray and Peterson, which has revolutionized steroid chemistry to an extent hardly foreseeable when these studies were begun. The comprehensive review by Peterson (24) provides the most recent summary of the accomplishments in this area. Figure 1 shows schematically the sites of the progesterone molecule at which hydroxylation has been

achieved, a solid line signifying the β- and a dashed line the α-orientation of
the hydroxyl group. There is hardly a position on the steroid nucleus that
cannot be hydroxylated by the proper choice of microorganism. Many
microorganisms possess enzymes capable of hydroxylating in more than one
position. Conspicuous for its absence is the hydroxylation in the 18-position,
known to occur in the adrenal gland and required in the synthesis of aldosterone. It is strange that this biologically important hydroxylation reaction
should not as yet have been observed to occur with microorganisms, although
it is not too bold to predict that it will be discovered in time. The newly
introduced hydroxyl groups can serve as handles for further chemical transformations. They can be oxidized, eliminated to give rise to double bonds,
or transformed to other functional groups. Other microbial transformations
are the important dehydrogenation in the 1,2-position; scission between
carbon atoms 9 and 10, 13 and 17, 17 and 20; and hydrogenation of the 4,5
as well as of the carbon-oxygen double bonds.

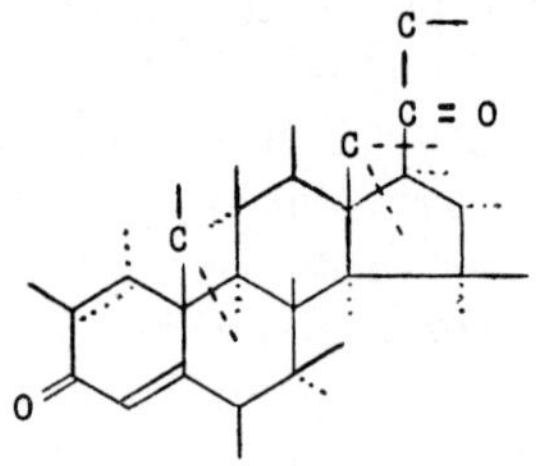

Fig. 1. Progesterone molecule: sites at which microbiological transformation has
been achieved. Solid line, β-orientation of the hydroxyl group; dashed line, α-orientation.

Attempts to prepare cell-free extracts and further purify the enzymes
involved in the various hydroxylation reactions have not as yet been successful. Cell-free extracts capable of performing the (irreversible) dehydrogenation in the 1,2-position and the reversible dehydrogenation-hydro-
genation reactions at the oxygen functions in positions 3 and 17 have become
available largely through the work of Talalay and his collaborators (20, 31).

Of interest to the proceedings of this conference are conversions observed
by us several years ago involving cleavage between carbon atoms 17 and 20
as well as 13 and 17 (12). I am referring to the formation of testololactone
and $\Delta^1$-testololactone from progesterone and other steroidal substrates (Fig.
2). The activity of $\Delta^1$-testololactone in human breast cancer is described by
Dr. Segaloff in another paper in this symposium. The significance of this
compound for future efforts derives from the fact that it has no demonstrable
hormonal activity per se. Some unusual effects of synergism with or antagonism toward some of the steroid hormones have recently been observed by

Lerner *et al.* (19). The experience with this compound suggests that some of the older, "inactive" steroids might be fruitful subjects for re-evaluation by the more recently developed biological assay methods. The existence of a hormonally inactive substance capable of modifying the course of breast cancer certainly provides a powerful stimulus for further work.

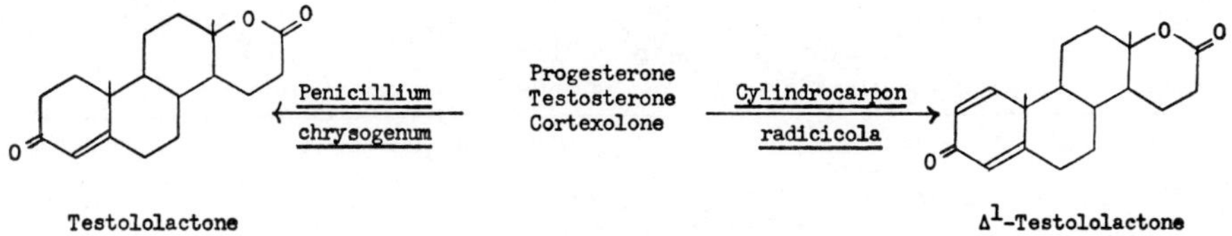

**Testolol actone**

Penicillium chrysogenum ← Progesterone Testosterone Cortexolone → Cylindrocarpon radicicola

$\Delta^1$-Testololactone

FIG. 2.  Oxidation  to  ring-D  lactones.

The hydroxylated compounds readily available by microbiological methods of easily accessible substrates provided the basis for our own work on 9α-halogenated steroids. Originally conceived as intermediates in the conversion of 11-epicortisol to cortisol, it soon became evident that the enhancement in activity achieved, particularly by 9α-fluorination of 11β-hydroxylated steroids, was of broader significance than could be visualized at the outset (10). Fluorination has since been achieved in other positions (Fig. 3),

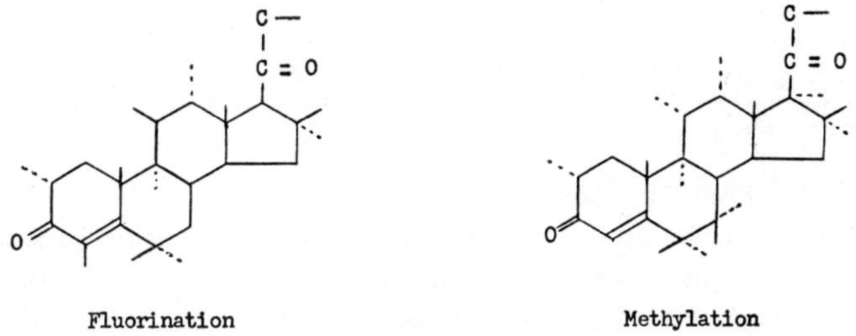

Fluorination                              Methylation

FIG. 3.  Positions  in  hydroxylated  compounds  at  which  fluorination  or  methylation has been achieved.

leading to compounds with interesting and unusual biological properties. The scope of chemical modification was enlarged when the Upjohn group showed that methylation in the 2- and 6-positions of adrenal steroids could also lead to compounds possessing enhanced or modified biological properties (16, 30). Figure 3 shows the positions that have been methylated to date.

In a recent review (8) we have characterized the unique structure-activity relationships in this field as being of a degree of consistency, both in qualitative and quantitative terms, not encountered in any other area of medicinal

chemistry. The conclusion was reached from available data that incorporation of the functional groups listed in the first column of Table I, either
alone or in arbitrary combinations with each other, into the basic 11β-
hydroxyprogesterone molecule would result in a molecule in which the glucocorticoid and anti-inflammatory activities could be calculated by multiply-
ing the appropriate "enhancement factors" for all the groups substituted in

TABLE I

ENHANCEMENT FACTORS FOR VARIOUS FUNCTIONAL GROUPS

| Functional group | Glycogen deposition, rat | Anti-inflammatory, rat | Effect on urinary sodium[a] |
|---|---|---|---|
| 9α-Fluoro | 10 | 7-10 | + + + |
| 9α-Chloro | 3–5 | 3 | + + |
| 9α-Bromo | 0.4 | . . . | + |
| 12α-Fluoro | 6–8 | . . . | + + |
| 12α-Chloro | 4 | . . . | . . . |
| 1-Dehydro | 3–4 | 3–4 | — |
| 6-Dehydro | 0.5–0.7 | . . . | + |
| 2α-Methyl | 3–6 | 1–4 | + + |
| 6α-Methyl | 2–3 | 1–2 | — — — |
| 6α-Fluoro | 2–4 | 2–4 | — — — |
| 16α-Hydroxyl | 0.4–0.5 | 0.1–0.2 | — — — — — |
| 16α-Methyl | 1–3 | 3–6 | — — — — — |
| 17α-Hydroxyl | 1–2 | 4 | — |
| 21-Hydroxyl | 4–7 | 25 | + + |
| 21-Fluoro | 2 | 2 | — — |

[a] + = Retention; — = excretion.

that molecule. Even as complex a biological event as salt retention could
be expressed in terms of the newly added functional groups by adding the
appropriate pluses and minuses. As an example Table II shows the calculation of the above three activities for triamcinolone, proceeding by stepwise
addition of the individual functional groups to the basic 11β-hydroxypro-
gesterone molecule and comparing the calculated values with those actually
found. It should be emphasized again that these enhancement factors apply
only to the particular activities for which they are listed.

Utilizing the above principle of cumulative activities, it has been possible
to synthesize substances that are extremely potent as glucocorticoids yet
possess no salt-retaining activity. The record bearers at this time are the
two substances shown in Fig. 4, in which the parent cortisol structure is
modified by the addition of four functional groups. The structure on the
left, 6α,9α-difluoro-16α-methylprednisolone (7, 29) has been reported to
possess seven hundred times the glucocorticoid activity of cortisol (F). The
compound shown on the right, 6α,9α-difluoro-16α-hydroxyprednisolone ace-

## TABLE II

### CALCULATION OF ACTIVITIES OF 9α-FLUORO-16α-HYDROXYPREDNISOLONE USING ENHANCEMENT FACTORS

| Functional group added | Resulting compound | Glycogen deposition | | Anti-inflammatory | | Effect on urinary sodium[a] | |
|---|---|---|---|---|---|---|---|
| | | Calculated | Found | Calculated | Found | Calculated | Found |
| ··· | 11β-Hydroxyprogesterone | ··· | 0.1 | ··· | < 0.01 | ··· | ··· |
| 9α-Fluoro | 9α-Fluoro-11β-hydroxy-progesterone | 1 | 0.85 | < 0.1 | < 0.1 | +++ | +++ |
| 21-Hydroxy | 9α-Fluorocorticosterone | 4–7 | 4.6 | < 2.5 | 2.7 | +++++ | +++++ |
| 17α-Hydroxyl | 9α-Fluorohydrocortisone | 4–14 | 11 | 11 | 13 | +++++++ | +++++++ |
| 1-Dehydro | 9α-Fluoroprednisolone | 12–56 | 28 | 33–44 | 20 | +++++ | ++++ |
| 16α-Hydroxyl | 16α-Hydroxy-9α-fluoro-prednisolone | 4.8–28 | 13 | 3.3–8.8 | 4 | — | — |

[a] + = Retention; — = excretion.

tonide (6, 22) possesses the more modest activity of four hundred times that of cortisol. Both compounds cause a net excretion of sodium and potassium.

Of particular interest to us was the fact that halogen in the 9α- and 12α-positions showed equal enhancement of glucocorticoid activity except when

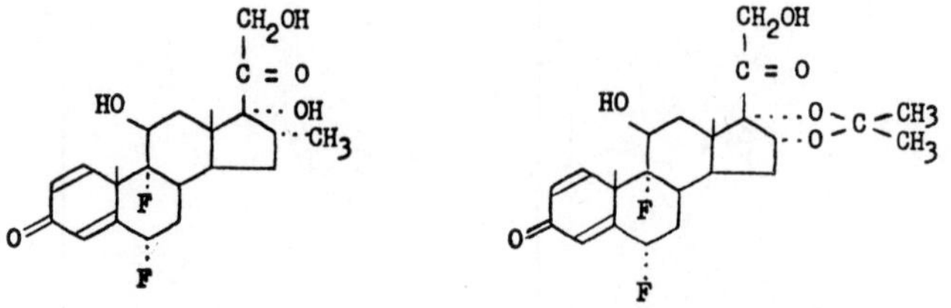

| Liver glycogen (rat): | 700 X F | 400 X F |
|---|---|---|
| Cotton pellet (rat) : | 120 X F | 100 X F |
| Urinary electrolytes (rat): | Na excretion | Na and K excretion |

FIG. 4. The most potent corticoids (as of October, 1959): (left) 6α,9α-difluoro-16α-methylprednisolone; (right) 6α,9α-difluoro-16α-hydroxyprednisolone acetonide.

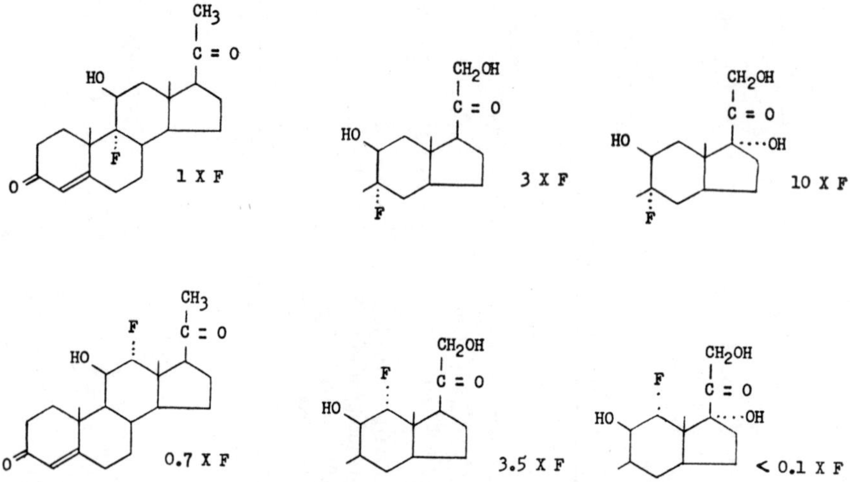

FIG. 5. Glucocorticoid activity of 9α- and 12α-fluorocorticoids.

a 17α-hydroxyl group was present. In that case 12α-halogenated compounds showed no appreciable activity (Fig. 5). We ascribed this lack of activity (8) to the enforced hydrogen bonding between the 12α-halogen atom and the nearby 17α-hydroxyl group (Fig. 6). In contrast, no such effect is possible between this latter group and the 9α-halogen atom. Confidence in the above interpretation would be greatly strengthened if it were possible to induce biological activity in a 12α-halo-17α-hydroxy steroid by abolishing

the hydrogen bonding. We were able to achieve this objective by employing
a chemical grouping capable of covering the 17α-hydroxyl group without
loss, in fact with a considerable gain, in corticoid activity (9). This grouping is the 16α,17α-isopropylidenedioxy grouping, which by substituting for
the hydrogen atom of the 17α-hydroxyl group precludes hydrogen bonding

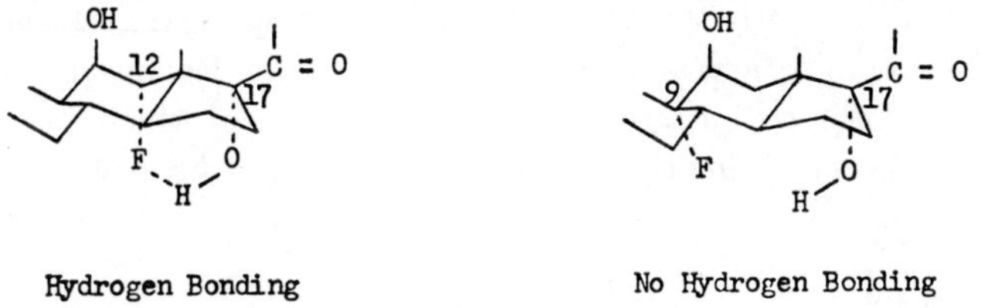

Hydrogen Bonding                    No Hydrogen Bonding

Fig. 6. Hydrogen bonding between 12α-halogen atom and 17α-hydroxyl group
(left) contrasted with lack of bonding between 9α-halogen atom and 17α-hydroxyl
group (right).

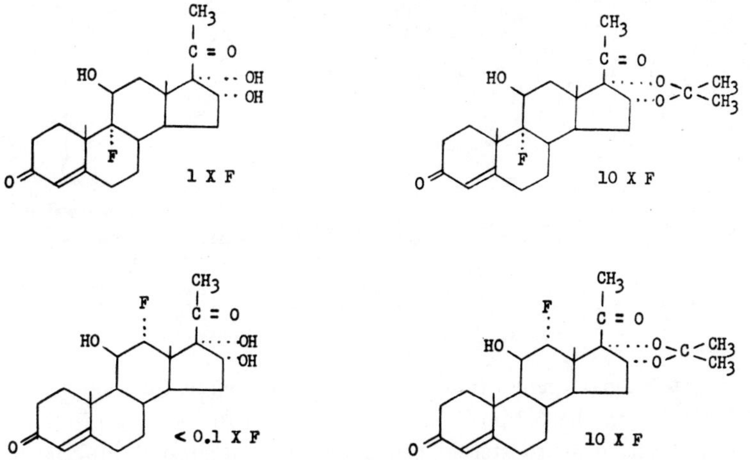

Fig. 7. Effect of hydrogen bonding on glucocorticoid activity of 12α-fluorosteroids.

toward the 12α-halogen atom. For the purpose of comparison we synthesized and assayed both the 9α- and the 12α-fluoro derivatives of 11β,16α,-
17α-trihydroxyprogesterone (Fig. 7). The 9-fluoro derivative had glucocorticoid activity equal to that of cortisol. The 12-fluoro derivative, as
expected, had no measurable activity. Then we prepared the isopropylidenedioxy derivatives of the two compounds and determined their glucocorticoid
activity. In full accord with the hydrogen-bonding hypothesis, both the
9- and the 12-fluoro derivative now showed equal activity, the enhancement
being tenfold as expected for the isopropylidenedioxy grouping. The restora-

tion of biological activity to an inactive yet potentially active molecule on the basis of a rational approach is indeed gratifying in a field that is still largely dominated by empiricism.

Efforts to fluorinate and methylate the steroid nucleus in new positions and to devise novel methods for the introduction of these groups are continuing. The activity-enhancing properties of the 6α-fluoro atom were discovered independently by the Upjohn (17) and Syntex (5) groups. Based on the fluorobromination method first described by Robinson *et al.* (27), Bowers (3), synthesized a series of 6-fluoro steroids, of which 6α-fluoro-17α-acetoxyprogesterone is singled out and shown in Fig. 8 because of its interest

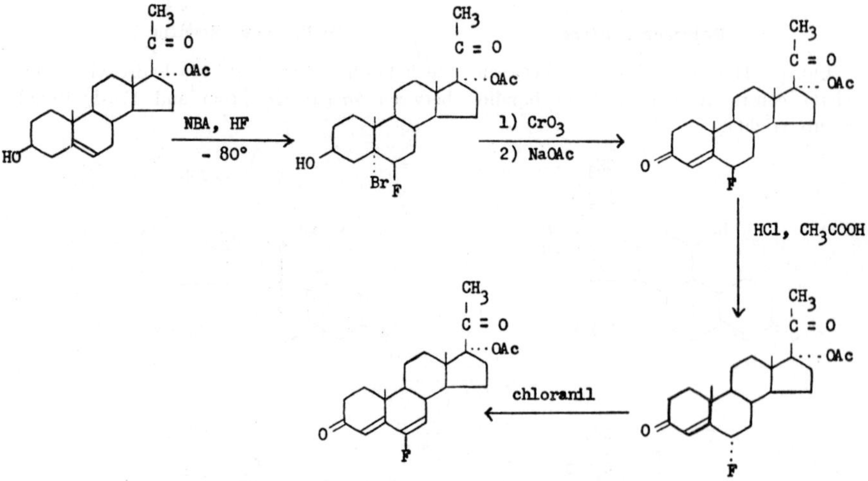

FIG. 8. Synthesis of 6α-fluorosteroids.

as a progestational agent. Bowers *et al.* (4) subsequently showed that dehydrogenation in the 6,7-positions enhances even further the progestational activity of this 6-fluoro steroid producing the potent oral progestogen, 6-fluoro-6-dehydro-17α-acetoxyprogesterone. The enhancement effected by dehydrogenation is still more pronounced in the corresponding 6-chloro derivative (25), which is one of the most potent oral progestogens. The structures and activities in the peroral Clauberg assay of these and two other potent progestogens are shown in Fig. 9.

Methods for the direct introduction of the 6-fluorine atom into a $\Delta^4$-3-ketone have been devised by Bloom *et al.* (2) and by Nakanishi *et al.* (23). The first-named authors convert the $\Delta^4$-3-ketone into the 3-enol acetate, which on reaction with perchloryl fluoride yields the 6β-fluoro-$\Delta^4$-3-ketone, isomerizable with acid to the 6α-epimer (Fig. 10). The use of perchloryl fluoride as a fluorinating agent in steroid chemistry was pioneered by Jensen

(13), who converted the 3-pyrrolidyl enamine of cholestenone into its 2α-fluoro derivative and later extended this reaction to the preparation of 2α-fluoro-4,5α-dihydrotestosterone (23) (Fig. 11). This latter compound is of

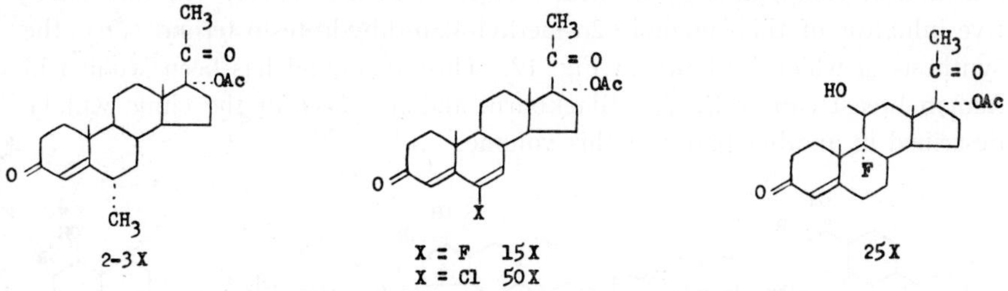

FIG. 9. New potent oral progestogens. Oral Clauberg assay: 17α-ethynyl-19-nor-testosterone = 1.

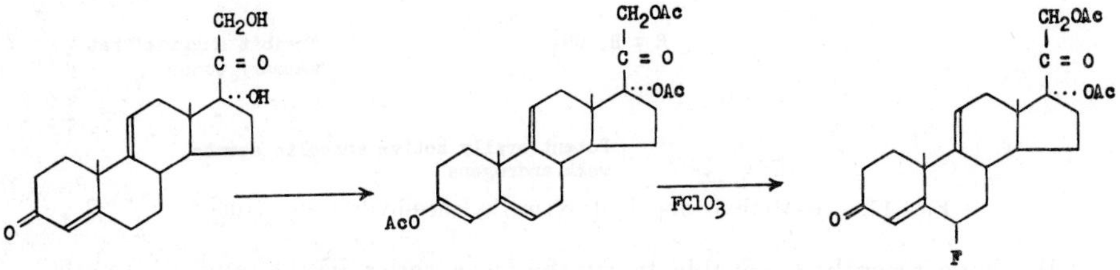

FIG. 10. 6-Fluorination with perchlorylfluoride (FClO₃).

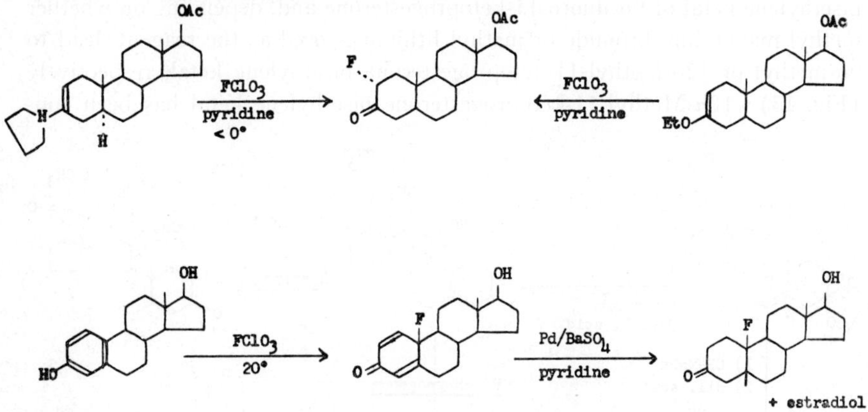

FIG. 11. Fluorination with perchlorylfluoride (FClO₃).

interest because of its ability to inhibit the methylcholanthrene-induced Huggins tumor in the rat. Another novel application of perchloryl fluoride as a fluorinating agent was described by Mills (21), who obtained 10β-fluoro-$\Delta^{1,4}$-androstadien-17β-ol-3-one from estradiol. Mild catalytic reduction of this 10-fluoro steroid produced 10β-fluoro-4,5-dihydrotestosterone (Fig. 11).

Inhibition of the Huggins mammary tumor is being used as a criterion for selection of compounds for clinical studies in breast cancer. Another effective inhibitor of this tumor is 2α-methyl-4,5α-dihydrotestosterone (26), the synthesis of which is shown in Fig. 12. This compound has been studied in human breast cancer by Dr. Blackburn, and its effect in the clinic will be described in another paper in this volume.

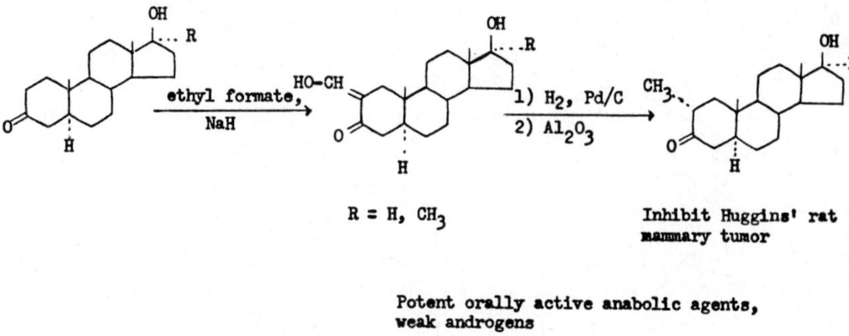

R = H, CH₃

Inhibit Huggins' rat mammary tumor

Potent orally active anabolic agents, weak androgens

FIG. 12. 2α-Methyl- and hydroxymethylenedihydrotestosterones.

We have recently been able to synthesize a series of 9α- and 12α-methylated derivatives of progesterone (33). These syntheses start with the bisethylene ketal of 9α-fluoro-11-ketoprogesterone and, depending on whether methyl magnesium bromide or methyl lithium is used as the reagent, lead to 9α-methyl or 12α-methyl-11-ketoprogesterone bisethylene ketal, respectively (Fig. 13). 12α-Methyl-11-ketoprogesterone bisethylene ketal has been con-

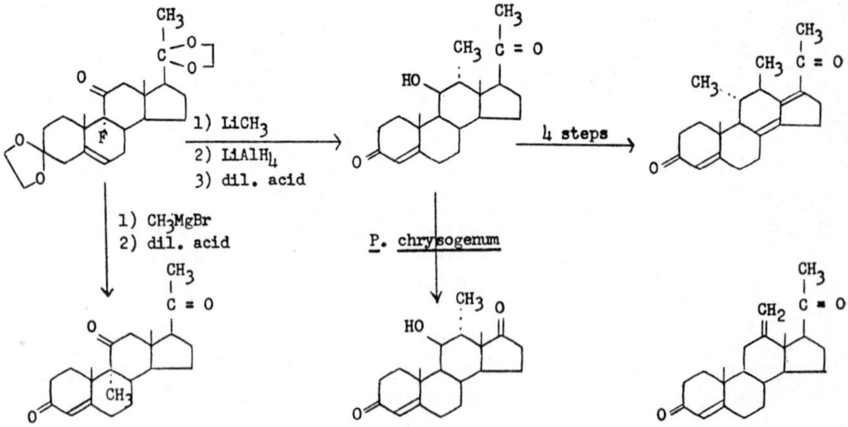

FIG. 13. 9α- and 12α-Methylprogesterones.

verted into a number of interesting products, some of which are shown in Fig. 13). Application of the above Grignard reaction to 9α-fluorocortisone bisethylene ketal leads after reduction of the 11-keto group to 9α-methyl-cortisol (11) (Fig. 14). This latter compound has also been prepared by Hoffman *et al.* (15) by the action of methyl magnesium iodide in the presence of excess methyl iodide on the 3-ethylenedioxy 17,20;20,21-bisdi-oxymethylene derivative of 9α-bromocortisone. Although similar in a formal sense, the two reactions proceed by different mechanisms. An interesting by-product in the reaction of 9α-fluorocortisone bisethylene ketal with methyl lithium is the 11α-methyl epoxide shown on the lower left, which on reaction

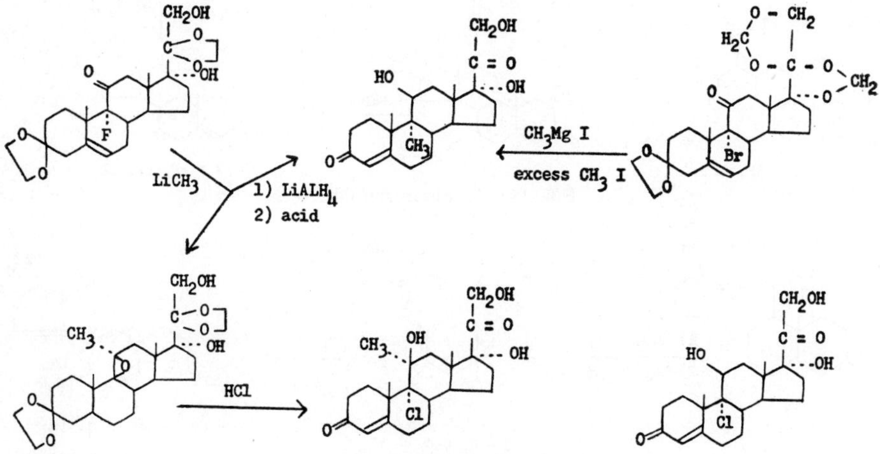

Fig. 14.   9α-Methylhydrocortisone.

with hydrogen chloride forms 11α-methyl-9α-chlorocortisol, a homolog of the biologically highly active 9α-chlorocortisol. Recently, this compound has also been prepared by Beyler *et al.* (1). Interestingly, it shows no significant gluco- or mineralocorticoid activity.

We have pursued the synthesis of 16-halogenated derivatives of andro-stenedione and testosterone because of our belief that halogen, adjacent to a vital oxygen function as in the case of the 9- and 12-halo derivatives of 11-oxygenated steroids, might lead to biologically interesting consequences (32). Our synthesis of such 16-halo androgens is shown in Fig. 15. Andro-stenedione is hydroxylated in the 16α-position by the microorganism *Strepto-myces roseochromogenus* followed by mesylation of the resulting 16α-hy-droxyandrostenedione. Substitution of the 16α-mesyloxy group by chloride ion leads to the 16β-chloro derivative, whereas reaction with potassium bi-fluoride in diethylene glycol yields both 16α- and β-fluoroandrostenedione.

The 17-keto group is then selectively reduced by sodium borohydride in methanol. Application of this sequence of reactions to 9α-fluoro-11β-hy-droxyandrostenedione likewise leads to the corresponding 16-halogenated derivatives.

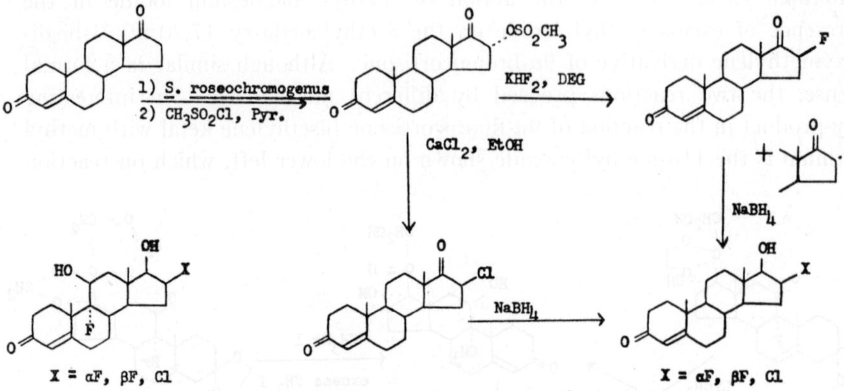

X = αF, βF, Cl

FIG. 15.  16-Fluorosteroids

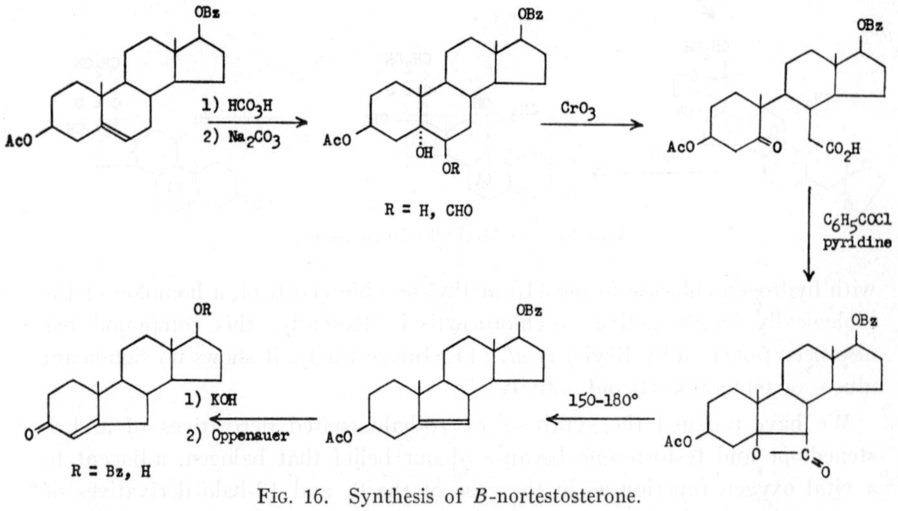

R = H, CHO

R = Bz, H

FIG. 16.  Synthesis of B-nortestosterone.

Considerable interest has recently been shown in steroids in which one of the six-membered rings has been contracted to a five-membered ring. Rull and Ourisson (28) have prepared B-nortestosterone by the procedure shown in Fig. 16, which proceeds via the interesting β-lactone shown on the lower right. The biological properties of this compound have not been reported. Hirschman et al. (14) synthesized A-norcortisol from prednisone (Fig. 17), utilizing a benzylic acid rearrangement for the contraction of ring A. Weisenborn and Applegate (34) converted progesterone into A-norprogesterone by the procedure shown in Fig. 18. This A-nor steroid was shown by

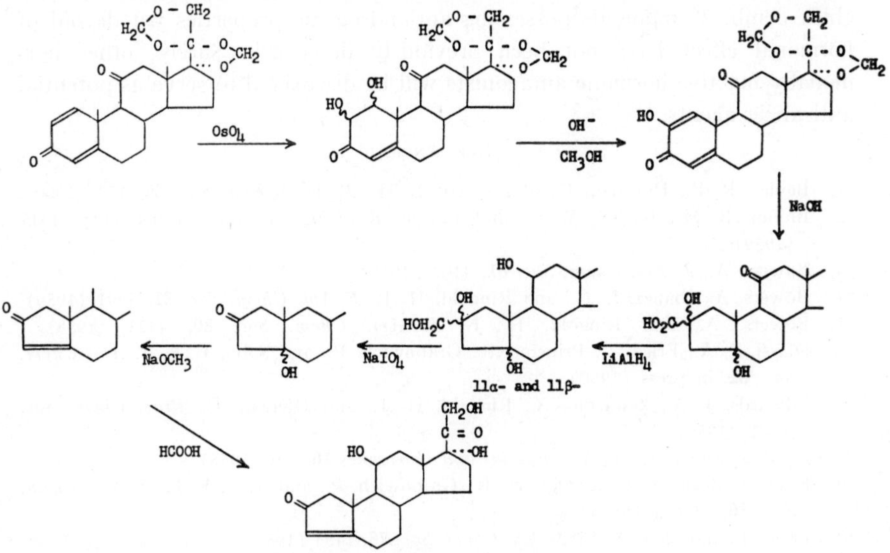

FIG. 17. Synthesis of A-norcortisol.

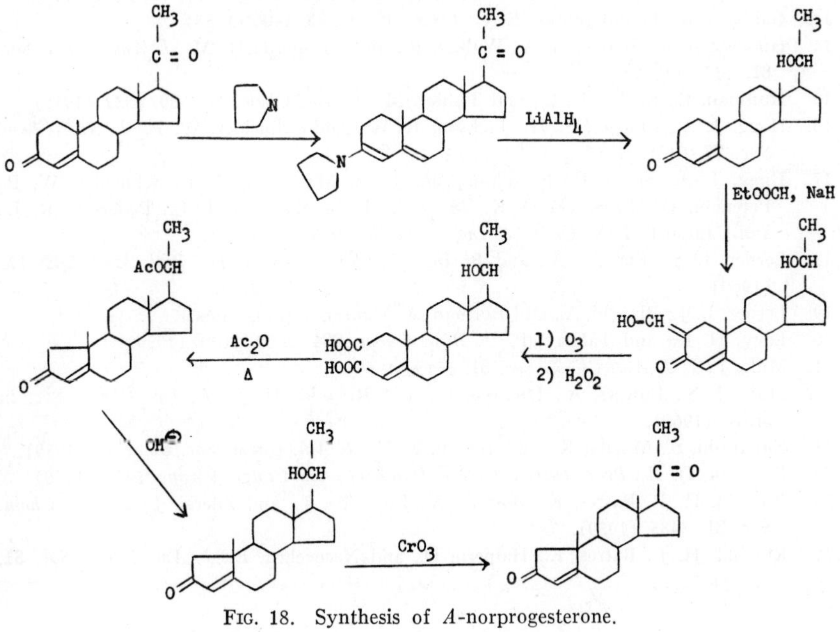

FIG. 18. Synthesis of A-norprogesterone.

Lerner and associates (18) to be devoid of progestational activity, in fact of any hormonal activity. Instead, $A$-norprogesterone was capable of inhibiting the effects of both exogenous and endogenous androgen on the seminal vesicles and ventral prostate of the rat, and of exogenous androgen on the chick comb. Compounds possessing antiandrogenic properties yet devoid of hormonal effect have not been previously described. Surely, other hormonally inactive hormone antagonists will be discovered to serve as potential anticancer agents.

REFERENCES

1. Beyler, R. E., Hoffman, F., and Sarett, L. H. *J. Am. Chem. Soc.* **82**, 178 (1960).
2. Bloom, B. M., Bogart, V. V., and Pinson, R. *Chem. & Ind. (London)* p. 1317 (1959).
3. Bowers, A. *J. Am. Chem. Soc.* **81**, 4107 (1959).
4. Bowers, A., Ibanez, L. C., and Ringold, H. J. *J. Am. Chem. Soc.* **81**, 5991 (1959).
5. Bowers, A., and Ringold, H. J. *J. Am. Chem. Soc.* **80**, 4423 (1958).
6. Diassi, P. A., Fried, J., Principe, P., Grabowich, P., and Sabo, E. F. *J. Am. Chem. Soc.* **81**, in press (1960).
7. Edwards, J. A., Zaffaroni, A., Ringold, H. J., and Djerassi, C. *Proc. Chem. Soc.* p. 87 (1959).
8. Fried, J., and Borman, A. *Vitamins and Hormones* **16**, 303 (1958).
9. Fried, J. Borman, A., Kessler, W. B., Grabowich, P., and Sabo, E. F. *J. Am. Chem. Soc.* **80**, 2338 (1958).
10. Fried, J., and Sabo, E. F. *J. Am. Chem. Soc.* **76**, 1455 (1954).
11. Fried, J., and Sabo, E. F. *J. Am. Chem. Soc.* in press.
12. Fried, J., Thoma, R. W., and Klingsberg, A. *J. Am. Chem. Soc.* **75**, 5764 (1953).
13. Gabbard, R. B., and Jensen, E. V. *J. Org. Chem.* **23**, 1406 (1958).
14. Hirschman, R., Bailey, G. A., Walker, R., and Chemerda, J. M. *J. Am. Chem. Soc.* **81**, 2822 (1959).
15. Hoffman, F., Beyler, R. E., and Tishler, M. *J. Am. Chem. Soc.* **80**, 5322 (1958).
16. Hogg, J. A., Lincoln, F. H., Jackson, R. W., and Schneider, W. P. *J. Am. Chem. Soc.* **77**, 6401 (1955).
17. Hogg, J. A., Spero, G. B., Thompson, J. L., Magerlein, B. J., Schneider, W. P., Peterson, D. H., Sebek, O. K., Murray, H. C., Babcock, J. C., Pederson, R. L., and Campbell, J. A. *Chem. & Ind. (London)* p. 1002 (1958).
18. Lerner, L. J., Bianchi, A., and Borman, A. *Proc. Soc. Exptl. Biol. Med.* **103**, 172 (1960).
19. Lerner, L. J., Bianchi, A., and Borman, A. *Cancer* in press (1960).
20. Levy, H. R., and Talalay, P. *J. Biol. Chem.* **234**, 2009, 2014 (1959).
21. Mills, J. S. *J. Am. Chem. Soc.* **81**, 5515 (1959).
22. Mills, J. S., Bowers, A., Djerassi, C., and Ringold, H. J. *J. Am. Chem. Soc.* in press, (1960).
23. Nakanishi, S., Morita, K., and Jensen, E. V. *J. Am. Chem. Soc.* **81**, 5259 (1959).
24. Peterson, D. H. *Proc. Intern. Congr. Biochem., 4th Congr. Vienna 1958* (1959).
25. Ringold, H. J., Batres, E., Bowers, A., Edwards, J., and Zderic, J. *J. Am. Chem. Soc.* **81**, 3485 (1959).
26. Ringold, H. J., Batres, E., Halpern, O., and Necoechea, E. *J. Am. Chem. Soc.* **81**, 427 (1959).

27. Robinson, C. H., Finckenor, L., Oliveto, E. P., and Gould, D. *J. Am. Chem. Soc.* **81**, 2191 (1959).
28. Rull, T., and Ourisson, G. *Bull. soc. chim. (France)* p. 1581 (1958).
29. Schneider, W. P., Lincoln, F. H., Spero, G. B., Murray, H. C., and Thompson, J. L. *J. Am. Chem. Soc.* **81**, 3167 (1959).
30. Spero, G. B., Thompson, J. L., Magerlein, B. J., Hanze, A. R., Murray, H. C., Sebek, O. K., and Hogg, J. A. *J. Am. Chem. Soc.* **78**, 6213 (1956).
31. Talalay, P. *Physiol. Revs.* **37**, 362 (1957).
32. Thomas, G. H., and Fried, J. U.S. Patents 2,857,403 (1958) and 2,901,494 (1959).
33. Thomas, G. H., Guiducci, M., Sabo, E. F., and Fried, J. Unpublished data.
34. Weisenborn, F. L., and Applegate, H. E. *J. Am. Chem. Soc.* **81**, 1960 (1959).

## DISCUSSION

**L. J. Lerner:** The antiandrogenic activity of $A$-norprogesterone, referred to by Dr. Fried, was demonstrated in the castrated immature male rat assay and the chick comb assay.

Weanling castrated male rats were subcutaneously administered seven daily injections of 25 µg. of testosterone propionate, various doses of $A$-norprogesterone and combinations of the $A$-norsteroid and the androgen. The animals were sacrificed 24 hours after the last injection, and the ventral prostate, seminal vesicles and coagulating gland, and levator ani were removed and weighed. $A$-norprogesterone at daily doses of 1 and 5 mg. markedly reduced, and 25 mg. completely prevented, the androgen-stimulated growth of the accessory sex organs and the levator ani. A daily dose of 5 mg. of this compound, administered to nonandrogen-treated castrates, slightly reduced the levator ani, seminal vesicle, and coagulating gland weights. This may be due to an inhibition of adrenal androgen.

Dr. Dorfman in a recent paper showed that a single subcutaneous injection of 0.5 mg. of testosterone enanthate in 2-day-old cockerels induced a 100% increase in comb weights over that of controls by the eighth day post injection. This procedure was utilized to induce comb growth, and $A$-norprogesterone in sesame oil was applied to the comb daily for 7 days in total doses of 0.04, 0.2, 1.0, and 5.0 mg. The androgen-induced comb growth was completely prevented by the 5-mg. dose of this compound and partially antagonized with the lower doses, relative to the size of the dose. The comb growth of nonandrogenized birds was retarded by a 1.0-mg. total dose of this antagonist.

Antiandrogenic activity of this compound was also demonstrated in both the chick and castrate rat assays when androsterone was employed as the stimulating androgen.

Intact male rats treated for 7 or 10 days with $A$-norprogesterone had significantly smaller accessory sex organs. This indicates that this norsteroid is effective against endogenous as well as exogenous androgen.

$A$-Norprogesterone is orally active but is less effective by this route than when parenterally administered.

This compound has no estrogenic, anti-estrogenic, antiprogestational, or glucocorticoid activity at the doses tested. It is practically inactive as a progestogen since 100 mg. is required to elicit even a minimal glandular response in the Clauberg assay.

**G. Pincus:** Is the relative oral to subcutaneous activity of a similar order to that for progesterone?

**L. J. Lerner:** No. *A*-Norprogesterone is orally active in much smaller doses than is progesterone; however, somewhat larger doses must be administered by this route than by the subcutaneous route for a similar degree of response.

**C. Chen:** We have prepared three estranolone isomers. In the baby-chick comb assay the simultaneous administration of 10 mg. of each of these three compounds with 2 mg. of androsterone for 7 days caused the reduction by 30% of comb growth normally induced by androsterone alone.

Compound I itself is completely nonandrogenic. Compound II is only slightly androgenic, but compound III is about one-fifth as androgenic as androsterone. Besides, all three compounds are antiestrogenic, as tested by vaginal smear and uterine weight methods. The compounds in question are estran-17β-ol-3-one: 5α,10α; 5β,10β; and 5α,10β isomers.

**H. J. Ringold:** We published recently the synthesis of a series of 19-nordihydro-allotestosterone derivatives prepared by lithium ammonia reduction of the corresponding $\Delta^4$-3-ketones. Dr. Chen and a group from Eli Lilly independently reported the preparation of a number of 19-noretiocholanolone derivatives by catalytic hydrogenation of estrogens. We have also observed the antiestrogenic activity of a number of these compounds, in particular 19-norandrostan-17β-ol-3-one, which is a rather potent anti-estrogen in our hands.

**E. V. Jensen:** I would like to say a word about the 2α-fluoroandrogens because I think they represent a very interesting point in the relation of structure to activity. Dr. Fried mentioned that introduction of the 2α-methyl group into dihydrotestosterone and similar compounds leads to very potent androgenic, anabolic, and anti-breast-tumor agents. The substitution of fluorine in the 2α-position differs from substitution of a methyl group, in that fluorine appears to knock out or greatly reduce the primary hormonal activity, even though fluorine is much closer in size to the original hydrogen atom than is the methyl group. In tests carried out by Dr. Stafford and his associates at Upjohn, 2α-fluorodihydrotestosterone acetate was inactive as an androgen, yet it was quite active in inhibiting Dr. Huggins' methylcholanthrene-induced rat mammary cancer as well as being a potent anabolic agent. Thus, we have a compound of practically the same molecular shape and size as an active androgen which shows low primary hormonal potency while retaining secondary actions.

**H. J. Ringold:** I wish to comment on the androgenic activity of 2α-fluorodihydro-testosterone and of 2α-fluorotestosterone as well as their 17α-methyl analogs. We did not find nearly as much separation of activity for this series of compounds as Dr. Jensen has found. We have found that the compounds are fairly potent androgens, although not as strong as testosterone; nor are they as potent myotropic agents as the 2α-methyl compounds. On the other hand, the 2α-fluoro compounds are potent anti-gonadotropic agents in the parabiotic rat.

# Physiology and Pharmacology of Steroids Affecting Tumor Growth

## Victor A. Drill

*Research Laboratories, G. D. Searle and Company, Chicago, Illinois*

The remissions caused by naturally occurring androgens and estrogens in patients with cancer of the breast or of the prostate have led to the study of related steroids for their effects on experimental tumors and human cancer. The present review will discuss: (1) the endocrine properties of steroids employed in the treatment of cancer, (2) the effect of natural and new synthetic steroids on the growth of experimental tumors, (3) the endocrine properties of newer synthetic steroids, and (4) structure-activity relationships where such data exist. An attempt has been made to correlate this information to determine as closely as possible the various mechanisms by which these steroids may act to affect tumor growth. The broad areas of activity discussed will include the androgens, estrogens, progestins, antiestrogens, and antiandrogens. Inasmuch as the steroids also affect pituitary function, a brief discussion of certain pituitary hormones is also included.

## I. Androgens

Androgens, such as testosterone propionate, are employed in the treatment of cancer of the breast. They were originally used on the basis that they antagonize estrogens, and evidence for this relationship may be summarized briefly as follows: (1) The incidence of spontaneous carcinoma of the breast in mice is decreased by castration. (2) Estrogens increase the incidence of carcinoma of the breast in certain strains of mice. (3) Testosterone decreases the incidence of carcinoma of the breast in susceptible strains of mice.

The above relationships are not as simple as previously supposed. First, such antagonisms are most clearly seen in specific strains of mice. Secondly, it is now known that certain patients can be treated by either androgen or estrogen. Lastly, androgens may produce a beneficial response in patients who have been subjected to castration and adrenalectomy to remove the endocrine sources of estrogen, thus eliminating estrogen antagonism as a means of action.

Androgens were first used in the treatment of mammary cancer with metastases by Ulrich (124) and Loesser (70, 71). Others have extended their initial studies to demonstrate that the best response is obtained in postmenstrual patients with osseous metastases. Approximately 80 % of all patients treated experience relief of pain, whereas objective improvement of lesions occurs in about 15–30 % of the patients. Marked subjective improvement is often reported concomitant with progression of the disease. The incidence of regression of bone metastases is 25 % or greater, whereas soft tissue lesions respond frequently. When remissions occur they are temporary, lasting an average of 7–8 months with a maximum duration of $1\frac{1}{2}$ to 2 years (90). However, the fact that testosterone can produce some effect in this disease has led to the study of a variety of steroids, both experimentally and clinically, in attempts to find better therapeutic agents.

### A.   Effect of Testosterone and Related Steroids on Tumor Growth

1.   *Testosterone Derivatives and Human Mammary Cancer.*   Gellhorn, Kennedy, Segaloff, and others have studied androgens related to testosterone for their effectiveness in patients with breast cancer. The work of Segaloff and associates has been particularly valuable as they have made a systematic investigation of a series of structurally related compounds that, as will be pointed out later, supplies basic information to a number of related areas of research. Compounds that have been active in producing temporary remissions are dihydrotestosterone (30, 61, 114), 17α-methyltestosterone (113), methylandrostenediol (60, 112), 17α-vinyltestosterone (111), and 19-nortestosterone (105). Androstenediol, androstanedione, etiocholanolone, or dehydroepiandrosterone did not induce remissions (104, 108, 110, 115). The relative effects of these and other steroids have been reviewed by Segaloff (102, 103). Of the compounds studied, it appears that a decrease in androgenicity is associated with a decreased clinical effectiveness. None of the compounds proved to be superior to testosterone propionate in the treatment of mammary cancer.

A halogenated compound, fluoxymesterone, has been reported by Lyster *et al.* (74) to be very active orally as an androgen in experimental studies. Chemically the compound is 9α-fluoro-11β-hydroxy-17α-methyltestosterone. Gordan (35) reported that 1.5–2.0 mg. per day orally over a period of 4–6 months produced full androgenic effects in 10 hypogonadal males. A number of investigators have found that fluoxymesterone, in oral doses of 10, 20, or 30 mg. per day, is as active as testosterone in producing remissions in patients with breast cancer (3, 29, 62, 63, 106). Various degrees of virilizing side effects were noted, particularly clitoral enlargement. However, despite the high doses, some reports indicate that the androgenic effects are not as great as those produced by testosterone propionate. Since fluoxymesterone is at least as active as testosterone propionate in producing remissions and can be administered orally, it may be the present drug of choice for the treatment of advanced breast cancer. Although ethynyltestosterone is inactive (13), the nor derivative has recently been reported to induce remissions (69).

Many of the steroids mentioned above have a lower androgenic potency than testosterone when compared in experimental animals. However, the clinical dose of testosterone propionate is far above the androgenic dose, so that when the weaker steroids are administered in such high doses androgenicity will occur in the patient. When androgenicity is very low, the androgenic side effects in patients have decreased concomitantly with a decrease in effectiveness.

2. *Androgens and Experimental Tumors.* The effect of testosterone and related steroids on different types of tumors in animals has received a moderate amount of study. In 1936 Heiman and Krehbiel (46) recognized that the growth of mammary fibroadenomas was associated in part with factors relating to sex and pregnancy and began to study the effect of the known steroids on tumor growth. Since then Heiman (42–44) and others have shown that castration or testosterone decreases the number of takes of transplants of the tumors and that testosterone decreases tumor growth in the unoperated rat.

If castration or hypophysectomy decreases tumor growth, the tumors are said to be hormone sensitive. Only hormonally sensitive tumors respond to testosterone. Illustration of some tumor responses to testosterone and the variation in effect on the rat fibroadenoma is shown in Table I. Noble (90)

TABLE I

RESPONSE OF CERTAIN MAMMARY TUMORS TO TESTOSTERONE

| Mammary tumor | Testosterone effect[a] | Reference |
|---|---|---|
| Fibroadenoma | — | 42 |
| Fibroadenoma | 0[b] | 83, 84 |
| Fibroadenoma | — or 0 | 80 |
| Fibroadenoma | — | 58 |
| Adenocarcinoma | 0 | 26 |
| Methylcholanthrene-induced | — | 116 |
|  | — | 54 |

[a] — = Inhibition; 0 = no effect.
[b] Ovariectomized.

has pointed out that, in the case of the rat mammary fibroadenoma, sensitivity to hormones will depend in part on the number of transplants and that older generations are more resistant. In the hormone-sensitive tumors the effect of testosterone usually is not greater than that of ovariectomy, and thus this steroid is inactive in the castrated rat. Other growths, such as spontaneous tumors which arise in various strains of mice possessing the milk factor, do not regress after ovariectomy, hypophysectomy, or testosterone (85).

*3. Effect of Steroids on Fibroadenoma Growth.* The development of hormonally dependent tumors in animals has led to studies on the effect of steroids structurally related to testosterone in attempts to develop more potent compounds for use in patients with mammary cancer. The mammary fibroadenoma in the rat is useful to the extent that changes in growth rate of the hormonally dependent tumor following steroid administration resemble the response of human mammary carcinoma to hormonal therapy. Huggins and Mainzer (58) have performed a series of detailed studies on the effect of steroids on fibroadenoma growth, utilizing mainly hormonally dependent tumors. The study is important because it encompasses a series of compounds sufficient in number so that relationships of structure to tumor inhibition may be concluded and, further, sufficient for correlation of tumor-inhibiting effects with the endocrine activity of the steroids.

TABLE II
EFFECT OF ANDROSTANE DERIVATIVES ON RAT FIBROADENOMA GROWTH (58)

| Compound | Effect[a] |
|---|---|
| Androstan-3-one | 0 |
| Androstan-17β-ol | — |
| Androstan-17β-ol-3-one (dihydrotestosterone) | — — |
| Etiocholan-17β-ol-3-one | 0 |
| Androstan-3α-ol-17-one (androsterone) | — — |
| 4-Androsten-17β-ol-3-one (testosterone) | — — |
| 4-Androsten-17α-ol-3-one (epitestosterone) | 0 |
| 4-Androstene-3,17-dione | — |

[a] 0 = No effect; — = inhibition.

Table II compares the effect of a series of androstane derivatives on fibroadenoma growth. It will be noted that slight changes in structure may increase inhibiting effects, or in other cases render the compound inactive. As roughly quantitated in this table, testosterone, androsterone, and dihydrotestosterone produce good inhibition of tumor growth. The 17β-hydroxy configuration is significant, for the 17α-hydroxy derivative (epitestosterone) is inactive.

The steric configuration of the hydroxyl group at position 3 is also important for compounds in the androstane series. As shown in Table III, the 3β-hydroxy derivatives either were weak inhibitors of tumor growth or actually increased the growth rate of the fibroadenoma, whereas α-hydroxy derivatives were depressants of tumor growth.

Because of the activity of dihydrotestosterone, a number of methyl derivatives were studied (Table IV). Although the $2\alpha,17\alpha$-dimethyl derivative is active, other substitutions decreased inhibiting activity and in one case appeared to increase the rate of tumor growth. The effects of other alkyl derivatives of androstane are summarized in Table V. $17\alpha$-Methyltestosterone and $17\alpha$-ethyl-19-nortestosterone (norethandrolone) showed good

TABLE III

3-HYDROXYSTEROIDS AND RAT FIBROADENOMA GROWTH (58, 59)

| | Substitution | | Effect on Tumor[a] | |
| | | | Normal | Ovariec- |
| Compound | 3 | 17 | rat | tomized |
|---|---|---|---|---|
| Androstan- (androsterone) | $\alpha$OH | 0 | — — | |
| Androstan- (epiandrosterone) | $\beta$OH | 0 | + | |
| 5-Androsten- (dehydroisoandrosterone) | $\beta$OH | 0 | + | 0 |
| 5-Androstene- | $\beta$OH | $\beta$OH | + | +? |
| 4-Androstene- | $\alpha$OH | $\beta$OH | — — | 0 |
| 4-Androstene- | $\beta$OH | $\beta$OH | — | 0 |

[a] — = Inhibition; + = stimulation; 0 = no effect.

TABLE IV

DIHYDROTESTOSTERONE DERIVATIVES AND RAT FIBROADENOMA GROWTH (58)

| Compound | Effect[a] |
|---|---|
| $2\alpha$-Methyldihydrotestosterone | — — |
| $2\alpha,17\alpha$-Dimethyldihydrotestosterone | — — |
| 2,2-Dimethyldihydrotestosterone | 0 |
| $2,2,17\alpha$-Trimethyldihydrotestosterone | + |
| 4,4-Dimethyldihydrotestosterone | 0 |

[a] 0 = No effect; — = inhibition; + = stimulation.

TABLE V

EFFECT OF ALKYL DERIVATIVES OF ANDROSTANE ON RAT
FIBROADENOMA GROWTH (58, 59)

| Compound | Effect[a] |
|---|---|
| $17\alpha$-Methyltestosterone | — — |
| $17\alpha$-Ethyl-19-nortestosterone | — — |
| $17\alpha$-Ethynyl-19-nortestosterone | + |
| $16\alpha$-Methylandrosterone | 0 |
| 16-Methyleneandrosterone | 0 |
| $3\alpha$-Methylandrostane-$3\beta,17\beta$-diol | 0 |
| $3\beta$-Methylandrostane-$3\alpha,17\beta$-diol | 0 |

[a] — = Inhibition; + = stimulation; 0 = no effect.

tumor-inhibiting effects. Simple changes in structure, such as in 17α-ethynyl-19-nortestosterone (norethyndrone), actually increased tumor growth in both normal and ovariectomized rats whereas other substitutions rendered the compound inactive (58, 59).

Dihydrotestosterone was studied more extensively than the other compounds and was observed to inhibit the stimulation of tumor growth produced by estradiol-17β or progesterone, reducing tumor weight to the level of or slightly below that obtained in ovariectomized, untreated rats (58). However, in tumors with a low degree of hormonal dependence, dihydrotestosterone failed to inhibit tumor growth. Dihydrotestosterone delayed but did not prevent the formation of mammary cancer in rats fed 7,12-dimethylbenz-α-anthracene. It produced regression of tumors induced by methylcholanthrene in 14 of 17 rats and increased tumor size in three animals (54).

After the demonstration that 2-methyldihydrotestosterone was a potent inhibitor of mammary tumors in rats, Blackburn and Childs (5) studied the compound clinically. They reported that the propionate of this compound administered intramuscularly three times a week produced a temporary regression of metastatic lesions of patients with cancer of the breast. The effect was equal to, and may have been superior to, that of testosterone.

4. *Effect of Steroids on Methylcholanthrene-Induced Mammary Tumors.* Mammary tumors induced in rats by methylcholanthrene may also be useful for studying the comparative action of steroids. Shay and co-workers (116, 117) and Huggins and associates (54) have studied the hormonal factors influencing the growth of mammary carcinoma induced in rats by the oral administration of methylcholanthrene. Most of the tumors induced are hormone dependent and the data to date indicate that steroids affect the growth of this tumor in a manner parallel to their effect on the rat mammary fibroadenoma.

## B. *Mechanism of Action of Androgenic Steroids*

The mechanism of action of testosterone and related chemicals in producing remission in patients with mammary cancer or in decreasing growth of tumor in experimental animals cannot be stated with certainty. The various means by which such steroids may act are outlined as follows: They may (1) affect tumor growth because of specific effects related to androgenicity; (2) inhibit pituitary function; (3) affect tumor growth because of specific anabolic effects, e.g., nitrogen retention, calcium retention, which may influence tumor metabolism; (4) affect other endocrine activities of steroids (progestational, antiestrogen); (5) act through metabolic products; (6) produce specific effects on tumor unrelated to endocrine activity.

* STEROID PHYSIOLOGY AND TUMOR GROWTH

*1. Androgenicity.* With regard to androgenicity and effectiveness, none of the steroids listed in Table VI, studied by Segaloff and co-workers, is more effective than testosterone. This is true even though all compounds are administered in doses in excess of those required to produce only androgenic maintenance effects. Segaloff (102, 103) has reviewed his studies and con-

TABLE VI

RELATION OF ANDROGENICITY TO CLINICAL EFFECTIVENESS OF STEROIDS
IN MAMMARY CANCER (102, 103)

| Compound | Clinical response[a] | |
|---|---|---|
| | Tumor | Androgen |
| Testosterone | − − | + + |
| Epitestosterone | 0 | 0 |
| Etiocholanolone | 0 | 0 |
| Dihydrotestosterone | − − | + + |
| Androstanedione | 0 | 0 |
| 5-Androsten-3β-ol-17-one | 0 | 0 |
| 5-Androstene-3β,17β-diol | 0 | + |
| 17-Methylandrostenediol | − | + |
| 17-Methyltestosterone | − − | + + |
| 17-Vinyltestosterone | − | + |
| 19-Nortestosterone | − | + |
| Fluoxymesterone | − − | +(? 2+) |

[a] − = Inhibition; + = stimulation; 0 = no effect.

cluded that these compounds appear to be effective in relation to androgenicity. It may be observed from the data that the potent steroids effective in causing remission produce androgenic effects, and, secondly, that a decrease in clinical androgenicity is associated with a decreased therapeutic effectiveness in patients with metastatic cancer of the breast. The effectiveness of fluoxymesterone also appears to be related to its androgenicity, as the dose employed is far above an androgenic maintenance dose, although the type of androgenic side effect is different from that of other androgens. With regard to 2-methyldihydrotestosterone, Blackburn and Childs (5) reported that this compound appeared to produce less androgenicity than testosterone in patients with metastatic mammary cancer, but cautioned that evaluation of this impression must await expanded clinical studies. Undoubtedly further information on this point will be presented in other papers at this meeting.

In their studies on the effect of various estrogens on the growth of fibroadenoma in the rat, Huggins and Mainzer (58) noted that the preputial glands of the female rats were enlarged and the vestigial ventral prostate, when present, was increased in size (Table VII). These changes in the

weights of the preputial glands and the vestigial ventral prostate are effects
characteristic of androgens. It is difficult though, from such measurements,
to quantitate the androgenic potency of these compounds. This is particularly true in endeavoring to use the preputial gland as a means of assay, for
during dissection a variable amount of fluid escapes from the gland. The
data in Table VII illustrate that compounds which depress tumor weight

TABLE VII

EFFECT OF STEROIDS ON AVERAGE FIBROADENOMA AND VESTIGIAL
VENTRAL PROSTATE WEIGHTS (58)

| Treatment | Tumor weight (mg.) | Vestigial prostate weight (mg.) |
|---|---|---|
| None | 677–1920 | 5.1 |
| Ovariectomy | 68–190 | — |
| 4-Androsten-17β-ol-3-one (testosterone) | 114 | 103 |
| 4-Androsten-3,17-dione | 873 | 116 |
| Androstan-17-one | 1731 | 0 |
| Androstan-17β-ol | 473 | 27 |
| Androstan-3α-ol-17-one (androsterone) | 258 | 94 |
| Androstan-17β-ol-3-one (dihydrotestosterone) | 76 | 271 |
| 2α-Methyldihydrotestosterone | 48 | 134 |

are androgenic, but the degree of androgenicity cannot be quantitated.
Additional data on the androgenic potency of some of these compounds, as
determined by seminal vesicle assay are given in Table IX.

   2. *Pituitary Inhibition.* Testosterone can depress pituitary function,
as indicated by the decrease in urinary gonadotropins, inhibition of ovulation, and decrease in ovarian weight which occur during treatment. Bottomly
and Folley (6) demonstrated that the reduction in ovarian weight induced
by testosterone is due to selective inhibition of the pituitary and does not
occur when gonadotropin is administered concurrently with testosterone.
Thus it has been thought that the ability of testosterone and related compounds to inhibit tumor growth may be related to an inhibition of gonadotropin secretion from the pituitary gland.

   Most of the patients studied by Segaloff and co-workers (Table VIII)
showed a decrease in urinary gonadotropins following treatment with
testosterone or other effective steroids, but not with inactive steroids.
Gonadotropins usually fell in both responsive and unresponsive patients. It
seemed for a while that a relationship may exist between active steroids and
their ability to depress gonadotropins. However, Segaloff *et al.* (106) have

recently reported that fluoxymesterone, although producing remissions, did not significantly lower urinary gonad-stimulating hormone. Blackburn and Alpert (4) have also found that 2-methyldihydrotestosterone failed to depress urinary gonadotropin. Van Eck and Chang (125) observed that, although testosterone propionate would depress pituitary gonadotropin in castrated and X-ray irradiated mice, ovarian tumors still occurred. It

TABLE VIII

EFFECT OF ANDROSTANE DERIVATIVES ON URINARY GONADOTROPIN, 17-KETOSTEROID EXCRETION, AND COMPARATIVE INHIBITION OF HUMAN AND ANIMAL TUMORS[a, b]

| | Clinical response | | Urine excretion | | Rat fibro-adenoma |
| --- | --- | --- | --- | --- | --- |
| | Tumor | Andro-genicity | 17-Keto-steroids | Gonado-tropins | |
| 4-Androsten-17β-ol-3-one (testosterone) | − − | + + | ↑ | ↓ | − − |
| 4-Androsten-17α-ol-3-one (epitestosterone) | 0 | 0 | 0 | ↓ | 0 |
| Etiocholan-17β-ol-3-one | 0 | 0 | ↑ | 0 | 0 |
| Androstan-17β-ol-3-one (dihydrotestosterone) | − − | + + | ↑ | ↓ | − − |
| Androstane-3,17-dione | 0 | 0 | ↑ | 0 | |
| 5-Androsten-3β-ol-17-one (dehydroisoandrosterone) | 0 | 0 | ↑ | 0 | 0 |
| 5-Androstene-3β,17β-diol | 0 | + | ↑ | 0 | + or 0 |
| 17α-Methyl-5-androstene-3β,17β-diol | − | + | 0 | 0 | |
| 17α-Methyltestosterone | − − | + + | 0 | ↓ | − − |
| 17α-Vinyltestosterone | − | + | 0 | 0 | |
| 19-Nortestosterone | − | + | ↑ | ↓ | |
| Fluoxymesterone | − − | + | 0 | 0 | |

[a] Clinical data from papers of Segaloff and experimental data from papers of Huggins.
[b] − = Inhibition; 0 = no effect; + = stimulation; ↑ = increase; ↓ = decrease.

would appear therefore, from both clinical and animal studies, that simple depression of gonadotropin is not the single factor responsible for inhibition of tumor growth and that there is not a correlation between steroid effectiveness and gonadotropin inhibition.

It is tempting to believe that steroids induce remissions of mammary cancer by depressing pituitary functions other than gonadotropins. Testosterone has, for example, been effective in an ovariectomized-adrenalectomized patient, which would indicate the possibility of an effect on the pituitary gland. The studies of Huggins and Mainzer (58) demonstrate that, although ovariectomy markedly reduces fibroadenoma growth in rats, maximum reduction in tumor weight is obtained following hypophysectomy. Inasmuch as the steroids did not decrease fibroadenoma growth more than hypophysectomy, the compounds *may* be acting by inhibiting pituitary function other than gonadotropins. However, fluoxymesterone has been observed to produce remission in some but not all hypophysectomized patients with mammary cancer (3, 63). One is led to conclude that although steroids may act by depressing pituitary function, and thus mimicking hypophysectomy, this may not be the basic mechanism of their action.

*3.  Anabolic Activity.*  The anabolic properties of testosterone, which have been known for a long time, may be a factor in producing remissions. Steroids have been synthesized that show a separation of anabolic and androgenic effects (15, 99a). The best example of such a compound is 17-ethyl-19-nortestosterone (norethandrolone), which has been reported to produce a gain in underweight patients of 10 or more pounds (33, 66, 128).

Many of the steroids studied by Segaloff and co-workers, as discussed above, are known to have anabolic effects. The compounds noted by Huggins and Mainzer (58) to decrease fibroadenoma growth in rats were also anabolic, as judged by the weight gain of the animals. Additional data on relative myotropic potency, as determined by the levator ani method, are given in Table IX. Further, the metabolic effects of 2-methyldihydrotestosterone have been observed in one patient and are reported to be qualitatively similar to those of testosterone (5). Such metabolic effects do not necessarily denote androgenicity, which must be separately evaluated. Sufficient comparative data, either experimental or clinical, are not available to determine whether the remissions produced by various steroids in women are related to their myotropic or anabolic properties.

*4.  Other Endocrine Activities.  a.  Progestational activity.*  The role of progesterone in breast growth and the effect of progestational compounds in general will be discussed later. It is, however, known that testosterone can cause proliferation of the mammary gland, and Huggins has observed that steroids inhibit growth of the mammary fibroadenoma transplants in rats and at the same time stimulate the mammary gland. The limited data available at our laboratory on progestational activity of the compounds being discussed in this section are summarized in Table IX.

*b.  Antiestrogenic activity.*  Testosterone has certain antiestrogenic properties, and such activity is a possible means of action in depressing growth of hormone-dependent tumors. Available antiestrogenic data, from our laboratory and from the Cancer Chemotherapy National Service Center, on the compounds being discussed are included in Table IX. The relative antiestrogenic potency of these steroids differs greatly between the two studies listed because of difference of methodology. The Cancer Chemotherapy National Service Center data would indicate no relationship between antiestrogenic potency and tumor inhibition of the androgen derivatives, whereas our own data are not extensive enough at this time to permit of drawing any conclusion. Other information concerning antiestrogenic steroids will be reviewed later in this presentation.

*5. Metabolism of Steroids.* The production of 17-ketosteroids is not related to clinical effectiveness. Segaloff has shown that steroids may increase urinary 17-ketosteroids independently of their ability to induce

TABLE IX

COMPARISON OF ANTIESTROGENIC POTENCY OF COMPOUNDS INHIBITING
TUMOR GROWTH

| Compound | Tumor Growth[a] | | Andro-genic[d] | Myotro-pic[d] | Proges-tational[e] | Anti-estrogenic[f] | |
|---|---|---|---|---|---|---|---|
| | Clinical[b] | Rat[c] | | | | A | B |
| 4-Androsten-17β-ol-3-one (testosterone) | — — | — — | 35 | 26 | . . . | 80 | 46 |
| Androstan-17β-ol-3-one (dihydrotes-tosterone) | — — | — — | 13 | 21 | . . . | . . . | 41 |
| 5-Androsten-3β-ol-17-one (dehydroiso-androsterone) | 0 | 0 | 8* | < 5* | . . . | . . . | 35 |
| 5-Androstene-3β,17β-diol | 0 | + or 0 | 14* | 9* | . . . | . . . | 25 |
| 17α-Methyltestos-terone | — — | — — | 24 | 26 | . . . | . . . | 41 |
| 17α-Vinyltestos-terone | — | — | 2 | 20 | . . . | . . . | |
| 19-Nortestoster-one | — | — | 6 | 100 | 0 | 40 | 26 |
| 17-Ethyl-19-nortestosterone (Nilevar) | . . . | — — | 6 | 100 | 750 | 1250 | 63 |
| 17-Ethynyl-19-nortestosterone (Norlutin) | . . . | + | 2 | 1 | 50 | 800 | 66 |

[a] — = Inhibition; 0 = no effect; + = stimulation; . . . = no data.
[b] Data of Segaloff
[c] Data of Huggins.
[d] Testosterone propionate = 100%. Data from Saunders and Drill (99) except data labeled (*), which is from Cancer Chemotherapy National Service Center.
[e] Data of R. L. Elton.
[f] A = Data of R. Edgren. B = Cancer Chemotherapy National Service Center data.

remissions (Table VIII). 2-Methyldihydrotestosterone also increases keto-steroid output (5). In general, 17-alkylated steroids do not increase 17-ketosteroid excretion.

A number of investigators have also suggested that the metabolism of testosterone to an estrogen may explain the exacerbation occasionally noted during androgen therapy. It has since been shown that estrogens can be isolated from the urine of ovariectomized, adrenalectomized patients receiving androgens (86). From the standpoint of studying new steroids, it would be extremely interesting to observe the effects on tumor growth of an androgenic steroid that is not metabolizable to an estrogen.

6. *Direct Effect on Tumor Growth.* The possibility that steroids may exert a direct effect on tumor growth, independently of an endocrine mechanism, must also be kept in mind. Steroids are not more effective in depressing tumor growth in animals than hypophysectomy. This is usually interpreted to mean that the steroid is acting by an endocrine mechanism. However, the apparent cause-and-effect relationship may not be real, and the steroid, even though not more effective than hypophysectomy, may be acting directly. In man there is some evidence that steroids may produce remission in hypophysectomized patients. If such is confirmed by more extensive study, it would certainly point to a direct steroid action. Testololactone, a steroid derivative without known endocrine effects, is discussed in other papers presented at this meeting (cf. paper by Segaloff *et al.*, in this volume).

## II. Estrogens

Compounds with estrogenic activity are used in the treatment of (1) cancer of the prostate and metastases, and (2) cancer of the breast and metastases.

With regard to the prostate, earlier data had shown that castration produces atrophy of the prostate gland. The studies of Huggins and co-workers extended this relationship considerably, demonstrating in the dog that (1) castration caused complete cessation of prostatic secretion; (2) testosterone propionate in the castrate dog increased prostatic size and secretion; (3) estrogen decreased prostatic size and secretion; (4) estrogen administration with androgen decreased or abolished prostatic secretion, and prostatic size decreased.

The above results then led Huggins and co-workers and others to employ estrogens and castration clinically.

The rationale for the initial use of estrogens in the treatment of disseminated breast cancer is not as concrete as that for prostate cancer. The incidence of breast cancer is highest in the 40–60-year age group concomitant with a decrease in ovarian function and an excess of FSH, LH, and prolactin, perhaps indicating, as some have thought, that estrogenic therapy might be employed. Further, as Haddow and associates (39) point out, estrogens can induce cancer in certain strains of animals, and carcinogens are often able to reduce tumor size and retard tumor growth in experimental animals. It was also observed by Farrow and Woodard (27) that estrogen acts similarly to testosterone propionate in affecting calcium metabolism in patients with mammary cancer and osseous metastases, again indicating that estrogens may be of value in treatment.

## A. Estrogens and Prostatic Cancer

*1. Steroids and Production of Prostatic Cancer.* Although prostatic cancer may be hormonally dependent at a certain stage in its growth, this does not necessarily mean that the tumor is directly induced by androgens. There is no evidence that prostatic cancer in man is caused by testosterone. First, prostatic cancer usually develops at an age when testicular function is declining, as measured by urinary bioassay and determination of 17-keto-steroid excretion. A survey of patients over 45 who had received intensive androgen therapy for noncancerous reasons did not demonstrate an increased incidence of prostatic cancer (68). Testosterone has also been administered in high doses for 3 months to patients with advanced prostatic cancer by Brendler *et al.* (9). Exacerbations were produced in some patients, although others experienced a palliative benefit, perhaps due to the anabolic properties of testosterone. Of most interest, however, the authors report that the majority of patients showed no change in their clinical picture even though serum acid phosphatase and urinary 17-ketosteroids rose considerably. Of further interest are the studies of Horning (50), who reported that prostatic carcinoma arose more frequently in mice receiving methylcholanthrene after pretreatment with stilbestrol rather than with testosterone.

Although there does not appear to be evidence implicating testicular androgens as a causative factor in prostatic cancer, the tumor, once it develops, is at least temporarily hormonally dependent, as it responds to castration. Castration removes not only testicular androgen, but also testicular estrogens, perhaps unknown materials, and, lastly, influences pituitary function.

*2. Experimentally Induced Prostatic Tumors.* In contrast to the study of experimentally induced mammary tumors, few studies have been made on the production of prostatic cancer. In the earlier work of Huggins benign tumors of the dog were employed to study the effect of castration and estrogen administration. Horning (50) has produced prostatic adenocarcinoma in the mouse by implanting methylcholanthrene into the prostate gland, and Kirschbaum (65) has also induced prostatic cancer with carcinogens. These tumors have not been employed, however, to study possibly inhibitory effects of steroid derivatives.

3. *Mechanism of Action of Estrogens on Prostatic Cancer.* The use of estrogens in the treatment of prostatic cancer was originally based on the known antagonism of estrogens to certain effects of androgens in experimental animals. Thus, if castration were effective because it removed androgens, estrogens might be effective because they would antagonize the effect of androgens in the noncastrated individual. Certain quantitative relationships between estrogens and testosterone do exist. The studies of Huggins and Clark (55) demonstrated a quantitative reciprocal relationship between stilbestrol and testosterone as measured by the secretory output of the prostate in castrate dogs. A similar antagonism can also be demonstrated on the serum acid phosphatase values of patients with prostatic cancer.

However, when other end points are used to assess estrogen-androgen antagonism, it is often found either that such an antagonism does not exist or that testosterone and the estrogen react in a similar manner. For example, Brendler (8) reported that in the intact, immature rat, testosterone in doses sufficient to maintain a castrate prostate completely prevent the usual effect of estradiol, even if the dose of estradiol was increased to five times that of testosterone. Similar results were obtained in the castrate animal undergoing maintenance replacement therapy with testosterone or in the castrate animal during attempts to restore the prostate from the atrophic state after a 1-week period without treatment. Saunders (98) has shown, over an extensive dose range, that estrone has no influence on the increase in ventral prostate weight in rats treated with testosterone. The effects of testosterone and estrone on seminal vesicle were additive. Thus, in these studies testosterone and estradiol were not antagonistic. Further, Gunn and Gould (38) demonstrated that castration impaired the uptake of zinc[65] by the dorsolateral lobes of the rat's prostate. This impairment of zinc uptake can be prevented by substitution therapy with testosterone or with estradiol within a specified dose range. It does not seem probable, therefore, that a simple physiological antagonism between testosterone and estrogens is sufficient to explain the inhibiting effects of estrogens on the prostate gland.

There is evidence to indicate that the estrogens may exert effects in prostatic cancer through a pituitary mechanism, as will be discussed in the following section. A direct effect of estrogens is not ruled out for McDonald and Latta (76) have demonstrated that natural and synthetic estrogens significantly inhibit anaerobic glycolysis of human prostatic adenoma slices.

## B. Estrogens and Mammary Tumors

*1. Effects of Estrogens on Experimental Tumors.* The work of Heiman in the 1930's began to point out that estrogens may stimulate tumor growth (42–46). Since that time a number of investigators have confirmed the finding that estrogens can stimulate mammary fibroadenoma growth. However, there are other reports in the literature indicating a lack of effect of estrogens on such tumors. Noble (90) has reviewed these data, pointing out that the positive effects of estrogen have usually been obtained with early generations of the tumor line, whereas the studies reporting no effect of estrogen on the tumors were usually performed with older generations of the tumor line.

Estrogens can have a biphasic effect on the growth of rat mammary fibroadenoma. Millar and Noble (80) reported in 1954 that low doses of stilbestrol may stimulate tumor growth in the normal female rat, whereas high doses will inhibit growth (Table X). Huggins and co-workers (59) have

TABLE X

EFFECT OF DOSAGE OF ESTROGEN ON RESPONSE[a] OF
RAT MAMMARY FIBROADENOMA (59, 80)

| Compound | Dosage (μg.) | Normal | Ovariectomized | Hypophysectomized |
|---|---|---|---|---|
| Stilbestrol | 5, 10 | + | | |
| | 200, 400 | — | | |
| Estrone | 1 | | + | 0 |
| | 50 | | — | |
| Estradiol | 0.1 | | + | |
| | 20 | | — | |
| Estriol | 10 | | + | |
| | 20 | | + | |
| | 100 | | — | |

[a] — = Inhibition; 0 = no effect; + = stimulation.

also carried out a series of studies with estrone, estradiol, and estriol, finding that small doses of these compounds promote tumor growth in the ovariectomized rat, whereas high doses inhibit tumor growth. In one study a small dose of estrone, which stimulated tumor growth in the ovariectomized rat, was without effect in the hypophysectomized animal (Table X).

Estrogens have also been reported to increase the incidence, decrease the incidence, or have no effect on the incidence of mammary tumors in rats induced by polycyclic hydrocarbons (31, 101, 116). In view of the data quoted above in the biphasic response to estrogens, the variation in response obtained in tumors induced by carcinogens may be related to the different doses of estrogen employed by the above investigators.

*2. Comparative Clinical Effectiveness of Estrogens.* When comparative studies of the effect of estrogens on cancer of the breast have been undertaken, they have generally demonstrated that materials such as diethylstilbestrol, ethynylestradiol, estradiol dipropionate, and estrone sulfate (Premarin) are approximately equally effective in producing subjective relief, primary tumor regression, soft tissue regression, and bone regression. The dosages of the materials employed have been quite high but have usually been in proportion to the estrogenic potencies of the compounds (88). Other materials, such as dienestrol, appear to be somewhat less effective than the above steroids.

Few derivatives of estrogens have been studied for their inhibiting effect on tumor growths, as contrasted with the large number of testosterone derivatives that have been evaluated. Huffman *et al.* (51) have shown that compounds such as 16-ketoestrone and 16-ketoestradiol are potent inhibitors of mitoses in *in vitro* studies. A related compound, mytatrienediol (16α-methylepiestradiol-3-methyl ether) has been reported by Spencer *et al.* (121) to produce improvement in patients with prostatic carcinoma, but also to produce a definite response in patients with multiple myeloma.

*3. Mechanism of Action of Estrogens.* The mechanism by which the estrogens act to decrease tumor growth and cause remissions in patients with mammary cancer is not known. The estrogens are powerful inhibitors of pituitary functions (as will be discussed later) and are generally thought to act by this means. The fact that high doses of estrogens do depress pituitary function and that simultaneous regression of tumor size occurs must mean that the large doses of estrogen do not act directly on the tumor to stimulate growth. Further, the possibility that large doses of estrogens directly depress tumor growth is not ruled out.

## III. Progestins

Progesterone and progestational compounds, in contrast to the androgens and estrogens, have received relatively little study in relationship to tumor growth. Further, studies on the effect of progesterone on tumor growth have produced contradictory results.

*1. Progesterone and Experimental Tumors.* Heiman (45) reported that progesterone inhibited the growth of mammary fibroadenoma in intact female rats, whereas Millar and Noble (80) did not obtain any effect when a smaller dose of progesterone was used. Variable results have been obtained in ovariectomized rats (Table XI). Progesterone increased the incidence of mammary tumors in animals fed a diet containing 2-acetylaminofluorine (11) or methylcholanthrene (54).

The variations in response to progesterone may be due to factors such as dosage and difference in tumor strains. It is possible that perhaps progesterone also produces a biphasic response, depending on dosage. A detailed study with various doses of progesterone must be undertaken in intact, ovariectomized, and hypophysectomized animals before the exact role of this hormone in tumor growth can be defined.

TABLE XI

EFFECT OF PROGESTERONE ON GROWTH OF RAT MAMMARY FIBROADENOMA

| Progesterone | | Tumor growth[a] | | |
|---|---|---|---|---|
| Reference | Dose (mg.) | Normal female | Ovariectomized | Hypophysectomized |
| (45) | 13 | — | 0 | |
| (80) | 5 | 0 | | |
| (59) | 1 | | 0 | 0 |
| | 4 | | + | |

[a] 0 = No effect; — = inhibition; + = stimulation.

2. *Effect of Estrogen and Progestin on Tumor Growth.* Estrogen-progesterone interrelationships are important in normal breast growth, as mentioned in the last section on pituitary function. It is perhaps pertinent, however, to mention at this time the effects of such combinations in the intact animal.

It is well established that estrogens can inhibit progesterone-induced endometrial proliferation (12), and Miyake and Pincus (81) have pointed out that this antagonistic effect of estrogen can be quantitated by determining the carbonic anhydrase activity of the endometrium. When estrogen-induced tumors were studied, progesterone had an antagonistic effect. Noble and Collip (91) reported that mammary tumors induced by estrone were depressed by progesterone. Mardones *et al.* (77) found that estrogen-induced uterine myofibromas were also depressed by progestins. They further observed that 19-norprogesterone was more active than progesterone in depressing the growth of these tumors in guinea pigs. The rat mammary fibroadenoma has also been studied, and Millar and Noble (80) noted that progesterone inhibited the stimulating effect of stilbestrol in intact animals (Table XII). Huggins *et al.* (59) reported that the stimulating effect of small doses of estriol on tumor growth was increased by progesterone. On the other hand, the effect of larger doses of progesterone was inhibited by a high dose of estrone (Table XII).

3. *Clinical Studies.* Gordon and associates (36) studied the effect of

progesterone on cancer of the breast and observed objective evidence of
remission in only 2 of 20 patients. 17-Ketosteroid excretion was increased
and urinary gonad-stimulating hormone was decreased. Recently Goldenberg and Hayes (32) studied the effect of a new compound with progestational effects, 9α-bromo-11-ketoprogesterone, in 49 patients with breast
cancer. The drug produced objective remission in 20 % of the patients compared with 25 % remission in patients receiving testosterone propionate.

TABLE  XII

EFFECT OF COMBINATIONS OF ESTROGEN AND PROGESTERONE ON
RAT MAMMARY FIBROADENOMA GROWTH

| | Treatment | | Fibroadenoma growth[a] | |
| | | | | |
| Reference | Estrogen (μg.) | Proges- terone (mg.) | Normal | Ovariec- tomized |
|---|---|---|---|---|
| (59) | Estriol, 20 | — | | + |
| | Estriol, 20 | 1 | | + + |
| | — | 1 | | 0 |
| (59) | Estrone, 100 | — | | 0 |
| | Estrone, 100 | 4 | | + |
| | — | 4 | | + + |
| (80) | Stilbestrol, 20 | — | + | |
| | Stilbestrol, 20 | 5 | 0 | |
| | — | 5 | 0 | |

[a] 0 = No effect; + = stimulation.

*4. New Progestins.* Progestational activity has been studied extensively
by ourselves (100), Miyake and Pincus (82), and others, and active compounds in this field have recently been reviewed (14). Representative
structures and potencies of some of these new compounds are illustrated in
Tables XIII, XIV, and XVI. It is of interest that a 17-spirolactone has
progestational activity (47). It should be noted that progestational potency
can at times differ quite significantly, depending on whether a 2+ or 3+
endometrial response (McPhail scale) is taken as the end point (Tables
XIII, XIV). Further, there is no direct relationship between progestational
potency and ability to inhibit the growth of rat mammary fibroadenoma;
in fact, two compounds stimulated tumor growth (Table XIV).

## IV.  ANTIESTROGENS AND ANTIANDROGENS

### A.  Definitions

It is well known that one drug may reduce the response produced by
another drug. Drugs having this effect are known as *antagonists,* and such
antagonism exists in a wide variety of fields, including the endocrine system.

The antagonistic effect is often described as an anti- effect and thus the terms *antiestrogen* and *antiandrogen* have crept into the endocrine literature. However, these titles are only descriptive and do not suggest the mechanism by which the antagonistic effect is produced. We should keep in mind that pharmacologically three major types of antagonism are known, namely, *physiological antagonism, chemical antagonism,* and *specific antagonism.* Specific antagonism may be subdivided into three groups: *competitive antagonism, irreversible competitive antagonism,* and *noncompetitive antagonism.* The principles underlying these different types of antagonism are well established in the pharmacologic literature. Before the terms can be correctly applied to the anti- effects of endocrine active chemicals, the drugs in question must receive careful study to define the receptor systems and the quantitative relationships of the antagonism. The different types of antagonism mentioned above will be briefly discussed.

*1. Physiological Antagonism.* This term is used to describe the situation in which two drugs act by different mechanisms, or on different organ systems, to produce effects that are mutually antagonistic. For example, nitroglycerin causes a fall in blood pressure and epinephrine causes a rise in blood pressure. If particular doses are chosen, these two agents may be given together without inducing a change in blood pressure. Numerous other examples of this type of antagonism may be found, and it is likely that many steroid interactions are on the basis of physiological antagonism.

*2. Chemical Antagonism.* In chemical antagonism the active drug combines chemically with another drug, its antagonist, to form a compound with either no activity or substantially less activity than the original. Only a few proved instances of chemical antagonism between drugs are known and there are no data to indicate that steroid antagonism occurs by this mechanism.

*3. Specific Antagonism.* This type of antagonism is of great interest because of the prevalence and usefulness of specific antagonists in medicine. Specific antagonists may be divided into three subgroups: competitive antagonists, irreversible competitive antagonists, and noncompetitive antagonists.

*a. Competitive antagonists.* The competitive antagonists are those agents which have as their characteristic action the ability to interfere with the eventual combination between the stimulus and the responding system. This interference exists in the form of a competition between the agonist and antagonist for a particular site of action for which both have an affinity. Ordinarily the antagonist does not elicit a response of a tissue with which it combines. An example of competitive antagonism is the relationship between histamine and an antihistamine drug. For increasing concentrations of histamine required to produce bronchial constriction, an increased amount of the competitive antagonist (antihistamine) is required. The antihistamine itself has no effect on bronchial smooth muscle; it serves only to block the effect of histamine. This relationship usually states that the dose of active drug necessary to cause maximum response increases in a linear fashion with the increasing doses of the antagonist. Although a quantitative relationship exists between the active drug and its antagonist, the relationships are not strictly linear, but rather are curvilinear. There are several possible explanations for the curvilinear result; one implies that more than one molecule of antagonist combines with the receptor and that this combination occurs in stages. Nevertheless, we need note at this time only the quantitative relationship between the active drug and its antagonist, and, secondly, that the antagonist is usually devoid of effects on the system being measured. Such competitive inhibition is reversible, for the inhibiting drug can be overcome by an increased supply of the active ingredient.

It may be expected that some antiestrogenic or antiandrogenic effects are explainable by this mechanism. The only steroids presently known to act as competitive antagonists are 17-spirolactones, steroids which block the effects of aldosterone on the excretion of sodium and potassium (59a, b).

*b. Irreversible competitive antagonism.* In certain instances the antagonist appears to compete with the active drug for a site of action, and the resulting combination between the antagonist and its receptor is so firm that the antagonist cannot be separated from its site of action. This is termed irreversible competitive antagonism. It may be illustrated by the effect of an adrenergic blocking agent, such as dibenamine, or by the irreversible inhibition of cholinesterase by a variety of organic phosphates, such as diisopropylfluorophosphate. At the present time there is no indication that steroids act by this mechanism.

*c. Noncompetitive antagonism.* The term noncompetitive antagonism has arisen from a more detailed consideration of the mode of action of certain enzyme inhibitors. It is known, for example, that some enzyme inhibitors act not by competition with a substrate, but rather by competition with coenzyme. An example of this type of antagonism exists in the case of disulfiram, a drug that inhibits the enzymes responsible for oxidation of acetaldehyde. Disulfiram competes not with acetaldehyde, but with reduced diphosphopyridine nucleotide, the coenzyme of the aldehyde oxidase. Thus, no amount of acetaldehyde can overcome the inhibition produced by disulfiram.

## B.  Antiestrogenic Activity of Steroids

1.  *Estrogen Antagonism by Estrogens.*  Several groups have reported that impeded estrogens, such as estriol and its relatives, can inhibit the actions of estradiol-17β and estrone on the uterus of rats and mice (22, 23, 48, 56). Huggins and Jensen (56) showed that this inhibition occurred only over a narrow range of doses. This was confirmed by Edgren and Calhoun (23), who also demonstrated that at dose levels below the narrow range of inhibitory effects estriol only added to the estrone-induced response. They further showed that estrogens produce simple additive effects when studied by the vaginal smear response of rats or mice (20). It would appear, therefore, that the ability of one estrogen to inhibit the effects of another occurs only over a narrow range of dosage and, as far as known, such an effect is not significant in attempting to explain the tumor-inhibiting activity of estrogens.

2.  *Estrogen Antagonism by Androgens.*  The androgens were first reported as estrogen antagonists by de Jongh and Korenchevsky and by Dennison (cf. 26a). Since then the degree of antagonism reported by various authors has varied considerably, depending in part on the organ response being measured, and one may conclude that androgens may antagonize certain, but not all, responses of estrogen.

With regard to the vaginal smear, it has been observed that testosterone will block the epithelial keratinization and leucocytic migration induced by estrone or by estriol (16, 17). The antagonistic effects of androgens and estrogens have recently been reviewed by Edgren (17).

Rat uterine weight has been used by a large number of investigators (126a) as an end point to determine the effects of combinations of estrogens and androgens. Most groups have found that androgens inhibit the effects of estrogens on uterine growth. However, over a narrow dose range of mixtures of testosterone propionate and estrone it can be demonstrated that testosterone propionate augments uterine growth produced by estradiol-17β and estriol. It might appear, therefore, that low doses of estrone are augmented by androgens whereas high doses are inhibited (25). Testosterone will also counteract the effect of estrogen on the mouse uterus (18). On the other hand, Szego (123) has reported that testosterone was ineffective in inhibiting the water-imbibition effects of estradiol-17β.

With regard to the pituitary, Albert (1) has shown that estrogen-induced pituitary hypertrophy can be prevented by the simultaneous administration of testosterone. Further, Hoogstra and Paesi (49) demonstrated that, although pituitary FSH was increased by testosterone propionate and decreased by estradiol benzoate, the estradiol did not modify the testosterone response.

Of particular interest are the results of Arhelger and Huseby (2), who demonstrated that the effects of estradiol and estrone on the mammary glands can be antagonized by endogenous androgens.

*3. Estrogen Antagonism by Progesterone.* There are numerous papers indicating that progesterone can inhibit the stimulating effects of estrogen on the uterus. In mice progesterone inhibits estrone-induced uterine weight changes (18, 21, 24), although estriol-induced growth is largely unmodified (22). When the vaginal smear response or changes in the chick oviduct are studied, both synergistic and antagonistic interactions of estrogens and progestins can be obtained (17, 67, 79). The growth of the mammary gland of intact animals is stimulated by a combination of estrogen and progesterone (40, 119), although an excess of estrogen will inhibit the response.

*4. Antiestrogenic Activity of Nortestosterones.* The 19-nortestosterones have been shown to be potent antiestrogens. These compounds, although derivatives of testosterone, show little effect as androgens. In addition to antiestrogenic activity, their greatest potency is in the progestational and, secondly, anabolic areas.

It was first demonstrated by Payne *et al.* (93) that 17-ethyl-19-nortestosterone antagonized the effects of estrogens on the ovary and uterus of hypophysectomized rats. Although much less potent an androgen than testosterone propionate, 17-ethyl-19-nortestosterone was about seventy times more effective than testosterone in blocking estrogen- induced uterine growth (18). Bowers *et al.* (7) have studied the blocking effects of a series of dihydro-19-nortestosterones, and recently Edgren and associates of our laboratory have reported on the estrogen antagonistic action of 29 compounds related to 19-nortestosterone (24). Both groups of investigators found several compounds to be very active, although potencies vary in the two studies, probably because of the different end points chosen.

The most active compounds in Edgren's study are listed in Table XIII. It may be noted that there is not a direct correlation between antiestrogenic and progestational potency, or with the other endocrine properties listed. The data on the *n*-butyl compound also demonstrates that a compound may be progestational without blocking the ability of estrone to increase uterine weight. It is of interest that an antiestrogenic activity of such steroids has also been obtained in women. Ferin (28) reported that 19-nortestosterone has an antiestrogenic action in castrated female patients treated with estrogen, and recently 17-ethyl-19-nortestosterone has been observed to have a similar effect (122).

The significance of an antiestrogenic effect of steroids in the treatment of human cancer is unknown. Table IX does not indicate any relationship between the effectiveness of steroids, as evaluated clinically by Segaloff, and their antiestrogenic potency. However, it is possible that the correct end point for the determination of antiestrogenic potency may not have been chosen. If such compounds were to depress tumor growth by an antiestrogenic action, one must assume that the tumor is estrogen dependent at the time of treatment.

TABLE XIII

COMPARISON OF ANTIESTROGENIC POTENCY OF 19-NORTESTOSTERONE DERIVATIVES WITH OTHER ENDOCRINE EFFECTS (24)

| Substituent | Antiestrogenic[a] | Progestational[a] 2 + | Progestational[a] 3 + | Estrogenic[b] Uterus | Estrogenic[b] Vaginal smear | Androgenic[c] | Myotropic[c] |
|---|---|---|---|---|---|---|---|
| Isopropyl | 2200 | 1000 | 1200 | — | — | < 1 | 2 |
| Ethyl | 1250 | 1000 | 750 | < 1 | 0 | 6 | 100 |
| Methyl | 880 | 500 | 30 | < 0.01 | — | 6 | 100 |
| Ethynyl | 800 | 50 | 50 | 0.01 | 0 | 2 | 1 |
| 2-Methallyl | 680 | 2500 | 1200 | 0.01 | 0 | 1 | < 5 |
| Propynyl | 500 | 300 | 500 | < 0.03 | 0 | 0.5–1 | Catabolic |
| n-Butyl | 0 | 150 | 100 | 0.01 | 0 | < 0.5 | < 1 |

[a] Progesterone = 100.
[b] Estrone = 100.
[c] Testosterone propionate = 100.

For further comparison, the endocrine properties of steroids that affect rat mammary fibroadenoma growth, as studied by Huggins and associates, are listed in Table XIV. Compounds were chosen for this table on the basis of available endocrine data. There is no indication of a correlation of the endocrine activities listed with effect on tumor growth.

## C. Antiandrogenic Compounds

A specific antiandrogenic compound would be of particular interest for study in the treatment of the hormonally dependent phase of prostatic cancer, even though our knowledge of the biological factors influencing growth of prostatic carcinoma is poor. A phenanthrene derivative has been reported to act as an antiandrogen, inhibiting the effect of testosterone on the seminal vesicle, prostate, and levator ani of the rat (95) and the action of testosterone on the cock's comb (12a). In an earlier paper at this conference, Fried observed that A-ring-norprogesterone was also antiandrogenic. These compounds apparently do not have other endocrine activities and may be acting specifically to block the effects of testosterone. Further experimental and eventually clinical data on these substances will be of interest, as they offer another theoretical approach to the treatment of cancer.

## V. Pituitary Function

Estrogens and androgens can inhibit the pituitary gland and there is evidence to indicate that many of the steroids producing remissions in patients with cancer are effective because they act through such a mechanism.

TABLE XIV

COMPARATIVE ENDOCRINE ACTIVITIES AND EFFECT OF STEROIDS ON
RAT MAMMARY FIBROADENOMA GROWTH

| Compound | Tumor weight[a] (mg.) | Andro- genic[b] | Myo- tropic[b] | Progesterone[c] | | Anti- estro- genic[c] |
|---|---|---|---|---|---|---|
| | | | | 2 + | 3 + | |
| 17-Ethynylnortestosterone | 3306 | 2 | 1 | 50 | 50 | 800 |
| 17-Propylnortestosterone | 2082 | < 1 | 10 | 250 | 250 | 300 |
| Control females | 917 | — | — | — | — | — |
| 17-Ethynyl-5(10)- estrenolone | 723 | 0 | 0 | 10 | 0 | 0 |
| Nortestosterone | 359 | 6 | 100 | < 1 | 0 | 40 |
| 17-Ethyl-5(10)- estrenolone | 195 | 1 | 10 | 50 | 50 | 20 |
| 17-Methylnortestosterone | 126 | 6 | 100 | 500 | 30 | 880 |
| 17-Ethylnortestosterone | 107 | 6 | 100 | 1000 | 750 | 1250 |
| Ovariectomized rats | 79 | — | — | — | — | — |

[a] Tumor weight data from Huggins et al. (58, 59).

[b] Androgenic and myotropic data from Saunders and Drill (99), testosterone propionate = 100 %.

[c] 2 + Progestational data from Dr. R. L. Elton (progesterone = 100 % in 2 + and 3 + response). 3 + Progestational data and antiestrogenic data from Edgren et al. (24).

*1. Pituitary Function and Prostate Gland.* Smith and Engle (118) demonstrated that hypophysectomy produces marked testicular changes together with changes in accessory organs, such as the prostate, which were similar to that seen after castration. Moore and Price (84a) observed similar testicular changes after the administration of estrogen. However, estrogen did not affect the testes if gonadotropic extract was simultaneously injected, and it was concluded that estrogen affects the testes indirectly by inhibiting pituitary gonadotropins. It was later shown that the administration of phenolic estrogens eliminated prostatic secretion in the dog, but, when estrogen and gonadotropin were administered simultaneously, prostatic secretion was preserved, although reduced in amount (52).

There is a fair amount of evidence implicating prolactin as an important factor in the control of prostate growth. For example, Grayhack et al. (37), noting that the prostate of the hypophysectomized castrate rat was less responsive to testosterone than that of animals subjected only to castration, found that the response to testosterone in the hypophysectomized castrate rat could be appreciably increased by the simultaneous administration of prolactin. It has also been demonstrated by Sonnenberg and associates (120) that an anterior pituitary preparation containing prolactin and labeled with radioactive iodine localized in a large concentration in the rat prostate. In these studies testosterone depressed the uptake of the radioactivity in the prostate, whereas castration and estradiol increased the concentration of radioactivity in the prostate. Prolactin administered alone apparently did not have any direct effect on the ventral prostate, as judged by size of the gland in the rat (107). Further, prolactin did not produce histological changes in human Leydig cells, although these cells were influenced by luteinizing hormone (75).

The above data indicate that testosterone and prolactin have a synergistic effect on the prostate gland. Estrogens may possibly exert their effect by interfering with this relationship by producing pituitary inhibition, perhaps by influencing prolactin production, or by affecting utilization at the end organ.

2. *Pituitary Hormones and the Mammary Gland.* The interrelationship between the steroids and pituitary hormones in causing ductal growth, lobular development, and finally lactation have been reviewed by Nelson (89), Lyons and associates (72, 73), and Hadfield (40, 41). Although estrogens can produce ductal growth and estrogens plus progesterone cause further development of the mammary gland in the *intact* rodent, such hormones are without effect on the mammary gland of the hypophysectomized animal. In the hypophysectomized rat good lobuloalveolar development can be induced by administering estrogen, progesterone, and prolactin (mammotropin). Lactation will occur if adrenocortical hormones are also administered. Growth hormone (somatotropin) synergizes both the lobuloalveolar development and lactation as described above, but is inactive in the absence of prolactin. However, in C3H mice, Nadine (87) observed that growth hormone produces mammogenic and lactogenic effects in the absence of prolactin.

3. *Pituitary-inhibiting Effect of Steroids.* Of the natural steroids, the estrogens are usually stated to be the most potent pituitary inhibitors, progesterone the least active, with testosterone being intermediate in effectiveness. Dr. F. J. Saunders, in unpublished studies, has obtained some comparative data on these steroids. Spayed rats were injected with the steroid at different dose levels for 30 days, the pituitary was removed and homogenized, and comparative assays were performed in immature rats using ovarian weight as an end point. Progesterone was ineffective at high doses (Table XV). Testosterone produced some pituitary inhibition at a dose of 0.2 mg. but did not completely inhibit the output of pituitary gonadotropins at a

dose of 1.0 mg. The estrogens, as expected, were quite effective, and the dose producing inhibition was in general proportional to the estrogenic activity of the compound.

TABLE XV

PITUITARY GONADOTROPIN-INHIBITING EFFECT OF STANDARD ESTROGENS, PROGESTERONE, AND TESTOSTERONE[a, b]

| Compound | Complete pituitary inhibition (mg.) | Slight pituitary inhibition (mg.) | Estrogenic potency[c] | |
|---|---|---|---|---|
| | | | Mouse uterus (%) | Rat vaginal (%) |
| Estrone | 0.02 | 0.01–0.02 | 100 | 100 |
| Estradiol-17β | 0.005–0.02 | 0.005 | 370 | 650 |
| Diethylstilbestrol | 0.005 | 0.001 | 625 | 478 |
| Estriol | 0.1 | 0.05–0.1 | 11 | 7 |
| Progesterone | (10) | (10) | — | — |
| Testosterone propionate | (1) | 0.2 | — | — |

[a] Unpublished data from Dr. F. J. Saunders.
[b] Doses listed without parentheses produced pituitary inhibition. Parentheses indicate an inactive dose of compound.
[c] Data from Dr. R. Edgren.

Saunders has also studied the pituitary-inhibiting effects of new steroids which have progestational, androgenic, and anabolic effects. The steroid derivatives which are potent progestational agents in the Clauberg test are still poor pituitary inhibitors (Table XVI). Both the ethyl and ethynyl derivatives of nortestosterone are active, with the latter compound being more potent. It is not surprising that 17-ethynyl-5(10)-estrenolone is the most active, as this steroid is also estrogenic (7 % activity of estrone). The data of Epstein et al. (26b) in parabiotic rats show a different series of pituitary-inhibiting potencies than Saunders' data. In parabiotic rats 17-ethyl-19-nortestosterone depressed gonadotropin hypersecretion at doses which were anabolic and not significantly androgenic (34). The compounds also inhibit pituitary function as judged by the blockade of ovulation in the rabbit (Table XVI).

*4. Depression of Pituitary Function as a Mechanism of Action of Steroids.* Hypophysectomy decreases tumor growth to a greater extent in experimental animals than ovariectomy (Table XVII), and there are some data demonstrating that a similar situation exists in man. Hypophysectomy is not only effective against growths such as the rat mammary fibroadenoma, but also decreases the incidence of mammary cancer induced by dibenzanthracene (80). Compounds decreasing tumor growth in animals mimic the effect of hypophysectomy. Further, androgenic steroids which inhibit the growth of rat fibroadenoma are not more effective than hypophysectomy.

TABLE XVI

PITUITARY-INHIBITING EFFECTS OF STEROIDS AND RELATIONSHIP TO PROGESTATIONAL POTENCY[a]

| | Complete pituitary inhibition[b] | Slight pituitary inhibition[c] | Parabiotic rats[d] | 50% Inhibition, ovulation[e] | | Progestational potency[f] |
|---|---|---|---|---|---|---|
| | | | | 1 | 2 | 2 + |
| Progesterone | (10) | (10) | (40) | 1–2 | 1–2 | 100 |
| 9α-F-11-Keto-17-acetoxyprogesterone | (2) | ? 2.0 | — | — | 0.1 | 2500 |
| 17-(2-Methallyl)-nortestosterone | (0.5) | (0.5) | — | 0.5 | 0.5 | 2500 |
| 17-Propynyl-nortestosterone | (0.5) | (0.5) | — | <2 | — | 500 |
| 17-Ethylnortestosterone | (2.0) | 1.0 | <0.01 | <0.2 | — | 1000 |
| 17-Ethynylnortestosterone | 0.5 | 0.5 / ? 0.2 | 0.3–0.6 | 0.1 | — | 50 |
| 17-Ethynyl-5(10)-estrenolone | 0.1–0.2 | 0.1 | 0.6 | 0.1 | — | 10 |
| 17-Methylnortestosterone | — | — | <0.1 | 0.1 | — | 500 |

[a] Parentheses indicate an inactive dose. Underline indicates active at dose used, but inactive at lower doses.

[b] Data of Dr. F. J. Saunders, unpublished, ovarian weight of recipient < 19 mg.

[c] Data of Dr. F. J. Saunders, unpublished, ovarian weight of recipient slightly reduced.

[d] Data of Epstein et al. (26b), active dose chosen as that which decreased ovarian weight > 30 %.

[e] Ovulation inhibition data; column 1 from Pincus et al. (94a); column 2 from Dr. R. L. Elton.

[f] Progestational potency, subcutaneous administration, progesterone = 100 %; data from Dr. R. L. Elton.

Since estrogens and androgens produce pituitary inhibition, it is tempting to assume that they may act by depressing prolactin output, although the studies of Segaloff with testosterone, other androgens, or estrogens, demonstrate that these steroids either show no effect on urinary prolactin or increase the urinary titer of prolactin. However, such data do not rule out a prolactin mechanism, as the steroids could affect prolactin response by other mechanisms. For example, estrogen and progesterone must be administered in a definite ratio to stimulate mammary growth in the *intact* rat. The effect is decreased when high doses of estrogen are employed, perhaps by interfering with prolactin response.

TABLE XVII

COMPARATIVE EFFECT OF OVARIECTOMY, HYPOPHYSECTOMY, AND TREATMENT
WITH TWO POTENT STEROIDS ON RAT MAMMARY FIBROADENOMA WEIGHT[a]

| | Tumor weight (mg) | | |
| Treatment | Intact | Overiecto-mized | Hypophysec-tomized |
|---|---|---|---|
| 1. None | 540 | 182 | 34 |
| 2. None | 318 | — | 47 |
| 3. None | 1464 | 163 | 46 |
| 4. None | 242 | 59 | — |
|    Testosterone | — | 50 | — |
| 5. None | 2217 | 186 | — |
|    Dihydrotestosterone | — | 101 | — |
| 6. None | 443 | 91 | — |
|    Dihydrotestosterone | — | 60 | — |

[a] Data from various papers of Huggins and co-workers.

*5. Pituitary Factors and Experimental Tumor Growth.* Some studies have been made on the effect of crude pituitary extract, growth hormone, and prolactin on the growth of rat mammary fibroadenoma (59, 80). Such data as are available are in a sense preliminary, and further work must be carried out before the role of the pituitary factors in tumor growth can be delineated.

## VI. SUMMARY

The endocrine properties of steroids that affect tumor growth in patients have been reviewed. These steroids, together with many newer steroids, have also been studied for their ability to depress growth of the rat mammary fibroadenoma. Although data on the rat mammary fibroadenoma have been reviewed in detail, this is not to imply that such a tumor is necessarily the one of choice for the experimental study of new steroid compounds. This tumor is at present of interest to the extent that it has been utilized to study a large number of steroids. It is, however, pertinent to note that apparently some correlation exists between rat and human tumors; for the androgens, estrogens, and their derivatives have been effective against both mammary cancer in patients and the rat mammary fibroadenoma. This correlation does not appear to hold in the case of progestational activity. It must be borne in mind that these compounds with progestational activity also have other endocrine properties, and thus the lack of correlation may not simply be related to progestational activity. When other experimental mammary tumors are studied a different set of relationships may be found. Sufficient data are not available on prostatic tumors to determine whether or not similar relationships exist between the response of experimental tumors and clinical tumors.

The mechanism by which the steroids act to depress tumor growth, either experimentally or clinically, is not known. It does not appear, however, that effective compounds are acting simply as physiological antagonists. That is to say, an androgen-dependent tumor is not simply depressed by the opposing types of actions that may be found in an estrogen. Similarly, androgenic steroids and derivatives are probably not acting simply as physiological antagonists to estrogen. Steroids which depress tumor growth are pituitary inhibitors, and there is indirect evidence to indicate that such compounds are acting to a large degree by depressing pituitary function. The possible relationships of prolactin, ACTH, and growth hormone, particularly in relation to cancer of the breast, require a great deal of further study before definitive statements of their relationship to tumor growth can be made. Preliminary evidence does, however, indicate that these or other pituitary factors may be important in the control of tumor growth. The androgenic derivatives that produce remissions in patients with cancer of the breast still appear to be active in proportion to their androgenicity. Data on the relative pituitary-inhibiting effects of these steroids are not available. Some of the steroids may act more directly on the tumor to depress growth, perhaps through the mechanism of competitive inhibition at the receptor site. The discovery of steroids with this type of activity would be most desirable, and $\Delta^1$-testololactone, should it continue to be active in patients, may direct efforts in this direction.

In view of our relative lack of knowledge, or even ignorance, concerning the mechanism of action of steroids which depress tumor growth, it is important that new steroids, which have activities in any one of the areas listed below, be further explored clinically: (1) compounds active in depressing growth of rat mammary fibroadenoma; (2) compounds which show high potency as androgens, estrogens, progestins, antiestrogens, antiandrogens, or as pituitary inhibitors, independent of effects on rat mammary fibroadenoma growth; (3) compounds with unusual mixtures of endocrine properties.

Such studies may lead to the finding of more beneficial drugs and will also provide additional data for the future correlation of experimental and clinical results and, hence, a better predictability for new compounds.

REFERENCES

1. Albert, S. *Endocrinology* **30**, 454 (1942).
2. Arhelger, S. W., and Huseby, R. A. *Proc. Soc. Exptl. Biol. Med.* **76**, 811 (1951).
3. Beckett, V. L., and Brennan, M. J. *Surg. Gynecol. Obstet.* **109**, 235 (1959).
4. Blackburn, C. M., and Albert, A. *J. Clin. Endocrinol. and Metabolism* **19**, 603 (1959).
5. Blackburn, C. M., and Childs, D. S., Jr. *Proc. Staff Meetings Mayo Clinic* **34**, 113 (1959).
6. Bottomly, A. C., and Folley, S. J. *J. Physiol. (London)* **94**, 26 (1938).
7. Bowers, A., Ringold, H. J., and Dorfman, R. I. *J. Am. Chem. Soc.* **79**, 4556 (1947).
8. Brendler, H. *Proc. 3rd Natl. Cancer Conf. 1956* p. 268 (1956).
9. Brendler, H. C., Chase, W. E., and Scott, W. W. *A.M.A. Arch. Surg.* **61**, 433 (1950).
10. Burchenal, J. H., Stock, C. C., and Rhoads, C. P. *Cancer Research* **10**, 209 (1950).
11. Cantarow, A., Stasney, J., and Paschkis, K. E. *Cancer Research* **8**, 412 (1948).
12. Courrier, R. *Vitamins and Hormones* **8**, 179 (1950).
12a. Dorfman, R. I. *Endocrinology* **64**, 464 (1959).
13. Douglas, M. *Brit. J. Cancer* **6**, 32 (1952).
14. Drill, V. A. *Federation Proc.* **18**, 1040 (1959).
15. Drill, V. A., and Riegel, B. *Recent Progr. in Hormone Research* **14**, 29 (1958).
16. Edgren, R. A. *Acta Endocrinol.* **25**, 365 (1959).
17. Edgren, R. A. *Ann. N.Y. Acad. Sci.* **83**, 160 (1959).
18. Edgren, R. A., and Calhoun, D. W. *Proc. Soc. Exptl. Biol. Med.* **94**, 537 (1957).
19. Edgren, R. A., and Calhoun, D. W. *Am. J. Physiol.* **189**, 38 (1957).
20. Edgren, R. A., and Calhoun, D. W. *Am. J. Physiol.* **189**, 355 (1957).
21. Edgren, R. A., and Calhoun, D. W. *Anat. Record* **128**, 542 (1957).
22. Edgren, R. A., and Calhoun, D. W. *Anat. Record* **34**, 558 (1959).
23. Edgren, R. A., and Calhoun, D. W. *J. Endocrinol.* **20**, 325 (1960).
24. Edgren, R. A., Calhoun, D. W., Elton, R. L., and Colton, F. B. *Endocrinology* **65**, 265 (1959).
25. Edgren, R. A., Calhoun, D. W., and Harris, T. W. *Anat. Record* **131**, 547 (1958).
26. Eisen, M. J. *Cancer Research* **1**, 457 (1941).
26a. Emmens, C. W., and Parkes, A. S. *Vitamins and Hormones* **5**, 233 (1947).
26b. Epstein, J. A., Kupperman, H. S., and Cutler, A. *Ann. N.Y. Acad. Sci.* **71**, 560 (1958).
27. Farrow, J. H., and Woodard, H. Q. *J. Am. Med. Assoc.* **118**, 339 (1942).
28. Ferin, J. *Ann. endocrinol. (Paris)* **16**, 895 (1955).
29. Field, J. B. *Proc. Am. Assoc. Cancer Research* **2** (3), 200 (1957).
30. Gellhorn, A., Holland, J., Herrmann, J. B., Moss, J., and Smelin, A. *J. Am. Med. Assoc.* **154**, 1274 (1954).
31. Geyer, R. P., Bryant, J. E., Bleisch, V. R., Pierce, E. M., and Stare, F. J. *Cancer Research* **13**, 503 (1953).
32. Goldenberg, I., and Hayes, M. A. *Cancer* **12**, 738 (1959).
33. Goldfarb, A. F., Napp, E. E., Stone, M. L., Zuckerman, M. B., and Simon, J. *Obstet. & Gynecol.* **11**, 454 (1958).
34. Goldman, J. N., Epstein, J. A., and Kupperman, H. S. *Endocrinology* **61**, 166 (1957).
35. Gordan, G. S. *J. Am. Med. Assoc.* **162**, 600 (1956).

36. Gordon, D., Horwitt, B. N., Segaloff, A., Murison, P. J., and Schlosser, J. V. *Cancer* **5**, 275 (1952).
37. Grayhack, J. T., Bunce, P. L., Kearns, J. W., and Scott, W. W. *Bull. Johns Hopkins Hosp.* **96**, 154 (1955).
38. Gunn, S. A., and Gould, T. C. *Endocrinology* **58**, 443 (1956).
39. Haddow, A., Watkinson, J. M., and Petersen, E. *Brit. Med. J.* **II**, 393 (1944).
40. Hadfield, G. *Ann. Roy. Coll. Surg. Engl.* **22**, 73 (1958).
41. Hadfield, G., and Young, S. *Brit. J. Surg.* **46**, 265 (1958).
42. Heiman, J. *Am. J. Cancer* **39**, 178 (1940).
43. Heiman, J. *Am. J. Cancer* **39**, 172 (1940).
44. Heiman, J. *Am. J. Cancer* **40**, 343 (1940).
45. Heiman, J. *Cancer Research* **3**, 65 (1943).
46. Heiman, J., and Krehbiel, O. F. *Am. J. Cancer* **27**, 450 (1936).
47. Hertz, R., and Tullner, W. W. *Proc. Soc. Exptl. Biol. Med.* **99**, 451 (1958).
48. Hisaw, F. L., Velardo, J. T., and Goolsby, C. M. *J. Clin. Endocrinol. and Metabolism* **14**, 1134 (1954).
49. Hoogstra, M. J., and Paesi, F. J. *Acta Endocrinol.* **24**, 353 (1957).
50. Horning, E. S. *Brit. J. Cancer* **6**, 80 (1952).
51. Huffman, M., Jones, R. W., and Katzberg, A. A. *Cancer* **10**, 707 (1957).
52. Huggins, C. *Harvey Lectures Ser.* **42**, 148 (1946-47).
53. Huggins, C. *Proc. Soc. Exptl. Biol. Med.* **92**, 304 (1956).
54. Huggins, C., Briziarelli, G., and Sutton, H., Jr. *J. Exptl. Med.* **109**, 25 (1959).
55. Huggins, C., and Clark, P. J. *J. Exptl. Med.* **72**, 747 (1940).
56. Huggins, C., and Jensen, E. V. *J. Exptl. Med.* **102**, 335 (1955).
57. Huggins, C., and Jensen, E. V. *J. Exptl. Med.* **102**, 347 (1955).
58. Huggins, C., and Mainzer, K. *J. Exptl. Med.* **105**, 485 (1957).
59. Huggins, C., Torralba, Y., and Mainzer, K. *J. Exptl. Med.* **104**, 525 (1956).
59a. Kagawa, C. M., Cella, J. A., and Van Arman, C. G. *Science* **126**, 1015 (1957).
59b. Kagawa, C. M., Sturtevant, F. M., and Van Arman, C. G. *J. Pharmacol. Exptl. Therap.* **126**, 123 (1959).
60. Kasdon, S. C., Fishman, W. H., Dart, R. M., Bonner, C. D., and Homberger, F. *J. Am. Med. Assoc.* **148**, 1212 (1952).
61. Kennedy, B. J., *Cancer* **8**, 488 (1955).
62. Kennedy, B. J. *Cancer* **10**, 813 (1957).
63. Kennedy, B. J. *New Eng. J. Med.* **259**, 673 (1958).
64. Kennedy, B. J., and Nathanson, I. T. *J. Am. Med. Assoc.* **152**, 1135 (1953).
65. Kirschbaum, A. *Proc. 3rd Natl. Cancer Conf. 1956* p. 331 (1957).
66. Kory, R. C., Watson, R. W., Bradley, M. H., and Peters, B. J. *J. Clin. Invest.* **36**, 907 (1957).
67. Lang, W. R. *Ann. N. Y. Acad. Sci.* **83**, 77-358 (1959).
68. Lesser, M. A., Vose, S. N., and Dixey, G. M. *J. Clin. Endocrinol. and Metabolism* **15**, 297 (1955).
69. Lewin, I., Spencer, H., and Herrmann, J. B. *Proc. Am. Assoc. Cancer Research* **3**, 37 (1959).
70. Loesser, A. A. *Acta Unio Intern. contra Cancrum* **4**, 375 (1939).
71. Loesser, A. A. *Lancet* **ii**, 698 (1941).
72. Lyons, W. R., Johnson, R. E., Cole, R. D., and Li, C. H. *In* "Hypophyseal Growth Hormone, Nature and Actions" (R. W. Smith, ed.), p. 461. McGraw-Hill, New York, 1955.

73. Lyons, W. R., Li, C. H., and Johnson, R. E. *Recent Progr. in Hormone Research* **14**, 219 (1958).
74. Lyster, S. C., Lund, G. H., and Stafford, R. O. *Endocrinology* **58**, 781 (1956).
75. Maddock, W. O., Epstein, M., and Nelson, W. O. *Ann. N. Y. Acad. Sci.* **55**, 657 (1952).
76. McDonald, D. F. and Latta, M. I. *Endocrinology* **59**, 159 (1956).
77. Mardones, E., Iglesias, R., and Lipschütz, A. *Proc. Soc. Exptl. Biol. Med.* **86**, 451 (1954).
78. Mardones, E., Jadrijevic, D., and Lipschütz, A. *Nature* **177**, 478 (1956).
79. Mason, R. C. *Endocrinology* **51**, 570 (1952).
80. Millar, M. J., and Noble, R. L. *Brit. J. Cancer* **8**, 495 (1954).
81. Miyake, T., and Pincus, G. *Proc. Soc. Exptl. Biol. Med.* **99**, 478 (1958).
82. Miyake, T., and Pincus, G. *Endocrinology* **63**, 816 (1958).
83. Mohs, F. E. *Am. J. Cancer* **38**, 212 (1940).
84. Mohs, F. E. *Proc. Soc. Exptl. Biol. Med.* **43**, 270 (1940).
84a. Moore, C. R., and Price, D. *Am. J. Anat.* **50**, 13 (1932).
85. Mühlbock, O. *In* "Endocrine Aspects of Breast Cancer" (A. R. Currie, ed.), p. 291. Livingstone, Edinburgh, 1958.
86. Myers, W. P. L., West, C. D., Pearson, O. H., and Karnofsky, D. A. *J. Am. Med. Assoc.* **161**, 127 (1956).
87. Nadine, S. *Science* **128**, 772 (1958).
88. Nathanson, I. T., Adair, F. E., Allen, W. M., and Engle, E. T. *J. Am. Med. Assoc.* **146**, 471 (1951).
89. Nelson, W. O. *Ciba Colloq. Endocrinol.* **4**, 402 (1952).
90. Noble, R. L. *Pharmacol. Revs.* **9**, 367 (1957).
91. Noble, R. L., and Collip, J. B. *Can. Med. Assoc. J.* **44**, 1 (1941).
92. Noble, R. L., and Walters, J. H. *Proc. Am. Assoc. Cancer Research* **1**, 35 (1954).
93. Payne, R. W., Hellbaum, A. A., and Owens, J. N., Jr. *Endocrinology* **59**, 306 (1956).
94. Pearson, O. H., Eliel, L. P., Rawson, R. W., Dobriner, K., and Rhoads, C. P. *Cancer* **2**, 943 (1949).
94a. Pincus, G., Chang, M. C., Zarrow, M. X., Hafez, E. S. E., and Merrill, A. *Endocrinology* **59**, 695 (1956).
95. Randall, L. O., and Selitto, J. J. *Endocrinology* **62**, 693 (1958).
96. Rawson, R. W., and Rall, J. E. *Recent Progr. in Hormone Research* **11**, 257 (1955).
97. Roberts, S., and Szego, C. M. *Physiol. Revs.* **33**, 393 (1953).
98. Saunders, F. J. *Endocrinology* **63**, 498 (1958).
99. Saunders, F. J., and Drill, V. A. *Endocrinology* **58**, 567 (1956).
99a. Saunders, F. J., and Drill, V. A. *Metabolism* **7**, 315 (1958).
100. Saunders, F. J., Colton, F. B., and Drill, V. A. *Proc. Soc. Exptl. Biol. Med.* **94**, 717 (1957).
101. Scholler, J., and Carnes, R. E. *Proc. Am. Assoc. Cancer Research* **2**, 243 (1958).
102. Segaloff, A. *Proc. 3rd Natl. Cancer Conf. 1956* p. 257 (1956).
103. Segaloff, A. *Cancer* **10**, 808 (1957).
104. Segaloff, A., Bowers, C. Y., Gordon, D. L., Schlosser, J. V., and Murison, P. J. *Cancer* **10**, 1116 (1957).
105. Segaloff, A., Bowers, C. Y., Rongone, E. L., and Murison, P. J. *Cancer* **12**, 735 (1959).

106. Segaloff, A., Bowers, C. Y., Rongone, E. L., Murison, P. J., and Schlosser, J. V. *Cancer* **11**, 1187 (1958).
107. Segaloff, A., Flores, A., and Steelman, S. L. *J. Clin. Endocrinol. and Metabolism* **15**, 847 (1955).
108. Segaloff, A., Gordon, D. L., Bowers, C. Y., Schlosser, J. V., and Murison, P. J. *Cancer* **6**, 1114 (1953).
109. Segaloff, A., Gordon, D., Carabasi, R. A., Horwitt, B. N., Schlosser, J. V., and Murison, P. J. *Cancer* **7**, 758 (1954).
110. Segaloff, A., Gordon, D., Horwitt, B. N., Murison, P. J., and Schlosser, J. V. *Cancer* **8**, 785 (1955).
111. Segaloff, A., Gordon, D., Horwitt, B. N., Murison, P. J., and Schlosser, J. V. *Cancer* **8**, 903 (1955).
112. Segaloff, A., Gordon, D., Horwitt, B. N., Schlosser, J. V., and Murison, P. J. *Cancer* **5**, 271 (1952).
113. Segaloff, A., Horwitt, B. N., Carabasi, R. A., Murison, P. J., and Schlosser, J. V. *Cancer* **6**, 483 (1953).
114. Segaloff, A., Horwitt, B. N., Carabasi, R. A., Murison, P. J., and Schlosser, J. V. *Cancer* **8**, 82 (1955).
115. Segaloff, A., Horwitt, B. N., Gordon, D., Murison, P. J., and Schlosser, J. V. *Cancer* **5**, 1179 (1952).
116. Shay, H., Gruenstein, M., and Harris, C. *Proc. Am. Assoc. Cancer Research* **2**, 146 (1956).
117. Shay, H., Harris, C., and Gruenstein, M. *J. Natl. Cancer Inst.* **13**, 307 (1952).
118. Smith, P. E., and Engle, E. T. *Am. J. Anat.* **40**, 159 (1927).
119. Smith, T. C., and Richterick, B. *Endocrinology* **68**, 89 (1958).
120. Sonnenberg, M., Money, W. L., and Rawson, R. W. *Endocrinology* **54**, 832 (1954).
121. Spencer, H., Samachson, J., and Laszlo, D. *Proc. Am. Assoc. Cancer Research* **2**, 252 (1957).
122. Stokes, P. E., Horwith, M., Pennington, T. G., and Clarkson, B. *Metabolism* **8**, 709 (1959).
123. Szego, C. M. *Endocrinology* **50**, 429 (1952).
124. Ulrich, P. *Acta Unio Intern. contra Cancrum* **4**, 377 (1939).
125. Van Eck, G. J. V., and Chang, C. H. *Cancer Research* **15**, 280 (1955).
126. Velardo, J. T. *Am. J. Physiol.* **186**, 468 (1956).
126a. Velardo, J. T. *Ann. N. Y. Acad. Sci.* **75**, 441 (1959).
127. Velardo, J. T., and Sturgis, S. H. *Proc. Soc. Exptl. Biol. Med.* **90**, 609 (1955).
128. Watson, R. W., Bradley, M. H., Callahan, R., Peters, B. J., and Kory, R. C. *Am. J. Med.* **26**, 238 (1959).

## DISCUSSION

**M. W. Woods:** I would like to ask Dr. Drill about the possible direct action of steroids on the fibroadenoma tumor. To what extent might the antitumor effect of the various steroids be correlated with a direct effect upon the tumor glycolysis? Is it possible that low concentrations of some of these steroids would stimulate glycolysis whereas high doses may produce inhibition?

**V. Drill:** I do not know what the effect of these steroids on glycolysis in the fibroadenoma might be and am not aware of any literature on this point.

**R. L. Noble:** I would like to congratulate Dr. Drill on his attempt to produce this degree of correlation in the results which he has given us. I am, however, a little worried that perhaps we are attempting to oversimplify the assay of steroids in rats with mammary tumors. The mammary tumors in the rat are, certainly in our experience, not at all standardized; they are not like mammary cancer in the mouse. This should be emphasized in attempting to evaluate chemotherapeutic studies. The spontaneous tumor in the rat is nearly always a fibroadenoma rather than an adenocarcinoma. With regard to induced tumors in the rat, they may be produced by female sex hormone, the use of aminofluorene, and, finally, the hydrocarbons. These substances all produce adenocarcinomas, but response of the tumor to steroids varies. For instance, in the estrogen-induced tumors progesterone tends to be inhibitory, whereas with the aminofluorene tumors estrogen is strongly stimulatory. Therefore it is important to state the origin of the rat tumor so that the response to these compounds can be correlated with the inducing agent. Obviously one has to start somewhere in the biological screening and it may well be that the effects of steroids on the fibroadenoma or on the hydrocarbon-induced tumors will be quite comparable to the effect obtained in humans. At this stage, however, I think it is simply a question of trial and error. Perhaps emphasis should be given to standardization of the mammary tumors in the rat for such chemotherapeutic studies.

**V. Drill:** Dr. Noble's comments and cautions are certainly appreciated as he has published a considerable amount of the original work in this field. Some of the points raised by Dr. Noble are discussed in the manuscript but were not presented orally because of the lack of time. The rat fibroadenoma and the methylcholanthrene-induced tumors were emphasized because of the comparative studies with steroids that are available. Interpretation of such data is at times difficult, as Dr. Noble points out, because of the variation in tumor growth rates. In grading the tumor response in the tables an attempt was made to determine significance of the response. Sometimes this was not simple. I am sure that there are other tumors that will show a different response to these steroids. As Dr. Noble suggests, it would be of great interest to standardize several mammary tumors and compare the effects of different steroids on their growth. It would also be of value if mean tumor weights and standard errors were reported.

**B. Hokfelt:** In the hypophysectomized rats there is no effect of estrogen and progesterone on tumor growth, but if prolactin and growth hormone are added there is an effect. I wonder if you had any information on the effect of insulin or thyroxine on tumor growth.

**V. Drill:** I do not have any information on the effect of these hormones on tumor growth.

**I. Lewin:** We have studied the effect of $17\alpha$-ethynyl-19-nortestosterone, which you referred to as Norlutin, on a series of patients with mammary carcinoma. The patients were randomized against similar patients receiving testosterone propionate, and we have observed that the number of regressions produced by Norlutin is about the same as that observed with testosterone propionate. Since this compound has been reported to increase the growth of the rat fibroadenoma, it would appear that in this instance there is no correlation between effect in the rat and in man.

**V. Drill:** Yes, I agree with you. This point, as I mentioned in the text, should be emphasized. I have, however, wondered about the estrogenicity of the sample of Norlutin used. Some of the earliest samples of this compound apparently contained variable amounts of an estrogen, as different degrees of estrogenic activity were reported in initial papers. I wondered if Dr. Huggins hadn't studied such a sample of the material wherein the estrogenicity may have accounted for the increase in tumor weight which was observed.

**I. Lewin:**    Vaginal smears, which were done concurrently as Norlutin was administered to the patients, did not demonstrate an estrogenic effect.

**H. J. Ringold:**  I would like to comment on the grade of Norlutin which Dr. Huggins tested in his tumor. This was a very carefully purified sample which, as far as we could tell, was completely free of estrogen.

**V. Drill:**  I am glad to know that. One other compound, 17-propyl-19-nortestosterone also stimulated growth of the rat fibroadenoma.

# III. STEROID METABOLISM AND BIOCHEMISTRY

# The Binding of Steroid Hormones by Plasma Proteins[1]

WILLIAM H. DAUGHADAY AND IDA KOZAK MARIZ

*Metabolism Division, Department of Medicine, Washington University School of Medicine, St. Louis, Missouri*

For many years one of the ultimate goals of the endocrine physiologist was the development of adequate methods for the measurement of hormones in blood. In thyroid and adrenocortical research, this goal has been largely achieved, but the arrival at this historic milestone has made it evident that, in understanding the activity of hormones in the blood, there are new complexities to plague us and stimulate our curiosity. It is now evident that measurements of hormonal levels are interpretable only in the light of knowledge concerning the physicochemical state of a hormone in blood.

The interaction of steroids and plasma proteins has been the subject of recent comprehensive reviews (5, 11). Only the development of certain concepts and methods need be mentioned here. It was early thought that the steroid hormones were associated with the lipoproteins of the plasma because of the lipophilic properties of the steroid hormones. Support for this hypothesis seemed to be provided by the report that plasma protein fraction III-0, prepared by the methods developed in the laboratory of E. J. Cohn, contained estrogenic activity. The significance of this observation remains in doubt because it is now recognized that protein fractionation using alcoholic solutions largely disrupts the labile bonds involved in the interaction of steroid hormones and plasma proteins.

Subsequent workers obtained information concerning steroid-protein interactions by comparing the solubility of steroids in solutions of plasma proteins to the solubility in simple buffers. More recently the availability of sensitive and specific methods for measuring steroids, of which the use of radioactive steroids has been the most important, has simplified the application of equilibrium dialysis, ultrafiltration, ultracentrifugation, and electrophoresis methods to the study of steroid-protein interactions.

## ALBUMIN BINDING OF STEROIDS

The extraordinary ability of albumin to bind a great number of chemical substances of diverse nature directed attention to its probable role in steroid binding. It has been found that human albumin does bind all the steroid

[1] This investigation was supported by research grant A-255, from the National Institute of Arthritis and Metabolic Diseases, Bethesda, Maryland.

hormones, but the strength of binding varies greatly. Table I presents the calculated association constants derived from the publications of Sandberg *et al.* (11). The binding of corticosteroids is comparatively weak, whereas the binding of the estrogenic hormones is much stronger. The binding of progesterone and testosterone lies between these two extremes.

TABLE I

The Calculated Association Constants for the Binding of Steroid Hormones by Human Albumin[a, b]

| Hormone | $nK \times 10^4$ [c] |
|---|---|
| 1. Cortisol | 0.5 |
| 2. Cortisone | 0.5 |
| 3. Corticosterone | 1.3 |
| 4. Testosterone | 3.4 |
| 5. Progesterone | 3.7 |
| 6. Estrone | 4.4 |
| 7. Estradiol | 16.1 |

[a] Data from Sandberg *et al.* (*11*).

[b] pH 7.0, 5° C., 4% albumin solutions.

[c] $nK = \dfrac{\text{(steroid albumin complex)}}{\text{(free steroid) (albumin)}}$

The binding capacity or the number of available binding sites on the albumin molecule is so great that saturation of the binding sites with steroid hormones is never achieved under physiologic conditions. Each human albumin molecule appears to have two primary binding sites for corticosterone and testosterone and only one binding site for progesterone and estrone (11). If this information is correct, albumin is capable of binding in excess of 40 mg. of corticosterone per 100 ml. of human plasma.

Little is known concerning the specificity of the binding sites of human albumin for individual steroids. Sandberg *et al.* (11) report that "saturation" of albumin with corticosterone did not alter the binding of estrone, progesterone, and testosterone. Likewise, an excess of progesterone did not alter the binding of estrone, testosterone, and corticosterone. Specificity of the binding sites is suggested by these results, but because of the limited solubility of the steroids in water it is possible that "saturation" of all the potential binding sites was never achieved.

## Corticosteroid-Binding Globulin (CBG)

Certain important differences between the binding of steroid hormones by human plasma and by albumin solutions are indicative of other important binding proteins in plasma. Albumin seems to be predominant in the reversible binding of estrogens by plasma and may play an important role in the binding of testosterone and progesterone. In contrast, the plasma binding of cortisol and corticosterone in physiologic concentrations greatly exceeds that attributable to the contained albumin (3). The high affinity of cortisol and corticosterone for albumin decreases when increasing amounts of these hormones are added to a dialysis system. The affinity of plasma for estrone, progesterone, and testosterone is much less influenced by the amount of these steroids in the dialysis system (Fig. 1). The presence of a second binding protein in plasma with limited binding capacity but with a high affinity for the corticosteroid hormones was first suggested by these observations. This protein will be referred to as the corticosteroid-binding globulin (CBG).

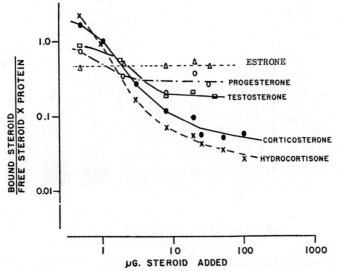

Fig. 1. The effect of steroid load on the binding of estrone, testosterone, progesterone, corticosterone, and cortisol by 10 ml. of plasma dialyzed against 80 ml. of phosphate-saline buffer pH 7.4 at 4° C. (3).

The partition of the cortisol of normal plasma into unbound, albumin-bound, and CBG-bound cortisol has been calculated at different concentrations of total cortisol from dialysis experiments at 4° C. (Fig. 2).[2] With additions of 0.5 µg. of cortisol per 10 ml. of normal plasma, between 98 and 99 % of the cortisol is bound to CBG and the contribution of albumin-bound cortisol to total bound cortisol is negligible. The plasma studied in Fig. 2

---

[2] An unexplained feature of this chart is that the fraction of cortisol bound by albumin in the presence of other plasma proteins (calculated as the difference between total bound cortisol and the CBG-bound cortisol) is less than would have been predicted on the basis of experiments with purified human albumin. This apparent loss of binding activity has been observed in other experiments with human plasma.

had corticosteroid-binding capacity equivalent to 16 µg. of cortisol per 100 ml. of plasma. Normally the binding capacity of CBG appears to be $20 \pm 5$ µg. of cortisol or $5 \times 10^{-7} M$, which is approximately twice the total normal resting cortisol concentration. The apparent association constant of the binding of cortisol by this protein has been calculated to be $5.4 \times 10^8$ in our experiments. This is considerably higher than the estimate of Slaunwhite and Sandberg (12) of $3 \times 10^7$. To emphasize the high affinity of this protein for cortisol, the association constant for the binding of thyroxine by thyroxine-binding protein (roughly $8 \times 10^9$) is only one order of magnitude greater (9) than we find for CBG.

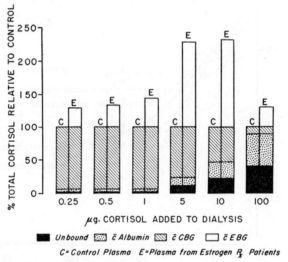

Fig. 2. The partition of plasma cortisol between unbound, CBG-bound, and albumin-bound cortisol at 4° C. The concentration of cortisol bound to CBG was calculated at the three lowest levels of cortisol loading, where the extent of albumin binding introduces little error.

The ability of related steroids to displace cortisol-$4$-$C^{14}$ and corticosterone-$4$-$C^{14}$ from CBG has provided information about the specificity of the corticosteroid binding site (3). The results indicate that cortisol and corticosterone share the same binding site and are bound more firmly to this site than are structurally related steroids. Certain minor structural alterations in the molecules of the active steroid hormones greatly decrease the ability of a steroid to displace the normal hormone from the CBG binding site. The configuration of the oxygen group at carbon-11 is critical. If the oxygen is present as a keto group or an 11α-hydroxy in place of the normal 11β-hydroxy group, there is a greatly decreased affinity for the CBG binding site. Other molecular alterations such as the introduction of a 9α-fluoro or an aldehyde group at carbon-19 (aldosterone) also greatly decrease the affinity for the binding site.

Continuous flow paper electrophoresis has been useful in characterizing CBG (4, 12). The strength of the steroid-protein bond is insufficient to prevent major dissociation during electrophoresis of a mixture of plasma and corticosterone or cortisol. Equilibration of the labeled hormone between plasma and buffer prior to electrophoresis prevents the artifacts of dissociation. A clean separation of the corticosteroid-binding globulin from albumin

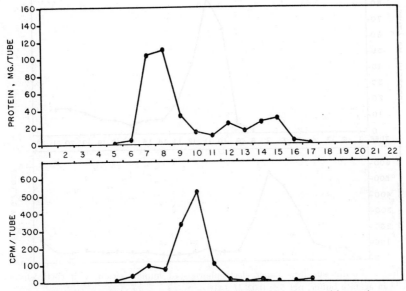

Fig. 3. Continuous flow paper electrophoresis of human serum with corticosterone-4-$C^{14}$ in barbital buffer pH 8.8, ionic strength 0.045 (4).

has been obtained in barbital buffer pH 8.8, ionic strength 0.045, in which CBG has the mobility of an α-globulin (Fig. 3). In 0.02 $M$ acetate buffer, pH 5.2, CBG migrates toward the anode whereas most of the plasma proteins exhibit no migration or migrate toward the cathode (Fig. 4). In general those proteins which migrate toward the anode are acid glycoproteins. Glucosamine and bound hexose are present in the tubes with CBG activity. As little protein is present in the tubes with CBG, purifications up to 400-fold have been obtained with a single continuous flow electrophoresis.

Other forms of fractionation have been less successful. Cohn fraction IV-4 contains the activity, but the lability of the protein has prevented significant concentration over the original plasma. Corticosteroid-binding globulin is precipitable between 35 and 55 % saturation with ammonium sulfate, but with considerable loss of activity.

Temperature has a great influence on the affinity with which CBG binds the corticosteroid hormones. Unlike albumin, the extent of binding of cortisol by CBG is very much less at 37° C. as compared to 4° C. (8, 12). As much as 5–10 % of plasma cortisol may be unbound at body temperature as compared to the 1 or 2 % unbound at 4° C. CBG is stable at 37°,

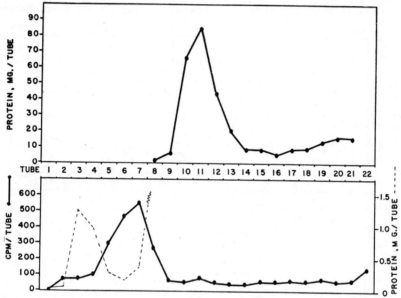

Fig. 4. Continuous flow paper electrophoresis of human serum with corticosterone-4-$C^{14}$ in acetate buffer, pH 5.2, 0.02 $M$ (4).

but if the temperature is raised to 60° C. binding activity is irreversibly lost. Lowering the pH to less than 5 results in loss of binding activity even at room temperature.

## Estrogen-Induced Binding Activity

Important alterations in corticosteroid metabolism occur in pregnancy or in individuals treated with large doses of estrogens. These include an increase in plasma cortisol concentration, an exaggerated response of plasma cortisol to ACTH, and a decrease in the removal rate of cortisol from the plasma (1, 2, 6, 7, 13). Although the total cortisol of plasma is elevated in these conditions associated with enhanced estrogenic activity, Mills and Bartter (8) could find no increase in the ultrafilterable cortisol and Slaunwhite and

Sandberg (10, 12), using equilibrium dialysis of diluted plasma samples, found evidence of increased protein binding. Most of the alterations of cortisol metabolism which have been reported in pregnancy and in patients treated with estrogens can be attributed to enhanced protein binding. Both groups of workers have postulated that an increase in corticosteroid-binding globulin (called "transcortin" by the Buffalo group) is responsible for the increased binding of cortisol.

Some observations which I will present have led us to a different conclusion, namely, that the increased binding activity in states of enhanced estrogenic activity is the result of an increase in a binding protein which can be differentiated from CBG.

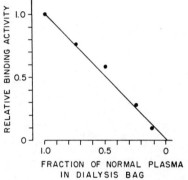

FIG. 5. The relative concentration of CBG in plasma dilutions as determined by multiple dialysis equilibrium.

It is difficult to compare the binding activity of normal plasma to the plasmas of pregnant or estrogen-treated patients by separate equilibrium dialysis because the intrinsic content of cortisol and other steroids differs greatly. A comparison of two plasmas in exactly the same environment of cortisol and other possible competing ligands is desirable. This is accomplished in multiple equilibrium dialysis in which two or more plasma samples in dialysis bags are equilibrated with the same buffer containing the desired amount of cortisol-$4$-$C^{14}$. An estimation of the relative concentration of CBG in the two plasmas is possible by measuring the ratio of the protein-bound cortisol in the two plasma samples under conditions of minimal cortisol loading. Under these conditions the contribution of albumin to total binding is insignificant.

The validity of this method is illustrated in the results obtained by multiple equilibrium dialysis of dilutions of normal plasma (Fig. 5). An accurate estimation of the relative concentration of CBG in the dialysis bags was possible without dependence on the inherent inaccuracy of measuring the high ratio of bound cortisol to free cortisol in individual dialysis experiments.

The CBG activity of plasma from normal men has been compared to that of pregnant or estrogen-treated patients in double dialysis equilibrium

TABLE II

DOUBLE EQUILIBRIUM DIALYSIS: COMPARISON OF PLASMA FROM ESTROGEN-TREATED PATIENTS AND CONTROLS[a]

| Number | Plasma 17-OHCS after est. $R_x$ | $\dfrac{\text{Bound F est. } R_x\ [b]}{\text{Bound F control}}$ |
|:------:|:---:|:---:|
| 1 | 35 | 1.36 |
| 2 | 22 | 1.07 |
| 3 | 50 | 1.15 |
| 4 | 57 | 1.04 |
| 5 | 24 | 1.27 |
| 6 | 46 | 0.93 |
| 7 | 39 | 1.29 |
| 8 | 77 | 1.01 |
| 9 | 27 | 1.24 |
| 10 | 19 | 1.48 |
| Mean: | 39.6 | $1.18 \pm 0.02$ |

[a] Conditions: 48-hour dialysis at 4° C; 0.5 µg. cortisol; 5 ml. plasma from estrogen-treated subjects; 5 ml. control plasma in separate dialysis bags.

[b] Ratio of bound cortisol in plasma from estrogen-treated patients to bound cortisol in control plasma.

TABLE III

DOUBLE EQUILIBRIUM DIALYSIS: PREGNANCY PLASMA COMPARED TO CONTROLS[a]

| Number | Duration of pregnancy (months) | $\dfrac{\text{Bound F preg.}[b]}{\text{Bound F control}}$ |
|:------:|:---:|:---:|
| 1 | 3 | 1.06 |
| 2 | 5 | 1.02 |
| 3 | 5 | 1.15 |
| 4 | 8 | 1.27 |
| 5 | 9 | 0.92 |
| 6 | Pool: 7½–9 | 1.06 |

[a] Conditions: 48-hour dialysis at 4° C.; 0.5 µg. of cortisol; 5 ml. control plasma; 5 ml. plasma from pregnant women in separate dialysis bags.

[b] Ratio of bound cortisol in plasma from pregnant women to bound cortisol in control plasma.

systems (Tables II and III). Only a small and often inconsistent increase in binding was evident. Under the conditions of dialysis most of the excess cortisol in the plasma of patients with enhanced estrogenic activity was transferred to the control plasma.

The hypothesis that alteration in the binding of cortisol in pregnancy and after estrogen treatment is related to a simple increase of the corticosteroid-binding globulin is incompatible with the results obtained with double equilibrium dialysis. In seeking an explanation for the apparent conflict of our results with those of other workers, a number of possibilities have been considered. A systematic analytic error in our hands appears to have been eliminated from consideration by having our experiments duplicated in another laboratory engaged in studies of protein binding.[3]

Attention to the experimental conditions used by others suggested certain important differences. Mills and Bartter (8) carried out their ultrafiltrations at 37° C. whereas 4° C. has been used for our equilibrium dialyses. We have

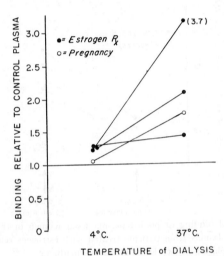

FIG. 6. The cortisol binding of pooled plasma of women in the last trimester of pregnancy and three plasmas from patients treated with estrogens relative to that of control plasma as determined in equilibrium dialysis at 4° and 37° C.

done double dialysis equilibrium experiments at each temperature and have found a differential effect of temperature on the relative binding of the two types of plasma (Fig. 6). At body temperature the binding of cortisol by the plasma of pregnant or estrogen-treated subjects became clearly predominant. The change in ratio of binding was largely the result of a decrease in the absolute binding in the normal control plasma.

The influence of cortisol loading on the relative binding of normal plasma and plasma from individuals with high estrogen levels has been investigated because Slaunwhite and Sandberg (12) had used a cortisol load equivalent to 5.5 µg. per 10 ml. of plasma to demonstrate the greater binding of the

---

[3] We are grateful to Dr. Avery Sandberg for his assistance in this control study.

latter type of plasma. We have compared the binding of cortisol by four plasmas of individuals with increased estrogenic activity directly to control plasma using our standard conditions of cortisol loading (0.5 μg. per 10 ml. of plasma) and also using 5.5 μg. of cortisol per 10 ml. of plasma (Fig. 7). The change in cortisol loading, which at first glance appears to be trivial, caused a major shift in the relative binding of the two types of plasma. This finding cannot be explained by an estrogen-induced increase in the corticosteroid-binding globulin; in such a situation the relative binding of cortisol would be greatest at the lowest level of cortisol loading.

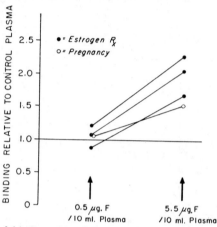

FIG. 7. The cortisol binding of pooled plasma from women in the third trimester of pregnancy and three plasmas from patients treated with estrogens relative to the binding of cortisol by control plasma at two levels of cortisol loading.

The relationship between cortisol loading and the relative binding of plasma from estrogen-treated patients has been examined over an extended range of cortisol loading (Fig. 8). The plasma pool from estrogen-treated patients used in this series of dialyses contained an initial concentration of 17-hydroxycorticosteroids of 65 μg. per 100 ml. With additions of cortisol up to 10 μg. per 10 ml. of plasma, there was an increase in the percentage of excess cortisol in the dialyzed plasma from the estrogen-treated patients. When 100 μg. of cortisol was added to the dialysis, the excess binding induced by estrogenic treatment became relatively smaller.

The absolute amount of excess cortisol bound by the plasma from estrogen-treated patients has been calculated from the specific activity of cortisol in each dialysis and plotted as a function of the unbound cortisol (Fig. 9). An S-shaped curve suggesting a titration curve is obvious although the intervals of free cortisol concentration are not ideal for this analysis. The excess

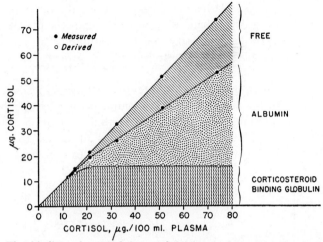

FIG. 8. The binding of cortisol by pooled plasma from estrogen-treated patients relative to the binding of cortisol by control plasma at different cortisol loads. One hundred per cent is considered to be the total number of counts in the control plasma. The observed concentration of unbound cortisol and the calculated amounts of cortisol bound to CBG and albumin are indicated on the assumption that they are the same in the two types of plasma. The excess binding of cortisol in the plasma of patients treated with estrogens is attributed to an independent binding system.

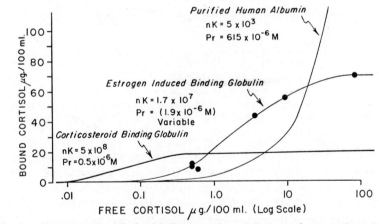

FIG. 9. The properties of the binding proteins of human plasma estimated from available data. The albumin curve is plotted from the data of Sandberg *et al.* (11). Albumin binding in plasma may be less than that of purified albumin. *Pr* is the concentration of binding protein. For CBG and estrogen-induced binding globulin, the number of binding sites per molecule is assumed to be 1. The concentration of estrogen-induced binding globulin is variable, probably dependent on the magnitude and duration of the estrogen effect. The value given is that observed in a pool of plasma from three patients treated with large doses of estrogens.

binding capacity of this plasma for cortisol was in the order of 70 µg of cortisol per 100 ml. greater than the control plasma. On the basis of the free steroid concentration necessary for half saturation of the enhanced binding sites of the plasma from estrogen-treated patients, an association constant of $1.7 \times 10^7$ was calculated.

Attempts have been made to separate the estrogen-dependent binding protein from CBG, but without success. Continuous flow electrophoresis at pH 8.8 in both barbital and tris-maleate buffers and at pH 5.2 in acetate buffer failed to demonstrate two distinct peaks of bound cortisol. The results of continuous flow electrophoresis of plasma from normal and estro-

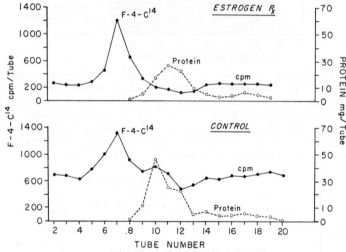

FIG. 10. Comparison of continuous flow paper electrophoresis of cortisol-4-$C^{14}$ in the presence of normal plasma and plasma from estrogen-treated patients. Preliminary equilibration was carried out with 10 ml. of plasma and 1500 ml. of electrophoretic buffer (0.02 $M$ acetate, pH 5.2).

gen-treated subjects at pH 5.2 with cortisol loading are presented in Fig. 10. The extent of protein binding apparent at the peak of radioactivity in the experiment with plasma from estrogen-treated subjects was greater, but the migration of the bound cortisol occurred at the normal position. Further evidence that the estrogen-induced binding activity has similar physical properties to CBG is the finding that both proteins are unstable at room temperature at pH 4.

We have little information concerning the specificity of the changes in steroid binding which occur after the administration of estrogens. Double dialysis equilibrium with progesterone failed to detect any increase in the binding of this steroid by plasma of patients treated with estrogens.

## SUMMARY

We have considered three proteins of human plasma that bind steroids. The first of these is albumin, which binds all steroid hormones but has the greatest affinity for the estrogens, less affinity for progesterone and testosterone, and least affinity for the corticosteroid hormones. It appears to have little significance in binding corticosteroid hormones under physiologic conditions.

Corticosteroid-binding globulin, an α-glycoglobulin, is the second steroid-binding protein. The concentration of this protein is so small that it can bind only about 20 µg. of cortisol per 100 ml. of plasma. The affinity of this protein for cortisol is much higher at 4° C. than at 37° C. The binding site(s) of the corticosteroid-binding globulin seem to be relatively specific for the corticosteroid hormones.

In pregnancy and after the administration of estrogens, there appears in the plasma a third binding protein which resembles corticosteroid-binding globulin in its electrophoretic behavior but can be differentiated from it on the basis of the comparative affinity for cortisol at 4° C. and the fact that the extent of cortisol binding is less influenced by temperature.

## REFERENCES

1. Christy, W. P., Wallace, E. Z., Gordon, W. E., and Jailer, J. W. *J. Clin. Invest.* **38**, 299 (1959).
2. Cohen, M., Stiefel, M., Reddy, W. J., and Laidlaw, J. C. *J. Clin. Endocrinol. and Metabolism* **18**, 1076 (1958).
3. Daughaday, W. H. *J. Clin. Invest.* **37**, 511 (1958).
4. Daughaday, W. H. *J. Clin. Invest.* **37**, 519 (1958).
5. Daughaday, W. H. *Physiol. Revs.* **39**, 885 (1959).
6. Martin, J. D., and Mills, I. H. *Clin. Sci.* **17**, 137 (1958).
7. Migeon, C. J., Bertrand, J., and Wall, B. E. *J. Clin. Invest.* **36**, 1350 (1957).
8. Mills, I. H., and Bartter, F. C. *J. Endocrinol.* **18**, v (1959).
9. Robbins, J., and Rall, J. E. *Recent Progr. in Hormone Research* **13**, 161 (1957).
10. Sandberg, A. A., and Slaunwhite, W. R., Jr. *J. Clin. Invest.* **38**, 1290 (1959).
11. Sandberg, A. A., Slaunwhite, W. R., and Antoniades, H. N. *Recent Progr. in Hormone Research* **13**, 209 (1957).
12. Slaunwhite, W. R., Jr., and Sandberg, A. A. *J. Clin. Invest.* **38**, 384 (1959).
13. Wallace, E. Z., Silverberg, M. I., and Carter, A. C. *Proc. Soc. Exptl. Biol. Med.* **95**, 805 (1957).

## DISCUSSION

**A. A. Sandberg:** In a much larger series of steroids which we have studied, we have been unable to demonstrate competition among the various steroids for the sites on human albumin. By that I mean that estrone, estradiol, progesterone, testosterone, and corticosterone, all seem to have peculiar sites on the albumin molecule. The saturation of the system by another steroid will not displace the bound steroid on the albumin. This does not hold true for cortisol. Of all the steroids, cortisol seems to be displaced very easily by estrogens, progesterone, and testosterone from the human albumin molecule.

My second comment is in relation to the possible existence of an estrogen-binding protein in human plasma. Experiments which we have carried out since our presentation at the Laurentian Conference in 1956 tend to support the previous evidence that there is no special plasma protein for the binding of estrogens, unless it resides in the albumin system, which binds estrogens in human plasma. Dr. Daughaday published, and we have confirmed, the fact that some animals do have a corticosteroid-binding protein. The dog, however, does not seem to have this protein in the plasma. We felt that since the levels of this protein were low in the dog plasma, the administration of estrogens would give us a very sensitive system for studying the changes in the corticosteroid-binding protein (transcortin) induced by the estrogen. Unfortunately we could not raise the levels of transcortin in the plasma of the dog, even with tremendous doses of estrogen.

My next comment is in relation to what appear to be differences in interpretation and methodology between Dr. Daughaday's laboratory and ours. Dr. Daughaday referred to a laboratory which repeated his experiments. This was our laboratory and, indeed, under the conditions of his dialysis we cannot find a difference in the binding between normal plasma and the plasma of pregnant women or subjects treated with estrogens. We tend to attribute this to the high equilibria constants of Dr. Daughaday's method. Repeating the experiments with the identical plasmas under our experimental conditions, we showed tremendous differences in the binding; that is, plasma from patients that have been treated with estrogens binds cortisol much more than does the control plasma. In addition we have repeated the competition equilibria-dialysis experiments to which Dr. Daughaday referred. Using our dilution method, differences between normal plasma and that from pregnant women receiving estrogen were substantiated. We also agree with Dr. Daughaday that this protein does not behave as two proteins, either electrophoretically or by chemical separation of the plasma. At least in our hands, it has been very difficult to show the existence of two binding systems, which Dr. Daughaday postulates.

**W. H. Daughaday:** Of course we have been watching what is going on in Dr. Sandberg's laboratory with great interest. The only question that I have about his ideas as to the specificity of albumin binding of individual steroids concerns the great difficulty inherent in trying to saturate albumin. In the case of corticosterone you have to add the equivalent of 40 mg. of corticosterone to saturate the binding sites in the albumin of 100 ml. of plasma and proportionately higher amounts of the other steroids. Perhaps the water solubility of these steroids will not permit this total saturation of any one binding site. Dr. Sandberg's original criticism of our observation, that there is no increase in corticosterone-binding globulin in pregnancy in which we used the ratio of bound to free steroid, was that this measurement was subject to error because of the large association constants. I don't want to belabor the point, but it's quite evident that in the double dialysis equilibrium system we do not measure the association constant, but only the proportion of bound steroid, this, in fact, is very easily done with considerable accuracy. His criticisms are not really pertinent to the problem of the double dialysis system because if you have twice as much corticosteroid-binding protein you should have twice as much bound steroid. I don't see how you can escape that conclusion.

**C. J. Migeon:** I would like to ask one question and make two comments.

The question is: I noted that Dr. Daughaday in his conclusion said that pregnancy and estrogen therapy induced the production in plasma of a protein slightly different from that found normally for the binding of cortisol. I was wondering if Dr Daughaday felt that in pregnancy the increase in cortisol-binding globulin was related to the increase of estrogens that occurs during pregnancy.

My first comment is related to the half-life of cortisol during pregnancy. We found that this half-life was prolonged [Migeon, C. J., Bertrand, J., and Wall, B. E. *J. Clin. Invest.* **36**, 1350 (1957)]; this appears to be due to the increased binding of cortisol. It would seem that an increase in protein binding of cortisol could decrease the rate of catabolism of the hormone. At the same time, there is evidence also that the rate of glucuronidation in pregnancy is slower than normal.

The second comment is related to some of our work on the cortisol levels in maternal and fetal circulations. We find quite regularly that maternal levels of cortisol are two to four times higher than the fetal levels [Migeon, C. J., Prystowsky, H., Grumbach, M. M., and Byron, M. C. *J. Clin. Invest.* **35**, 488-493 (1956)].

I think it is of interest that Dr. Sandberg and his group have reported that the corticosteroid-binding globulin is increased in the maternal circulation while it is lower than normal in the fetal circulation. Consequently, one could conceive of the transplacental passage of steroids as an *in vivo* dialysis, the placenta being the dialysis membrane between maternal and fetal circulation; because of the large amounts of corticosteroid-binding globulin in maternal blood and the small amounts in the fetal blood, at equilibrium the cortisol levels of the mother would be higher than those of the fetus.

**W. H. Daughaday:** It would appear from the excretion of estrogens that the levels in pregnancy are comparable to those that are given to patients with carcinoma, and for that reason the first assumption would be that the estrogens of pregnancy are responsible for producing this pattern of steroid-protein bindings. There is no question that there is increased binding—the real problem is the question whether this is the same protein or an altered corticosteroid-binding globulin. It has different properties that permit its separation.

**L. L. Engel:** I'd like to make one comment on the state of estrogen in plasma. Some years ago Dr. Oncley, Mr. Purdy, and I decided to examine the binding of estrogens by various purified plasma protein fractions, as prepared in Dr. Oncley's laboratory. After reviewing the literature we came to the sad conclusion that there was no really good information available on what the circulating estrogen was. Hence the nature of our problem changed and we embarked on an attempt to identify some circulating plasma estrogens by reasonable chemical criteria. Two types of experiments were done: In one $C^{14}$-estradiol was injected into patients and after a suitable time interval blood was drawn and processed. In the second type of experiment, blood was drawn from women in the last trimester of pregnancy and the method of isotope dilution was used. In both sets of experiments we obtained concordant results, namely, that the most abundant circulating estrogen was estrone sulfate. There were also minor amounts of estrone glucosiduronate. I mention this simply to point out that it is a little bit risky to assume that free estrogen is the principal circulating compound and to base physiological conclusions on this assumption.

**D. L. Berliner:** I would like to comment on what Dr. Migeon mentioned in relation to the increased half-life of cortisol in pregnant women. I do not think that the only cause of this increased half-life is the binding of cortisol in blood. We have found that there are other compounds normally circulating or during stress, which will inhibit the conjugating capacity for cortisol in the liver. ACTH in adrenalectomized animals

[Berliner, D. L., Nabors, C. J., Jr., and Dougherty, T. F. *41st Meeting Endocrinol. Soc.*, p. 20 (1959)] and animals treated with estrogens will inhibit conjugation of corticosteroids by the liver, and this influences the half-life of cortisol in blood.

**G. Pincus:** I'd like to ask two questions. First of all, have you any idea of the origin of your estrogen-induced protein; where does it come from? Secondly, is there any indication that in patients with cancer, particularly breast cancer, there is any alteration in the cortisol-binding capacity or any steroid-binding capacity in the blood? This would be extremely interesting in terms of studies of cancer. Finally, what about the binding capacity of the cell on which the hormones act? Have you, or has anybody here, studied the tissues in terms of their possible binding constituents?

**W. H. Daughaday:** We have a hard enough time deciding where the normal corticosteroid binding protein arises. We have made measurements in patients with liver disease. One patient who had virtually total hepatic necrosis had essentially no ability to bind cortisol. Patients with severe cirrhosis have some decrease in their binding ability. Dr. Sandberg has attempted the same measurements, having more trouble finding any decrease in liver disease. The liver would be the most suspicious organ of origin. The derivation of the estrogen-induced binding activity remains completely in doubt, and as far as we can tell the untreated patient with carcinoma has no alteration. In regard to tissue binding of steroids, we got into this problem very optimistically by looking at tissue binding first and made studies of fixation of cortisol onto liver slices. Actually the system is really extraordinarily difficult for any definitive work. Although we published on this, the interpretations remain in doubt.

**A. C. Carter:** In answer to Dr. Pincus' second question, Dr. Sandberg and I have some preliminary data which would indicate that the transcortin levels are elevated above normal in patients with progressive metastatic carcinoma.

**P. Troen:** The increased levels of circulating corticosteroids in pregnant and estrogen-treated patients, respectively, have been referred to without distinction. However, some of our experiments, which are still in progress, indicate that the human placenta, at least during *in vitro* perfusion, has the capacity to produce corticosteroids. This may be another variable to be considered in study of the pregnant patient.

**A. A. Sandberg:** Just two short comments regarding Dr. Pincus' questions. We have been unable to find differences in the levels of transcortin in patients with liver disease, including patients with severe liver disease. I wonder whether Dr. Daughaday's single patient with a substantial decrease in binding due to liver necrosis, actually did not have a greatly increased plasma cortisol level because of the severe illness, the high cortisol levels encroaching upon the ability of the protein to bind. We have some evidence which indicates that the level of transcortin is fairly high in the lymph of the thoracic duct of patients with cancer. We do not know what levels would be in normal lymph. Our hypothesis at the moment is that the protein (transcortin) comes from the reticuloendothelial (RE) system. We have found that in the human in some diseases involving the RE system the transcortin levels are decreased. It is known that estrogen stimulates the RE system. We wonder whether this may not be a possible explanation for the elevated transcortin levels induced by estrogen. We are also studying the binding of the various cellular fractions of the uterus, ovary, and liver for the binding of cortisol. Unfortunately, the results are too preliminary to say anything.

# The Effects of Steroids on the Levels of the Plasma 17-Hydroxycorticosteroids and the Serum Protein-Bound Iodine[1]

ANNE C. CARTER, ELAINE BOSSAK FELDMAN, AND ELEANOR Z. WALLACE

*The State University of New York, College of Medicine at New York City, and the Medical Service (Division II) Kings County Hospital, Brooklyn, New York*

The studies to be presented concern the alterations induced in the levels of plasma 17-hydroxycorticosteroids (17-OHCS) and serum protein-bound iodine (PBI) by the administration of various steroid hormones to human subjects. The possible mechanisms by which exogenous estrogens elevate the plasma levels of 17-OHCS and androgens depress the levels of serum PBI will be discussed in detail. These studies were performed for the most part in our laboratory. Data made available by Drs. R. A. Huseby and F. H. Tyler have been included in this report.

## METHODS

The patients studied were postmenopausal women, most of whom had progressive metastatic carcinoma of the breast. Unless otherwise indicated, in the studies performed in our laboratory the following methods were used: plasma and urinary 17-OHCS were measured by the method of Peterson *et al.* (20), urinary 17-ketosteroids by the Norymberski (12) modification of the method of Drekter *et al.*, urinary creatinine by the method of Bonsnes and Taussky (2), and serum PBI by a modification of the method of Zak *et al.* (1, 27). Twenty-four-hour thyroidal $I^{131}$ uptakes were performed by conventional methods using 10 µg. $I^{131}$ as a tracer dose. Basal metabolic rates were performed using a Sanborn Metabolator. Transcortin levels were determined by the method of Slaunwhite and Sandberg (23). Levels of thyroid-binding protein (TBP) were determined by the method described by Robbins (21). Studies performed by Drs. Huseby and Tyler utilized the following methods: plasma 17-OHCS by the method of Eik-Nes (7); free and conjugated plasma 17-OHCS by the methods of Nelson and Samuels (18) and Helmreich *et al.* (15), respectively; free and conjugated urinary 17-OHCS by the method of Glenn and Nelson (13) and Helmreich (14), respectively; and urinary 17-ketosteroids by the method of Callow *et al.* (3).

[1] This work was supported in part by grants CY3601 and CY3358 from The National Cancer Institute, The National Institutes of Health, United States Public Health Service.

## THE INFLUENCE OF STEROIDS ON THE LEVELS OF THE PLASMA 17-HYDROXYCORTICOSTEROIDS

### *Estrogens*

Previous studies have shown that adequate doses of various oral estrogen preparations raised the levels of plasma 17-OHCS (Table I) (24, 26). Observations in a small group of patients indicated that lower doses of conjugated equine estrogen (Premarin®) did not elevate the levels of plasma

TABLE I*

EFFECT OF VARIOUS ESTROGEN PREPARATIONS ON PLASMA 17-HYDROXYCORTICOSTEROIDS

| Therapy | Dose (mg./day p.o.) | Number of subjects | Plasma 17-OHCS (µg./100 ml.) | |
|---|---|---|---|---|
| | | | Control | After therapy |
| Ethynyl estradiol | 0.1 | 5 | $23 \pm 5.0^a$ | $46 \pm 12.2$ |
| Ethynyl estradiol | 0.5 | 18 | $15 \pm 6.0$ | $58 \pm 18.1$ |
| Stilbestrol | 15.0 | 8 | $19 \pm 4.1$ | $54 \pm 10.1$ |
| Conjugated estrogens (Premarin) | 10.0 | 5 | $24 \pm 4.8$ | $42 \pm 5.0$ |

[a] Mean ± standard deviation.

* From Wallace and Carter, *J. Clin. Invest.* **39**, 601 (1960).

17-OHCS (4). The administration of parenteral estradiol resulted in variable elevations of the levels of plasma 17-OHCS (Table II). The levels of plasma 17-OHCS, after the administration of estradiol benzoate, either 5 mg. thrice weekly or 3 mg. daily, were not as striking as those seen in patients treated with oral estrogenic preparations. It is of interest that the levels of total urinary 17-OHCS fell even at the lower dose levels, although these dose levels did not produce elevations of the levels of plasma 17-OHCS. The administration of estrogens in amounts sufficient to elevate morning plasma 17-OHCS levels did not alter the normal diurnal change in the plasma levels of 17-OHCS (4, 16).

Previous studies have shown that ethynyl estradiol augmented the response of the plasma 17-OHCS to exogenous ACTH (Table III) (26). 17α-Ethyl-19-nortestosterone, 30 mg. per day by mouth failed to increase the resting levels of plasma 17-OHCS and did not alter the response of the adrenal to exogenous ACTH (5).

Peterson has reported that the elevated levels of plasma 17-OHCS seen during estrogen therapy represented an increase in authentic hydrocortisone as judged by isotope dilution and by isotope derivative assays of the plasma hydrocortisone (19). Employing these methods, he has found that the synthesis of cortisol was decreased. By utilizing paper chromatography in

TABLE  II

EFFECT OF PARENTERAL ESTRADIOL PREPARATIONS ON PLASMA AND
URINARY 17-HYDROXYCORTICOSTEROIDS[a]

| Therapy | Number of days | Plasma 17-OHCS (µg./100 ml.) | | Urinary 17-OHCS (mg./24hr) | |
|---|---|---|---|---|---|
| | | Pre-therapy | Post-therapy | Pre-therapy | Post-therapy |
| Estradiol, 1.0 mg./day | 18 | 5 | 16 | 4.3 | 1.8 |
| Estradiol benzoate, 5 mg. t.i.w. | 34 | 15 | 16 | 6.3 | 4.1 |
| Estradiol benzoate, 5 mg. t.i.w. | 42 | 12 | 17 | 3.7 | 1.7 |
| Estradiol benzoate, 5 mg. t.i.w. | 41 | 15 | 27 | 2.4 | 2.5 |
| Estradiol benzoate, 3 mg./day | 32 | 17 | 32 | 5.0 | 2.8 |
| Estradiol benzoate, 3 mg./day | 34 | 14 | 28 | 2.8 | 1.9 |

[a] Studies performed by Dr. R. A. Huseby.

TABLE  III

EFFECT OF ORAL STEROIDS ON PLASMA 17-HYDROXYCORTICOSTEROIDS AND
ON THEIR RESPONSE TO ACTH

| Steroid | Number of patients | Plasma 17-OHCS (µg./100 ml.) | | | |
|---|---|---|---|---|---|
| | | Pretherapy | | Posttherapy | |
| | | Pre-ACTH | Post-ACTH | Pre-ACTH | Post-ACTH |
| Ethynyl estradiol, 0.5 mg./day | 9 | $15 \pm 5$[a] | $42 \pm 6$ | $65 \pm 16$ | $118 \pm 34$ |
| 17α-Ethyl-19-nor-testosterone, 30 mg./day | 5 | $21 \pm 5$ | $48 \pm 19$ | $21 \pm 7$ | $53 \pm 18$ |

[a] Mean ± standard deviation.

a Bush I system, at least the major portion of the elevated Porter-Silber chromogens (84, 109, 110, 110 %) have been found by Huseby to have the same mobility and color reactions as authentic cortisol, and no other areas of chromogenic material could be found (16). These findings indicate that the elevated levels of plasma 17-OHCS measured by the Porter-Silber method after the administration of estrogens, represent authentic hydrocortisone.

Administration of ethynyl estradiol for periods of 2–4 weeks resulted in a significant decrease in the mean excretion of total urinary 17-OHCS in 9 patients studied (Table IV). There was a significant decrease in the excre-

TABLE IV*

URINARY STEROID EXCRETION BEFORE AND AFTER ETHYNYL ESTRADIOL

(0.5 MG. PER DAY P.O.)

| Steroid | Number of patients | Control excretion (mg./24 hr) | Post-estrogen excretion (mg./24 hr) | $p^a$ |
|---|---|---|---|---|
| Total urinary 17-OHCS | 9 | 4.3 ± 1.4[b] | 3.1 ± 1.5 | < 0.01 |
| Free urinary 17-OHCS | 8 | 0.51 ± 0.19 | 0.67 ± 0.46 | > 0.05 |
| Urinary 17-KS | 6 | 8.2 ± 3.5 | 7.7 ± 2.3 | > 0.05 |

[a] $p$ Determined by Student's $t$ test.
[b] Mean ± standard deviation.
* From Wallace and Carter, *J. Clin. Invest.* **39**, 601 (1960).

TABLE V

LEVELS OF FREE AND CONJUGATED PLASMA AND URINARY 17-HYDROXYCORTICOSTEROIDS

BEFORE AND AFTER STILBESTROL IN 6 SUBJECTS[a]

(15 MG. PER DAY P.O.)

| | Number of patients | Control | Posttherapy | $p^b$ |
|---|---|---|---|---|
| Free plasma 17-OHCS (µg./100 ml.) | 6 | 12 ± 4.9[c] | 44 ± 10.3 | < 0.001 |
| Conjugated plasma 17-OHCS (µg./100 ml.) | 6 | 12 ± 5.5 | 10 ± 4.4 | > 0.1 < 0.2 |
| Free urinary 17-OHCS (mg./24 hours) | 6 | 0.2 ± 0.11 | 0.28 ± 0.1 | N.S. |
| Conjugated urinary 17-OHCS (mg./24 hours) | 6 | 4 ± 1.1 | 2 ± 0.9 | < 0.001 |

[a] Studies performed by Dr. R. A. Huseby.
[b] $p$ Determined by Student's $t$ test.
[c] Mean ± standard deviation.

tion of the conjugated 17-OHCS and no change in the excretion of the free 17-OHCS. These findings were confirmed by Dr. Huseby. In plasma the levels of free 17-OHCS rose significantly with the administration of stilbestrol, but no real change occurred in the conjugates (Table V).

A marked delay in the rate of clearance of exogenous hydrocortisone from plasma of estrogen-treated subjects has also been demonstrated (Table VI)

TABLE VI

CLEARANCE FROM PLASMA OF INTRAVENOUS HYDROCORTISONE

| Subject | Plasma 17-hydroxycorticosteroids (µg./100 ml.) | | | |
|---|---|---|---|---|
| | Control | 4 Hr. | 6 Hr. | 8 Hr. |
| Normal postmenopausal subject | 24 | 48 | 33 | — |
| Postmenopausal subject after ethynyl estradiol 0.5 mg./day p.o. | 49 | — | 142 | 108 |

(26). The rate of disappearance of intravenously administered tetrahydrocortisone from plasma of 4 control subjects and 7 patients in whom plasma 17-OHCS levels had been elevated by the administration of diethylstilbestrol or ethynyl estradiol was different (Fig. 1) (25). The estrogen-treated

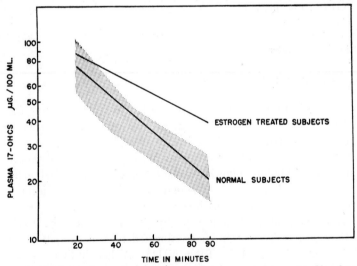

FIG. 1. Comparison of tetrahydrocortisone clearance rates in control and estrogen-treated subjects. Solid lines indicate calculated means for the 4 control and 7 estrogen-treated subjects. Stippled area indicates the extreme limits of variation for the control group. The mean percentage decreases of plasma 17-OHCS levels per minute for estrogen-treated subjects is significantly less than that for control subjects at the 1% level. From Wallace and Carter (25).

patients cleared intravenously administered tetrahydrocortisone from blood at a significantly slower rate than did the control group ($p < 0.01$).

It was found that estrogens produced: (a) a sustained elevation above normal resting levels of plasma 17-OHCS associated with augmented increase in the plasma levels of these steroids following the administration of exogenous ACTH; (b) a marked delay in the rate of clearance of exogenous hydrocortisone and tetrahydrocortisone from plasma; and (c) a decrease in the excretion of total urinary 17-OHCS due to a decrease in the conjugated fraction, but estrogens did not induce hyperadrenalcorticism. These findings suggested that the normal metabolism of endogenous hydrocortisone had been altered. If estrogens produced an alteration in the specific cortisol-binding protein, transcortin, most of the above findings could then be explained.

The effect of administration of estrogen to humans on the binding of cortisol to transcortin was studied in 12 patients (Table VII) (25). There

TABLE VII

EFFECT OF ESTROGEN THERAPY ON BINDING OF CORTISOL
TO TRANSCORTIN IN 12 PATIENTS

|  | Before therapy | During therapy |
|---|---|---|
| Plasma 17-OHCS (µg./100 ml.) | $20 \pm 5.7$[a] | $50 \pm 11.8$ |
| Cortisol binding before 1 µg. F (% bound) | $90 \pm 4.1$ | $97 \pm 1.4$ |
| Decrease in % bound after 1 µg. F | $23 \pm 3.9$ | $12 \pm 2.6$ |

[a] Mean ± standard deviation.

was an increase in the percentage of cortisol bound to transcortin; the mean level was $90 \pm 4.1$ % bound before therapy and $97 \pm 1.4$ % after therapy when the levels of plasma 17-OHCS had become elevated. There was also a significant increase in the transcortin-binding capacity when determined by the suppression of binding following the addition of 1 µg. cortisol. There was a mean decrease of $23 \pm 3.9$ % bound in the control subjects and of $12 \pm 2.6$ % in patients treated with estrogens ($p < 0.01$).

The increased protein-binding capacity for hydrocortisone might also explain the marked decrease in the conjugated plasma 17-OHCS following the administration of ACTH (Table VIII). Although the free levels of plasma 17-OHCS were elevated by exogenous estrogen, 17-OHCS would be bound to transcortin while the actual amount of hormone available to be metabolized would decrease under acute stress. Thus, there would be a decrease in the levels of the conjugated plasma 17-OHCS.

The data presented indicate that the administration of estrogen to man results in a significant increase in the percentage of hydrocortisone bound to transcortin and in transcortin-binding capacity. This elevation in the specific cortisol-binding protein, transcortin, would explain the euadrenal clinical state, the elevated resting levels of the plasma 17-OHCS, the delayed rate of clearance of exogenous hydrocortisone from plasma, and the decreased

TABLE VIII*

EFFECT OF 12-HOUR ACTH TEST ON PLASMA AND URINE 17-HYDROXYCORTICOSTEROIDS[a]
(100 I.U. ACTH I.V.)

| Therapy | Number of subjects | Plasma 17-OHCS[b] (µg./100 ml.) | | Urinary 17-OHCS[c] (µg./hour) | |
|---|---|---|---|---|---|
| | | Free | Conjugates | Free | Conjugates |
| None | 4 | 50 | 71 | 429 | 1924 |
| | | (48–54) | (57–79) | (270–544) | (1758–2180) |
| Stilbestrol, 15 mg./day p.o. | 3 | 91 | 26 | 273 | 821 |
| | | (85–97) | (18–35) | (164–362) | (708–940) |

[a] Studies performed by Dr. R. A. Huseby.
[b] Mean of values obtained at 9 and 12 hours after start of infusion.
[c] Excretion between the 9th and 12th hour.
* From Wallace and Carter, *J. Clin. Invest.* **39**, 601 (1960).

excretion of total urinary 17-OHCS of patients treated with estrogens, but would fail to explain the delay in clearance from plasma of tetrahydrocortisone. Tetrahydrocortisone is not significantly bound to transcortin. At present there is no explanation for the delayed clearance from plasma of tetrahydrocortisone.

## Nonestrogenic Steroids

The effect of administration of various nonestrogenic steroids on the levels of plasma and urinary 17-OHCS has been studied (Tables IX and X). 17α-Methyl-19-nortestosterone did not alter the levels of the plasma 17-OHCS, although the excretion of urinary 17-OHCS was decreased significantly. The 17-ketosteroid excretion was also decreased significantly in patients receiving 17α-methyl-19-nortestosterone (11). No further investigations have been carried out to elucidate the mechanism of these observed changes; however, one might speculate that 17α-methyl-19-nortestosterone suppresses the adrenal cortex. In our laboratory, a lowering of uncertain statistical significance in the levels of plasma 17-OHCS was observed in patients receiving testosterone propionate while there was no change in the excretion of urinary 17-OHCS. Drs. Huseby and Tyler, employing the method of Eik-Nes (7), observed no alteration in the levels of the plasma 17-OHCS.

The administration of 6α-methyl-17α-acetoxyprogesterone and 6α-fluoro-17α-acetoxyprogesterone resulted in elevated levels of plasma 17-OHCS when

## TABLE IX

EFFECT OF VARIOUS STEROID PREPARATIONS ON PLASMA 17-HYDROXYCORTICOSTEROIDS

| Steroid | Dose (mg./day p.o.) | Number of subjects | Plasma 17-OHCS (µg./100 ml.) | | $p^a$ |
| | | | Pre-therapy | Post-therapy | |
| --- | --- | --- | --- | --- | --- |
| 17α-Methyl-19-nortestosterone | 30 | 8 | $20 \pm 6.3^b$ | $21 \pm 9.0$ | N.S. |
| 17α-Ethyl-19-nortestosterone | 30 | 5 | $21 \pm 2.6$ | $21 \pm 6.5$ | N.S. |
| Testosterone propionate | $300^c$ | 6 | $23 \pm 6.9$ | $17 \pm 2.9$ | $> 0.05 < 0.1$ |
| Testosterone propionate[d] | $300^c$ | 5 | $18 \pm 4.9$ | $17 \pm 4.0$ | N.S. |
| Progesterone[d] | 2000 | 7 | $20 \pm 7.1$ | $20 \pm 8.3$ | N.S. |
| 9α-Bromo-11-keto-progesterone[d] | 300 | 4 | $16 \pm 4.9$ | $19 \pm 4.8$ | N.S. |

[a] $p$ Determined by Student's $t$ test.
[b] Mean $\pm$ standard deviation.
[c] Testosterone propionate 100 mg. thrice weekly intramuscularly.
[d] Studies performed by Drs. F. H. Tyler and R. A. Huseby.

## TABLE X

EFFECT OF VARIOUS STEROID PREPARATIONS ON URINARY 17-HYDROXYCORTICOSTEROID EXCRETION

| Steroid | Dose (mg./day p.o.) | Number of subjects | Urinary 17-OHCS (mg./24 hr.) | | $p^a$ |
| | | | Pre-therapy | Post-therapy | |
| --- | --- | --- | --- | --- | --- |
| 17α-Methyl-19-nortestosterone | 30 | 15 | $4.6 \pm 2.8^b$ | $2.0 \pm 0.99$ | $< 0.001$ |
| Testosterone propionate | $300^c$ | 8 | $3.9 \pm 1.9$ | $3.0 \pm 2.0$ | N.S. |
| Testosterone propionate[d] | $300^c$ | 5 | $4.1 \pm 2.0$ | $3.7 \pm 1.8$ | N.S. |
| Progesterone[d] | 2000 | 7 | $3.5 \pm 1.3$ | $4.7 \pm 1.9$ | N.S. |
| 9α-Bromo-11-keto-progesterone[d] | 300 | 4 | $4.8 \pm 2.2$ | $7.2 \pm 4.3$ | N.S. |

[a] $p$ Determined by Student's $t$ test.
[b] Mean $\pm$ standard deviation.
[c] Testosterone propionate 100 mg. thrice weekly intramuscularly.
[d] Studies performed by Drs. F. H. Tyler and R. A. Huseby.

measured by the method of Peterson *et al.* (20). No change in levels of plasma 17-OHCS was observed by Dr. Huseby employing the method of Eik-Nes (7) to follow the administration of these steroids. The administration of both these progesterone derivatives caused increased excretion of 17-OHCS (4, 16) when measured either by the method of Peterson *et al.* (20) or of Glenn and Nelson (13). Further studies are indicated to determine the significance of these findings.

## THE EFFECT OF VARIOUS STEROIDS ON THE LEVELS OF PROTEIN-BOUND IODINE IN SERUM

It has been reported previously that alterations in the levels of serum protein-bound iodine (PBI) and thyroxine-binding protein (TBP) in the absence of signs or of symptoms of thyroid dysfunction occur following the administration of estrogens and androgens (6, 8–10, 17). The effect of various steroids on the levels of serum PBI are shown in Table XI. Administration

TABLE XI
EFFECT OF VARIOUS STEROIDS ON SERUM PROTEIN-BOUND IODINE

| Steroid | Dose (mg./day p.o.) | Number of subjects | Serum PBI (µg./100 ml.) | | $p^a$ |
|---|---|---|---|---|---|
| | | | Pre-therapy | Post-therapy | |
| 17α-Methyl-19-nortestosterone | 30 | 16 | $7.7 \pm 1.1^b$ | $3.3 \pm 0.6$ | $< 0.001$ |
| Testosterone propionate | $300^c$ | 9 | $7.2 \pm 1.4$ | $4.6 \pm 1.2$ | $< 0.01$ |
| 6α-Methyl-17α-acetoxyprogesterone | 40–200 | 5 | $7.6 \pm 1.1$ | $6.2 \pm 1.9$ | $> 0.05 < 0.1$ |
| 6α-Fluoro-17α-acetoxyprogesterone | 200 | 5 | $6.5 \pm 0.8$ | $8.2 \pm 2.5$ | $> 0.1 < 0.2$ |
| Stilbestrol | 15 | 8 | $6.1 \pm 1.9$ | $8.6 \pm 2.3$ | $< 0.01$ |
| Conjugated estrogens (Premarin) | 10 | 3 | $6.1 \pm 1.2$ | $6.5 \pm 1.4$ | N.S. |
| Conjugated estrogens (Premarin) | 5 | 2 | 6.1 | 7.6 | N.S. |

[a] $p$ Determined by Student's $t$ test.
[b] Mean $\pm$ standard deviation.
[c] Testosterone propionate 100 mg. thrice weekly intramuscularly.

of testosterone propionate 100 mg. thrice weekly resulted in significant lowering of the serum PBI, as reported previously (17). Administration of stilbestrol in doses of 15 mg. per day was accompanied by increased levels of serum PBI. This dose was one-half the amount employed by Dowling *et al.* (6), who found significant increases in the levels of the serum PBI. Premarin® in the doses employed did not alter the serum PBI. A striking finding was the marked lowering of the serum PBI following the administration of 30 mg. per day by mouth of 17α-methyl-19-nortestosterone (17-MNT). The effect was more marked than that induced by testosterone propionate in a comparable group of patients treated in this study (11) and in studies reported by others (8, 10, 17).

Although there was a marked decrease in the serum PBI, there was no change in the thyroidal $I^{131}$ uptake in subjects receiving 17-MNT (Table XII). The basal metabolic rate was followed serially in 2 patients on 17-

### TABLE XII

EFFECT OF 17α-METHYL-19-NORTESTOSTERONE AND TESTOSTERONE PROPIONATE ON THYROID FUNCTION

| | Number of patients | Pre-therapy | Post-therapy | $p^a$ |
|---|---|---|---|---|
| **17-MNT** | | | | |
| PBI μg./100 ml. | 16 | $7.7 \pm 1.1^b$ | $3.3 \pm 0.6$ | $< 0.001$ |
| Thyroidal $I^{131}$ Uptake (% in 24 hours) | 11 | 25 | 22 | |
| **TP** | | | | |
| PBI (μg./100 ml.) | 9 | $7.2 \pm 1.4$ | $4.6 \pm 1.2$ | $< 0.01$ |
| Thyroidal $I^{131}$ Uptake (% in 24 hours) | 7 | 38 | 35 | |

[a] $p$ Determined by Student's $t$ test.
[b] Mean ± standard deviation.

MNT. Control values of $+13\%$ and $+4\%$ rose to peaks of $+40\%$ and $+32\%$ after 2 and 6 months of therapy, respectively.

Serum thyroxine-binding protein was studied in 3 patients and in all instances fell after 17-MNT therapy (Table XIII). The mean control level was 0.44 μg. thyroxine bound per milliliter serum with a range of 0.33–0.61. The mean level after 5–9 weeks of therapy was 0.074 μg. per milliliter with a range of 0.063–0.089. Concentrations of free thyroxine during therapy were increased threefold over control values.

A more detailed study was carried out before and after administration of 17-MNT 30 mg. daily by mouth to a healthy 36-year-old woman who was two years post menopause (Table XIV). By the second day of therapy, the level of PBI fell and continued to diminish throughout the period of study. The first detectable fall of the level of the TBP was noted on the fourth day of therapy and had diminished to one-third the control level by the four-

TABLE XIII

THYROXINE-BINDING PROTEIN

(17α-METHYL-19-NORTESTOSTERONE, 30 MG. DAILY, P.O.)

| Patient | Total dose (mg.) | PBI (μg./100 ml.) | TBP Capacity[a] (μg./ml.) |
|---|---|---|---|
| F.Mi. | None | 7.2 | 0.37 |
| | 1410 | 3.5 | 0.089 |
| R.C. | None | 5.9 | 0.33 |
| | 1020 | 3.9 | 0.067 |
| P.P. | None | 8.3 | 0.61 |
| | 2040 | 3.4 | 0.063 |
| Control | — | 4.8 | 0.26 |

[a] Studies were performed by Dr. J. Robbins.

TABLE XIV

ELECTROPHORESIS BY REVERSE FLOW WITH 0.1 M AMMONIUM CARBONATE, pH 8.5[a]

| Days therapy | PBI (μg./100 ml.) | TBP Capacity[b] (μg./100 ml.) | $T_4$ in Prealbumin[b, c] (μg./100 ml.) | BMR (%) | Plasma 17-OHCS (μg./100 ml.) | Cholesterol (mg./100 ml.) |
|---|---|---|---|---|---|---|
| 0 | 5.8 | 0.16 | 1.3 | −5 | 14 | 287 |
| 1 | 5.1 | 0.16 | — | — | — | — |
| 4 | 5.0 | 0.094 | 1.2 | — | — | — |
| 6 | 4.7 | — | — | — | — | — |
| 9 | 4.2 | — | — | +18 | — | — |
| 11 | 3.9 | — | — | — | — | — |
| 14 | 3.7 | 0.064 | 1.2 | +20 | 12 | 270 |
| Normal | — | 0.18 | 1.1 | — | — | — |

[a] Subject D. H., 36-year-old woman, two years post menopause. Therapy: 17α-methyl-19-nortestosterone, 30 mg. daily per os.

[b] Studies were performed by Dr. J. Robbins.

[c] Added $T_4$ concentration = 2.6 μg. per milliliter serum.

teenth day of therapy. There was no significant change in the prealbumin-binding protein as determined by the method of Robbins (21). The basal metabolic rate (BMR) rose from a control level of −5 % to +20 % after 14 days of therapy, although the level of free thyroxine was not increased.

There was no change in the thyroidal I[131] uptake. Clinically the patient showed no evidence of thyroid dysfunction. Studies of thyroxine disappearance rates, thyroidal iodide clearance, iodine pools, and iodine degradation are being undertaken in order to delineate the direct effects of 17-MNT on the thyroid and on extrathyroidal mechanisms.

Similar studies in patients given methyl testosterone for 4 weeks revealed increased thyroxine disappearance with increased absolute degradation of hormonal iodine and no change in iodide metabolism (10). It has been suggested that the primary effect of methyl testosterone is first to cause a profound decrease in the concentration of TBP in serum with resultant changes in thyroid function. These changes include elevated free thyroxine, increased thyroxine metabolism, suppression of thyrotropin with decreased thyroxine secretion and a fall in serum PBI. When a steady state is reached, thyroxine levels, thyroid iodide clearance, thyroid hormone secretion, and thyroxine degradation are all normal (10). Administration of testosterone propionate resulted in no change in thyroxine survival time nor consistent change in TBP levels although the levels of the serum PBI decreased significantly (8). Since the administration of 17α-methyl-19-nortestosterone is accompanied by rapid and significant lowering of the levels of the serum PBI and TBP, the mechanism involved in altering these levels may be elucidated more readily than those changes accompanying treatment with other steroids.

## SUMMARY

From the data presented, the following conclusions are drawn:

1. Estrogen administration to humans in adequate doses produces: (a) an elevation above normal of levels of plasma 17-OHCS and augmented increases of these steroids in plasma after intravenous ACTH, without hyperadrenalcorticism. (b) elevation of levels of plasma 17-OHCS due to authentic cortisol; (c) a decrease in urinary excretion of conjugated 17-OHCS; (d) a delay in the rate of clearance from plasma of exogenous hydrocortisone and tetrahydrocortisone; (e) an increase in hydrocortisone binding to transcortin and transcortin-binding capacity. This alteration could explain all the above findings (a–d) except the diminished rate of clearance from plasma of exogenous tetrahydrocortisone.

2. The nonestrogenic steroids administered fail to alter consistently the levels of plasma 17-OHCS.

3. 17α-Methyl-19-nortestosterone administration leads to a profound fall in the serum PBI and in the thyroxine-binding capacity and to a rise in the calculated levels of free thyroxine without altering the 24-hour thyroidal I[131] uptake.

4. Administration of testosterone propionate results in lowering of the levels of serum PBI.

5. Administration of adequate doses of estrogen is accompanied by elevation of the levels of serum PBI.

6. The other steroids administered fail to alter the levels of serum PBI.

## ACKNOWLEDGMENTS

The authors are indebted to Dr. Avery A. Sandberg, Roswell Park Memorial Institute, for the transcortin-binding determinations, and to Dr. Jacob Robbins, National Institute of Arthritis and Metabolic Diseases, National Institutes of Health, for the thyroxine-binding protein determinations.

Estinyl® and Premarin® were generously supplied by the Schering Corporation and Ayerst, McKenna and Harrison, respectively. All other steroids were supplied by the Cancer Chemotherapy National Service Center. Tetrahydrocortisone was generously supplied by Merck, Sharp and Dohme and The Upjohn Company.

The technical assistance of James McCarrick, B.S., M.S.; Harold L. Schwartz, B.S.; and Joel Spivak, B.S., is gratefully acknowledged.

## REFERENCES

1. Bodansky, O., Benua, R. S., and Pennacchia, G. *Am. J. Clin. Path.* **30**, 375 (1958).
2. Bonsnes, R. W., and Taussky, H. H. *J. Biol. Chem.* **158**, 581 (1945).
3. Callow, N. H., Callow, R. K., and Emmens, C. W. *Biochem. J.* **32**, 1312 (1938).
4. Carter, A. C., and Wallace, E. Z. Unpublished data.
5. Carter, A. C., Weisenfeld, S., and Goldner, M. G. *Proc. Soc. Exptl. Biol. Med.* **98**, 593 (1958).
6. Dowling, J. T., Freinkel, N., and Ingbar, S. H. *J. Clin. Endocrinol. and Metabolism* **16**, 1491 (1956).
7. Eik-Nes, K. *J. Clin. Endocrinol. and Metabolism* **17**, 502 (1957).
8. Engbring, N. H., and Engstrom, W. W. *J. Clin. Endocrinol. and Metabolism* **19**, 783 (1959).
9. Engstrom, W. W., Markhardt, B., and Liebman, A. *Proc. Soc. Exptl. Biol. Med.* **81**, 582 (1952).
10. Federman, D. D., Robbins, J., and Rall, J. E. *J. Clin. Invest.* **37**, 1024 (1958).
11. Feldman, E. B., and Carter, A. C. *J. Clin. Endocrinol. and Metabolism* **20**, 842 (1960).
12. Gibson, G., and Norymberski, J. K. *Ann. Rheumatic Diseases* **13**, 59 (1954).
13. Glenn, E. M., and Nelson, D. H. *J. Clin. Endocrinol. and Metabolism* **13**, 911 (1953).
14. Helmreich, M. L. Unpublished data.
15. Helmreich, M. L., Jenkins, D., and Swan, H. *Surgery* **41**, 895 (1957).
16. Huseby, R. A. Unpublished data.
17. Keitel, H. G., and Sherer, M. G. *J. Clin. Endocrinol. and Metabolism* **17**, 854 (1957).
18. Nelson, D. H., and Samuels, L. T. *J. Clin. Endocrinol.* **12**, 519 (1952).
19. Peterson, R. E. *Recent Progr. in Hormone Research* **15**, 231 (1959).
20. Peterson, R. E., Wyngaarden, J. B., Guerra, S. L., Brodie, B. B., and Bunim, J. J. *J. Clin. Invest.* **34**, 1779 (1955).
21. Robbins, J. *Arch. Biochem. Biophys.* **63**, 461 (1956).

22.  Robbins, J. Unpublished data.
23.  Slaunwhite, W. R., Jr., and Sandberg, A. A. *J. Clin. Invest.* **38**, 384 (1959).
24.  Taliaferro, J., Cobey, F., and Leone, L. *Proc. Soc. Exptl. Biol. Med.* **92**, 742 (1956).
25.  Wallace, E. Z., and Carter, A. C. *J. Clin. Invest.* **39**, 601 (1960).
26.  Wallace, E. Z., Silverberg, H. I., and Carter, A. C. *Proc. Soc. Exptl. Biol. Med.* **95**, 805 (1957).
27.  Zak, B., Willard, H. H., Meyers, G. B., and Boyle, A. J. *Anal. Chem.* **24**, 1345 (1952).

DISCUSSION

**W. H. Daughaday:**   Dr. Carter has chosen to use the unitarian theory of changes after estrogens that Dr. Sandberg has proposed. However, it should be noted that there is nothing incompatible with their observations and our results presented earlier The decrease in the urinary conjugates bothers me a little bit if we accept the idea that Dr. Sandberg in particular envisages, that the elevation of the total hydrocortisol is a compensatory mechanism to maintain a normal plasma level of unbound steroid—one would expect that the amount being degraded by liver would be normal. We can't really escape completely the possibility that there is a secondary effect on the rate of degradation by liver. In reference to the apparent decrease in the rate of disappearance of tetrahydrocortisone, this is the same observation that Christy *et al.* had made in pregnancy. It is possible that this could be evidence in favor of the estrogen-induced binding activity that I described.

**A. C. Carter:**   In regard to Dr. Daughaday's comment about the decrease in urinary 17-hydroxycorticosteroid conjugates, preliminary observations by Dr. Sandberg and myself indicate that the levels of transcortin rise before the plasma levels of 17-hydroxycorticosteroids following administration of estrogen. We have no direct evidence to exclude the possibility that estrogens interfere with metabolism of cortisol by the liver.

**E. H. Tyler:**   I would like to turn your attention to the situation at physiologic doses of estrogen in contrast to the superphysiologic dose used here. In normal females the rate of removal of hydrocortisone is delayed as compared to that in males, and this same delay can be induced in normal young males by the administration of estrogens in very small amounts. These amounts do not affect the plasma level of cortisol (17-hydroxycorticosteroid), nor the binding protein or proteins, presumably. So I think there is evidence of a primary effect on removal rate in addition to the evidence presented here for a change in binding protein.

**D. L. Berliner:**   In relation to the work which was presented here, it should be pointed out that perhaps the reason why tetrahydrocortisone is not normally being removed from the blood in your study is because there is some lack in the formation of the conjugated derivative and that this action might be a direct liver effect.

The 17-hydroxycorticosteroid determination by the Porter-Silber reaction, in our hands, reflects not only the levels in blood of cortisol, but also of tetrahydrocortisol, tetrahydrocortisone, and other compounds. During stress or during treatment with ACTH there is also an increase of these tetrahydro compounds in blood. T. E. Weichselbaum and H. W. Margraf [*J. Clin. Endocrinol. and Metabolism* **19**, 1011 (1959)] have isolated and identified tetrahydrocortisone from blood of normal individuals.

**S. J. Mellette:**   I would like to inquire a bit more about the time relationships in this phenomenon of increased plasma levels of 17-hydroxycorticoids following administration of stilbestrol or other estrogenic substances. As you will remember, in 1956 Dr Isabel Taliaferro, from our institution, reported elevations in plasma corticoids in association with the administration of stilbestrol. In this study, the first plasma levels were measured some 3 days after the stilbestrol had been initiated. After treatment was discontinued, however, it took approximately 10 days for the levels to return to normal. If we are to assume that transcortin or some such protein is involved, it would be expected that changes in the levels of such a substance would be parallel. This in itself should not, however, mean very much because, as we all know, the levels of many proteins are altered by estrogen administration and such changes may be incidental. We have been interested, for example, in plasminogen and related proteins. This is a group of plasma substances with which Dr. Pincus has also done some work in relation to their possible role in the degradation of pituitary hormones. For other reasons, we determined levels of these proteins on samples obtained in the study done by Dr. Taliaferro which I have just mentioned. We found that, at some points, after the administration of stilbestrol, changes in 17-OH corticoids and in these substances were parallel. There were, however, discrepancies. A rise in blood fibrinolytic activity occurred early, along with the rise in 17-OH corticoids, but the proenzyme, plasminogen, required several more days to reach peak levels. We have also thought it of some interest to follow the remarkable elevations of plasma 17-OH corticoids which may be obtained in the hypophysectomized patient who is receiving estrogens, by the administration of small doses of cortisone. In such a patient, who had received no maintenance cortisone for about 28 hours, plasma levels of around 9 μg. % were obtained. Levels of 90 μg. % and above could be reached at 1 hour after the small 25-mg. oral dose of cortisone.

**A. C. Carter:** In answer to your last observation, we previously reported that patients with untreated adrenal insufficiency did not have plasma level rises in the 17-hydroxycorticosteroids following the administration of ethynyl estradiol. However, in patients with some adrenal function, levels of plasma 17-OHCS could be elevated. In answer to your first question, the levels of transcortin were altered by the second day and the levels of 17-OHCS steroid levels were elevated by the third day. At present we are studying the changes after withdrawal of estrogens. I cannot make any comments about plasminogen, but there are certain points of interest regarding thy-

TABLE A

SERUM PROTEIN-BOUND IODINE LEVELS IN HEALTHY POSTMENOPAUSAL WOMEN AND POSTMENOPAUSAL WOMEN WITH CARCINOMA OF THE BREAST

| Group | Number of subjects | Mean age | Mean years post-menopause | Mean years post-surgery | PBI[a] (μg./100 ml.) |
|---|---|---|---|---|---|
| 1. Healthy controls | 20 | 56 | 9.5 | — | 6.5 ± 1.2 |
| 2. "Cured" breast carcinoma | 27 | 66 | 12.9 | 10.1 | 6.3 ± 1.0 |
| 3. Progressive metastatic mammary carcinoma | 46 | 60 | 10.7 | 4.5 | 7.4 ± 1.3 |

[a] p, Not significant between groups 1 and 2 (> 0.95); p < 0.01 between groups 3 and 1 and < 0.001 between groups 3 and 2.

roxine-binding protein (TBP) and transcortin. As you may note, larger doses of estrogens are required to alter the levels of PBI. Administration of steroid which lowers the levels of TBP does not alter transcortin levels. These two proteins apparently respond to different steroids.

**A. Segaloff:**  Do the values on the patients before you treated them differ from those on patients that didn't have breast cancer?

**A. C. Carter:**  Table A will answer your question. Serum levels of PBI were studied in three groups of patients of comparable age and years postmenopause. The mean levels of serum PBI were, respectively, 6.5, 6.3, and 7.4 mg. per 100 ml. for healthy controls (Group 1), patients with "cured" breast carcinoma (Group 2), and patients with untreated progressive metastatic mammary carcinoma (Group 3). There is a statistically significant difference in the mean levels of serum PBI in patients with metastatic carcinoma of the breast and the control groups. There was no correlation between the levels of PBI and the site of dominant metastases or survival.

# The Metabolism of Dehydroisoandrosterone

R. VandeWiele and S. Lieberman

*Departments of Obstetrics and Gynecology and of Biochemistry, College of Physicians and Surgeons, Columbia University, New York, New York*

Of the hormonally active classes of compounds known to be secreted by the adrenal cortex, three are shown in Fig. 1. The most important member of one of these classes is hydrocortisone. A second class of hormones is that typified by aldosterone; and the third category is that product or products

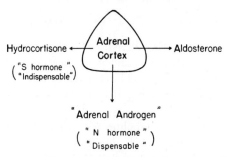

Fig. 1. Representative members of three hormonally active classes of compounds known to be secreted by the adrenal cortex.

to which the name "adrenal androgen" has been assigned. Albright (1) once called this latter product the N hormone, in contrast to hydrocortisone which he named the S hormone. Similarly Gallagher (6) has recently distinguished it from hydrocortisone by dubbing it "dispensable," since, unlike hydrocortisone, it is not necessary for the maintenance of life. Little if anything is known about the identity of the adrenal androgen, or, for that matter, about its true biological significance.

Evidence for the existence of this third class of compounds is mainly indirect, partly biochemical and partly biological. From the virilization present in patients with adrenal hyperplasia and adrenal cancer, it is evident that the adrenal can secrete products that are strongly androgenic, and from this it has been inferred that *in the normal individual* the adrenal secretes an androgen, albeit at lower levels. Better evidence for the secretion of this third class of products by the normal adrenal is derived from the presence in the urine of three $C_{19}$-11-deoxy-17-ketosteroids: dehydroisoandrosterone (D)—or 3β-hydroxy-$\Delta^5$-androsten-17-one; androsterone (A)—or 3α-hydroxyandrostan-17-one; and etiocholanolone (E)—or 3α-hydroxyetiocholan-17-one. Since these metabolites are found in the urine of male castrates and eunuchoids and in the urine of normal women, there is little doubt that they derive at least partly from adrenal precursors. Consequently, in describing this third class of hormones, it may be more precise to refer to these adrenal secretions as the progenitors of the three urinary 17-ketosteroids shown in Fig. 2 than to describe them by their possible biological consequence, as is implied by the term "adrenal androgen." Indeed, it is well

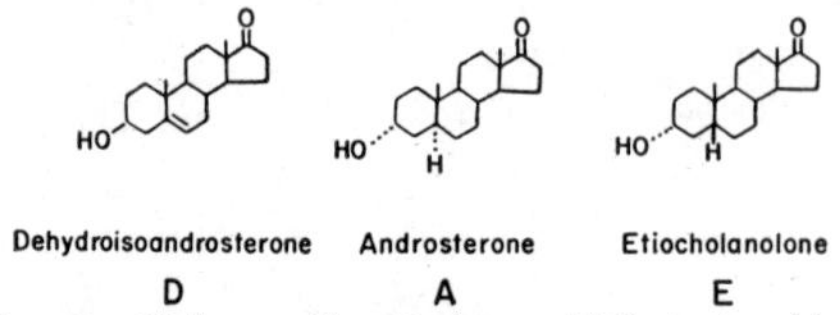

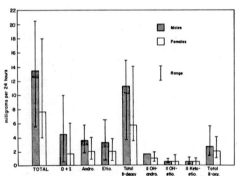

| Dehydroisoandrosterone | Androsterone | Etiocholanolone |
|:---:|:---:|:---:|
| D | A | E |

FIG. 2.   Urinary $C_{19}$-11-deoxy-17-ketosteroids.

known that the secretion of the adrenals of male castrates cannot maintain secondary male sex characteristics, and it is unnecessary to recall the situation that exists in women. It would seem, therefore, that at physiological levels this third class of compounds does not possess significant androgenic potency.

Our interest in these three metabolites was stimulated by the fact that less is known about their origin and significance than about most of the other steroids excreted in human urine. This is true even though these three metabolites were isolated from urine about a quarter of a century ago and

FIG. 3. Urinary levels of 17-ketosteroids measured in a group of normal young females (13) and males (8).

comprise about 75% of the total urinary 17-ketosteroids. In Fig. 3 are summarized the urinary levels of the 17-ketosteroids we have measured in a group of normal young males and females. On the left are given the values for the 11-deoxy compounds and on the right those of the 11-oxygenated compounds, about which nothing further will be said. The height of each bar represents the mean of about ten determinations and the range of these determinations is indicated by the vertical line within each bar. These values are in general similar to those reported by several other investigators (10–12). This figure is reproduced here for two purposes. The first is to indicate the magnitude of the 11-deoxy-17-ketosteroid excretion, particularly that of dehydroisoandrosterone. The second is to point out the large scatter of dehydroisoandrosterone excretion levels, which, in our male subjects, ranged from 0.1 mg. to 8.8 mg. per 24 hours, with a mean of 2.7 mg. Serial determinations on the same individual, on the other hand, revealed remarkably constant urinary levels of dehydroisoandrosterone.

The origin of these three steroids is an important problem, for if their occurrence in normal urine as well as in the urine of patients with various clinical syndromes is to be understood, it is essential that their precursors and their glandular source be known. Previous studies have indicated that urinary androsterone and etiocholanolone can be derived from more than one precursor, and consequently variations that occur in the urinary levels of these metabolites may reflect, in terms both of secretory mechanisms and catabolic transformations, very different processes.

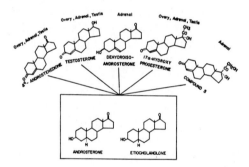

FIG. 4. Structures of possible precursors of androsterone and etiocholanolone.

Figure 4 illustrates the structures of some of the possible precursors of androsterone and etiocholanolone. All the compounds shown are capable of serving as precursors of androsterone and etiocholanolone, and since some of these possess considerably different biological potencies or biogenetic significance than others, it is essential to know which, in fact, is the true precursor in any specific instance. Obviously, the biological consequences of the secretion of a weak androgen, such as dehydroisoandrosterone, would be enormously different from that of testosterone or androstenedione. The situation is further complicated by the fact that some of these precursors may be produced either in normal or abnormal situations, not only by the adrenals, but also by the ovaries or testes, and therefore a mere analysis of the urinary levels of androsterone and etiocholanolone would not distinguish among an ovarian, testicular, or adrenal origin for these steroids.

This presentation concerns itself with our efforts to determine the *adrenal* precursors of these three metabolites as they occur in the urine of normal male and normal female subjects. It is unlikely that the adrenal precursor of the androsterone and etiocholanolone present in the urine of the normal male or female is a strong androgen such as testosterone or androstenedione. The atrophy of secondary sex characteristics in male castrates and the absence of virilization in females precludes the adrenal secretion of a potent androgen in amounts which would be consistent with the urinary levels of androsterone and etiocholanolone in such individuals.

Neither are 11-deoxy-$C_{21}$ precursors, such as 17α-hydroxyprogesterone, compound S, and related compounds likely to be important contributors to urinary androsterone and etiocholanolone in normal individuals. Three kinds of evidence support this conclusion. Catabolic studies of such precursors have demonstrated that the ratio of androsterone to etiocholanolone found after the administration of these compounds is different from that found in normal urine (5). Moreover, since the yield of 17-ketosteroids from such precursors is small, it would be expected that the principal metabolites of these precursors, pregnanetriol, tetrahydro-S, etc., would be present in normal urine in much larger amounts than are actually found. Furthermore, 11-deoxy-$C_{21}$-steroids have not been isolated in significant amounts from normal peripheral plasma.

From the foregoing, it would appear that the major adrenal precursor of androsterone and etiocholanolone present in normal urine is not identical with testosterone, androstenedione, 17α-hydroxyprogesterone, or compound S. This leaves dehydroisoandrosterone as a principal contender.

What are the previously known facts about dehydroisoandrosterone that suggest that it may be an important precursor of urinary androsterone and etiocholanolone? It is an adrenal product, for it has been isolated from adrenal tissue by Plantin *et al.* (19) and has also been isolated from adrenal vein blood by Lombardo and co-workers (13). The urinary excretion of dehydroisoandrosterone increases after the administration of ACTH (4) and decreases after hydrocortisone administration (9). Its urinary excretion is elevated, sometimes enormously, in patients with various diseases of the adrenal (14). That dehydroisoandrosterone can serve as an efficient precursor of urinary androsterone and etiocholanolone has been known for some fifteen years (15). Another characteristic of dehydroisoandrosterone that would be consistent with its secretion in appreciable amounts by the adrenal is its weak androgenic potency. It is conceivable that no visible androgenic effects would be apparent even if dehydroisoandrosterone were secreted by the normal adrenal in milligram amounts or, in other words, in amounts that would account for the urinary levels of androsterone and etiocholanolone, which together amount to from 4 to 10 mg.

In order to determine the magnitude of the contribution that the adrenal secretion of dehydroisoandrosterone could make for the urinary levels of androsterone and etiocholanolone, several phases of the metabolism of dehydroisoandrosterone have been studied in this laboratory. A sample of this compound, labeled with tritium at carbon 7, was obtained from the New England Nuclear Corporation. Since the validity of the results is dependent upon the degree of radiochemical homogeneity of the injected substance, a special effort has been made to establish the purity of the starting material. A detailed description of these procedures will be published elsewhere. After purification, this material having a specific activity of $30 \times 10^6$ counts per minute per milligram, was injected intravenously in trace amounts into several normal individuals, and the results obtained bear upon the following aspects: (1) the disappearance of radioactivity from the plasma; (2) the appearance of radioctivity in the urine; and (3) the incorporation of radioactivity into the urinary metabolites dehydroisoandrosterone, androsterone, and etiocholanolone.

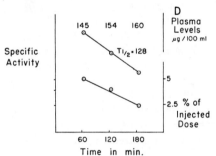

Fig. 5. Fate of tritiated dehydroisoandrosterone in plasma.

The fate of tritiated dehydroisoandrosterone in plasma following the intravenous injection of a tracer dose is illustrated in Fig. 5. The lower line describes the percentage of the injected dose present in peripheral plasma as dehydroisoandrosterone sulfate 1, 2, and 3 hours after administration. The upper line reveals, on a semilog plot, the decline in the specific activity of the dehydroisoandrosterone present as dehydroisoandrosterone sulfate during this time. From this determination it was possible to estimate a 128-minute half-life for dehydroisoandrosterone sulfate. In another subject, the value for $T_{1/2}$ was found to be 98 minutes. The values at the top indicate the absolute plasma levels of dehydroisoandrosterone sulfate, 1, 2, and 3 hours after injection.

Figure 6 illustrates a typical example of the manner in which radioactivity appears in urine after the injection of tritiated dehydroisoandrosterone. Urine was collected in this experiment for 3 days. On the ordinate
is the percentage of the administered dose. The radioactivity appearing in
the acid-hydrolyzed fractions, presumably occurring as conjugates of sulfuric
acid, is shown in the first three shaded bars. That which appeared in the
glucuronidase-hydrolyzed fraction is shown by the open bars and that which
appeared cumulatively in all 3 days is shown at the right. The solid bar
represents the total recovered radioactivity. In this experiment 72 % of
the administered dose was present in the urine although the usual recovery
is about 50 %. Two things are noteworthy from these data. The first is
that of the radioactivity appearing in the urine in the first 3 days, 35 %
probably occurred as sulfates and 65 % as glucuronidates. Secondly, and

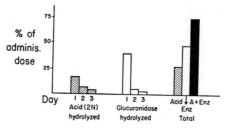

FIG. 6. Tritium in acid- and glucuronidase-hydrolyzed urinary fractions after intravenous administration of tritiated dehydroisoandrosterone.

most significantly for our experiments, these data show that the glucuronidates appear in the urine more rapidly than do the sulfates. This, of course,
confirms the previous observations of Bongiovanni and co-workers (3):
83 % of the glucuronidates appeared in the first day, whereas only 60 %
of the sulfates did.

The experiments carried out involve the isolation and identification of
three metabolites of dehydroisoandrosterone, namely, dehydroisoandrosterone, androsterone, and etiocholanolone. However, before describing the results,
it is necessary to explain the thought behind these experiments. We have
had two objectives. The first was to determine the secretory rate of dehydroisoandrosterone, that is, the amount of dehydroisoandrosterone manufactured daily by normal individuals. The second objective was to compare
the amount of radioactivity that was incorporated into each of the three
metabolites.

Figure 7 outlines the procedure employed to determine the secretory
rate. In principle, this technique is very old, but the recent introduction of
isotope dilution techniques have facilitated its application and ensured its

reliability. It has been used by Pearlman (16) to measure progesterone production, by Cope (4) and by Ayres (2) and their colleagues to measure hydrocortisone production, and by Peterson (17) and Ayres (2) and their co-workers and by us (21) to measure the secretory rate of aldosterone.

$$\text{Secretory rate} \atop \text{(mg/day)} = \frac{\text{Cpm of radioactive precursor injected}}{\text{Specific activity of urinary metabolite}}$$

**Procedure**

1. Inject intravenously tracer amount of radioactive precursor.
2. Collect urine for appropriate time.
3. Isolate urinary metabolite and determine specific activity.

FIG. 7.   Outline of procedure and equation employed to determine the secretory rate.

The procedure involves the intravenous injection of a tracer dose of tritium-labeled steroid, collection of an appropriate urine sample, and isolation and determination of the specific activity of a urinary metabolite that is derived only from the administered substance. From the total counts administered and the specific activity of the metabolite, it is possible to calculate the secretory rate in a manner which depends merely upon the dilution of the isolated metabolite by endogenously produced, unlabeled metabolites.

The validity of the results obtained by this technique depends upon some important assumptions. The urinary metabolite must be derived only from the administered precursor, which in turn must mix rapidly with the endogenous precursor. The complete sample of the radioactive metabolite must be in the urine specimen from which the metabolite is isolated. It is preferable to carry out the determination when steady state conditions hold, that is, when the rate of secretion of the precursor equals its rate of removal. Lastly, the fraction of the precursor converted to the metabolite should not be altered appreciably during the study. In connection with what follows, one of the above considerations deserves special emphasis. It will be recalled that the sulfates are excreted into the urine at a slower rate than are the glucuronidates. Since the fate of the metabolites must be decided by the end of the experiment, differences in excretion rate must be kept in mind in order to ensure that the proper sample of the metabolite has been collected.

Our second objective was to compare the tritium content of each of the three metabolites. As Fig. 8 attempts to illustrate, a comparison of the specific activities (SA) of the three metabolites should provide an indication of the amount of urinary androsterone (A) and etiocholanolone (E) which is derived from dehydroisoandrosterone and the amount which may be derived from other precursors. The endogenous precursors, dehydroisoandrosterone (D) and other possibilities designated X, are shown on top. Since only dehydroisoandrosterone can serve as a precursor of all three metabolites, only that fraction of androsterone and etiocholanolone derived from radio-active dehydroisoandrosterone will be labeled. That fraction arising from other precursors will not be radioactive. Thus the difference between the specific activity of the urinary dehydroisoandrosterone ($SA_D$) and those of urinary androsterone ($SA_A$) and etiocholanolone ($SA_E$) is a measure of the contribution of precursors other than dehydroisoandrosterone to the urinary metabolites androsterone and etiocholanolone. This comparison of specific activities gives *no* information about the secretory rate of other precursors; it is merely a measure of the magnitude of their contribution to the urinary metabolites.

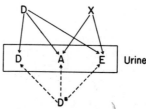

FIG. 8. Schematic representation of the factors determining the specific activity of the metabolites of dehydroisoandrosterone after the administration of radioactive dehydroisoandrosterone.

The equations describe the factors which determine the specific activities of the metabolites dehydroisoandrosterone and androsterone.

$$SA_D = \frac{c.p.m._D}{wt._D^D + wt._{D*}^{D*}}$$

$$SA_A = \frac{c.p.m._A}{wt._D^A + wt._{D*}^{A*} + wt._X^A}$$

$$SA_D = SA_A \text{ only when } wt._X^A = 0$$

The term $wt_D^D$ refers to the amount of urinary dehydroisoandrosterone derived from endogenously produced dehydroisoandrosterone and the term $wt_{D*}^{D*}$ equals the amount of the radioactive dehydroisoandrosterone found in the urine, which is derived from the administered tracer. This latter term is, of course, of negligible magnitude. The term $wt_D^A$ refers to the amount of urinary androsterone derived from endogenously produced dehydroisoandrosterone and the term $wt_{D*}^{A*}$ is self evident. The term $wt_X^A$ equals the amount of the unlabeled androsterone derived from endogenously produced precursors other than dehydroisoandrosterone. The specific activity of that portion of androsterone that was derived from dehydroisoandrosterone must, by definition, be equal to the specific activity of dehydroisoandrosterone ($SA_D$). As a result, the observed specific activities ($SA_D$ and $SA_A$) differ by virtue of the contribution of that portion of androsterone that was derived from X. Vice versa, the specific activities will be equal only when the amount of androsterone derived from X is zero.

Using this approach, the three metabolites found in each of the following experiments were isolated and their specific activities were determined. A detailed description of the experimental procedures used to isolate and purify these urinary catabolites will be published elsewhere. In a typical experiment the metabolites were isolated from the urine following mild acid hydrolysis or hydrolysis with β-*glucuronidase*. They were separated from each other first by chromatography on alumina, using a gradient elution technique, and then by paper chromatography, using the Bush A system. In every instance reported below, the specific activity of the metabolite was determined from materials isolated in this manner. In many instances, additional chemical processes were carried out to ensure the constancy of specific activity. After such purification it was found that in a normal young female individual, age 18, the specific activity of dehydroisoandrosterone was 16 counts per minute per microgram, the specific activity of androsterone was 17 counts per minute per microgram, and the specific activity of etiocholanolone 16 counts per minute per microgram.

From this experiment two facts have been established. The first is that the secretory rate of dehydroisoandrosterone, calculated from the specific activity of that metabolite by the equation shown in Fig. 7 amounts to 25 mg. per day. The second is that comparison of the specific activities of the three metabolites reveals that they are, within the experimental error of the method, identical. Therefore, if there are precursors of androsterone and etiocholanolone other than dehydroisoandrosterone, their contribution in the normal person to the urinary metabolites is small in comparison to that of dehydroisoandrosterone.

To obtain an experimental check of these theoretical considerations, an artificial situation was set up in which a known precursor of androsterone and etiocholanolone* was supplied exogenously. The results are shown in Fig. 9. The substance fed to one of our normal subjects was androstenedione, which serves as a precursor of only androsterone and etiocholanolone and therefore should decrease the specific activity of these urinary metabolites without altering that of dehydroisoandrosterone. The results are given in the bar graph at the bottom. The results of the control experiment are shown by the open bars and those of the androstenedione experiment by

---

* A known precursor other than dehydroisoandrosterone was supplied.

the shaded bars. The specific activity of dehydroisoandrosterone is the same whether or not androstenedione was administered. On the other hand, the specific activities of androsterone and etiocholanolone, as well as that of isoandrosterone which was isolated in this experiment, were significantly diminished by the exogenous administration of 10 mg. per day of this pre-

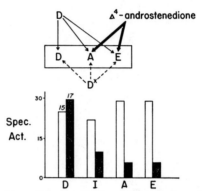

FIG. 9. Specific activities of the metabolites of dehydroisoandrosterone isolated from the urine of a normal individual before (open bars) and after (shaded bars) administration of $\Delta^4$-androstenedione.

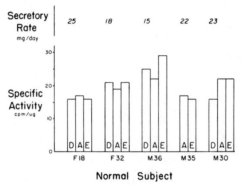

Normal  Subject

FIG. 10. Below: Specific activities of dehydroisoandrosterone (D), androsterone (A), and etiocholanolone (E) isolated from the urine of five normal subjects (sex and age indicated beneath abscissa). Above: Calculated secretory rates.

cursor. The numbers 15 and 17 at the top of the first two bars indicate the secretory rate of dehydroisoandrosterone in this individual as calculated from the specific activity of dehydroisoandrosterone.

Figure 10 summarizes the results obtained on five normal individuals; their sex and age are indicated at the bottom. The specific activities of dehydroisoandrosterone, androsterone, and etiocholanolone of these subjects are essentially equal to each other. The calculated secretory rates are given at the top. Owing to an accident, dehydroisoandrosterone was not isolated in one instance (M35). However, the specific activities of androsterone and etiocholanolone are shown, and the secretory rate of dehydroisoandrosterone was calculated from the specific activity of the androsterone, assuming of course that this value was identical with that of the dehydroisoandrosterone which was lost.

In conclusion, our results indicate that dehydroisoandrosterone is quantitatively an important secretory product of the adrenal. To emphasize this, Fig. 1 has been redrawn in the manner shown in Fig. 11. The daily produc-

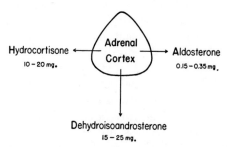

FIG. 11.   Daily production of adrenal hormones. Redrawn from Fig. 1 to demonstrate the quantitative importance of dehydroisoandrosterone.

tion of the three important secretory products of the adrenal is given. Within the experimental error of our method the data also make it apparent that the dehydroisoandrosterone, androsterone, and etiocholanolone excreted in the urine of the normal subjects studied were derived from one precursor and that this precursor was dehydroisoandrosterone. Other possible precursors of urinary androsterone and etiocholanolone, such as testosterone, androstenedione, 17α-hydroxyprogesterone, or compound S, contributed only a minor amount, if any, to the total urinary androsterone and etiocholanolone.

It is important to remember that this situation holds in the female individual as well as in the male. The amount of androstenedione and testosterone secreted by the testes must therefore be small in comparison to the amount of dehydroisoandrosterone produced by the adrenal. In support of this conclusion it can be added that some time ago Dr. Gallagher (7) estimated the daily production of testicular testosterone to be less than 3 mg per day, which is small compared to the above-mentioned secretory rate of dehydroisoandrosterone. The small contribution of the testicular secretion to the urinary ketosteroids in the male is a rather surprising finding and confirms an impression held by us and by others that, as an index of testicular function, the 17-ketosteroids have little, if any, value. In this respect these studies may well have a bearing on certain pathological conditions in women in whom the ovary has become the cause of extreme virilization. It has always been difficult to understand why the urinary 17-ketosteroids of patients with virilizing arrhenoblastomas are customarily within normal limits or even at the lower limit of the normal. It is evident from our studies that, even if the ovary of such patients secretes amounts of testosterone or androstenedione equivalent to those of the normal testicles, no elevation of the urinary 17-ketosteroids would be expected.

As mentioned before, our data do not give any information about the magnitude of other adrenal secretory products, such as 11-deoxy-17-hydroxy-20-ketopregnane compounds. Nevertheless, it can be concluded that, regardless of the quantity of such compounds made by the adrenal, they contribute little or nothing, in the normal individual, to the urinary androsterone and etiocholanolone. In diseased states, of course, urinary androsterone and etiocholanolone may be derived from any of the aforementioned precursors, and changes in their excretion pattern may reflect very different processes in terms of glandular secretion. Any rationalization about pathogenesis or glandular origin is impossible unless the precursors of these metabolites are dissociated from each other.

If the results reported here have supplied answers to one or two questions, they have also raised many other important ones. For example, what is the significance of the adrenal secretion of dehydroisoandrosterone? Does this compound possess some biological property other than its weak androgenicity? Or is it merely a biogenetic "waste" product of the adrenal, which fortuitously possesses weak androgenic potency? What are the factors, physiological or pathological, which control the adrenal secretion of dehydroisoandrosterone? The 11-deoxyketosteroids, dehydroisoandrosterone, androsterone, and etiocholanolone are virtually absent from the urine before puberty. The increase in the excretion of the 17-ketosteroids that occurs at this time, both in girls and in boys, is due predominantly to an increase in dehydroisoandrosterone, androsterone, and etiocholanolone. On the other hand, at the other end of the age scale, there is a progressive decrease in the 11-deoxy-17-ketosteroids, again in both males and females, with little, if any, change in the level of 11-oxyketosteroids (18). Furthermore, a similar pattern of excretion prevails in disease and under surgical stress (6, 8).

Lastly, what is the place of dehydroisoandrosterone in the biogenesis of the adrenal steroids? Figure 12 shows one known pathway. Dr. Samuel Solomon (20) in our laboratory has recently demonstrated that in a patient with a malignant tumor of the adrenal, $17\alpha$-hydroxypregnenolone can serve as precursor of urinary dehydroisoandrosterone. A similar conversion could also be demonstrated in *in vitro* experiments using homogenates of the excised tumor (see Discussion below). Thus the scheme shown in Fig. 12 appears to be reasonable. The factors that determine what fraction of pregnenolone serves as a precursor for hydrocortisone and aldosterone and what fraction is diverted to dehydroisoandrosterone remain to be determined.

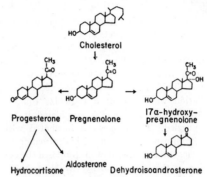

FIG. 12. Biogenesis of dehydroisoandrosterone.

REFERENCES

1. Albright, F. *Harvey Lectures Ser.* **38**, 123, (1943).
2. Ayres, P. J., Garrod, O., Simpson, S. A., and Tait, J. F. *Biochem. J.* **65**, 639 (1957).
3. Bongiovanni, A. M., and Eberlein, W. R. *J. Clin. Endocrinol. and Metabolism* **17**, 328 (1957).
4. Cope, C. L., and Black, F. *Brit. Med. J.* **I**, 1020 (1958).
5. Dorfman, R. I. *Recent Progr. in Hormone Research* **9**, 4 (1954).
6. Gallagher, T. F. *Harvey Lectures Ser.* **52**, 1 (1958).
7. Gallagher, T. F. Personal communication.
8. Herrman, W. L., Hayes, M. A., Holdenberg, I. S., and Schindl, I. K. *J. Clin. Endocrinol. and Metabolism* **19**, 849 (1959).
9. Jailer, J. W. and VandeWiele, R. *Gynaecologia* **138**, 276 (1954).
10. Kappas, A., and Gallagher, T. F. *J. Clin. Invest.* **34**, 1566 (1955).
11. Kappas, A., and Gallagher, T. F. *J. Clin. Invest.* **34**, 1599 (1955).
12. Kellie, A. E., and Wade, A. P. *Biochem. J.* **66**, 490 (1957).
13. Lombardo, M. E., McMorris, C., and Hudson, P. B. *Endocrinology* **65**, 426 (1959).
14. Mason, H. L., and Engstrom, W. W. *Physiol. Revs.* **30**, 321 (1950).
15. Mason, H. L., and Kepler, E. J. *J. Biol. Chem.* **16**, 255 (1945).
16. Pearlman, W. H. *Biochem. J.* **67**, 1 (1957).
17. Peterson, R. E. *Recent Progr. in Hormone Research* **15**, 230 (1958).
18. Pincus, G., Dorfman, R. I., Romanoff, L. P., Rubin, B. L., Bloch, E., Carlo, J., and Filmore, H. *Recent Progr. in Hormone Research* **11**, 307 (1955).
19. Plantin, L. O., Diczfalusy, E., and Birke, G. *Nature* **179**, 421 (1957).
20. Solomon, S., Carter, A. C., and Lieberman, S. *J. Biol. Chem.* **235**, 351 (1960).
21. Ulick, S., Laragh, J. H., and Lieberman, S. *Trans. Assoc. Am. Physicians* **71**, 225 (1958).

DISCUSSION

**R. I. Dorfman:**  Dr. M. Goldstein has incubated adrenal adenoma tissue, from a patient with Cushing's syndrome, with pregnenolone-$H^3$, and demonstrated the formation of dehydroepiandrosterone-$H^3$. In a second experiment involving a masculinized woman with a massive adrenal adenoma, the intravenous administration of pregnenolone-$H^3$ resulted in the excretion of dehydroepiandrosterone-$H^3$. Thus the pathway from pregnenolone to dehydroepiandrosterone seems to be well established.

**L. L. Engel:**   May I cite some experiments that were carried out in our laboratory over the last few years by Dr. Bagget in collaboration with Dr. Dorfman and Dr. Savard, and also my brother in North Carolina? We studied steroid biogenesis in testicular tumors taken from young boys. The first was an interstitial cell tumor of the testis. On incubation of this tissue with $C^{14}$-acetate we were able to isolate labeled dehydroisoandrosterone. This steroid is therefore not exclusively adrenal in origin. A second, similar incubation was done of a testicular tumor that was highly undifferentiated and malignant. Some pathologists considered it to be adrenal in origin and others were frankly puzzled. The tissue was incubated with $C^{14}$-acetate, and labeled pregnenolone, 17-hydroxypregnenolone, and dehydroisoandrosterone were isolated. These findings support the biosynthetic mechanism proposed by Dr. Lieberman and provide evidence for production of this compound by two tissues other than the normal adrenal cortex. I should like to ask Dr. Lieberman how the removal of the label from his tritiated dehydroisoandrosterone in 7 position, by formation of 7-hydroxy- or 7-ketodehydroisoandrosterone, would affect his calculation of the amount of the secretory product?

**S. Lieberman:**   Any metabolic removal of tritium from the precursor would result in an apparent secretory rate higher than the true value. But the question of removal of tritium from C-7 during the formation of, say 7-ketodehydroisoandrosterone, is not at stake in this analysis. The analysis is independent of the numerous catabolic pathways dehydroisoandrosterone may undergo. In this instance, we are concerned only with dehydroisoandrosterone reisolated from the urine. The secretory rate depends merely upon the difference between the specific activities of the injected precursor and the isolated metabolite.

One of the assumptions referred to the necessity that the urine specimen contain the entire sample of the radioactive metabolite whose specific activity is to be measured. It is of no consequence if other radioactive metabolites are excreted at some later time or, indeed, if they are accounted for at all. For example, in the instance I gave, the radioactivity that appeared as urinary dehydroisoandrosterone was only about 1–2 % of the administered tritium. In other words, most of the radioactivity had gone elsewhere. Nevertheless, the secretory rate could be estimated from the specific activity of the isolated dehydroisoandrosterone.

**S. Solomon:**  I would like to describe our experimental evidence for the biosynthesis of dehydroisoandrosterone as shown on Dr. Lieberman's last slide. These experiments were conducted with the assistance of Dr. Anne Carter. Tritium-labeled 17α-hydroxypregnenolone-3-monoacetate was administered intravenously to a 26-year-old female who had adrenal carcinoma and who was excreting large amounts of dehydroisoandrosterone. Urine was collected for 3 days following administration of the labeled precursor. Then the patient underwent surgery for the removal of a metastatic mass from the flank and from the pelvic region. One portion of flank tumor was incubated with cholesterol-$4$-$C^{14}$ and the second half was incubated with tritium-labeled 17α-hydroxypregnenolone-3-monoacetate. The pelvic tumor mass was also incubated with tritiated 17α-hydroxypregnenolone acetate.

The results obtained are as follows: From the neutral fraction of the first 2 days' urine collections, tritium-labeled dehydroisoandrosterone, androsterone, and etiocholanolone were isolated. Radioactive isoandrosterone was also detected. From the radioactivity present in the isolated 17-ketosteroids the conversion from the injected 17α-hydroxypregnenolone was 3.4 %, 64 % of which could be accounted for by dehydroisoandrosterone. When 17α-hydroxypregnenolone acetate was administered to a normal young male, the conversion to urinary dehydroisoandrosterone, androsterone, and etiocholanolone was only 0.1 %. This finding is in agreement with the results obtained by other investigators who have administered 21-deoxy C-21 steroids to humans and found only minute conversions to urinary 17-ketosteroids.

From the homogenate of the flank tumor incubated with cholesterol-4-$C^{14}$, radioactive dehydroisoandrosterone, pregnenolone, and 17α-hydroxypregnenolone were isolated after their addition as carriers. It was also demonstrated that tritiated 17α-hydroxypregnenolone was converted by the flank tumor to radioactive dehydroisoandrosterone. In the case of the pelvic tumor incubated with tritiated 17α-hydroxypregnenolone acetate, no carrier steroids were added at the end of the incubation. Here radioactive dehydroisoandrosterone and 17α-hydroxypregnenolone were isolated. From the lowered specific activity of the isolated 17α-hydroxypregnenolone it was calculated that 0.133 mg. of this steroid was being produced endogenously per hour per gram of tumor tissue during the incubation. Thus, from the results obtained by us and from the results cited by Drs. Dorfman and Engel, it seems that a biosynthetic pathway leading to dehydroisoandrosterone has been established. Whether this is the only pathway remains to be demonstrated.

**M. E. Lombardo·** In a recent publication we reported the results of the analysis of twelve samples of human adrenal vein blood. Each sample consisted of approximately 200–250 ml. In every case we isolated cortisol, and from the amounts isolated the secretion rates were roughly 25–50 mg. a day. On the other hand, we isolated dehydroisoandrosterone only in a special case: in addition to having carcinoma of the breast, this patient was a psychotic. This was the first and only time we isolated dehydroisoandrosterone from human adrenal vein blood. On the other hand 17α-hydroxyprogesterone was isolated in at least a third of the samples that we analyzed. Reichstein's compound S was found in over one-third of the samples. Our results don't agree with the assumption that approximately 25 mg. of dehydroisoandrosterone are secreted by the human adrenal. In addition we have done a number of biosynthetic studies with the human adrenal using 5-pregnenolone, progesterone, and 17α-hydroxyprogesterone as substrates. In no case were we able to isolate $C_{19}$-ketosteroids from these studies. When 5-pregnenolone was used as substrate, progesterone and 17α-hydroxyprogesterone were isolated as intermediates and cortisol as the main product. However, 17α-hydroxypregnenolone was never isolated.

**S. Lieberman:** The incubation studies mentioned by Dr. Lombardo in the second part of his discussion do not seem to me directly pertinent to the subject presented tonight, so I limit my comments to the first part of his discussion. There are in fact two reports in the literature of the isolation of dehydroisoandrosterone from adrenal vein blood. The first one is the one by Dr. Lombardo, already mentioned in our presentation. The second one was by Bush, who measured dehydroisoandrosterone in the adrenal vein blood of a patient with virilization. We did not mention this study since no complete characterization of the isolated dehydroisoandrosterone was made.

In this study it was Dr. Bush's purpose to determine whether the amounts of dehydroisoandrosterone found in adrenal vein blood could account for the patient's urinary dehydroisoandrosterone. He came to the conclusion that the amount of dehydroisoandrosterone in the adrenal vein blood could account for the daily excretion of dehydroisoandrosterone on the not unlikely assumption that 10 % of the manufactured dehydroisoandrosterone was excreted unchanged into the urine. We are not surprised by the failure of Dr. Lombardo to find dehydroisoandrosterone in the adrenal vein blood from 11 of his 12 patients. We have already mentioned in the talk that the $C_{19}$-11-deoxyketosteroids are decreased by age, disease, and surgical stress. There are many reports in the literature of low 17-ketosteroids in patients with metastatic carcinoma. These, as we understand it, were the kind of patient from whose adrenal effluent Dr. Lombardo attempted to isolate dehydroisoandrosterone. We have studied a group of patients with metastatic prostatic carcinoma and found only insignificant amounts of 11-deoxy-17-ketosteroids in their urine. It can therefore be inferred that the secretion of dehydroisoandrosterone by such patients must be very low.

**F. C. Greenwood:** Dr. Lieberman, I wonder if you would like to comment on our experiences with the 11-deoxy-17-ketosteroids in the urine of patients after adrenalectomy. We used the occurrence of dehydroepiandrosterone, androsterone, and etiocholanolone in the urine of patients after adrenalectomy as additional evidence for residual or accessory adrenal tissue. These were cancer patients who had been previously oophorectomized. Etiocholanolone has been isolated from pooled urine, kindly characterized for us by Dr. Gallagher. We have chromatographic evidence only for androsterone, but as I recall we have never been able to pick up dehydroisoandrosterone. You stressed in your talk that your work applied to normal individuals. I wonder if perchance you have used an adrenalectomized patient for your metabolic studies on dehydroisoandrosterone.

**S. Lieberman:** We have not injected this material into an adrenalectomized patient. I would have thought that the finding of etiocholanolone in the urine of an adrenalectomized patient merely means that another precursor arising from some other gland has served as a source of this metabolite.

**H. Wilson:** The biosynthetic pathway to dehydroisoandrosterone (DHA) in the adrenal cortex which Drs. Lieberman and Solomon have demonstrated obviously presupposes that considerable amounts of 17-hydroxy-$\Delta^5$-pregnenolone are regularly formed. If this is so, some of it should appear in the urine as $\Delta^5$-pregnene-3β,17α,20α-triol (5PT). This would be analogous to the metabolism and excretion of 17-hydroxyprogesterone in the form of pregnane-3α,17α,20α-triol. Other workers have found 5PT in the urine in isolated instances, first in subjects with an adrenal carcinoma, and recently in one or two normal persons.

We have estimated the excretion of both DHA and 5PT in 18 subjects of various types. It turns out that 5PT is a very common urinary constituent. Of 8 subjects without adrenocortical dysfunction, 6 excreted this metabolite to the extent of about 100–200 µg. per day. This finding indicates that $\Delta^5$-17-hydroxypregnenolone is commonly formed in the adrenal cortex, and secreted unchanged in small amounts. 5PT was also found in the urine of 1 of 2 subjects having Cushing's disease, and in 2 young women presenting symptoms of hirsutism and obesity. In 6 patients with adrenal carcinoma 5PT was uniformly elevated to between 3 mg. and 50 mg. per day.

In comparing these findings with the excretion of DHA in the same individuals we were interested to see that there was no consistent relationship. For example, there were some who had essentially no DHA (and we believe this unusual result to be correct), but they did excrete 5PT. Others had only DHA and no 5PT, and some excreted both steroids, but their relation to each other was different in each subject. Most of the adrenal carcinoma patients had larger amounts of DHA than of 5PT. We would therefore agree with Dr. Lieberman's remark that elevated DHA is quite characteristic of malignant adrenocortical disease; but 5PT may be another good indicator.

The absence of a consistent relationship between urinary DHA and 5PT led us to think there might be another source of DHA beside 17-hydroxy-$\Delta^5$-pregnenolone. However, the convincing experiments which have just been presented make this an unlikely hypothesis. The amount of DHA in the urine of any one individual would now seem to depend on the efficiency with which it is converted to androsterone and etiocholanolone.

**C. J. Migeon:** I would like to go back to Dr. Engel's question. I agree with Dr. Lieberman that the metabolic fate of dehydroisoandrosterone does not affect the calculation of the rate of production of the hormone. However, I would like to ask what is known of the possible exchange of the tritium with nonisotopic hydrogen in the body; this would affect the measurement of the production rate. A second question: I think that the half-life of dehydroisoandrosterone in the plasma reported by Dr. Lieberman was actually for the sulfate fraction. Does Dr. Lieberman have data on the half-life of the free compound?

**S. Lieberman:** To answer the last question first, it is true that the rate studies reported were estimated from the dehydroisoandrosterone sulfate fraction. We have, on one occasion, made an effort to measure the rate of disappearance of free dehydroisoandrosterone in plasma, but the sample collected 1 hour after the administration of the tracer contained an insignificant amount of radioactivity in the free fraction. The question of the exchangeability of tritium is very pertinent and important. As I stated earlier, had we lost tritium spuriously by virtue of exchange, we would have estimated secretory rates greater than they truly are. It is our intention to carry out this type of experiment in an adrenalectomized patient who presumably is not making any dehydroisoandrosterone. In this case, the specific activity of the isolated dehydroisoandrosterone would be identical with the administered dehydroisoandrosterone if no tritium were lost from the molecule by metabolic processes. A similar experiment has already been carried out by Stanley Ulick in our laboratory with tritiated aldosterone. A sample of aldosterone which had been labeled by the Wilzbach procedure was administered to an adrenalectomized patient. The isolated tetrahydro metabolite had the same specific activity as the injected hormone. This demonstration of the stability of tritium in a sample of aldosterone, labeled by the Wilzbach method, does not quite bear upon the question of the stability of tritium in the dehydroisoandrosterone we employed. This radioactive dehydroisoandrosterone was prepared by the New England Nuclear Corporation, by a chemical process which introduces most of the isotope in C-7. To remove exchangeable tritium, they subjected the sample to alkaline saponification twice. We saponified the sample once again before purifying it further. I believe that such processing is more drastic than any metabolic reaction is likely to be and, therefore, that it is improbable that isotope has been lost merely by exchange.

**K. Savard:** I should like to add a little further evidence to the melancholy case of relegating the testis to a secondary role as a contributor to urinary 17-ketosteroids. We have had occasion to evaluate the total androgen in the spermatic venous blood of large breeding bulls supplied to us by Dr. F. X. Gassner of Colorado. After extraction, bioassay (in the chick-comb androgen assay) revealed that the level of 4-androstene-3,

17-dione plus testosterone was rarely in excess of 10–15 μg. per 100 ml. of plasma in testicular effluent from nongonadotropin-treated animals. This low level taken together with the low volume of blood flow through the testes of the bull, and for that matter of man, points to a rather small 24-hour secretion of urinary 17-ketosteroid precursors; this extrapolation gives us values not too far removed from the value of 3–5 mg. of testosterone produced per 24 hours by the human male reported by Dr. Gallagher.

Finally, may I compliment Dr. Lieberman on his preoccupation with the purity of the radioactive starting material? Far too often the commercially procured radioactive substances, particularly steroids, have been used in apparent gay abandon, without concern for possibility of radioactive contamination. One such material appeared to be homogeneous in two different paper chromatographic systems and one adsorption chromatogram, but on dilution with carrier material and crystallization was found to contain a contaminant in apparently 20 % amounts. The use of several physical-chemical parameters in the evaluation of radiochemical homogeneity, like those utilized by Dr. Lieberman, cannot be overdone.

# Recent Studies on Estrogen Metabolism[1]

LEWIS L. ENGEL[2]

*The John Collins Warren Laboratories of the Collis P. Huntington Memorial Hospital of Harvard University at the Massachusetts General Hospital, and the Department of Biological Chemistry, Harvard Medical School, Boston, Massachusetts*

It is rather difficult to discuss some of the newer aspects of estrogen metabolism without including the subject matter assigned to some of the other speakers at this symposium. Therefore, an attempt will be made to limit this discussion to those areas which *a priori* seem to be excluded by the other titles. Furthermore, in order to achieve a more satisfactory perspective on the work which has been occupying the attention of workers in the field of estrogens for the last few years, it is appropriate to examine the main lines that have led to the present areas of interest.

## HISTORICAL

The earliest work on estrogens was that which derived from the discovery of the biological effects of crude extracts of ovarian tissue and later the effects of extracts of the urine of gravid and nongravid women on the

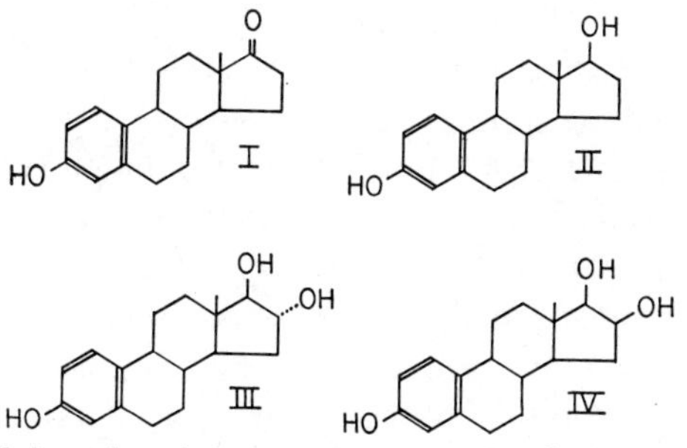

FIG. 1. Structural formulas of estrone (I), estradiol-17β (II), estriol (III), and 16-epiestriol (IV).

vaginal mucosa and on the uteri of immature and castrate rodents. These studies led to the establishment of quantitative techniques for the measurement of estrogenic activity and paved the way for the isolation of the three estrogenic substances (Fig. 1), from urine and from tissues, which occupied

[1] This is Publication No. 1003 of the Cancer Commission of Harvard University. This work was supported by grants from the National Cancer Institute, United States Public Health Service, a grant from the American Cancer Society, Inc., and a grant from the Jane Coffin Childs Memorial Fund for Medical Research.

[2] Permanent Faculty Fellow of the American Cancer Society.

a central position for the next twenty years. The isolation of estrone $(I)^3$ (11, 12, 17), estradiol-17β (II) (39), and estriol (III) (18, 40) (Fig. 1), the first of which was the first crystalline steroid hormone to have been isolated, was accomplished during the early 1930's, and for nearly twenty years these three compounds were thought to be the only steroidal estrogens that had any role in human physiology. During the same period, the work of Dodds (13–16) and his associates and of others led to the discovery of several series of organic compounds that did not possess the steroid skeleton, but that had biologic effects indistinguishable from those of estrone and estradiol. The large-scale commercial production of diethylstilbestrol and its relatives very soon made available for physiologic and pharmacologic studies and for clinical use highly potent estrogens whose effects mimicked those of the natural products. The advantages of the synthetic estrogens insofar as cost of production and availability are concerned were such as to divert attention from the natural products, which could be obtained only by expensive extractions from natural sources and on a relatively small scale. These considerations, combined with the low concentrations of estrogens present in tissues and body fluids and the difficulties in handling them, impeded progress in this area.

### The Isolation of New Urinary Metabolites

It was not until the postwar era, with its tremendous development of delicate and efficient separation methods, of specific and precise detection methods, and of new synthetic procedures, that interest once again turned toward the natural compounds. In large part the impetus for this renaissance of interest came from workers in the cancer field who observed the effects of estrogens on human breast and prostatic cancer (45).

The efforts of Brown (8, 9) and of Bauld (4) to develop highly sensitive and specific methods for the chemical estimation of estrone, estradiol, and estriol in the urine of nonpregnant individuals, in conjunction with the newer separation methods, revealed for the first time new phenolic steroids structurally and biochemically related to the three compounds known at that time (Figs. 1–3). The first of these new compounds to be isolated was 16-epiestriol (IV) (42), an estriol epimer with considerably less biologic activity. Its discovery was followed in short order by that of the ring D ketols, 16α-hydroxyestrone (V) (43) and 16β-hydroxyestrone (VI) (7, 32), as well as the isomeric 16-ketoestradiol (VII) (32) and the diketone 16-ketoestrone (VIII) (52).

An unusual and unexpected metabolite was 18-hydroxyestrone (IX) (37,

---

[3] Roman numerals refer to structural formulas in the figures.

38), also isolated from human pregnancy urine. Its close relation to aldo-sterone, which also bears an aldehyde group at C-18, has suggested that it may be formed in the adrenal cortex.

The administration of estradiol-$C^{14}$ to a patient led to the discovery of representatives of a new class of metabolites in the urine. The first member was 2-methoxyestrone (X), discovered by the Gallagher group (29, 30).

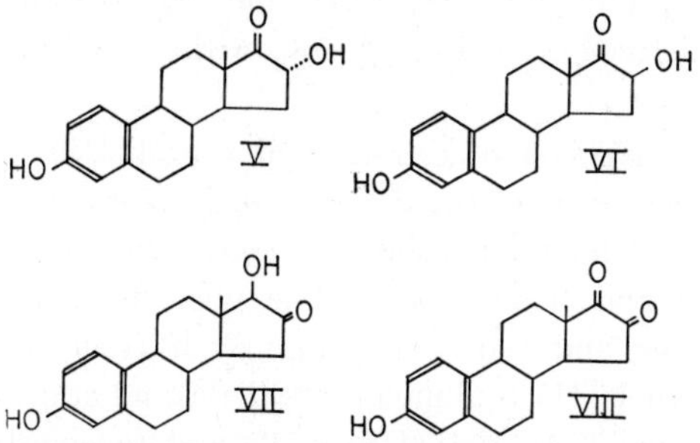

FIG. 2. Structural formulas of 16α-hydroxyestrone (V), 16β-hydroxyestrone (VI), 16-ketoestradiol-17β (VII), and 16-ketoestrone (VIII).

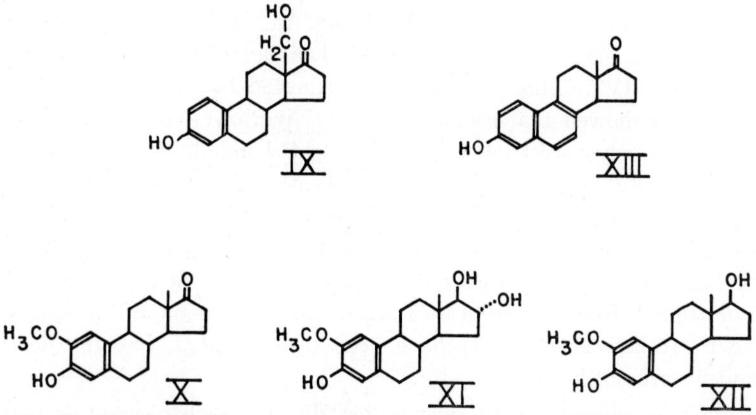

FIG. 3. Structural formulas of 18-hydroxyestrone (IX), 2-methoxyestrone (X), 2-methoxyestriol (XI), 2-methoxyestradiol (XII), and equilenin (XIII).

This finding was soon confirmed (19), and later 2-methoxyestrone was isolated from human pregnancy urine (36). More recently 2-methoxyestriol (XI) (22) and 2-methoxyestradiol (XII) (24) were isolated.

The last compound which has been added to this list is equilenin (XIII), a naphtholic steroid which had been known for many years as an important urinary metabolite in the pregnant mare (26), but which had, prior to its isolation from an adrenal cortical carcinoma (49), not been thought to be of interest in human physiology.

## METABOLIC INTERRELATIONS

The technical advances which led to the isolation of these substances have also made it possible to perform experiments designed to uncover the metabolic relations between them. The administration of suspected precursors, either isotopically labeled or unlabeled, and the identification of transformation products in the urine have provided a first approximation. More definitive information on individual reactions and the enzymes and cofactors involved may be derived from experiments with isolated tissues and more refined systems.

The ready interconversion of estrone and estradiol by human liver and other tissues has been demonstrated (46), and in recent years it has been possible to isolate from human placenta soluble enzymes requiring diphosphopyridine nucleotide and triphosphopyridine nucleotide, which effect interconversion of estrone and estradiol (31). As a result of studies on the metabolism of estradiol (II) by human fetal liver and adult human liver, the conversion of estradiol to estriol (III) (21) and to epiestriol (IV) (20a) has also been demonstrated. It is likely that estrone (II) plays the role of an intermediate and is hydroxylated at carbon 16 in either the α- or the β-configuration to give the two α-ketols (V and VI) which have been isolated from urine (Fig. 4). These ketols could then be reduced to the epimeric triols (III and IV). This pathway was suggested by Brown and Marrian (10, 41), who showed that administered 16α-hydroxyestrone was recovered in the urine largely as estriol. On the basis of double-labeling experiments, Fishman et al. (23) also concluded that estrone rather than estradiol was a more direct precursor of estriol. Evidence for the occurrence in placental extracts of enzymes capable of carrying out the reduction of 16α-hydroxyestrone has recently been presented by Ryan (48). The *in vivo* formation of 16-ketoestradiol from estradiol (33) and the conversion of administered estrone to 16-ketoestrone (52) have been demonstrated, but the detailed mechanisms are not known.

No solid experimental data exist as yet for the mechanism of formation of the methoxy derivatives of estrone, estradiol, and estriol, but by analogy with other hydroxylating enzymes (reviewed in 44), it may be presumed that an aromatic hydroxylase which requires molecular oxygen and reduced triphosphopyridine nucleotide (TPNH) serves to introduce the hydroxyl group at carbon 2. The formation of the methyl ether could occur through the action of a catechol *O*-methyl transferase which transfers the methyl group of *S*-adenosylmethionine. Such a mechanism has been demonstrated for the methylation of epinephrine metabolites (2).

Evidence has been obtained from incubation experiments that 18-hydroxyestrone may be formed in the adrenal gland (38), and it may be presumed that a specific steroid hydroxylase is involved.

The position of equilenin in this series is not understood, and indeed it has been suggested on the basis of experiments in a pregnant mare (27) that the naphtholic estrogens are formed by a route independent of that generally accepted for the phenolic estrogens in the same species (51).

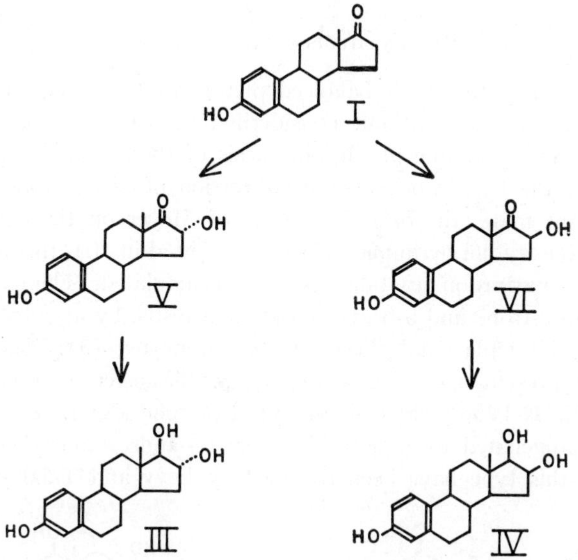

FIG. 4.   Postulated pathways for the formation of estriol (III) and epiestriol (IV).

In assessing the significance of this complex array of metabolites, a number of questions present themselves. Of primary importance is the question whether these substances constitute metabolic degradation products having little intrinsic interest save as a measure of the amount of the primary secretory product formed or whether they have specific physiologic functions. In this connection it should be noted that all the compounds described, except for estrone, estradiol, and estriol, have extremely low estrogenic potency. The observations of Hisaw and his associates on the antagonism between estradiol and estriol in their action upon the rat uterus* indicate that these substances have qualitatively different actions and perhaps specific physiologic functions. Recently Kappas et al. (28) have found that etiocholanolone, a metabolite of testosterone, which had long been regarded as biologically inactive, had a remarkable pyrogenic activity, a

---

* Reviewed in Velardo (53).

phenomenon apparently unrelated to the androgenic activity of its precursor. One must therefore consider the possibility that each of the estradiol metabolites described above may have its own specific biologic action which is unrelated to, and cannot be inferred from, the biologic activity of the precursor substance. Here indeed is a new area for investigation and one in which the fortunate accident may play a role as important as that of the deliberately designed experiment.

## BIOSYNTHESIS OF ESTROGENS

It is not possible to give a balanced picture of the recent work on the metabolism of estrogens without considering, at least briefly, the current status of our understanding of the biogenesis of these hormones. Since the publication of the basic work on the conversion of testosterone to estrone in the pregnant mare, the *in vitro* studies of Meyer on the conversion of testosterone to estradiol by human ovaries (reviewed in 20), further information on the aromatization reaction has been accumulated. The conversion of testosterone to estrone and estradiol by stallion testis, by an adrenal cortical carcinoma, and by placental slices has been reported (3). The pathways postulated at present are outlined in Fig. 5. Testosterone (XIV) is first hydroxylated at C-19 to yield 19-hydroxytestosterone (XV). This compound can be dehydrogenated to 17β,19-dihydroxy-1,4-androstadien-3-one (XVI). Reactions of this type have been reported by Levy and Talalay (34, 35).

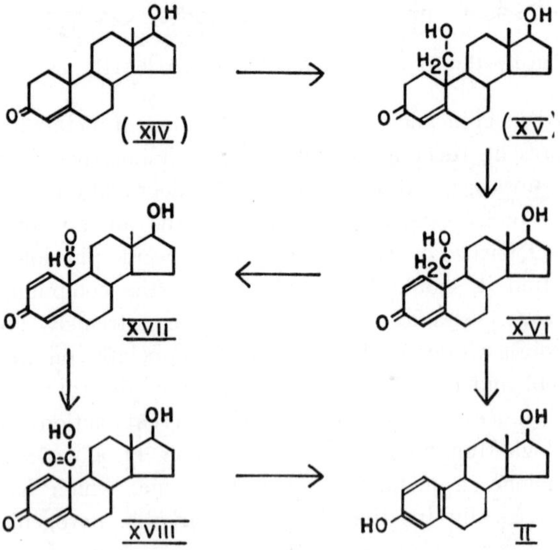

FIG. 5.　Postulated pathways for the aromatization of testosterone (XIV).

Estradiol (II) can then be formed by loss of formaldehyde in a reverse aldol condensation or by successive dehydrogenation to the aldehyde (XVII) and the carboxylic acid (XVIII), which can then be decarboxylated to estradiol. More recently, Ryan (47) has shown that in placental tissue effective conversion of testosterone and androstenedione to estradiol and estrone, respectively, can be achieved with the microsomal fraction fortified with reduced triphosphopyridine nucleotide. In pursuing this work further (48), he made the additional important discovery of an alternative route for the formation of estriol (Fig. 6). He found that 5-androstene-3β,16α,17β-triol was converted in good yield by placental microsomes and TPNH to estriol, that 16α-hydroxytestosterone was converted to 16α-hydroxyestrone,

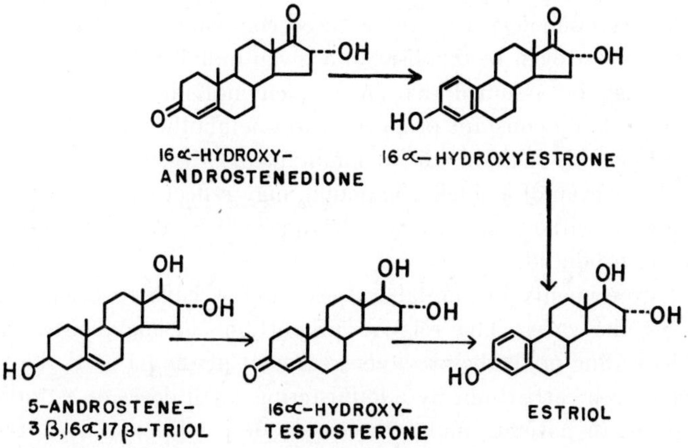

16α-HYDROXY-ANDROSTENEDIONE

16α-HYDROXYESTRONE

5-ANDROSTENE-3β,16α,17β-TRIOL

16α-HYDROXY-TESTOSTERONE

ESTRIOL

Fig. 6. Alternative mechanism for the formation of estriol according to Ryan (48).[4]

and that the last-mentioned compound was readily reduced to estriol. Thus a second mechanism, for the formation not only of estriol, but also of the ring D ketols, is possible. The relative importance of these two mechanisms remains to be determined.

The formation of estrogens from testosterone does not require the presence of either gonads or adrenal cortex. The experiments of West et al. (54) have demonstrated this conversion in castrate adrenalectomized cancer patients. The extent of the transformation is quite small and its physiologic significance unknown.

## DISCUSSION

As a consequence of the increased complexity of the pattern of estrogen metabolism, the task of the analyst who is asked to provide some measure

[4] The author wishes to thank Dr. Ryan and the *Journal of Biological Chemistry* for permission to reproduce this figure.

of estrogen production by an examination of blood and urine has been rendered much more difficult. At the outset, it must be stated that there is no analytical method available at the present time which will accomplish the desired objective of measuring all the known urinary metabolites in the concentrations in which they are present in the normal male, the normal premenopausal and postmenopausal woman, or even in pregnancy. The two methods which are generally regarded as being the most satisfactory at the present time are those of Brown (8, 9) and of Bauld (4). The method of Brown in particular has been subjected to a most rigorous scrutiny, including careful checking by isotope dilution methods (25), and may be expected to yield results of a high order of reliability. However, only estrone, estradiol, and estriol are measured by this method. It is legitimate to inquire to what extent the excretion levels of these three compounds are representative of the pattern of estrogen metabolism in a given individual. As a first approximation, it may be assumed that in a given individual the metabolites are excreted in roughly constant proportion to one another and that in a steady state situation, this relation will be maintained. Measurement of one or two compounds, or even of a single compound, may reflect the level of production of the hormone without giving any quantitative information as to the amount of hormones produced.

Recent experiments in our laboratories (11a) have revealed that this is not always the case. The relative proportions of metabolites may vary widely, depending upon the previous treatment of the patient. These experiments have been carried out by administering small doses of estradiol-$16$-$C^{14}$ intravenously to patients under three sets of conditions: first, the control state; second, after previous administration of relatively large doses of unlabeled estradiol; and third, after the administration of an antibiotic which sterilizes the gastrointestinal tract. Urine from these patients is collected in 8-hour periods for 24–48 hours after the administration of the radioactive hormone. The urinary conjugates are hydrolyzed with $\beta$-glucuronidase, and a lipid extract is prepared. From this crude extract a phenolic fraction is isolated and individual metabolites are separated on a gradient elution partition chromatogram based upon the systems of Aitken and Preedy (1). With these chromatographic columns, it is possible to separate and measure quantitatively by radioactivity five compounds: 2-methoxyestrone, estrone, estradiol, epiestriol, and estriol.

The results of the experiments are presented in Figs. 7 and 8. In the case of the patient who was given a test dose of radioactive estradiol after a course of pretreatment with estradiol benzoate, significant changes in the rates of excretion of several metabolites have been noted (Fig. 7). Although the rates for methoxyestrone and estradiol did not change significantly, the rate of excretion of estrone was slightly higher and that of epiestriol distinctly higher than in the control state. The most dramatic effect, however, was upon the rate of excretion of estriol. These results suggest that under conditions of pretreatment with the hormone, an adaptive change had occurred in the individual which lead to a more rapid and effective disposal of the estradiol load.

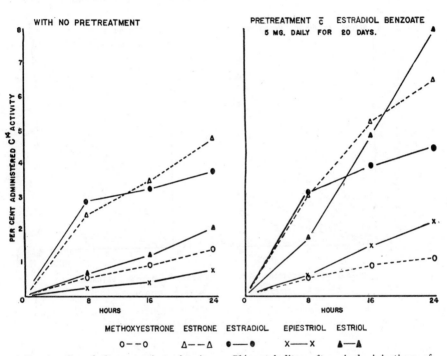

Fig. 7. Cumulative excretion of urinary $C^{14}$-metabolites after single injections of 200 μg. of estradiol-$16$-$C^{14}$ in the control state (left) and after 20 days' pretreatment with a daily dose of 5 mg. of estradiol benzoate.

The situation with regard to the patient pretreated with an intestinal antibiotic (Neomycin) was quite different. In this instance the effect was a general decrease in the rate of excretion of all the metabolites measured (Fig. 8).

These experiments bring to the fore an aspect of estrogen metabolism which is not usually considered within the framework of studies on urinary excretion. This is, of course, the enterohepatic circulation, in which estrogens are involved to a significantly greater extent than the other steroid hormones.

The enterohepatic circulation of estrogens has been known for many years and has most recently been studied by Sandberg and Slaunwhite (50), who showed that when estradiol-$C^{14}$ was injected intravenously approximately half of the radioactivity appeared in the bile. Since only about 7 % of the injected dose appears in the feces, most of the biliary radioactivity must be resorbed. The results of the experiment with Neomycin are thus subject to one of two possible explanations. The decreased urinary excretion of radio-activity during the first 32 hours after administration of estradiol may be the

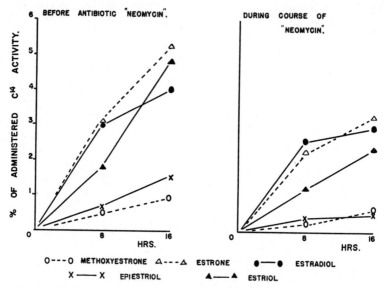

FIG. 8. Cumulative excretion of urinary $C^{14}$-metabolites before (left) and after (right) treatment of a patient with Neomycin. The patient had been pretreated with estradiol benzoate.

result of increased fecal excretion or of diminished resorption of the radio-activity, which would lead to its being excreted over a longer period of time than in the normal subject. For present purposes the explanation is not important, since these experiments are cited merely to indicate some of the factors that may play a role in the metabolism of estrogens and may influence the outcome of experiments in which urinary excretion alone is measured.

In considering the metabolism of estrogens in relation to the problem of breast cancer, certain very difficult questions are always asked and are usually either evaded completely or answered in a most unsatisfactory manner. I shall not depart from the usual pattern. The first question is: Are there sources of estrogens other than the gonads and the adrenal cortex?

This question arises as a consequence of finding material in the urine of gonadectomized and adrenalectomized individuals which gives a positive Kober reaction, the color test employed as the final step in the Brown procedure. These Kober chromogens are present, usually, in extremely low concentrations which preclude their identification as bona fide estrogens by any procedure available at the present time. In some patients residual adrenal tissue may be present, but it is hard to see how it could be responsible for the production of an amount of estrogen compatible with the presumed urinary level in the face of the doses of cortisone or similar compounds required to maintain these patients. This amount of cortisone would certainly be expected to reduce pituitary ACTH secretion to a low level, and thus reduce function of the residual adrenal tissue.

The conversion of cortisone or other corticosteroids used for maintenance of adrenalectomized patients to estrogen has been suggested, but no convincing evidence for such a transformation has yet been produced.

When biological assay of urinary extracts is employed for the detection of estrogens, exogenous sources of estrogen must be considered. The widespread use of diethylstilbestrol and other synthetic estrogens for fattening steers and for caponizing fowl introduces the hazard of contamination of foodstuffs with estrogenic material. The occurrence of plant estrogens (5), either in the native state or as a result of fermentations of plant material, is also well known. Experiments to exclude these possible sources of estrogen must be very carefully controlled. In addition, interactions between estrogens present in mixtures may give false results (53). The effects of inhibitors and synergists are also possible sources of error.

In considering possible relations between estrogen metabolism and the development, maintenance, and inhibition of mammary cancer (reviewed in 45), a great deal of attention has been given to the aspect of the problem which relates to the effect of the tumor-host complex upon the hormone. Many attempts have been made to detect differences in excretion levels of endogenous estrogens by normal postmenopausal women and women with breast cancer, by women with breast cancer who respond to hormonal alteration and those who do not. Similarly, the disposal of test doses of estrogens by patients in the above categories has been studied. In no cases have any useful differences been detected.

Attempts to detect differences in metabolism of estrogens by normal and cancerous breast tissue have been less extensive. The difficulties of interpreting data obtained from morphologically heterogeneous material are readily appreciated. Nevertheless this area should be explored more extensively. Breuer and Nocke (6) have attempted to correlate the ability of various normal and malignant tissues to metabolize estrogens with the level of oxidative metabolism as measured by $Q_{O_2}$ but the tissues varied so much that no clear conclusions could be drawn.

Another aspect of the problem is the action of the estrogens upon the various tissues. This phase is now undergoing rapid expansion as a consequence of the development of methods and systems for the study of hormone action at the molecular level.

### SUMMARY

Recent developments in our knowledge of estrogen metabolism have been described. The discovery of new urinary metabolites of estradiol and of new biosynthetic pathways has been discussed. Some implications of these findings for the cancer problem have been considered.

### REFERENCES

1. Aitken, E. H., and Preedy, J. R. K. *Biochem. J.* **62**, 15P (1956).
2. Axelrod, J., and Tomchick, R. *J. Biol. Chem.* **233**, 702 (1958).
3. Baggett, B., Engel, L. L., Balderas, L., Lanman, G., Savard, K., and Dorfman, R. I. *Endocrinology* **64**, 600 (1959).
4. Bauld, W. S. *Biochem. J.* **63**, 488 (1956).
5. Bradbury, R. B., and White, D. E. *Vitamins and Hormones* **12**, 207 (1954).
6. Breuer, H., and Nocke, L. *Acta Endocrinol.* **31**, 69 (1959).
7. Brown, B. T., Fishman, J., and Gallagher, T. F. *Nature* **182**, 50 (1958).
8. Brown, J. B. *Biochem. J.* **60**, 185 (1955).
9. Brown, J. B., Bulbrook, R. D., and Greenwood, F. C. *J. Endocrinol.* **16**, 49 (1957).
10. Brown, J. B., and Marrian, G. F. *J. Endocrinol.* **15**, 307 (1957).
11. Butenandt, A. *Naturwissenschaften* **17**, 879 (1929).
11a. Cameron, C. B., Trofimow, N., and Engel, L. L. Unpublished data.
12. Dingemanse, E., De Jongh, S. E., Kober, S., and Laqueur, E. *Deut. med. Wochschr.* **56**, 301 (1930).
13. Dodds, E. C. "Biochemical Contributions to Endocrinology." Stanford Univ. Press, Stanford, California, 1957.
14. Dodds, E. C., Golberg, L., Lawson, W., and Robinson, R. *Nature* **141**, 247 (1938).
15. Dodds, E. C., Campbell, N. R., and Lawson, W. *Nature* **141**, 78 (1938).
16. Dodds, E. C., Golberg, L., Lawson, W., and Robinson, R. *Nature* **142**, 34 (1938).
17. Doisy, E. A., Veler, C. D., and Thayer, S. *Am. J. Physiol.* **90**, 329 (1929).
18. Doisy, E. A., Thayer, S. A., Levin, L., and Curtis, J. M. *Proc. Soc. Exptl. Biol. Med.* **28**, 88 (1930).
19. Engel, L. L., Baggett, B., and Carter, P. *Endocrinology* **61**, 112 (1957).
20. Engel, L. L. *Cancer* **10**, 711 (1957).
20a. Engel, L. L., Baggett, B., and Halla, M. Unpublished data.
21. Engel, L. L., Baggett, B., and Halla, M. *Biochim. et Biophys. Acta* **30**, 435 (1958).
22. Fishman, J., and Gallagher, T. F. *Arch. Biochem. Biophys.* **77**, 511 (1958).
23. Fishman, J., Bradlow, H. L., and Gallagher, T. F. *J. Am. Chem. Soc.* **81**, 2273 (1959).
24. Frandsen, V. A. *Acta Endocrinol.* **31**, 603 (1959).
25. Gallagher, T. F., Kraychy, S., Fishman, J., Brown, J. B., and Marrian, G. F. *J. Biol. Chem.* **233**, 1093 (1958).

26. Girard, A., Sandulesco, G., Fridenson, A., Gaudefroy, C., and Rutgers, J. J. *Compt. rend. acad. sci.* **194**, 1020 (1932).

27. Heard, R. D. H., Jacobs, R., O'Donnell, V., Peron, F., Saffran, J. C., Solomon, S. S., Thompson, L. M., Willoughby, H., and Yates, C. H. *Recent Progr. Hormone Research* **9**, 383 (1954).

28. Kappas, A., Hellman, L., Fukushima, D. K., and Gallagher, T. F. *J. Clin. Endocrinol. and Metabolism* **18**, 1043 (1958).

29. Kraychy, S., and Gallagher, T. F. *J. Am. Chem. Soc.* **79**, 754 (1957).

30. Kraychy, S., and Gallagher, T. F. *J. Biol. Chem.* **229**, 519 (1957).

31. Langer, L. J., and Engel, L. L. *J. Biol. Chem.* **233**, 583 (1958).

32. Layne, D. S., and Marrian, G. F. *Biochem. J.* **70**, 244 (1958).

33. Levitz, M., Spitzer, J. R., and Twombley, G. H. *J. Biol. Chem.* **222**, 981 (1956).

34. Levy, H. R., and Talalay, P. *J. Biol. Chem.* **234**, 2009 (1959).

35. Levy, H. R., and Talalay, P. *J. Biol. Chem.* **234**, 2014 (1959).

36. Loke, K. H., and Marrian, G. F. *Biochim. et Biophys. Acta* **27**, 213 (1958).

37. Loke, K. H., Watson, E. J. D., and Marrian, G. F. *Biochim. et Biophys. Acta* **26**, 230 (1957).

38. Loke, K. H., Marrian, G. F., and Watson, E. J. D. *Biochem. J.* **71**, 43 (1959).

39. MacCorquodale, D. W., Thayer, S. A., and Doisy, E. A. *J. Biol. Chem.* **115**, 435 (1936).

40. Marrian, G. F. *Biochem. J.* **24**, 435 (1930).

41. Marrian, G. F. *Cancer* **10**, 704 (1957).

42. Marrian, G. F., and Bauld, W. S. *Biochem. J.* **59**, 136 (1955).

43. Marrian, G. F., Loke, K. H., Watson, E. J. D., and Panattoni, M. *Biochem. J.* **66**, 60 (1957).

44. Massart, L., and Vercauten, R. *Ann. Rev. Biochem.* **28**, 527 (1959).

45. Nathanson, I. T., and Kelley, R. M. *New Engl. J. Med.* **246**, 135, 180 (1952).

46. Ryan, K. J., and Engel, L. L. *Endocrinology* **52**, 287 (1953).

47. Ryan, K. J. *J. Biol. Chem.* **234**, 268 (1959).

48. Ryan, K. J. *J. Biol. Chem.* **234**, 2006 (1959).

49. Salhanick, H. A., and Berliner, D. L. *J. Biol. Chem.* **227**, 583 (1957).

50. Sandberg, A. A., and Slaunwhite, W. R., Jr. *J. Clin. Invest.* **36**, 1266 (1957).

51. Savard, K., Andrec, K., Brooksbank, B. W. L., Reyneri, C., Dorfman, R. I., Heard, R. D. H., Jacobs, R., and Solomon, S. S. *J. Biol. Chem.* **231**, 765 (1958).

52. Slaunwhite, W. R., Jr., and Sandberg, A. A. *Arch. Biochem. Biophys.* **63**, 478 (1956).

53. Velardo, J. T. *Ann. N. Y. Acad. Sci.* **75**, 441 (1959).

54. West, C. D., Damast, B. L., Sarro, S. D., and Pearson, O. H. *J. Biol. Chem.* **218**, 409 (1956).

## DISCUSSION

**M. J. Finkelstein:** I should like to make a few comments on Dr. Engel's excellent paper. To the best of my knowledge estrogens, including the "classical" estrogens which Dr. Engel showed on the screen, were never isolated from urine of normal women, outside pregnancy, unless natural estrogens had previously been injected. Actually, as Dr. Engel pointed out, nobody knows exactly the estrogenic content of the urine. All we know of estrogens in normal women is through indication, never isolation. The best chemical methods available operate on the sensitivity level which is below the expected normal estrogen excretion. So the problem is really very difficult.

During recent years we elaborated a method which may in part help those who want to analyze urinary estrogens in normal conditions. We came to our fluorometrical method in trying to identify the urinary estrogens, because this method is much more sensitive than one can expect any colorimetric method to be. But, as pointed out in our various publications, there are many problems involved in applying fluorometry to urinary assay. The main problem was how to purify the urinary extracts to obtain fractions that would be clean enough not to interfere with estrogenic substances of urine. And I think that we succeeded in part in elaborating a method which can estimate very low quantities of the estrogens in urine. For example, if to a 24-hour sample of urine, 1 μg. of any of the three "classical" estrogens is added it may be recovered at about 80 % yield, or more; but that of course does not say anything about the endogenous estrogen. Our method involves partition between solvents and separation of the individual estrogens by paper chromatography. The separated estrogens are estimated by means of fluorometry.

Since in the fluorometric procedure about 0.01 μg. can be accurately estimated we need for the estimation of the urinary estrogens only about one-fiftieth of a 24-hour urine specimen period. To make sure that the actual estrogens are being estimated, we have tried to identify the products obtained through paper chromatography by comparing their fluorescence spectrum, recorded with an automatic spectrofluorometer, with the authentic respective estrogens. We started to work on extracts of urine obtained from late pregnancy and had no difficulty in obtaining fluorometrically pure estrogens. Then we went to early pregnancy, 2 weeks after the first missed menstruation. Here too, estrone, estradiol, and estriol could be isolated in pure form. Then we went to normal urine, and we could obtain fractions that were almost spectrofluorometrically pure, but quantitatively we found that the content of estradiol was much less than 1 μg. in 24 hours. Estrone was also excreted at the level of about 1 μg. or less. We could not until now obtain fractions which would show pure estriol. To show the difficulty, I would like to point out one case. We tried a urine from a pseudohermaphrodite with congenital adrenal hyperplasia in which, on the basis of bioassays and of the original fluorometric method, we suspected high concentrations of all three estrogens, even more than in early pregnancy. We were unable by this method to show the presence of any of the "classical" estrogens in this urine. Instead we obtained material which showed entirely different fluorescence spectra. So it seems to us that the method may be used for the estimation of estrone, estradiol, and perhaps of estriol in normal cases. In addition it may be used for the detection of unknown urinary compounds showing the fluorescence reaction and occurring in normal and pathological urines. I am fully aware that our method does not solve all the problems of estimation of urinary estrogens referred to by Dr. Engel. I would not recommend using it for routine procedure.

**S. Kushinsky:** I should like to ask Dr. Engel several questions. The first is whether the example given, where the subject was under estrogen therapy and the estriol was elevated compared with the "base-line" study, is representative of other cases which you studied. Also, I wonder if you have expressed the data in terms of not only the cumulative excretion of these various metabolites, but also in terms of that amount of radioactivity excreted on a particular day and in terms of the fraction hydrolyzed to see whether different correlations may be possible. Presumably you did not obtain a constant amount of enzymatic hydrolysis, nor did you find the over-all rate of excretion to be constant—or did you? Certainly each of these factors would influence your results. And finally, what quantity of Neomycin was used in your antibiotic studies?

**L. Engel:** The answer to the first question is: Yes, we did try various ways of calculating these data; but it seemed that expressing them in terms of the cumulative excretion showed the relations between the metabolites and the differences in the behavior of the metabolites most clearly. These extracts were all prepared after hydrolysis with bacterial β-*glucuronidase,* which is extraordinarily effective in cleaving the estrogen glucosiduronates. In a number of instances we tried the solvolytic procedure after glucuronidase, but this usually afforded us only a very small increase in the amount of radioactivity converted to a lipid-soluble form. The recovery of radioactivity after glucuronidase did vary from individual to individual but was rather constant within a given individual and varied from about 60 % to 80 % of the total radioactivity. I am afraid I do not happen to have at my finger tips the answer to your question about the dose of Neomycin.

**F. C. Greenwood:** I'd like to thank Dr. Engel for his balanced review of the problem of the nature and source of estrogens after adrenalectomy. I would like to comment on some of the points he has raised.

First, we consider that the cortisone administered after operation is essentially a maintenance dose and is not designed to inhibit pituitary or adrenal function. It is possible that residual or accessory adrenal tissue could secrete estrogens even under long-term maintenance doses. We interpreted Lemmon's work on the break-through of estrogen secretion, after initial suppression by cortisone, to indicate that the pituitary and adrenal can adjust to the administered cortisone.

Second, as regards exogenous estrogen as a source of the urinary estrogens we have estimated: We have never had the courage to extract hospital diet for estrogen, but indirect evidence suggests that this is not a source. We got an association between the presence of biologically active estrogen and etiocholanolone in the urine of some patients after adrenalectomy. We took this as evidence for secretory residual or accessory adrenal tissue in these patients rather than steroid contamination of some hospital diets.

Third, if one finds estrogens and/or etiocholanolone in some urines after hypophysectomy, the results seem more acceptable to the steroid field than the same situation after adrenalectomy. Classically, pituitary removal is followed by adrenal and ovarian atrophy and presumably steroid secretion should be abolished. We interpreted our findings of steroid excretion after this operation as evidence for incomplete removal or accessory tissue when we attempted to correlate the steroid findings with the clinical course of the disease.

Finally, if I may quote Dr. Pincus—"so what?" This was a clinical hormonal research problem in cancer. Are the amounts detected of any clinical significance in the failure of some patients to benefit from adrenalectomy? After four years in this area we came to the conclusion that there wasn't a simple correlation between the clinical and hormonal events.

**S. Lieberman:** I should like to comment upon the explanation Dr. Engel gave of the results of one of his experiments. I refer to that experiment in which the pattern of urinary estrogen metabolites found in an untreated woman was compared with that existing after treatment with exogenous estradiol benzoate. The amount of excreted estriol, relative to four other estrogen metabolites, rose about fivefold after estrogen treatment. One explanation offered by Dr. Engel for this finding was that the catabolic mechanism had been altered by some adaptive process due to exposure to above-normal amounts of estradiol. Implied in this explanation is that alterations in the concentration of the enzymes responsible for the conversion of estradiol to estriol had occurred as a result of the experimental procedure and that these alterations led to an increased secretion of estriol.

This is an important point because similar explanations have been given in the literature to account for an observed difference in the ratio of two or more urinary metabolites caused by some abnormal situation (e.g., disease, stress). Such an explanation may indeed be true; but there is another, which I believe to be more likely, especially when elevated amounts of the hormonal precursor are present. It is true, however, that this alternative explanation is less glamorous.

Suppose precursor $A$ gives rise, on one hand, to metabolite $B$ and, on the other, to metabolite $C$ through the intervention of the enzymes, $b$ and $c$. By means of some experimental procedure, the ratio of $B:C$ is altered. Instead of accounting for this alteration by assuming a change in the concentrations of $b$ or $c$, it can probably be explained as a result of the variation in the concentration of the substrate (precursor $A$). The velocity of enzyme reactions is also dependent upon substrate concentrations, and it is conceivable that variations in this parameter alone could produce the observed change in B:C (Fig. A).

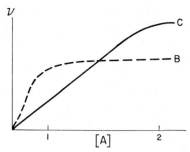

Fig. A. Two possible curves which describe the rate of formation of metabolite $B$ from precursor $A$ (dashed line) and of metabolite $C$ from precursor $A$ (solid line). It is obvious that the ratio of $B:C$ at concentration $1$ is very different than it is at concentration $2$, even though there has been no change in the concentrations of the enzymes.

**L. Engel:** This is an interesting speculation, but we cannot really test its validity or the validity of the explanation I offered by this type of *in vivo* experiment.

**G. Pincus:** One objective of this meeting is to see whether there is any relationship between steroids and cancer. Dr. Huggins spoke of estrogen-dependent tumors and estrogen-independent tumors; and if we are going to apply his logic to human breast cancer there should be evidence of estrogen dependence and estrogen independence. It seems to me that if there are active estrogens circulating in women with dependent tumors or if estrogens are absent, the tumor should go up or down correspondingly. So far as I know, Dr. Greenwood is the only one who has given evidence on this point. Do you have any?

**F. C. Greenwood:** I was more pessimistic than the results warrant, mainly because I have recently left this field to try to parallel our previous studies by measuring protein rather than steroid hormones. My colleague, Dr. Bulbrook, is to extend the work in the steroid-clinical area. I shall try to summarize the work we carried out before we went our separate ways.

We have determined the effect of endocrine ablation for breast cancer on the classic urinary estrogens and tried to correlate the changes with the clinical course of the disease. In prostatic cancer we studied estrogen, ketosteroid, and ketogenic steroid changes through castration or stilbestrol treatment. In all we had 91 incidents where the simple hypothesis of hormone dependence could be tested because we had both the clinical and hormonal effects of treatment. This is a crude test but better than a study of regression rates in which the effect on hormone levels is inferred, not measured. In the total of 91 incidents, 65 were in accord with the simple hypothesis of the dependence of breast and prostatic cancer on steroid hormones; the remainder could not be explained on this basis. We feel that this affords direct evidence that treatment based upon the hypothesis is rational and that the clinical effects could be due to the alteration in steroid levels on treatment.

Finally, we have estimated an array of urinary hormones in, so far, 40 patients *before* adrenalectomy or hypophysectomy and tried to correlate preoperative levels with the subsequent clinical effect. Estrogen, pregnanediol, and gonadotropin levels did not correlate.

There was a significant correlation between success and a high preoperative etiocholanolone level and a suggestion that a high 17-hydroxycorticoid level was associated with subsequent failure. We are continuing this series to see whether these statistical differences could become clinically useful in prognosing for adrenalectomy and hypophysectomy.

**J. T. Velardo:** Dr. Greenwood made the statement that the pituitary gland adjusts to the dose of cortisone. I was wondering how he came to this conclusion and about the quantitative aspects of his conclusion.

**F. C. Greenwood:** I should not have sounded so dogmatic—it was an opinion, not a statement. We considered the cortisone administered to be a maintenance dose and not designed to inhibit the pituitary. Adjustment to long-term steroid therapy by the endocrine system is a general finding, and we have extrapolated this to a particular situation. I did cite Lemmon's work in support and could add the escape from cortisone therapy in adrenal hyperplasia and resistance to the anabolic effects of testosterone.

**P. Troen:** Dr. Greenwood has referred to the possible importance of the influence of protein hormones on breast tissue as well as the influence of steroid hormones on this tissue. I should like to add a third aspect, namely, the effect of protein hormones on the metabolism of steroid hormones with the possibly different net result on the part of sensitive tissue. For example, we have recently shown that estradiol-17$\beta$ can be converted to estriol by human placental tissue, but apparently only when human chorionic gonadotropin is added to the perfusing medium. Further, using the perfused human placenta [Troen, P., and Gordon, E. E. *J. Clin. Invest.* **37**, 1516 (1958)], we have obtained an increased rate of citrate utilization only with the addition of estradiol and human chorionic gonadotropin together, and not from the addition of estradiol alone as might be expected from other studies with more purified placental preparations.

# Biochemical Parameters of Estrogen Action[1, 2]

GERALD C. MUELLER[3]

*McArdle Memorial Laboratory, University of Wisconsin, Medical School,
Madison, Wisconsin*

It is the goal of studies on the mechanism of action of estrogens, as well
as other hormones, to describe in molecular terms *both* the primary interaction of the hormone with the specific acceptor of the target cell and the
ensuing chain of biochemical alterations which account for the physiological
response of the intact tissue. In view of the range and complexity of the
problem, it is not surprising that studies on the mechanism of estrogen
action have attacked the problem from both ends. In the first instance some
investigators have attempted to pursue the hormone itself: to trace the
metabolism of the estrogen and the interaction of the molecule with constituents of cell-free biochemical systems. This has been done in the hope
of uncovering the specific molecular reaction responsible for the primary or
triggering effect of the hormone. Although many interesting biochemical
observations have been made in such enzyme preparations (4, 7, 9, 12, 17,
18, 19), their significance with respect to the physiological action of the
hormone remains to be demonstrated in all cases. A major barrier to their
evaluation has been a lack of exact information as to the molecular processes
which are altered in the response of the tissue to the hormone.

It is the purpose of this paper to present studies, attacking the problem
from the other end, directed at the biochemical dissection of the early
changes in the estrogen-stimulated rat uterus. Starting with the earliest
compositional changes, attempts have been made to elucidate the sequence
of metabolic alterations underlying the tissue response. The studies have
been particularly concerned with tracing these events back to their origin,
the primary action of the hormone. Though the latter destination has not
been achieved, it is hoped that the findings en route will help provide biochemical parameters by which the mechanism of action of estrogens will
ultimately be recognized and understood.

--------

[1] Experimental work reported in this presentation has been supported by a grant
from Alexander and Margaret Stewart Trust Fund; Grant No. 1897 from the United
States Public Health Service; and an Institutional Grant from the American Cancer
Society.

[2] In making this presentation the author wishes gratefully to acknowledge the spirited
collaboration of past and present associates; he is particularly indebted to Drs. Ailene
Herranen, Kristian Jervell, Yoshio Aizawa, and Jack Gorski.

[3] Lasker Professor of Cancer Research.

## GENERAL PROCEDURE

In the studies to be presented, evidence of early alterations of various areas of uterine metabolism by estrogenic hormones will be described. The data are largely derived from experiments with isotopic precursors designed to show the magnitude and sequence of changes in certain metabolic pathways with respect to time and degree of estrogen treatment. Routinely, ovariectomized rats (same age, weight, and time post ovariectomy) have been injected with a single dose of estradiol via the tail vein. The hormone is dissolved in buffered saline (13). After varying periods the rats are sacrificed and the uterine horns removed for *in vitro* experimentation. For metabolic studies with intact tissue, the uterine horns are opened longitudinally and cut into small equal segments. These segments are incubated at 37° C. in a medium containing the specific radioactive precursor for the metabolic pathway under study. In earlier studies the medium has been a glucose-balanced salt solution with an oxygen atmosphere (13). In later experiments, Eagle's tissue culture medium (3) and a 5 % $CO_2$ in oxygen atmosphere have been used with significantly better results. After the indicated incubation period, the enzymatic processes are stopped with acid and the tissue is separated into the following fractions: acid soluble, lipid, nucleic acid, and protein (14). Specific isolations are carried out where indicated.

In a number of studies enzymatic analyses have been carried out on estrogen-treated tissues; in such cases the segments have been homogenized either in isotonic sucrose or hypotonic (0.05 $M$) KCL solution, as indicated.

### EARLY CHANGES IN UTERINE COMPOSITION IN RESPONSE TO ESTROGENS

In response to a single physiological dose of a natural estrogen, the atrophic uterus of an ovariectomized female rat is rapidly converted to an actively growing organ. Histologically the first evidence of estrogen action is a generalized hyperemia of the tissue as early as 1 hour after the administration of the hormone (11). This is followed by an intracellular imbibition of water and salts which reaches a maximum within 4–6 hours (2, 16). After 12 hours the dry weight of the uterus begins to accumulate in reflection of the anabolic processes which have been mobilized by the hormone (16).

To characterize the nature of the anabolic response further, the composition of uteri after varying periods of estrogen treatment has been determined. Changes in the phospholipid, ribonucleic acid (RNA), protein, and deoxyribonucleic acid (DNA) were plotted in Fig. 1 as per cent deviation from the control level. All data were calculated per unit of DNA to reflect the average change per cell. The most rapid alteration in composition so far observed took place in the phospholipid fraction. Coincident with the water imbibition during the first few hours, gross increases in the phospholipid content occurred. Although the chart illustrates only the relative level of ethanolamine phospholipids, it has been demonstrated that corresponding and coincident increases also occurred with the choline- and inositol-containing phospholipids (1). Analysis of tissues after longer times of estrogen

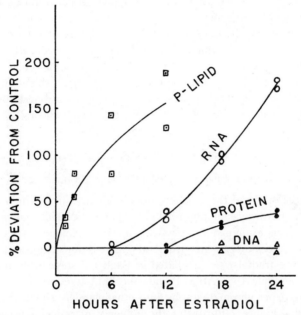

FIG. 1. Alterations in uterine composition following a single dose of estradiol. Ten micrograms estradiol was injected at zero time. DNA was measured in micromoles of thymine per uterus; RNA was measured as micromoles of uridine and calculated as the ratio of uridine to thymine. The phospholipid was measured as micromoles of ethanolamine phosphate. For purposes of comparison all data are expressed as per cent deviation from the control during the first 24 hours after hormone treatment.

treatment show that a peak level of phospholipid was reached by 12 hours and that the level remained the same or declined slightly during the ensuing 12 hours.

The next gross change in composition involved the average RNA content of the uterine cell. It is of interest that the RNA remained at the control level for the first 6 hours and then accumulated rapidly over the rest of the 24-hour period (8). In connection with current concepts in which RNA is considered to play the role of a template in protein synthesis, it is of interest that the RNA accumulation occurred prior to gross changes in average protein content per uterine cell. Figure 1 also illustrates the fact that no significant DNA synthesis per uterus takes place in the first 24 hours. Other experiments have demonstrated that DNA increases (per uterus) were measurable only after 40 hours of estrogen treatment. Thus we see that the early estrogen-induced changes in rat uterine composition are those of an initial hypertrophy rather than hyperplasia; it is possible that they reflect a restoration of those entities which are disproportionately depleted during the uterine atrophy following ovariectomy.

It should, however, be obvious that any description of estrogen action in molecular terms must account ultimately for the observed early changes in uterine composition. Conversely, it is evident that any molecular description of the events underlying these changes in composition should provide not only an understanding of what constitutes an estrogen response, but also the biochemical parameters for identifying or recognizing the initial triggering action of the hormone.

EARLY ALTERATIONS IN UTERINE METABOLISM IN RESPONSE TO ESTROGENS

### Early Effects of Phospholipid Synthesis[4]

To trace the origin of the estrogen-induced changes in uterine composition the metabolic pathways for phospholipid, ribonucleic acid, and protein synthesis have been examined in surviving uterine segments. In the case of phospholipids uterine segments from rats treated for various times with a single dose of estradiol were incubated in Eagle's tissue culture medium (3) containing inorganic $P^{32}$. After 1 hour the lipid fraction was isolated and separated by paper chromatography into ethanolamine, choline, and inositol phospholipids. Figure 2 illustrates the influence of previous estrogen treatment on the rate of incorporation of $P^{32}$ into the ethanolamine phospholipid fraction. It appears that the accumulation of this phospholipid can be correlated with an increased rate of synthesis. Since the other phospholipids responded in the same manner it seems most likely that the estrogen effect was mediated at some site common to all three classes of phospholipids.

In view of the remarkable stimulation of phospholipid metabolism in uterine segments from estrogen-treated rats, experiments were carried out with the *in vitro* addition of the hormone to control uterine segments. The results of four experiments testing the effect of various levels of estradiol *in vitro* are shown in Table I. The data indicate that the addition of 0.05 µg. of estradiol to 2.0 ml of Eagle's tissue culture medium gives a highly significant stimulation of the incorporation of $P^{32}$ into the ethanolamine

---

[4] The studies on phospholipid metabolism have been carried out in collaboration with Dr. Yoshio Aizawa.

phospholipids; when the dose of estradiol is either too high or too low the stimulatory action was not demonstrable (1). Although these results are of a preliminary nature, they encourage a search for their explanation in sub-cellular systems. Accordingly current investigations are concerned with the influence of estrogen on acetate activation as related to fatty acid synthesis and possible alterations in the metabolism of cytidine nucleotides and

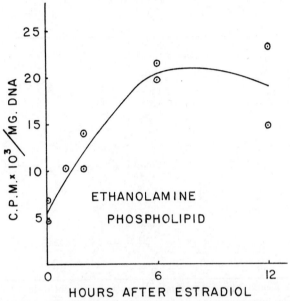

FIG. 2. Effect of pretreatment with estradiol on the incorporation of $P^{32}$ into etha-nolamine phospholipids. Rats were injected with 10 μg. of estradiol at zero time. After varying periods uterine segments were incubated with 200 microcuries of $P^{32}$ in 2 ml. of Eagle's tissue culture medium for a period of 1 hour at 37° in a 5 % $CO_2$, 95 % oxygen atmosphere. The ethanolamine phospholipid fraction was isolated by paper chromatography. The data are expressed as counts per minute in ethanolamine phospho-lipids per milligram of cellular DNA.

phosphatidic acid. It is of the utmost importance to ascertain the site of estrogen influence and to determine whether or not estrogen stimulation of phospholipid metabolism can be accounted for by changes in the level of the enzymes involved in phospholipid synthesis as has been demonstrated for amino acid incorporation into protein (10) and "one carbon" metabolism (6).

### Early Effects on Nucleic Acid Metabolism

Although the accumulation of ribonucleic acid could not be demonstrated prior to 6 hours of hormonal treatment, studies with radioactive precursors showed a striking acceleration of the incorporation of formate-$C^{14}$, glycine-2-$C^{14}$, serine-3-$C^{14}$, $C^{14}O_2$, and adenine-8-$C^{14}$ into nucleic acid purines by this time (5, 8, 14, 15). The results of two typical experiments in which radioactive formate and glycine were used as nucleic acid precursors is shown in Fig. 3. This response is also characteristic of the results with the other precursors.

TABLE I

*In Vitro* EFFECT OF ESTRADIOL ON THE INCORPORATION OF $P^{32}$ INTO ETHANOLAMINE PHOSPHOLIPIDS OF THE RAT UTERUS[a]

| Expt. | Estradiol added (μg.) | C.p.m./mg. DNA |
|---|---|---|
| A | Control | 81,700 |
| | 0.03 | 123,200 |
| | 0.1 | 108,000 |
| | 0.3 | 69,500 |
| | 1.0 | 79,800 |
| B | Control | 336,500 |
| | 0.001 | 316,500 |
| | 0.01 | 317,000 |
| | 0.1 | 435,000 |
| C | Control | 140,000 |
| | 0.05 | 208,000 |
| D | Control | 37,200 |
| | 0.05 | 96,500 |

[a] Uterine segments from ovariectomized rats were incubated in 2.0 ml. of Eagle's tissue culture medium containing 200 microcuries of $P^{32}$ and the indicated amounts of estradiol. The incubation period was 6 hours for experiments A, B, and C; 3 hours for experiment D. The ethanolamine phospholipid was isolated by paper chromatography. Data are expressed as counts per minute in ethanolamine phospholipids per milligram of uterine DNA.

In the case of nucleic acid synthesis, it could be demonstrated that the estrogen effect was exerted primarily on reactions leading to the labeling of the acid-soluble pool of nucleotides. As early as 1 hour following estrogen administration the incorporation of $C^{14}O_2$ into acid-soluble guanine nucleotides was stimulated significantly (Table II). The incorporation of this precursor into the uridylic acid nucleotide pool is similarly stimulated (8). Thus in a chronological sense, the reactions leading to the synthesis of the nucleotides are stimulated prior to any net accumulation of RNA. It would appear that the estrogen-induced accumulation of ribonucleic acid is secondary to the hormonal effect on the acid-soluble nucleotide pools.

In the investigation of the acid-soluble fraction from control and stimulated tissues it was also demonstrated that the nucleotide pools expanded under the influence of the hormone; in the case of the uridine nucleotides this could amount to as much as a fivefold increase after 6 hours of estrogen

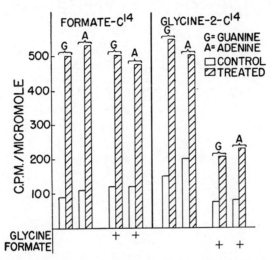

FIG. 3. The effect of pretreatment with estradiol on the incorporation of labeled formate and glycine into nucleic acid purines of surviving uterine segments. Uterine segments were from rats pretreated for 6 hours with a single 10-μg. dose of estradiol. Incubation period was 2 hours with labeled formate or glycine. Data are expressed as counts per minute per micromole purine and are taken from a publication by Mueller and Herranen (14).

TABLE II

EFFECT OF ESTRADIOL ON THE LABELING OF GUANINE IN THE ACID-SOLUBLE FRACTION[a] (8)

| In vivo pretreatment (hours) | Control[b] | Plus estrogen[b] |
|---|---|---|
| 1 | 95 | 105 |
|   | 84 | 100 |
| 3 | — | 263 |
|   | — | 136 |
| 6 | 75 | 359 |
|   | 78 | 368 |

[a] Ten micrograms estradiol injected intravenously at zero time. Segments from three uterine horns were incubated 1 hour with 5 μmoles $C^{14}O_2$; 0.58 μmole guanosine monophosphate carrier added to aliquot of acid-soluble fraction. Acid-soluble fraction was hydrolyzed 25 minutes at 90° C. in 4 % perchloric acid; guanine was isolated chromatographically (8).

[b] Data are expressed as total counts per minute in guanine per micromole thymine.

treatment (Table III). In the course of future investigation it will be important to ascertain whether these pool expansions result from new synthesis or degradation of existing nucleic acids as this observation constitutes another biochemical parameter of the tissue response to the estrogen.

TABLE III

EFFECT OF ESTROGEN ON LABELING OF ACID-SOLUBLE NUCLEOTIDES AND THE SIZE OF THE NUCLEOTIDE POOLS[a] (8)

| Data | b | Experiment I[c] | | Experiment II[d] | Experiment III[d] | |
|---|---|---|---|---|---|---|
| | | Adenine | UMP | Adenine | Adenine | UMP |
| μMoles isolated | C | 0.470 0.490 | 0.0060 | — — | 0.238 — | 0.0037 — |
| | E | 0.565 0.540 | 0.011 | — — | 0.282 — | 0.024 — |
| Specific activity (c.p.m. μmole) | C | | | 2465 | 2270 | 30,600 |
| | E | | | 6465 | 9630 | 26,700 |
| Total c.p.m. incorporated | C | | | 1080 945 | | 141 |
| | E | | | 4260 4560 | | 783 |

[a] Uterine segments incubated with NaHC$^{14}$O$_3$ (except Experiment I). Acid-soluble fraction was hydrolyzed 25 minutes at 90° C. in 4% perchloric acid. Adenine and uridine monophosphate (UMP) were isolated by ion exchange and paper chromatographic techniques. For the determination of total c.p.m., 1 μmole each of adenosine monophosphate (AMP) and UMP were added as carriers to an aliquot of the acid-soluble fraction. The data are expressed as micromoles adenine or UMP per micromole thymine, c.p.m. per micromole adenine or UMP, and total c.p.m. incorporated per micromole thymine.

[b] C = controls; E = 6 hours' pretreatment in vivo with 10 μg. estradiol.

[c] Experiment I: The data are obtained from 6 control and 6 estrogen-treated rats. No radioactivity measurements.

[d] Experiments II and III: Data obtained from 12 control and 12 estrogen-treated rats which had been incubated 1 hour with C$^{14}$O$_2$.

## Early Effects on Protein Synthesis

The effect of a single injection of estradiol (10 μg.) on the rate of incorporation of glycine-2-C$^{14}$ into the proteins of surviving segments is shown in Fig. 4. It is of interest that whereas the net accumulation of protein was not demonstrable prior to 12 hours (Fig. 1), the rate of incorporation of glycine was accelerated in a linear manner over the first 12 hours; thereafter the stimulatory process gradually subsided, resulting in a peak incorporation rate at 20 hours. In the ensuing 20 hours the rate of glycine incorporation declined towards the control level unless a second administration of estradiol was given to the animals; in which case protein labeling was stimulated again in a similar manner (13).

The stimulation of amino acid incorporation into the protein of surviving uterine segments occurred with all amino acids tested (13, 15). In addition it was observed (Fig. 5) that the incorporation of formate into protein was more responsive to the action of the estrogen than the incorporation of serine (5, 14). This was demonstrated to be due to the enhancement of serine

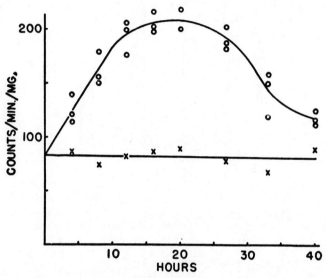

Fig. 4. The effect of a single dose of estradiol on the rate of incorporation of glycine-2-$C^{14}$ into protein of surviving uterine segments. Ten micrograms estradiol was injected intravenously at zero time. At the indicated times uterine segments were incubated with glycine-2-$C^{14}$ for 2 hours. Data are presented in counts per minute per milligram protein and are taken from a publication by Mueller (13).

synthesis from formate by estrogen treatment. In fact it was observed that the glycine ⇌ serine interconversion was accentuated in estrogen-stimulated tissues in whichever direction the interconversion was studied (5, 14).

In order to gain a better insight into the nature of the stimulating action of estrogens on protein synthesis, preliminary attempts have been made to measure the level of the enzymes catalyzing the various steps in protein synthesis. As evident from the diagram (Fig. 6) the first step in protein synthesis involves the carboxyl activation of amino acids with the energy contained in adenosine triphosphate (ATP). Since the reaction is a reversible one, the level of the individual amino acid-activating enzymes can be assayed by measuring the rate of incorporation of radioactive pyrophosphate into ATP.

In Fig. 7 the influence of estrogen treatment on the level of four amino acid-activating enzymes is shown. It is evident that acceleration of protein

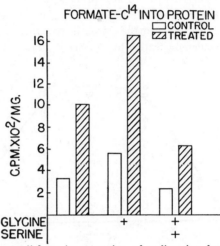

Fɪɢ. 5. Effect of estradiol on incorporation of radioactive formate into protein of surviving uterine segments. Rats were pretreated with 10 µg. of estradiol 6 hours prior to a 2-hour incorporation study. Data are expressed as counts per minute per milligram of protein and are taken from a publication by Mueller and Herranen (14).

$$
\underset{\substack{\text{NH}_2 \\ \text{(A.A.)}}}{\text{R-C-C}}\overset{\text{H} \quad \text{O}}{\underset{\text{OH}}{}} + \text{ATP} \underset{}{\overset{\text{Sol.E}}{\rightleftharpoons}} \left[ \underset{\substack{\text{NH}_2 \\ \text{(Active A.A.)}}}{\text{R-C-C}}\overset{\text{H} \quad \text{O}}{\underset{\text{AMP-Enzyme}}{}} \right] + \text{PP}^*
$$

Active A.A. + Sol. RNA $\rightleftharpoons$ RNA–AA

$$
\text{RNA-AA} + \underset{\text{(Acceptor)}}{\text{Peptide-NH}_2} \xrightarrow[\text{GTP}]{\text{Microsomes}} \underset{\text{NH}_2}{\text{Peptide-N-C-C-R}}\overset{\text{H O H}}{}
$$

Fɪɢ. 6. A diagram of reactions involved in protein synthesis. PP* = radioactive pyrophosphate; A.A. = amino acids; ATP = adenosine triphosphate; GTP = guanosine triphosphate.

synthesis as shown in Fig. 4 can be accounted for in part by the increases in activity of these enzymes. Assays for the response of the individual enzymes revealed that they all responded independently to estrogen treatment. It was also demonstrated in the case of leucine activation that the second step in protein synthesis, the transfer of the activated amino acid to the soluble RNA, was stimulated correspondingly by the estrogen treatment as might be expected. Analysis of the reactions concerned with the third step of protein synthesis, the actual formation of the peptide bond, remains to be investigated.

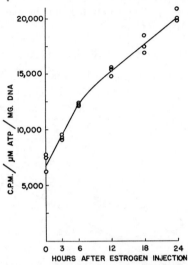

FIG. 7. Time curve on the combined response of four amino acid-activating enzymes following a single 10-μg. dose of estradiol. A mixture of leucine, methionine, tryptophan, and valine was used as substrate for the $PP^{32}$-ATP exchange system. Data are expressed as counts per minute per micromole of ATP by the enzyme from an amount of tissue containing 1.0 mg. of DNA. Data taken from a publication by McCorquodale and Mueller (10).

## Estrogen-Induced Alterations in Serine Aldolase Activity

As indicated in the preceding sections on nucleic acid and protein metabolism both the synthesis of serine from glycine and a one-carbon precursor, and the reverse cleavage reaction were found in uterine segments to be

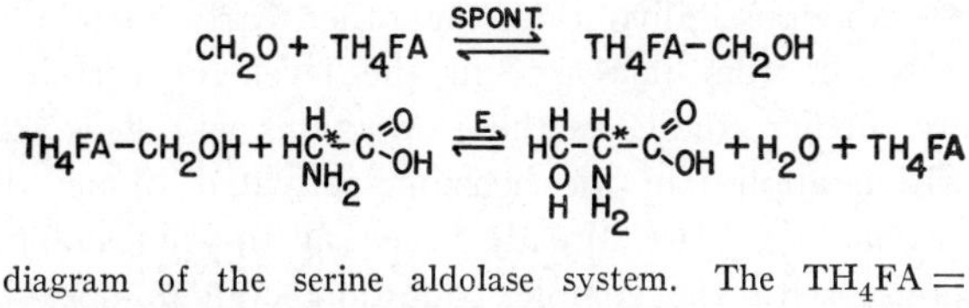

$$CH_2O + TH_4FA \xrightleftharpoons{\text{SPONT.}} TH_4FA-CH_2OH$$

$$TH_4FA-CH_2OH + HC^*\underset{NH_2}{\overset{H}{\underset{}{|}}}C\overset{\nearrow O}{\underset{OH}{}} \xrightleftharpoons{E} HC-\underset{N}{\overset{H}{\underset{|}{}}}\underset{N}{\overset{H}{\underset{|}{}}}C^*\overset{\nearrow O}{\underset{OH}{}} + H_2O + TH_4FA$$

FIG. 8. A diagram of the serine aldolase system. The $TH_4FA$ = tetrahydrofolic acid. The first reaction proceeds spontaneously; the second reaction is catalyzed by serine aldolase (E).

facilitated by estrogen treatment. Since the basic reaction (Fig. 8) is catalyzed by serine aldolase the level of this enzyme was assayed in homogenates of stimulated tissues by following the conversion of glycine-$2$-$C^{14}$ to serine-

2-$C^{14}$. The effect of varying degrees of estrogen treatment on the level of serine aldolase is shown in Fig. 9. As in the case of protein synthesis it would appear that the estrogen enhancement of "one carbon" metabolism in the pathways studied can be accounted for in part by increases in the activity of a participating enzyme.

### COMMENTS ON ESTROGEN ACTION

The observation that the early estrogen-induced alterations in two pathways (i.e., serine synthesis and amino acid incorporation into protein) can be accounted for by increases in the level of activity of participating en-

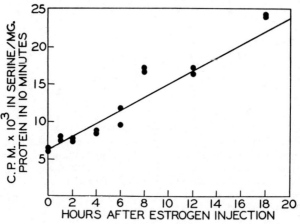

FIG. 9. Effect of estradiol pretreatment on the levels of serine aldolase in the rat uterus. Ten per cent homogenates were prepared from uterine horns of rats pretreated with 10 μg. estradiol for the indicated time. Data are expressed as counts per minute in serine per milligram protein residue of enzyme aliquot and are taken from a publication by Herranen and Mueller (6).

zymes suggests the possibility that the other early metabolic alterations reported also result from increases in the levels of certain rate-limiting enzymes. Only further studies in these directions will show whether or not this generalization applies in the hormone-activated tissue. But with the observations at hand we are already faced at the molecular level of the hormone response with the complex question: Where does the increased enzyme activity come from and what is the role of estrogen in its appearance? To approach the central problem it must be determined whether the increases in enzyme activity result from the *de novo* synthesis of new enzyme or reflect the activation of existing proenzymes.

Tackling primarily the simplest of these possibilities, our laboratory group has performed a large number of experiments with cell-free systems from the uterus in the effort to obtain some evidence for the possible activation of pre-existing, serine aldolase and the various amino acid-activating enzymes. To date the results have been completely negative. In these studies all attempts to apply the concepts of Villee (18) and Talalay (17) on estrogen- catalyzed transhydrogenation and to make use of the findings of Hollander (7) on the phenol-activated oxidase of rat uterus have failed to provide evidence for an enzyme activation. Accordingly these attempts also have failed to provide any evidence for the relevance of their observations to the molecular action of the hormone in the rat uterus.

At this point it seems most likely that the observed increases in enzyme activity result from a selective *de novo* synthesis of these entities. To prove this possibility is a more difficult task since it necessitates isolation and isotopic studies on the pure enzyme. However, if the explanation for the observed results does lie in *de novo* protein synthesis, it will become appropriate to inquire as to the participation of estrogens in this process. Possibly our attention will be directed to the alteration of intracellular factors that promote protein synthesis, or to changes in the metabolic state of the RNA templates; or perhaps the subcellular investigation into the early alterations in lipid metabolism will provide an explanation for these results. While at the very least it is anticipated that this approach will accrue information basic to the understanding of many cellular responses, it is more optimistically expected to provide the score card for recognizing those reactions that play relevant roles in the molecular mechanisms of action of estrogenic hormones.

### REFERENCES

1. Aizawa, Y., and Mueller, G. C. Unpublished data.
2. Astwood, E. B. *Endocrinology* **23**, 25 (1938).
3. Eagle, H. *J. Exptl. Med.* **102**, 37 (1955).
4. Hagerman, D. D., and Villee, C. A. *J. Biol. Chem.* **234**, 2031 (1959).
5. Herranen, A., and Mueller, G. C. *J. Biol. Chem.* **223**, 369 (1956).
6. Herranen, A. M., and Mueller, G. C. *Biochim. et Biophys. Acta* **24**, 223 (1957).
7. Hollander, V. P., Hollander, N., and Brown, J. D. *J. Biol. Chem.* **234**, 1678 (1959).
8. Jervell, K. F., Diniz, C. R., and Mueller, G. C. *J. Biol. Chem.* **231**, 945 (1958).
9. Langer, L. J., and Engel, L. L. *J. Biol. Chem.* **233**, 583 (1958).
10. McCorquodale, D. J., and Mueller, G. C. *J. Biol. Chem.* **232**, 31 (1958).
11. McLeod, J., and Reynolds, S. R. M. *Proc. Soc. Exptl. Biol. Med.* **37**, 366 (1938).
12. Marcus, P. I., and Talalay, P. *Proc. Roy. Soc.* **B144**, 116 (1955).
13. Mueller, G. C. *J. Biol. Chem.* **204**, 77 (1953).
14. Mueller, G. C., and Herranen, A. *J. Biol. Chem.* **219**, 585 (1956).
15. Mueller, G. C., Herranen, A. M., and Jervell, K. F. *Recent Progr. in Hormone Research* **14**, 95 (1958).
16. Szego, C. M., and Roberts, S. *Recent Progr. in Hormone Research* **8**, 419 (1953).

17. Talalay, P., Hurlock, B., and Williams-Ashman, H. G. *Proc. Natl. Acad Sci. U.S.* **44**, 862 (1958).
18. Villee, C. A., and Gordon, E. E. *Bull. soc. chim. Belges* **65**, 186 (1956).
19. Williams-Ashman, H. G., Cassman, M., and Klavins, M. *Federation Proc.* **18**, 352 (1959).

DISCUSSION

**E. V. Jensen:** All your observations, Dr. Mueller, are extremely interesting and your observation of the early increase in the phospholipids is especially striking. This is interesting to me in relation to some work that I had the opportunity to do last year in the laboratory of Professor Adolf Butenandt in Munich. We attempted to determine whether an early effect of testosterone administration is either to increase the amount of a particular nucleotide in rat prostate or to increase the rate of incorporation of radioactive phosphate into the nucleotides. Although we found that there was no effect of testosterone on either the specific activity or the amounts of the nucleotides in the immature rat prostate 4 hours after testosterone administration, two side observations were made which may bear on your findings. First, testosterone caused a marked increase in a single compound in prostate which appears to be a phosphorylated sugar. Of more direct relevance to your observations on the phospholipids is the relatively high concentration of cytidine nucleotides we observed in rat prostate. As you know, Kennedy and Weiss have shown that the cytidine nucleotides are the coenzymes for phospholipid synthesis, so that the abundance of these in prostate suggests that this may be involved in a phospholipid response to steroid hormone stimulation. Of course this is all in the rat prostate with testosterone, and your remarks are concerned with the rat uterus with estradiol, but still both are tissues that grow in response to steroid hormones. Therefore I think these facts should be used as a basis for further consideration. I would like to ask whether you have observed any marked preponderance of cytidine nucleotides in rat uterine tissue.

**G. C. Mueller:** I don't have this information at hand, Dr. Jensen. The analyses which we carried out earlier excluded the cytidine nucleotides. It is now important to investigate both their pool sizes and metabolic activities.

**W. H. Daughaday:** I am interested in this paper because Dr. Kipnis and Dr. Reiss, who are associated with me in St. Louis, are studying early actions of growth hormone on protein synthetic mechanisms. In your talk you gave no consideration to the possibility of transport mechanisms being involved in the early changes following estrogens. As I remember, Noall and Christianson have shown major change in amino acid transport of the uterus with estrogen. Do you think these changes in transport are important? Secondly, in your experiments on amino acid incorporation, have the amino acid pools been measured and the specific activity in amino acid pools calculated?

**G. C. Mueller:** We have tried to evaluate the amino acid pool sizes in the estrogen-stimulated and control uteri. So far as we can ascertain, there is no significant early change. I believe this has been confirmed by Dr. Kalman. With reference to the work of Christianson, in which he shows a stimulation of amino acid transporting activity following estrogen administration, I can only say that we have no data on this subject. I feel it may reflect the increased levels of amino acid-activating enzymes.

I would like to say this about the responses discussed here: I think they characterize the changes taking place in a tissue being induced to grow, which as such might well occur in other tissues mobilized for growth, whatever the stimulus. These studies are still far removed from the initial hormonal stimulus. I think that some interesting correlations will come out of the comparison of this tissue with the uterine tissue.

**V. P. Hollander:** I would like to ask Dr. Mueller whether he has studied the effect of histamine *in vitro* on the early synthesis of phospholipid, in view of the observations by Szego and colleagues that this substance may be implicated in the early phase of uterine weight gain due to estrogen.

**G. C. Mueller:** We haven't studied histamine effects on phospholipids, but we did study them earlier with reference to the nucleic acid- and protein-synthesizing pathways. In these cases histamine, if it did anything at all, was toxic to the system.

**H. G. Williams-Ashman:** If I understand your Fig. 7 correctly, you have estimated the activity of amino acid-activating enzymes in uterus by measurements of amino acid-dependent exchange of $P^{32}$ from labeled inorganic pyrophosphate into ATP. In relation to these experiments, have you determined the concentration of endogenous inorganic pyrophosphate in the uterus before and after treatment with estrogens? Also, have you information concerning the pool of inorganic pyrophosphate under the conditions of your experiments to determine the activity of amino acid-activating enzymes?

**G. C. Mueller:** We have studied the survival of pyrophosphate in these systems to evaluate the possibility that a pyrophosphatase might interfere with our determinations, and found that there is an extremely low pyrophosphatase activity in the system. We have also studied the reaction going both ways by measuring the transfer of the activated amino acid, and also from the standpoint of the amino acid accepting RNA. The same estrogen effect was obtained. Therefore I think there is no reason to begin to worry about the issues which you present.

**K. E. Paschkis:** I wonder, Dr. Mueller, whether you have used any antimetabolites in these studies? The reason for asking this is that we have recently studied various hormone-induced growth processes and other growth processes under the influence of antimetabolites, chiefly 5-fluorouracil, but also 6-azauracil and some others not yet completed. This goes back to our original studies of the use of an alternate pathway of RNA synthesis, utilizing preformed uracil, in rapidly growing tissues, both malignant and nonmalignant. Heidelberger *et al.*, as well as Welch *et al.*, synthesized uracil analogs. Normal growth processes are inhibited as one would expect in a rapidly growing tissue, but there evolves a curious dissociation of certain phases of growth processes. For instance, the initial early hydration of tissues incident to growth, induced by estrogens in the uterus or with androgens in the seminal vesicles, is not inhibited at all by 5-fluorouracil. The inhibition of mitosis far exceeds the inhibition of weight increment of the organs. With 5-fluorouracil one can show such dissociation of growth processes. Have you used any antimetabolites in your studies? And if so, how do they affect the various phases of estrogen-induced growth?

**G. C. Mueller:** I agree with Dr. Paschkis that there is something unusual in these systems. The original observations of Dr. Hertz on the aminopterin blocking of estradiol action (the hyperplastic response) prompted us to look for similar toxicity on the early biochemical responses. We were surprised and lost interest in that area when we found that animals which had received lethal doses of the aminopterin and were in a moribund condition still responded to estrogen treatment with an acceleration of protein synthesis similar to that seen in the controls. We haven't looked specifically at the nucleic acid aspects of this thing; this might be more interesting. With reference to 5-fluorouracil and related compounds, we have not used them in the estrogen experiments. However, we have worked with other antimetabolites, such as analogs of amino acids. These substances also do not block the initial responses. These observations prompted us initially to think first of enzyme activation in explaining our increased enzyme activities. I think it possible, however, that sufficient templates are available in the absence of new RNA synthesis to take care of the needs of protein synthesis during the first few hours of the hormonal response. Possibly the early estrogen response is concerned with an activation or conversion of these materials into a state of competence for protein synthesis.

**R. Grinberg:** Have you tried estrogen and progesterone together? Also, have you used uterine fibroids, instead of normal uterine tissue?

**G. C. Mueller:** All the studies so far performed with progesterone have concerned *in vitro* effects on surviving uterine segments. In such work progesterone has turned out to be exceedingly toxic. At the level of 10 µg. per reaction mixture (3 ml.) amino acid, incorporation into surviving segments was suppressed 50–75 %. However it did not show any selective effect with respect to whether the tissues were derived from estrogen-treated or control animals.

**A. White:** As I recall, you indicated that the animals you used were of the same age and were castrated on the same day. Did you indicate how old the animals were which you used? Secondly, have you examined the effect of estradiol on the uteri of noncastrated animals, or have you studied only atrophic uteri? I ask this question because there seems to be fairly general acceptance of the idea that in most tissues the enzymes that have been studied are present in concentrations far exceeding available substrates, and yet here you do get this apparent stimulation of new enzyme synthesis. It is rather interesting that progesterone in our hands, and in lymphoid tissue rather than those you used, is a most effective inhibitor of respiration, glucose oxidation, the incorporation of amino acids into protein, and the incorporation of glycine into nucleic acids. Finally, could a similar stimulation, perhaps of metabolic activity, be observed in uteri into which estradiol was directly placed?

**G. C. Mueller:** As to your last question, we have not worked with the installation of the estrogen into the uterus itself. The rats were originally from Sprague-Dawley strain; they were all born on the same day, and ovariectomized on the same day, at approximately three months of age. They weighed around 200 gm. at the time they were ovariectomized. All rats in any one experiment were of the same vintage. It is very important to take these precautions to limit the biological variation to very narrow range. In addition to these preparations, when we carry out experiments which involve comparisons of the *in vitro* factors, we do pool the segments from a group of animals and use them at random for individual flasks. This also reduces the variation to a very low level.

In reference to your second question, we have not done very much with intact animals because it is too difficult to standardize their physiological state. However, as time passes after ovariectomy we have noted that the estrogenic effect increases up to about one month. At 1 week post ovariectomy the estrogen effects appear but there is a higher base line; it seems that as the tissue atrophies, the base-line reactions decline. Accordingly we do all experiments with rats between one month and two months after ovariectomy.

**R. A. Huseby:** There has been a lot of work dealing with the RNA synthetic pathways within the cell that has indicated that nuclear RNA may be the precursor of cytoplasmic RNA. As you may know, Dr. Barnum and I studied this problem and felt that we had evidence that this was not so. In FIG. 1, you indicated that the soluble RNA in the cytoplasm initiated the reaction and this then proceeded to the particulate

RNA. This is the sort of thing Dr. Barnum and I thought we had seen. Have you studied the nuclear RNA in these preparations?

**G. C. Mueller:** We have not. The nucleus is extremely difficult to purify from uterine tissue. I think your question may have some bearing on a subject that Dr. Paschkis was talking about earlier. It is quite possible that certain reactions in the estrogen-treated tissues could be initiated in the nucleus. It has been observed histologically that estrogen treatment causes an increase in the amount of nuclear material as measured by tyrosine reaction for protein. This occurs without an increase in DNA content.

**J. T. Velardo:** Has Dr. Mueller any information at all on the so-called biochemical score card for the estrous cycle of the rat, that is taking the whole estrous cycle as a physiological unit? Also, has he any data on the transition from the immature state to the mature state in the rat; that is, the biochemical events during the first estrous cycle between the 35th and 45th day in the life of the female rat? I think such data would provide an excellent series of base-line controls.

**G. C. Mueller:** We have not studied this situation.

# Enzymatic Transport of Hydrogen by Estrogenic Hormones

H. G. Williams-Ashman, Shutsung Liao, and P. Talalay

*The Ben May Laboratory for Cancer Research, and Department of Biochemistry, The University of Chicago, Chicago, Illinois*

Recent studies from this laboratory have shown that certain enzyme systems which oxidize gonadal hormones also catalyze the transfer of hydrogen or electrons between biochemically important molecules in the presence of *catalytic* levels of these hormones. This paper will describe some aspects of the biochemistry of these reactions, in which certain estrogenic substances transport hydrogen or electrons at concentrations commensurate with those at which they exert physiological action. In some of these reactions, the active group of the hormones appears to be a secondary alcohol or ketone, while in others, a phenolic hydroxyl group is implicated in their carrier action. The possible relationship of these model studies to the mechanism of action of estrogens will be considered only in brief.

## Hydrogen Transfer between Pyridine Nucleotides

### Placental enzyme

Villee and his collaborators (6, 39) found that the reduction of DPN[1] catalyzed by soluble extracts of human placenta incubated with isocitrate was accelerated by the direct addition of microgram quantities of estradiol-17β. They proposed that estradiol-17β, and related steroidal estrogens, activated a soluble, DPN-specific isocitric dehydrogenase in placenta by converting an inactive form of the enzyme into an active one (8, 39). Talalay and Williams-Ashman (33) showed that this hypothesis was incorrect and that, under these conditions, estradiol-17β mediated a transfer of hydrogen from TPNH to DPN. The apparent activation of a DPN-linked isocitric dehydrogenase could be accounted for by the operation of a coupled reaction between a soluble, TPN-specific, isocitric dehydrogenase and a pyridine nucleotide transhydrogenase system according to the following equations:

$$\text{Isocitrate} + \text{TPN} \rightleftarrows \alpha\text{-ketoglutarate} + CO_2 + \text{TPNH}$$
$$\underline{\text{TPNH} + \text{DPN} \rightleftarrows \text{TPN} + \text{DPNH}}$$
$$\text{Isocitrate} + \text{DPN} \rightarrow \alpha\text{-ketoglutarate} + CO_2 + \text{DPNH}$$

---

[1] The following abbreviations are used in this paper: DPN = diphosphopyridine nucleotide; DPNH = dihydrodiphosphopyridine nucleotide; TPN = triphosphopyridine nucleotide; TPNH = dihydrotriphosphopyridine nucleotide; NMNH = dihydronicotinamide mononucleotide.

It was demonstrated that in this coupled reaction, the TPN-specific iso-citric dehydrogenase could be replaced by several TPN-reducing systems (e.g., glucose-6-phosphate dehydrogenase), or by TPNH added as such (30, 33). The action of estradiol-17β in this system was solely to stimulate the transhydrogenase reaction and was in no particular way related to the oxidation of isocitrate. That the estrogen-sensitive reaction in soluble extracts of human placenta is a transhydrogenation between pyridine nucleotides, rather than a DPN-specific isocitric dehydrogenase, has been confirmed by Villee and Hagerman (40) and by Hollander et al. (12, 13). Using partially purified enzyme preparations, Talalay and associates (30) showed that estradiol-17β mediated the transfer of hydrogen from DPNH to TPN, as well as from TPNH to DPN. The reversibility of this trans-hydrogenase reaction was shown to depend critically upon the relative con-centrations of pyridine nucleotides in the reaction mixture. Talalay et al. (30, 34) observed that, in the presence of low levels of estradiol-17β, this placental enzyme system catalyzed the reduction of a number of analogs of DPN by TPNH and DPNH.

Talalay and Williams-Ashman (33) proposed that the estradiol-17β-medi-ated transfer of hydrogen between pyridine nucleotides is catalyzed by a placental 17β-hydroxysteroid dehydrogenase, first described by Langer and Engel (21), which reacts at comparable rates with both DPN and TPN, as follows:

$$\text{Estrone} + \text{TPNH} + \text{H}^+ \rightleftarrows \text{estradiol-17β} + \text{TPN}$$
$$\text{Estradiol-17β} + \text{DPN} \rightleftarrows \text{estrone} + \text{DPNH} + \text{H}^+$$
$$\overline{\text{TPNH} + \text{DPN} \rightleftarrows \text{TPN} + \text{DPNH}}$$

This formulation implies that during the course of the transhydrogenase reaction, estradiol-17β undergoes alternate oxidation and reduction, and thereby transports hydrogen in virtue of the change steroid alcohol $\rightleftarrows$ steroid ketone. The evidence in support of this hypothesis has been documented in full (30, 33, 34) and may be summarized as follows: (a) Both dehydro-genase and transhydrogenase activities, when measured with a number of pyridine nucleotides, parallel one another during purification of the enzyme. (b) The specificity for both steroids and pyridine nucleotides is identical in both reactions. (c) Estradiol-17β and estrone become interconverted during the course of the transhydrogenase reaction. (d) The action of various inhibitors, or inactivating procedures, does not provide evidence for separate enzymes catalyzing dehydrogenation and transhydrogenation, provided that proper attention is paid to the relative affinities (and protective actions) of different pyridine nucleotides. (e) The stereospecificity of the placental enzyme for hydrogen transfer to DPN and TPN is the same as the stereospecificity for the transhydrogenase reaction for DPN [side II of the reduced pyridine nucleotides (31)]. These facts do not accord with the report of Hagerman and Villee (9) that, in human placenta, the estrogen-sensitive transhydrogenase can be separated from two distinct estradiol dehydrogenases, specific for DPN and TPN, respectively. Hagerman and Villee (9) believe that estrogenic steroids stimulate a soluble placental transhydrogenase by converting, in an unspecified manner, an inactive form of the enzyme into an active one. Unequivocal proof that oxidation of estradiol-17β by DPN and TPN, and estradiol-17β-mediated transhydrogenase reactions in placenta are catalyzed by one or three enzymes must await isolation of the catalytic protein(s) in a crystalline and/or homogeneous form.

### Soluble Hydroxysteroid Dehydrogenases of Liver and Bacteria

Hurlock and Talalay (16) found that the soluble 3α-hydroxysteroid dehydrogenase of rat liver catalyzes the transfer of hydrogen from TPNH to DPN upon the addition of catalytic concentrations of its steroid substrates, for example:

$$\text{Androstane-3,17-dione} + \text{TPNH} + \text{H}^+ \rightleftarrows \text{androsterone} + \text{TPN}$$
$$\underline{\text{Androsterone} + \text{DPN} \rightleftarrows \text{androstane-3,17-dione} + \text{DPNH} + \text{H}^+}$$
$$\text{TPNH} + \text{DPN} \rightleftarrows \text{TPN} + \text{DPNH}$$

Similarly, this enzyme will catalyze steroid-dependent transhydrogenations between DPNH and pyridine nucleotides of higher oxidation-reduction potential, such as the 3-acetylpyridine analog of DPN.

The adaptive 3α- and β-hydroxysteroid dehydrogenases of *Pseudomonas testosteroni,* which were isolated in a highly purified state by Talalay and his co-workers (23, 28, 32), react with DPN and a number of analogs thereof, but are inert toward TPN. Recent experiments by Talalay and Adams (29, 34) revealed that these bacterial enzymes catalyze hydrogen transfers from DPNH to the 3-acetylpyridine, 3-pyridine aldehyde, and thionicotinamide analogs of DPN in the presence of minute concentrations of their appropriate steroid substrates.

Holzer and Schneider (15) reported that two pyridine nucleotide-linked enzymes with dual nucleotide specificity (lactic and glutamic dehydrogenases) which do not react with steroids also catalyze some transfer of hydrogen from TPNH to DPN upon the addition of their substrates. But in these experiments, the rates of transhydrogenation were slower than those of dehydrogenation by two to three orders of magnitude. Moreover, such hydrogen transfers were demonstrated only with concentrations of carrier (substrate) molecules that were much greater than the total amount of hydrogen which passed from one pyridine nucleotide to another during the course of the reaction. The peculiar properties of hydroxysteroid dehydrogenases which enable them to catalyze efficient transfer of hydrogen between pyridine nucleotides appear to be: (1) high affinities for steroids, (2) favorable equilibrium constants for the oxidoreduction of steroids by pyridine nucleotides, and (3) comparable rates of reaction with DPN and TPN (in the case of the placental 17β- and hepatic 3α-hydroxysteroid dehydrogenases).

## Physiological Implications

Talalay and Williams-Ashman (30, 33) suggested that at least some of the physiological actions of estradiol-17β and estrone might result from their mediation of hydrogen transfer between TPN and DPN. Villee (38, 40) has discussed this hypothesis in relation to his original postulate that estrogens speed up the tricarboxylic acid cycle by virtue of activating a DPN-linked isocitric dehydrogenase (8). Stimulation of the soluble placental transhydrogenase system can be demonstrated with concentrations of steroidal estrogens ($10^{-8}\ M$) that are physiological rather than pharmacological. But proof that estrogen-mediated transhydrogenations represent even one of the primary mechanisms by which estrogenic hormones promote areal growth and function will require much more experimental evidence than is available at present.

## Synthetic Estrogens

The ability to induce cornification of the vagina in spayed animals is not confined to steroids. Thus, hydroxylated stilbenes such as diethylstilbestrol and hexestrol, substituted triphenylethylenes, doisynolic acids, isoflavones like genistein, dibenzanthracene diols, and even simple monophenols such as 4-*tert*-amylphenol, all exert estrogenic action (4). Many of these synthetic estrogens are devoid of either secondary alcohol or ketone groups. For this reason, it would not be expected that they could transport hydrogen in the presence of the placental 17-hydroxysteroid dehydrogenase or of any other enzymes of this class. Diethylstilbestrol does not activate the soluble placental transhydrogenase reaction (33, 37), although high concentrations of this synthetic estrogen compete with the action of estradiol-17β in this system (8, 37). It is of interest that Talalay and Marcus (32) found that the β-hydroxysteroid dehydrogenase of *Pseudomonas testosteroni* was strongly inhibited by diethylstilbestrol.

Two types of interaction of synthetic estrogens with enzyme systems have been reported. First, high concentrations of diethylstilbestrol, and certain related substances, were found to inhibit some oxidizing enzymes (3, 25), and to disrupt the coupling between oxidation and phosphorylation (27, 42), in animal mitochondria. Secondly, Hochster and Quastel (10, 11) reported that diethylstilbestrol functioned as an hydrogen carrier for some enzymatic oxidations and competed with the carrier action of cytochrome c and methylene blue in others. Hochster and Quastel (10) suggested that diethylstilbestrol exerts these actions by undergoing reversible oxidation to the corresponding quinone.

We have studied two different model enzymatic reactions in which catalytic levels of many synthetic and natural estrogens will transport hydrogen. In both model systems, the phenolic hydroxyl group of the estrogens is implicated in their carrier action. Many nonestrogenic phenols also mediate the oxidation of various hydrogen donors under these conditions. However, the insight into the mechanism of action of the placental estrogen-sensitive transhydrogenase reaction (30, 33, 34) which was gained from previous model studies with bacterial hydroxysteroid dehydrogenases (23, 28, 32) suggested that model enzymatic reactions in which synthetic estrogen transported hydrogen may be of heuristic value for an understanding of their mode of physiological action.

## PHENOLASE-CATALYZED OXIDATIONS

Phenolases are copper proteins that catalyze both the hydroxylation of monophenols to $o$-diphenols, and the oxidation of $o$-diphenols to $o$-quinones, at the expense of molecular oxygen. Otto Warburg (20) showed that in addition to catalyzing these reactions, phenolases promoted the oxidation of a number of hydrogen donors (including reduced pyridine nucleotides) upon the addition of catalytic quantities of $o$-diphenolic substrates:

$$2\ o\text{-diphenol} + O_2 \rightarrow 2\ o\text{-quinone} + 2\ H_2O$$
$$\underline{2\ DPNH + 2\ H^+ + 2\ o\text{-quinone} \rightarrow 2\ DPN + 2\ o\text{-diphenol}}$$
$$2\ DPNH + 2\ H^+ + O_2 \rightarrow 2\ DPN + 2\ H_2O$$

Three reasons prompted a study of the possible hydrogen-transporting activity of catalytic levels of phenolic estrogens in the presence of phenolases. First, the pioneer studies of Westerfield (41), Graubard and Pincus (7), and Bergstrom *et al.* (2) showed that copper oxidases isolated from potatoes and mushrooms "inactivated" steroidal estrogens. Recent experiments by Jellinck (17) indicate that the action of mushroom phenolases on estrone involves primarily an attack upon ring A of the molecule. Secondly, Mueller (26) reported that 2-hydroxy- and 4-hydroxyestradiol-17β stimulated the incorporation of formate into the proteins of isolated uterine horns *in vitro*, under conditions where the parent estradiol-17β was inactive. Thirdly, it appears that steroidal estrogens are hydroxylated in ring A *in vivo*, since Gallagher (5, 19) has isolated 2-methoxyestrone and 2-methoxyestriol from the urine of women.

In collaboration with Cassman (34, 43, 44) we found that low levels $10^{-5}$ to $10^{-6}M$) of estradiol-17β mediated the oxidation of ascorbic acid, DPNH and TPNH, ferrocytochrome c, and ferrocyanide by purified preparations of potato phenolase. The estradiol-17β-stimulated oxidation of DPNH proceeded to completion with the uptake of one atom equivalent of oxygen. The oxidations were inhibited by cyanide, but they were unaffected by catalase. The optimum pH for the reaction was in the vicinity of pH 6.5. The concentration of estradiol-17β required to promote 50 % of the maximal rate of oxidation of DPNH was $3 \times 10^{-6}M$. At low enzyme concentrations, a marked induction period was noted when estradiol-17β was used as carrier, but no such lag was apparent with 4-hydroxyestradiol-17β. If purified potato phenolase was incubated with DPN, ethanol, yeast alcohol dehydrogenase, and small amounts of estradiol-17β, a rapid consumption of oxygen ensued. Under these conditions, some of the estrogen was converted into products which when chromatographed on paper migrated close to the 2-hydroxy and 4-hydroxy derivatives of estradiol-17β. The phenolic hydroxyl group of estradiol-17β was essential for its carrier action. Thus, nearly equivalent activity was found with estradiol-17α and -17β, estrone, estriol, equilenin, and 17-deoxyestradiol, while 3-deoxyestradiol-17α was inactive. Neither 2-nitroestrone nor 4-nitroestrone was active in this system, and 1-methylestradiol-17β was also inert. These findings suggested that estradiol-17β was hydroxylated by the phenolase to an o-diphenolic product, which then transported hydrogen by undergoing a reversible, phenolase-catalyzed oxidation to the corresponding quinone.

Many synthetic phenolic estrogens functioned as hydrogen carriers in the presence of potato phenolase, e.g., hexestrol, diethylstilbestrol, bisdehydrodoisynolic acid, and genistein. A free phenolic hydroxyl group was necessary for substances to transport hydrogen in this system. However, the nature of the hydrogen-transporting intermediates responsible for the carrier action of these synthetic estrogens has not been determined. A variety of androgenic and adrenal cortical, nonphenolic, steroids were inert in this system.

Estradiol-17β and a number of synthetic phenolic estrogens also acted as hydrogen carriers for the oxidation of DPNH by mushroom phenolases. But these reactions were not catalyzed by copper sulfate, or crystalline hemocyanin, or a soluble phenolase isolated from spinach leaves.

The rather narrow distribution of phenolases in animal tissues makes it improbable that the transport of hydrogen or electrons by o-diphenolic derivatives under the action of these copper oxidases is related to the mechanism of action of estrogens.

## Model Experiments with Peroxidases

Akazawa and Conn (1) have shown that a number of phenols mediate the oxidation of DPNH, and other hydrogen donors, by horse-radish peroxidase in the presence of low levels of $Mn^{++}$ ions and molecular oxygen. Using purified preparations of either horse-radish peroxidase or lactoperoxidase, we found (34, 43, 44) that many estrogenic phenols stimulate the oxidation of DPNH, TPNH, and NMNH under these conditions. These oxidations proceeded to completion without the addition of hydrogen peroxide, and one atom of oxygen was utilized per mole of DPNH oxidized. Estradiol-17β did not mediate the oxidation of DPNH in the presence of $Mn^{++}$ ions, oxygen, and either cytochrome c or catalase. The peroxidase-$Mn^{++}$ catalyzed oxidations mediated by estradiol-17β were inhibited by cyanide and also by crystalline catalase. Only those estrogenic substances possessing a free phenolic hydroxyl group transported hydrogen in this system. Many types of synthetic estrogen were active. In marked contrast to the phenolase-catalyzed systems described above, certain o-diphenols (e.g., epinephrine and norepinephrine) did not mediate the oxidation of DPNH by the peroxidase-$Mn^{++}$ system, and inhibited the action of estradiol-17β therein. The concentration of estradiol-17β required to promote 50 % of the maximal rate of oxidation of DPNH was found to be $8 \times 10^{-6} M$.

The stimulation of the oxidation of DPNH by estradiol-17β in the peroxidase-$Mn^{++}$ system was also observed by Klebanoff (18), who found that thyroxine functioned in the same manner as this estrogen. The effects of thyroxine and estradiol-17β were additive.

The simplest explanation for this catalytic effect of phenolic estrogens is that suggested by Akazawa and Conn (1) for the action of many simple phenols. The peroxidase may catalyze the oxidation of the phenol (ROH) to an oxidized product (RO·) and hydrogen peroxide. This product is, presumably, of a free radical nature, and may act as the oxidant for the hydrogen donor. The hydrogen peroxide generated in the first reaction may oxidize the phenol, by a peroxidatic reaction, to the oxidized product. According to this formulation, the phenol-dependent oxidation of DPNH would proceed as follows:

$$2 \ ROH + O_2 \rightarrow 2 \ RO· + H_2O_2$$
$$2 \ ROH + H_2O_2 \rightarrow 2 \ RO· + 2 \ H_2O$$
$$\underline{4 \ RO· + 2 \ DPNH + 2 \ H^+ \rightarrow 4 \ ROH + 2 \ DPN}$$
$$2 \ DPNH + 2 \ H^+ + O_2 \rightarrow 2 \ DPN + 2 \ H_2O$$

This mechanism accounts for the following facts: (a) the stoichiometry of DPNH oxidation and oxygen consumption; (b) hydrogen peroxide is not required for, and does not accumulate during, the reaction; and (c) under these experimental conditions, hydrogen peroxide does not oxidize DPNH in the absence of an appropriate phenol. Moreover, if estradiol-17β is incubated with horse-radish peroxidase, Mn++ ions, and an excess of hydrogen donor (DPN, ethanol, and yeast alcohol dehydrogenase), it can be recovered from the reaction mixture virtually unchanged. The evidence available is consistent with the view that with monophenolic estrogens, the oxidized products (RO·) which transport hydrogen are phenoxy radicals, possibly stabilized as enzyme-phenoxy radical complexes. Of the compounds we examined, only diethylstilbestrol appears to undergo extensive chemical transformation under the conditions of these experiments. Isodienestrol (36) appears to be one of the products formed from diethylstilbestrol.

## OXIDATION OF REDUCED PYRIDINE NUCLEOTIDES BY UTERINE CYTOPLASMIC PARTICLES

Hollander and Stephens (14) have described a DPNH oxidase system bound to uterine cytoplasmic particles which bears a remarkable similarity to the horse-radish peroxidase-catalyzed model reactions just described. This uterine enzyme system oxidized DPNH and TPNH by molecular oxygen, required catalytic amounts of Mn++ ions and an appropriate phenol, and was inhibited by cyanide and by catalase. The activity of this oxidase system was negligible in uterine extracts prepared from spayed animals, but increased tremendously soon after the injection of either estradiol-17β or diethylstilbestrol. In this response to estrogens *in vivo*, the uterine oxidase system of Hollander and Stephens (14) resembled the uterine peroxidase discovered and characterized by Stotz and his collaborators (22, 24).

In collaboration with Libby (45), we have confirmed and extended the observations of Hollander and Stephens (14). In our experiments 3, 4-dimethylphenol was used as a carrier for the oxidation of DPNH. The phenol-activated oxidase system can be removed from uterine cytoplasmic particles by extraction with 1.2 M NaCl, and purified about threefold by further fractionation with ammonium sulfate. We found that the activity of this oxidase system in the uterine particles of spayed animals was increased approximately 150-fold seven days after the injection of diethylstilbestrol. Parallel measurements of the DPNH-cytochrome c reductase levels, and also of the aerobic oxidation of DPNH in the presence of cytochrome c, showed that these activities increased not more than twofold after estrogen administration. Our experiments suggest, but do not prove, that this uterine, phenol-activated, oxidase system is identical with the uterine peroxidase described by Stotz et al. (22, 24), as Hollander and Stephens (14) have considered.

Recent experiments by Temple and Hollander (35) show that under certain experimental conditions, estradiol-17β and other phenolic estrogens directly stimulate the uterine DPNH oxidase system in a similar manner to that which we observed in our model reactions with horse-radish peroxidase.

### REFERENCES

1. Akazawa, T., and Conn, E. E. *J. Biol. Chem.* **232**, 403 (1958).
2. Bergstrom, S., Theorell, H., and Westman, A. *Arkiv Kemi Mineral. Geol.* **19B** (6), 1-17 (1945).
3. Case, E. M., and Dickens, F. *Biochem. J.* **43**, 418 (1948).
4. Dodds, E. C. "Biochemical Contributions to Endocrinology." Stanford Univ. Press, Stanford, California, 1957.
5. Fishman, J., and Gallagher, T. F. *Arch. Biochem. Biophys.* **77**, 511 (1958).
6. Gordon, E. E., and Villee, C. A. *J. Biol. Chem.* **216**, 215 (1955).
7. Graubard, M., and Pincus, G. *Endocrinology* **30**, 265 (1942).
8. Hagerman, D. D., and Villee, C. A. *J. Biol. Chem.* **229**, 589 (1957).
9. Hagerman, D. D., and Villee, C. A. *J. Biol. Chem.* **234**, 2031 (1959).
10. Hochster, R. M., and Quastel, J. H. *Nature* **164**, 865 (1949).
11. Hochster, R. M., and Quastel, J. H. *Ann. N. Y. Acad. Sci.* **54**, 626 (1951).
12. Hollander, V. P., Hollander, N., and Brown, J. D. *J. Biol. Chem.* **234**, 1678 (1959).
13. Hollander, V. P., Hollander, N., and Brown, J. D. *Proc. Soc. Exptl. Biol. Med.* **101**, 475 (1959).
14. Hollander, V. P., and Stephens, M. L. *J. Biol. Chem.* **234**, 1901 (1959).
15. Holzer, H., and Schneider, S. *Biochem. Z.* **330**, 240 (1958).
16. Hurlock, B., and Talalay, P. *J. Biol. Chem.* **233**, 886 (1958).
17. Jellinck, P. H. *Biochem. J.* **71**, 665 (1959).
18. Klebanoff, S. J. *J. Biol. Chem.* **234**, 2480 (1959).
19. Kraychy, S., and Gallagher, T. F. *J. Biol. Chem.* **229**, 519 (1957).
20. Kubowitz, F. *Biochem. Z.* **292**, 32, 221 (1937).
21. Langer, L., and Engel, L. L. *J. Biol. Chem.* **233**, 583 (1958).
22. Lucas, F. V., Neufeld, H. A., Utterback, J. G., Martin, A. P., and Stotz, E. *J. Biol. Chem.* **214**, 775 (1955).
23. Marcus, P. I., and Talalay, P. *J. Biol. Chem.* **218**, 661 (1956).
24. Martin, A. P., Neufeld, H. A., Lucas, F. V., and Stotz, E. *J. Biol. Chem.* **233**, 206 (1959).
25. Meyer, R. K., and McShan, W. H. *Recent Prog. in Hormone Research* **5**, 465 (1950).
26. Mueller, G. C. *Nature* **176**, 127 (1955).
27. Salmony, D. *Biochem. J.* **62**, 411 (1956).
28. Talalay, P. *Physiol. Revs.* **37**, 362 (1957).
29. Talalay, P., and Adams, J. A. Unpublished observations.
30. Talalay, P., Hurlock, B., and Williams-Ashman, H. G. *Proc. Natl. Acad. Sci. U. S.* **44**, 862 (1958).
31. Talalay, P., and Levy, H. R. "Steric Course of Microbiological Reactions" (Ciba Foundation Study Group No. 2), p. 53. Churchill, London, 1959.
32. Talalay, P., and Marcus, P. I. *J. Biol. Chem.* **218**, 675 (1956).
33. Talalay, P., and Williams-Ashman, H. G. *Proc. Natl. Acad. Sci. U. S.* **44**, 15 (1958).

34. Talalay, P., and Williams-Ashman, H. G. *Recent Progr. in Hormone Research* **16**, 1 (1960).
35. Temple, S., and Hollander, V. P. *Abstr. 136th Natl. Meeting Am. Chem. Soc. Atlantic City, New Jersey* p. 76C (1959).
36. Vanderlinde, R. E., Vasington, F. D., and Westerfeld, W. W. *J. Am. Chem. Soc.* **77**, 4176 (1955).
37. Villee, C. A. *Cancer Research* **17**, 507 (1957).
38. Villee, C. A. *Perspectives in Biol. Med.* **2**, 290 (1959).
39. Villee, C. A., and Gordon, E. E. *J. Biol. Chem.* **216**, 203 (1955).
40. Villee, C. A., and Hagerman, D. D. *J. Biol. Chem.* **233**, 42 (1958).
41. Westerfield, W. W. *Biochem. J.* **34**, 51 (1940).
42. Williams-Ashman, H. G. *Abstr. 3rd Intern. Congr. Biochem. Brussels* p. 64 (1955).
43. Williams-Ashman, H. G., Cassman, M., and Klavins, M. *Federation Proc.* **18**, 352 (1959).
44. Williams-Ashman, H. G., Cassman, M., and Klavins, M. *Nature* **184**, 427 (1959).
45. Williams-Ashman, H. G., and Libby, P. Unpublished observations.

## DISCUSSION

**V. Hollander:** I would like to comment briefly on the phenol-activated oxidase system in rat uterus referred to by Dr. Williams-Ashman. This system has many properties of an induced enzyme system. Homogenates of uteri from spayed rats contain little or no phenol-activated reduced pyridine nucleotide oxidase. The administration of small quantities of estradiol, stilbestrol, or hexestrol to these animals produces a prompt response with a very remarkable increase in oxidase activity. Estradiol and hexestrol may function as *in vitro* phenolic cofactors for DPNH oxidation. The administration of estradiol to the rat results in the appearance of an enzyme in the uterus which uses this phenol as a cofactor for the oxidation of an important metabolite. Whether or not this DPNH oxidase is in fact uterine peroxidase is not known. I think that considerable work on this system will be necessary before its mechanism is elucidated, and at the time I don't believe anyone would be willing to speculate about its possible physiological role.

**G. C. Mueller:** Dr. Hollander, have you tried different nonestrogenic phenolic compounds for this enzyme induction?

**V. Hollander:** We have given phenol and 2,4,-dichlorophenol to animals in an effort to induce the enzyme, and no effect was seen.

**G. C. Mueller:** I had been interested in this work for a long time, in fact, ever since it appeared that Dr. Talalay could grow microorganisms on testosterone as the sole source of carbon. It doesn't surprise me that one finds steroid dehydrogenase arising in organisms which are submerged in steroid hormones as their sole source of carbon growth. In this connection it is also of interest to me that in the case of the placenta the situation is somewhat analogous. Similarly there are estrogens present during the development of the mammary gland tissue and, again, Dr. Hollander has found the transhydrogenase to be present. The thing that bothers me is that when we come to a hormonally responsive tissue like the rat uterus we have been unable to show any evidence for this so-called transdehydrogenation. I'm wondering whether this suggests that this particular tissue, not having been submerged in estrogen for a long period of time, has had no need for adaptively developing degradative metabolic pathways for the estrogen.

**H. G. Williams-Ashman:** Dr. Mueller's comment is most appropriate. If these estrogen-stimulated hydrogen transfers are indeed responsible for any of the physiological actions of estrogens, then the enzymes that catalyze them should be present in estrogen-sensitive tissues. However, the estrogen-activated transhydrogenase reactions we have studied are relatively slow compared with those of many other pyridine nucleotide-linked dehydrogenases (although this does not necessarily imply that they have no relation to the mode of action of estrogens). It is sometimes difficult to demonstrate these reactions in crude tissue extracts because of the presence of interfering enzymes. For example, enzyme systems that oxidize TPNH and DPNH, and also enzymes that degrade pyridine nucleotides at various positions in the molecule, are particularly active in certain accessory sexual tissues. Thus, negative evidence relating to the presence of estrogen-activated transhydrogenase systems in tissues which are particularly responsive to gonadal hormones should be interpreted cautiously.

**G. C. Mueller:** One simple question, Dr. Williams-Ashman: Have you looked for this transhydrogenase reaction in rat uterus?

**H. G. Williams-Ashman:** Gerald Gotterer, Shutsung Liao, and I have spent nearly six months looking for estradiol- and testosterone-stimulated transhydrogenations between pyridine nucleotides in rodent male accessory sexual tissues such as the prostate gland and seminal vesicle. We were unable to obtain evidence for such enzyme systems. However, our experiments were complicated by the fact that these tissues degrade pyridine nucleotides, and especially TPN and TPNH, at extremely rapid rates. We have not looked for estrogen-sensitive transhydrogenase reactions in the tissues of the female genital tract of the rat.

**V. Hollander:** We have failed to find estradiol-sensitive transhydrogenase in rat placenta. The explanation for this may be that the 17$\beta$-hydroxysteroid dehydrogenase is present in the particulate fraction in this species. If this enzyme is implicated in transhydrogenation, its presence in this fraction may make it technically difficult to demonstrate transhydrogenation when the other factors required are in the soluble fraction.

**Y. J. Topper:** I would like to ask Dr. Hollander whether there is any evidence which would implicate any of the thyroid hormones in the activation of these oxidases.

**V. Hollander:** Dr. Klebanoff has been interested in model systems somewhat similar to those described by Dr. Williams-Ashman in which thyroxine and triiodothyronine are used as the phenolic cofactors. Very similar coenzyme activities of these phenols can be demonstrated in Dr. Klebanoff's systems.

**P. Ofner:** Was an attempt made to demonstrate the dual role of the system as a steroid oxidoreductase and a phosphopyridine nucleotide transdehydrogenase by following the enzymatic transfer of labeled hydrogen and its distribution after addition of all participating substrates? In comment, I should like to suggest that the 2-, 3-, and 4,5-dione enols may act as $C_{19}$ analogs of the $o$-diphenols which Dr. Williams-Ashman showed to be potential hydrogen carriers in the presence of phenolase or peroxidase. The triterpenoid $\alpha$-Elaterin contains this functional group.

**H. G. Williams-Ashman:** The stereospecific transfer of hydrogen from estradiol-17$\beta$ to both DPN and TPN in the dehydrogenase reaction, and also from DPNH to the 3-acetylpyridine analog of DPN in the transhydrogenase reaction, has been demonstrated with the human placental enzyme system by Talalay and Jarabak. In regard to your second question, we have chemical evidence which suggests that, in the case of estradiol-17$\beta$, this compound transports hydrogen in the presence of certain phenolases by undergoing an initial hydroxylation to an *o*-diphenolic derivative(s), which, in turn, is reversibly oxidized to the corresponding *o*-quinone. We have not tested compounds of the type you mention for their ability to transport hydrogen in these phenolase-catalyzed reactions.

**G. Pincus:**   One of the consequences of the action of the estrogens is the growth of tissue. I would like to ask whether there is any indication that the enzyme systems by you and by Dr. Hollander in any way might be concerned with growth. Now I know there is a facile answer, i.e., you get TPNH and that sets many processes in motion; but that leaves me rather unsatisfied intellectually. Somewhat more technical and probably easier to answer is the question of the action of compounds that act as antagonists to estrogens, e.g., familiar hormones such as progestins or corticoids. What are the effects of such compounds in the systems which you have studied?

**H. G. Williams-Ashman:**   The mere demonstration of hormone-dependent oxido-reductions of the type I have described does not necessarily mean that such reactions are involved, in any way, in the stimulation of growth and function by gonadal hormones. Our philosophy has been that it is first necessary to understand the chemistry of these reactions, and the properties of the enzymes which catalyze them, before one can undertake meaningful experimentation which relates to their wider physiological significance.

We have not studied the possible inhibitory action of other classes of steroid hormones upon these estrogen-mediated reactions. However, a considerable amount of interesting work in this area has been performed by Dr. Villee and his collaborators. Villee has shown, for example, that certain analogs of stilbestrol, which were synthesized by Barany in Sweden, antagonize the action of estradiol-17β in the placental transhydrogenase system.

**C. Chen:**   Dr. Sam Koide in our laboratory has prepared the rat liver enzyme or enzymes according to the procedure of Dr. Williams-Ashman and others and has found that the androsterone-mediated transhydrogenation is inhibited by a catalytic amount of testosterone. I wonder what it all means, since testosterone is generally considered the primary androgen.

**H. G. Williams-Ashman:**   I was most interested to hear about these experiments performed by Dr. Chen. I presume you are referring to the soluble 3α-hydroxysteroid dehydrogenase of rat liver. Hurlock and Talalay showed that a variety of 3α-hydroxy- and 3-ketosteroids mediate the transfer of hydrogen between pyridine nucleotides in the presence of this enzyme. The steroids which are active in this system vary greatly in the degree and type of their physiological activities. It is unlikely that this enzyme is the only hydroxysteroid dehydrogenase with dual nucleotide specificity which catalyzes transhydrogenations mediated by androgenic steroids. But it seems to me that it is of the utmost importance that the interaction of different types of physiologically active steroids with such transhydrogenase systems be studied with relatively pure enzyme preparations.

**F. C. Greenwood:**   Have you determined whether high levels of hormones inhibit the transhydrogenase reactions? Perhaps this might bridge the gap between the hypothesis of one mechanism of hormone action and the role of estrogen in cancer. A reduction in estrogens after the present methods of endocrine surgery has been shown, and if regressions are due to this, then one would assume that a reduction in transhydrogenation in the body would follow. I am just wondering how this would be manifested, if at all, and whether any steroids, say cortisone, would replace estrogen in this transhydrogenation reaction. I must apologize for pushing you on the cancer side, but workers in clinical research are always interested in integrating fundamental research into the mosaic of the cancer problem.

**H. G. Williams-Ashman:** If I may answer Dr. Greenwood's second question first, we have tested the action of a number of steroid hormones on the placental transhydrogenase system which is activated by estradiol-17β and found that cortisone does not mediate hydrogen transfers in the presence of this enzyme. Previously, Dr. Villee observed that cortisone was inert in this system.

In regard to the first question, there is evidence for the inhibition of the rate of reduction of pyridine nucleotides by high concentrations of certain steroids in oxidations catalyzed by some hydroxysteroid dehydrogenases. Talalay found that this was the case when testosterone was used as a substrate for the β-hydroxysteroid dehydrogenase of *Pseudomonas testosteroni*. The action of quite a number of pyridine nucleotide-linked dehydrogenases is, in fact, depressed at high substrate concentrations, and the degree of inhibition often varies with the nature of the substrate and/or pyridine nucleotide which is present in the reaction mixture. To my knowledge, none of the steroids which mediate transhydrogenation in the presence of the soluble placental enzyme system depresses the rate of hydrogen transfer from TPNH to DPN at high concentrations. I may add that Villee has shown that large amounts of diethylstilbestrol inhibit estradiol-17β-mediated transhydrogenations catalyzed by the placental system, and also that Talalay and Marcus have shown that both diethylstilbestrol and hexestrol are potent inhibitors of the oxidation of testosterone by the β-hydroxysteroid dehydrogenase of *Pseudomonas testosteroni*.

**S. Kushinsky:** I should like to ask Dr. Mueller if he would expand on the point he made about the concentration of estrogens in breast, following the statement that there is a rather high concentration of estrogens in placenta.

**G. C. Mueller:** I didn't say there is a high concentration of estrogens in the breast; I simply said that the breast tissue in order to be physiologically perpetuated required a continuing source of this hormone and this might be involved in adaptive changes. I have no chemical analysis on breast tissue for estrogens.

**L. L. Engel:** I would like to come back to this question of inhibition. In our laboratory, Mr. Cowan has recently shown that estradiol-17α is a competitive inhibitor of the DPN-mediated estradiol-17β dehydrogenase. I wondered if it had the same effect on the transhydrogenase.

**H. G. Williams-Ashman:** We have not studied the possible inhibition of estradiol-17β mediated transhydrogenations by estradiol-17α. However, Dr. Villee showed originally that estradiol-17α did not stimulate hydrogen transfers in the human placental transhydrogenase system, and perhaps I might ask him whether he has observed any inhibitory action of estradiol-17α under these conditions.

**C. A. Villee:** We had some estradiol-17α that we got three or four years ago from Paul Munson, which I believe was the inactive isomer. This does indeed inactivate or competitively inhibit the transhydrogenase; but more recently we have bought some material said to be estradiol-17α from a commercial firm, and it is just as good as estradiol-17β in stimulating transhydrogenation.

**K. Thompson:** I have had some experience with the supplies of the so-called inactive estradiol. One should bear in mind that this material is obtained from urine and it is possible that impurities in some of the early samples might very well be a serious problem. If there is some interest in this particular compound, as there seems to be, it ought to be possible to get a sample that would be very highly purified. I believe the latest samples which have been used have been prepared with greatest care, but if there is any doubt the sample should be subjected to further purification.

**A. White:**    In another way I would like to underline what Dr. Williams-Ashman indicated in response to efforts to push him into interpreting the physiological significance of his data. I think it is fair to say that studies of the type which he has described, as well as other programs by members of this audience, are studies of the effects of steroids *in vitro* on either crude, semipurified, or more highly purified enzyme systems. There perhaps should be an extra word of caution against efforts to transfer the information from these studies to clinical situations. I make these comments for the following reasons. There are tissues in which estradiol may inhibit the utilization of a substrate, whether one studies this inhibition in an *in vitro* system or whether one rejects the steroid and then from the injected animal removes the tissue and examines its capacity to utilize a specific substrate, e.g., glucose, *in vitro* in the absence of additional steroid. Dr. Villee's observations have certainly supported and provided evidence for the concept that small amounts of estradiol will catalyze the activity of isocitric dehydrogenase in soluble extracts of placenta as well as other tissues. We have observed that estradiol added *in vitro* may inhibit the utilization by lymphoid tissue of pyruvate or succinate, which are also members of the tricarboxylic acid cycle. These data then emphasize that augmentation or inhibition of different enzyme systems may be obtained by addition of the same steroid *in vitro* to different tissues. It would thus seem highly premature to attempt to infer possible physiological significance of such data.

As another example, steroids which, insofar as we know, have no demonstrable morphological effect upon lymphoid tissue have very profound influences upon the enzymatic processes in this tissue, whether one incubates the tissue *in vitro* with the steroid or injects the steroid and then examines the tissue *in vitro* without additional steroid. It is very striking indeed to inject into one animal cortisol, a well-known involutor of lymphoid tissue, and to inject into another animal deoxycorticosterone, which ostensibly has no effect on lymphoid tissue structure or size, to prepare from each of these two lymphoid tissue sources a cell-free extract, and to study the capacity of these extracts to utilize glucose, succinate, or pyruvate and find that the degree of inhibition of the utilization of these substrates is just as striking when the tissue is prepared from the deoxy steroid-injected animal as from the cortisol-injected animal. This again re-emphasizes that we are studying the effects of steroids on specific or multienzyme systems. The possible physiological significance of such data is certainly not clear at the present time.

**H. G. Williams-Ashman:**    I would like to agree with the sentiments expressed by Dr. White. The utmost caution must be taken in attributing physiological significance to the demonstration of any effects of hormones upon isolated enzyme systems, especially when the enzymes used are rather impure. However, I would like to point out that the types of reaction I described this morning are of a somewhat different character from many of the reported actions of steroid hormones *in vitro* upon the action of various enzyme systems. In these reactions the amounts of hormones required to *stimulate* hydrogen transfers may be as much as four orders of magnitude lower than those usually required to *inhibit* the action of certain enzymes. Also, in the studies I presented, the hormones appear to transport hydrogen by undergoing alternate oxidation and reduction, and hence *participate* in these reactions.

# Fate of Steroid Estrogens in Target Tissues[1]

ELWOOD V. JENSEN AND HERBERT I. JACOBSON[2]

*The Ben May Laboratory for Cancer Research, The University of Chicago, Chicago, Illinois*

Through the fog which envelops our understanding of the general problem of growth and its physiological control, the steroid sex hormones stand out as agents whose participation in specific growth processes is clearly recognized. What these substances can do in promoting and restraining growth is well established. But how they do it is quite another matter. And, as you can see from the preceding presentations, the biochemical mechanism of steroid hormone action is a field which currently is receiving considerable attention.

Now when the organic or physical chemist talks about a "mechanism," it goes without saying that he knows the identity both of the reactants and of the final products, so that his concern is with the intermediate processes by which the transformation takes place. In many biological systems, unfortunately, the state of our knowledge is not so favorable, and, in the case of hormonal promotion of tissue growth, we really know neither the reactants nor the products. We administer what presumably is one of the reactants, the steroid, at a point far removed from the reaction site, and what happens to it on its way to the target tissue, how much of it actually gets there, what it reacts with when once there, and what happens chemically to the steroid as it stimulates growth, all are subjects known mostly by inference, speculation, or hypothesis.[3]

This is not to say that much valuable knowledge has not been secured concerning the metabolic transformation of steroids by mammalian organisms. The major part of such information comes from the elegant and detailed investigations of urinary steroids, and this is logical, for the urine is a rich source of steroid metabolites. Further knowledge concerning steroid metabolism has been obtained by incubating tissue slices or homogenates with steroid substrates and identifying the transformation products formed. Yet all this information, valuable as it is in the over-all endocrine picture, does not bear directly on the question of what takes place in the tissue which grows under hormonal stimulation. It is difficult to be sure whether

[1] This investigation was supported by a research grant from the National Institutes of Health, United States Public Health Service (CY-2897).

[2] The experiments here reported were carried out by G. N. Gupta, J. W. Flesher, L. Closs, A. Bhattacharya, M. E. Pont, S. Hennix, and C. Fernandez. We are grateful to Dr. Katherine Sydnor for valuable assistance in the animal experiments.

[3] Recently, information concerning the incorporation of the synthetic estrogen, hexestrol, into tissues of the goat has been obtained by Glascock and Hoekstra (4).

the urinary steroid metabolites result from reactions involved in growth processes, or whether they reflect transformations occurring in the course of degradation, transport, and excretion. And while tissue incubation studies tell us what a tissue or organ *can* do when presented with a certain steroid, they do not necessarily tell us what it *does* do in the physiological situation.

In considering these limitations on the present status of our knowledge about steroid-controlled growth, it seemed to us that information concerning the chemical fate—in the *specific target tissues*—of physiological amounts of steroid sex hormones should prove of value in the ultimate understanding of growth mechanisms. One difficulty with such studies is the relatively small dose of sex hormone required for physiological activity, and this is especially serious in the case of the estrogens. In our mind it is quite important that no more than physiological amounts of steroid hormone be administered if conclusions as to chemical fate are to be related to growth processes. Thus, it appeared that to get the information we desired, we would need special tools including radioactive steroids of unusually high specific activity. The highest activity possible with $C^{14}$ appeared insufficient for the purpose, so we turned to the use of tritium, which can be obtained carrier-free with a specific activity of about 60 curies per millimole of gas. And we began with the steroid estrogens.

## TRITIATION OF STEROID ESTROGENS

I shall say only a brief word about the preparation of tritiated estrogens. We obtained estradiol labeled in the 6,7-position by the catalytic reduction of 6-dehydroestradiol (Fig. 1). Reduction with a mixture of 10 % tritium

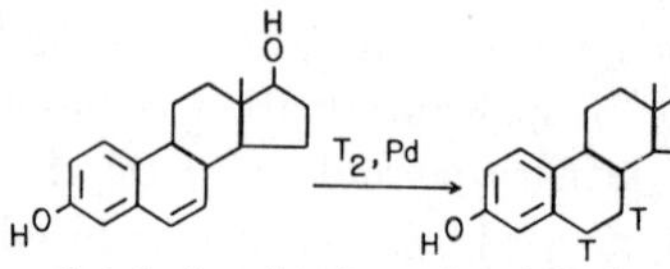

FIG. 1.   Catalytic tritiation of 6-dehydroestradiol.

in hydrogen gave a product with specific activity of 20 mc./mg., whereas reduction with carrier-free tritium gas gave estradiol of 117–195 mc./mg. This means that one can measure 1 μμg. of the substance. Thus, if the dose administered to a rat is 0.1 μg. one has the activity needed to track down 1/100,000 part of the administered steroid. We prepared 6,7-tritiated estrone by enzymatic oxidation of the tritiated estradiol using the bacterial enzyme of Hurlock and Talalay (7), and 9,11-tritiated estrone by catalytic reduction of 9(11)-dehydroestrone.

The apparatus developed for the tritiation of 3–5-mg. amounts of steroids is shown in Fig. 2. It is a microhydrogenation apparatus consisting of a reaction vessel, a mercury piston, and a sensitive horizontal null-point manometer designed so as to permit complete recovery of the excess gas. As tritium is absorbed by the magnetically stirred steroid solution (in ethylene glycol dimethyl ether with palladium black catalyst), the pressure in that part of the apparatus falls and the mercury droplet in the horizontal manometer moves to the left. One determines the volume of tritium absorbed by measuring the amount of mercury which must be added through a syringe operated by a screw micrometer to bring the pressure back to the original level as indicated by movement of the mercury drop back to its original position. The total gas volume of 20 ml. means that one works with about 50 curies of tritium, of which about 1 curie is incorporated into the steroid. Since 50 curies is more activity than one is allowed to bring to the University

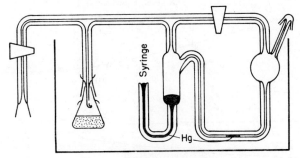

FIG. 2.  Tritiation apparatus.

of Chicago campus, the tritiations were carried out at the Argonne National Laboratory, and we are grateful to Drs. Kenneth Wilzbach and Louis Kaplan for making their facilities available to us.

It is interesting that there is no adverse isotope effect in the tritiation of the steroid double bond; in fact, the reduction appears to go a little faster with tritium than with hydrogen and is complete in 12–14 minutes. Complete reduction is confirmed by paper chromatography of an aliquot of the product. The reaction mixture obtained from 10 % tritium in hydrogen contains estradiol as the only nonvolatile radioactive material, and a benzene stock solution of this substance shows no appreciable decomposition after one year's storage. With the high-level estradiol, obtained with carrier-free tritium, there are other nonvolatile radioactive substances present, and there is gradual radiochemical decomposition on storage in solution (Fig. 3). The estradiol content (Fraction IV) gradually decreases to about 50 % after one year and to 25 % after 18 months. Thus, such highly radioactive steroids are usable at least a year and a half after preparation; but, at all stages, the material taken for an animal experiment should be purified by simple paper chromatography (Bush B-3) to insure that only estradiol is being administered.

## INCORPORATION PATTERN OF RADIOACTIVE ESTROGENS

The first question we wished to answer with our radioactive hormone was how much actually goes to the tissues which grow. In the young rat, a single dose of estradiol which gives a well-defined but not maximal uterine growth response is 0.1 µg.; so we set out to determine the amount of radioactivity present in various organs and tissues at different times intervals after the administration of this dose by both intravenous and subcutaneous

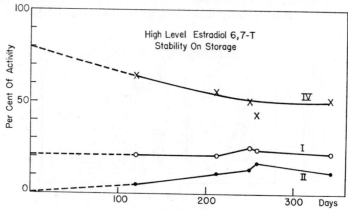

FIG. 3. Radioactivity in various paper chromatogram fractions on paper chromatography (Bush B-3) of aliquots of high-level stock solution. Fraction I = origin; Fraction IV = estradiol.

routes. To do this it was necessary to develop a method for the routine assay of tritium in tissues and blood; this assay works well and a detailed report will appear in the literature soon (8).

Following the single intravenous administration of 0.1 µg. of estradiol (in this case with specific activity of about 9 mc./mg.) to 24-day-old female rats, a maximum of radioactivity was observed in the uterus and cervix between 15 minutes and 1 hour. The amount present represents 0.2 % of that administered or 200 µµg. (Fig. 4). Vagina showed a similar pattern with about half as much incorporation, but ovary obtained its maximum radioactivity immediately, with more rapid decrease thereafter. The same relationship in incorporation patterns of uterus, vagina, and ovary following intravenous estradiol were observed repeatedly. When ten times as much hormone (1.0 µg.) was administered, about five times the radioactivity was present in the uterus in the early stages, but rapid clearance of the excess hormone took place, so that after 2 hours about 1.5 as much activity was present with the larger dose (Fig. 5).

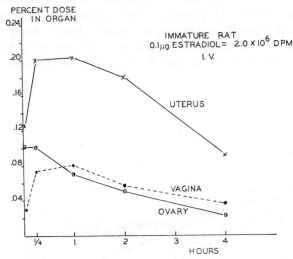

FIG. 4. Radioactivity in various organs after single intravenous administration of medium-level estradiol. Each point is the median value for samples from six animals. Uterus includes cervix.

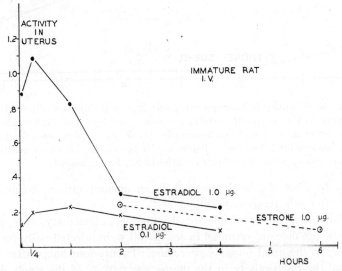

FIG. 5. Radioactivity in uterus after single intravenous administration of different doses of medium-level estradiol and high-level estrone. Each point is the median value of samples from six animals.

A roughly similar pattern was observed in the rat uterus when more highly radioactive estradiol was administered in doses of the order of 0.1 μg. (Fig. 6). After subcutaneous injection the maximum radioactivity was present in the uterus at 15 minutes to 2 hours, corresponding to about 0.15 % of the amount injected, or 150 μμg. of steroid. After 6 hours this activity had declined to about 0.08 % of the amount administered, or 80 μμg. After intravenous administration the initial radioactivity in the uterus was some-

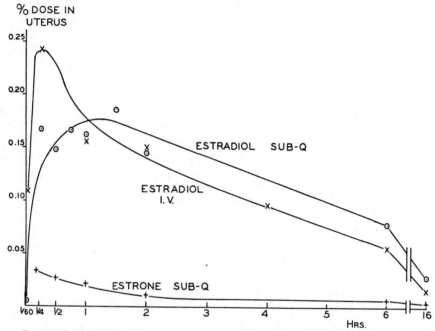

FIG. 6. Radioactivity in immature rat uterus after single injection of steroid in saline. Intravenous (I.V.) estradiol: 0.094 μg. (specific activity 96 μc./μg.); subcutaneous (Sub-Q) estradiol: 0.098 μg. (specific activity 117 μc./μg.); subcutaneous estrone: 0.10 μg. (specific activity 135 μc./μg.). Points for intravenous injections are median values for eight animals; points for subcutaneous injections, for six animals.

what higher, but the level soon fell to an amount rather similar to that present after subcutaneous injection.

Similar orders of magnitude for the uterine radioactivity were observed when 0.05-μg. doses of estradiol in sesame oil were injected daily for 7 days according to the usual bioassay procedure. Twenty-four hours after the last injection, the radioactivity in the uterus was 0.07 % of the single dose (or 0.01 % of the total dose), equivalent to 35 μμg. of steroid. Thus, it would appear that, whether administered intravenously or subcutaneously, the amount of steroid present in the uterus during the period when growth is being induced is a very small fraction of the already small administered dose, and is of the order of 30–150 μμg. These amounts are even smaller than those found by Mühlbock (10) and by Emmens (2) to stimulate cornification when applied directly on the vaginal epithelium.

It is interesting to compare the incorporation patterns of uterus and vagina with those of tissues which do not exhibit the marked growth response to

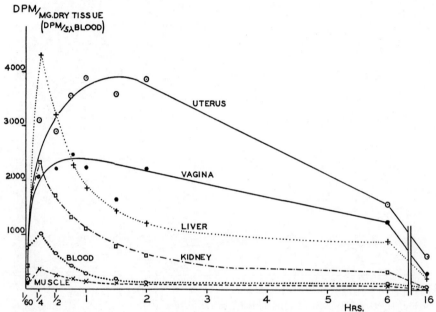

Fig. 7. Concentration of radioactivity in rat tissues after single subcutaneous injection of 0.098 μg. of estradiol (specific activity 117 μc./μg.) in saline. Liver and kidney points are mean values of 3 aliquots of dried pooled tissue; other points are median values of individual samples from six animals.

estrogens. In Fig. 7, the data from the foregoing single subcutaneous injection experiment are plotted in terms of radioactivity per milligram of dry tissue; since for most tissues 1 mg. dry weight is equivalent to about 5 μl. of fresh tissue volume, the values for blood are expressed in terms of DPM per 5 μl. Two facts are clear from these measurements. First, the incorporation patterns of liver, kidney, muscle, and blood (and for adrenal and bone not illustrated) are different from those of uterus and vagina, in that the former tissues reach their maximum activity very early with rapid decrease thereafter, whereas uterus and vagina continue to incorporate and retain steroid for a much longer period. Second, with the exception of muscle, the concentration of steroid in the tissues is considerably higher than that in the blood, although, the decrease in radioactivity in all tissues except uterus and vagina appears to parallel the fall in blood level.

The difference in steroid incorporation pattern of uterus and vagina from that of the other tissues is more pronounced when lower doses of estradiol are given (Fig. 8). Following a single subcutaneous dose of 0.01 µg. of estradiol in saline, the ability of uterus and vagina to incorporate and retain

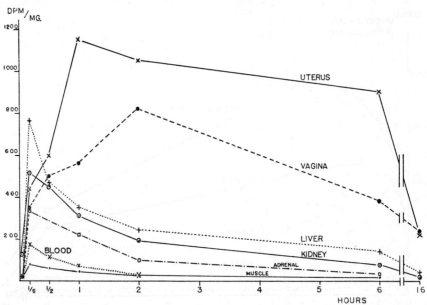

FIG. 8. Concentration of radioactivity in rat tissues after single subcutaneous injection of approximately 0.01 µg. of estradiol (specific activity 195 µc./µg.) in saline. Values are expressed as in Fig. 7. Liver and kidney points are mean values of 4 aliquots of dried pooled tissue; other points are median values of individual samples from six animals.

steroid, when the activity in the other tissues has markedly declined, is quite striking.

One other tissue I would like to mention is the pituitary, and here we have done just one experiment so what I say must be taken as only tentative. Following intravenous administration of 0.1 µg. of estradiol, Dr. Sydnor separated the anterior and posterior lobes of the pituitaries which were then assayed for radioactivity (Fig. 9). In contrast to the previous graphs, where each point represents the median value of samples from six or eight animals assayed separately, in the case of pituitary, eight lobes for each time point were pooled, the pools assayed, and each result divided by eight. The anterior pituitary, which is known to be influenced by steroid hormones, shows an incorporation pattern quite similar to that of uterus and vagina reaching a maximum radioactivity which corresponds to 2.5 μμg. of estradiol per pituitary. The posterior lobe, on the other hand, which is not known to be concerned with steroid hormones, showed maximum radioactivity immediately with rapid decrease thereafter. If this preliminary observation can be repeated and confirmed, I think it demonstrates an interesting difference between the two portions of the hypophysis.

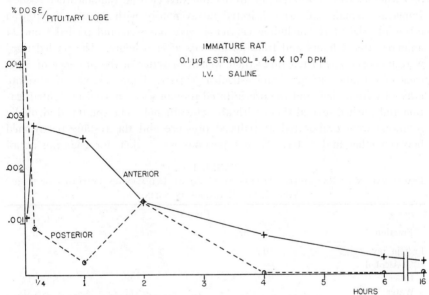

FIG. 9. Radioactivity in different pituitary lobes after single intravenous administration of high-level estradiol. Each point was calculated from single assay of eight pooled organs.

In examining these incorporation curves of estradiol into rat uterus, we wondered whether such studies could furnish information concerning the relation of estrogen structure and activity. It has always been an interesting question as to why it takes ten times as much estrone as estradiol to bring about the same uterine growth response. After intravenous administration of a physiological dose of estrone (1.0 μg.), there was only slightly more radioactivity in the uterus at 2 and 6 hours than from 0.1 μg. of estradiol (Fig. 5); this might suggest that estrone is only one-tenth as efficient in getting into the uterus, if it were not for the fact that administration of 1.0 μg. of estradiol did not give rise to much more activity in uterus during this period. When 0.1 μg. of estrone was administered subcutaneously, however, the amount of radioactivity reaching the uterus was only about one-tenth as much when the same amount of estradiol was given (Fig. 6). If this observation can be repeated and confirmed under different conditions of dose and administration, it may serve to explain the lower physiological activity of estrone as compared to estradiol.

### Nature of Radioactive Material in Uterus and Liver

The next problem is the nature of the radioactive material in the tissues and whether this is different in uterus and vagina from that in other tissues. Immature female rats were injected intravenously with 0.1 µg. of tritiated estradiol; the uteri (including cervices) were removed and pooled from 24 animals after 2 hours and from 36 animals after 6 hours. The pooled uteri were homogenized in ten times their weight of water in the presence of 5 µg. each of estradiol, estrone, and estriol as carrier. Four volumes of absolute ethanol were added, and the precipitated protein was removed by centrifugation and washed several times with absolute ethanol. The combined alcoholic solutions were evaporated at reduced pressure and the residue partitioned between ether and water. Aliquot portions were taken for counting at all

TABLE I

FRACTIONATION OF RADIOACTIVE TISSUES AFTER SINGLE INTRAVENOUS INJECTION OF 0.1 µG. HIGH-LEVEL ESTRADIOL IN SALINE[a]

| Fraction | Uterus | | Liver |
| | 2 hr. | 6 hr. | 2 hr. |
| --- | --- | --- | --- |
| Protein ppt. | 0.7 | 1.5 | 38 |
| 80% Alcohol | 99 | 98 | 47 |
|   Ether | 90 | 78 | 12 |
|   Water | 8 | 17 | 31 |

[a] As per cent of total radioactivity in homogenate.

stages, and the results are summarized in Table I, expressed as percentage of the total radioactivity in each homogenate. It is clear that, in uterus, very little radioactive material is bound to the alcohol-insoluble protein and that relatively little is in a water-soluble form. The picture is quite different in liver taken at 2 hours, when about half the radioactive material is bound to the protein precipitate and, of the unbound protein portion, about three-fourths is in a water-soluble form becoming ether-soluble after acid hydrolysis.

When the ether-soluble fractions, representing most of the radioactive material from the 2-hour and 6-hour uteri, were chromatographed on paper in a slightly modified Bush B-5 system, practically all the radioactivity moved with the estradiol fraction (Table II). Elution and rechromatography in a Bush B-3 system confirmed this identification. There was a very small amount of activity in the estrone fraction from the 6-hour uteri, which has yet to be rechromatographed and identified with certainty. In the same table are the results with the ether fraction from an experiment in which 0.1 μg. of estrone was administered intravenously. Although the latter is a single preliminary experiment which should be considered as only tentative, it suggests that administered estrone may be converted to a variety of products. It is interesting to note that Gallagher (3) has reported recently that the common urinary estrogen metabolites appear to arise from estrone rather than from estradiol.

TABLE II

CHROMATOGRAPHY OF ETHER-SOLUBLE FRACTION FROM UTERUS[a]

(0.1 μG. STEROID, I.V.)

| Fraction | Estradiol | | Estrone |
|---|---|---|---|
| | 2 hr. | 6 hr. | 2 hr. |
| 1 | 0.4 | 0.5 | 13 |
| 2 (Estriol) | 0.4 | 0.4 | 12 |
| 3 | 0.3 | 0.8 | — |
| 4 | 1.1 | 0.6 | 3 |
| 5 (Estradiol) | 96.2 | 93.2 | 29 |
| 6 (Estrone) | 1.3 | 3.9 | 22 |
| 7 | 0.3 | 0.3 | 21 |

[a] As per cent of activity recovered. Chromatography in modified Bush B-5 system in presence of carrier estradiol, estrone, and estriol.

TABLE III

FRACTIONATION OF RADIOACTIVE TISSUES AFTER SEVEN DAILY SUBCUTANEOUS INJECTIONS OF 0.05 μG. HIGH-LEVEL ESTRADIOL IN SESAME OIL[a]

| Fraction | Uterus | Liver |
|---|---|---|
| Protein ppt. | 0.9 | 41 |
| 80% Alcohol | 99.9 | 42 |
| Ether | 74 | 33 |
| Water | 6 | 9 |

[a] As per cent of total radioactivity in homogenate. Tissues taken 24 hours after the last injection.

A somewhat similar pattern was seen when 0.05 μg. of estradiol in sesame oil was administered daily for 7 days with the uteri and livers taken 24 hours after the last injection (Table III). On fractionation as previously described, again there was practically no binding of the steroid to the alcohol-insoluble protein of uterus and the major portion of the radioactive material was soluble in ether. In the liver, on the other hand, a substantial amount of radioactive substance was bound to protein, although in this 7-day experiment relatively little water-soluble metabolite was present. On paper chromatography, most of the radioactivity of the ether soluble fraction from uteri moved with estradiol, although in this case, there appeared to be two other significant components, one more polar than estradiol and one less polar (Table IV). Chromatography of the ether -soluble material from liver gave no predominant radioactive fraction; further work is necessary for the identification of the substances present.

TABLE IV

CHROMATOGRAPHY OF ETHER-SOLUBLE FRACTION[a]

(7 × 0.05 μG. ESTRADIOL, SUBCUTANEOUSLY IN OIL)

| Fraction | Uterus | Liver |
|---|---|---|
| 1 | 14 | 11 |
| 2 (Estradiol | 2 | 12 |
| 3 | 2 | 15 |
| 4 | 3 | 17 |
| 5 (Estradiol) | 69 | 23 |
| 6 (Estrone) | 10 | 22 |

[a] As per cent of activity recovered. Chromatography in modified Bush B-5 system in presence of carrier estradiol, estrone, and estriol.

Thus, it is clear that the chemical nature of the radioactive material present in rat uterus following the administration of tritiated estradiol differs considerably from that present in liver, and the uterine steroid would appear to be predominantly unchanged estradiol under all the conditions investigated.

The final and, perhaps most important, question we should like to answer is whether there is a selective intracellular localization of the radioactive steroid in the mitochondria, microsomes, nuclei, cytoplasm, or perhaps cell membranes. At present, we can merely pose the question and state that we are investigating the problem by means of our tritiated estrogen, using both fractionation and autoradiographic techniques.

## HORMONE ANTAGONISM

As discussed in some detail by Dr. Drill, it is well established that certain steroids can exert a marked inhibitory effect on the physiological actions of other steroids. One such example is the ability of progestational hormones to inhibit the uterine and vaginal responses to estrogens (1, 5, 9). In a study which Dr. Huggins and I carried out a few years ago (6), 9α-fluoro-11β-hydroxyprogesterone (FHP) was particularly effective in this regard. Conceivably, the FHP might antagonize the estrogen either by preventing its incorporation into the responsive tissue or else by interfering with its action at the receptor level. As a preliminary approach to this problem, we determined the amount of radioactivity incorporated into the uteri both of immature and of hypophysectomized rats following seven daily subcutaneous injections of 0.1 µg. of tritiated estradiol in sesame oil, with and without the simultaneous injection of 1.0 mg. of fluorohydroxyprogesterone. As seen in Table V, in the immature rat the inhibited uterus is about half as large

TABLE V

EFFECT OF 9α-FLUORO-11β-HYDROXYPROGESTERONE ON INCORPORATION
OF ESTRADIOL INTO RAT UTERUS[a]

| | Uterine weight (mg.) | | DPM/organ | DPM/mg. (dry) |
|---|---|---|---|---|
| | Wet | Dry | | |
| *Immature* | | | | |
| Estradiol alone | 197 | 52 | 1375 | 27 |
| Estradiol + FHP | 110 | 26 | 760 | 30 |
| Control | 54 | 15 | — | — |
| *Hypophysectomized* | | | | |
| Estradiol alone | 245 | 37 | 2020 | 55 |
| Estradiol + FHP | 82 | 18 | 888 | 49 |
| Control | 17 | 6 | — | — |

[a] 0.1 µg. Estradiol (20 µc./µg.) and 1.0 mg. FHP administered daily for 7 days by subcutaneous injection in sesame oil. Tissues assayed on eighth day. Each figure is the mean value of samples from six animals.

as the noninhibited uterus (on either a wet or dry weight basis), and incorporates about half as much radioactive steroid. A roughly similar pattern is seen with the hypophysectomized animals. One might conclude that the inhibited uterus grows only half as big because the FHP reduces by a factor of two the amount of estradiol incorporated, or one may argue that, if the total amount of estradiol taken up depends on the size of the organ, the similar concentration of radioactivity in both cases signifies that the inhibitor has no effect on estradiol incorporation. But no matter how one wishes to interpret the result, it is interesting that the rat uterus incorporates half as much estrogen and grows to half the size when the inhibitor is present.

SUMMARY

Tritiated estradiol and estrone have been prepared with specific activity sufficient to permit measurement of 1µµg. of steroid; a method has been developed for the routine assay of tritium in animal tissues. These tools have made possible the accurate determination of the amount and nature of radioactive steroid present in various tissues of the immature rat at different time intervals after the administration of physiological amounts of steroid estrogens. Two to six hours after the injection of 0.1 μg. of estradiol, the amount of steroid present in the uterus is of the order of 50 to 150 μμg.

Uterus and vagina differ from other tissues, such as liver, kidney, muscle, adrenal and blood, in that the radioactive steroid reaches a higher concentration and continues to be incorporated and retained in these growth-responsive tissues at a time when the radioactivity in the other tissues has declined to a low level. In uterus the major portion of the radioactive material is free estradiol, with practically no water-soluble or protein-bound activity being observed, whereas in liver the free steroid appears to be a mixture of substances, and, in addition, appreciable protein-bound and water-soluble radioactivity is present. Thus, both by steroid incorporation pattern and by the chemical fate of the estrogen in the tissue, one can distinguish between two types of tissues, illustrated by uterus, on the one hand, and by liver on the other. Whether these should be designated as "target" and "metabolizing" tissues, respectively, is a matter of individual opinion, but the phenomena here described, in addition to the classical growth-response behavior, afford criteria for the clear differentiation of the two types of tissues.

REFERENCES

1. Dessau, F. *Acta Brev. Neerl. Physiol. Pharmacol. Microbiol.* **7**, 126 (1937).
2. Emmens, C. W. *J. Endocrinol.* **2**, 444 (1941).
3. Fishman, J., Bradlow, H. L., and Gallagher, T. F. *J. Am. Chem. Soc.* **81**, 2273 (1959).
4. Glascock, R. F., and Hoekstra, W. G. *Biochem. J.* **72**, 673 (1959).
5. Hisaw, F. L., and Lendrum, F. C. *Endocrinology* **20**, 228 (1936).
6. Huggins, C., and Jensen, E. V. *J. Exptl. Med.* **102**, 347 (1955).
7. Hurlock, B., and Talalay, P. *J. Biol. Chem.* **227**, 37 (1957).
8. Jacobson, H. I., Gupta, G. N., Fernandez, C., Hennix, S., and Jensen, E. V. *Arch. Biochem. Biophys.* **86**, 89 (1960).
9. Korenchevsky, V., and Hall, K. *J. Pathol. Bacteriol.* **50**, 295 (1940).
10. Mühlbock, O. *Acta Brev. Neerl. Physiol. Pharmacol. Microbiol.* **10**, 42 (1940).

DISCUSSION

**C. A. Villee:** I have one question to ask before the general discussion: Do those numbers in your table on the blackboard represent the percentage of the total injected dose recovered in each tissue?

**E. V. Jensen:** Yes.

**C. A. Villee:** So you have accounted for a little more than 2 % of the total dose. Would you comment on where the rest of it is?

**E. V. Jensen:** The only indication we have is that a considerable part of it is in the kidney and urine. In this experiment we do not have the kidneys assayed yet, but from previous experiments we know the kidney is relatively rich, and we know qualitatively that the urine is also.

I think that this rapid falling off of the blood and liver levels signifies a rapid clearance of the administered hormone, even though we administer no more than what we think is a physiological dose. The actual physiological dose appears to be much less than that administered, and a major part of the radioactivity may appear in the kidney and urine, and also in the enterohepatic system, which we have not yet studied.

**A. A. Sandberg:** This might clear up the point for Dr. Villee: within 10 minutes after the injection of small amounts of $C^{14}$-estrone we have found nearly 90 % of the radioactivity in the bile of the rat.

**E. V. Jensen:** This might very well be the case in our rats, and it is something we will have to look into. Thank you for clearing up this point.

**L. L. Engel:** It may be hazardous to draw the conclusion that the behavior of a relatively large dose of the steroid is the same as that of the extremely minute dose given here. It may well be that the biliary excretion is an overload phenomenon when physiological limits are exceeded.

**S. Solomon:** In your hydrogenation with tritium gas, how much nonspecific exchange is there? This is important to know in view of the minute amount of tritium that is measured in the tissues. The point that Dr. Engel just made is substantiated by the experiments done in mice by Dr. R. D. H. Heard and his collaborators in 1951. They injected 1 mg. of estrone-$16$-$C^{14}$ per mouse intramuscularly and found $C^{14}O_2$. When these experiments were repeated by others using much smaller doses of labeled estrone, no $C^{14}O_2$ was detected.

**E. V. Jensen:** In answer to your question about the preparation of the material, both we and Dr. Wilzbach, with whom we have discussed this, feel that there is very little exchange during this tritiation. As you know, Wilzbach exchange is carried out by exposing an organic compound without any catalyst to carrier-free tritium gas usually over a period of at least a week and one gets random or semirandom labeling with tritium. Our tritium gas is removed after 15 minutes, so the opportunity for Wilzbach exchange is quite limited. Secondly, the specific activities obtained by Wilzbach exchange are many hundred times smaller than what we have here. Therefore, even if exchange took place in these 15 minutes, the tritium thus introduced should be negligible in comparison to that resulting from double-bond reduction.

**K. E. Paschkis:** I have one question and one comment. The question is with regard to localization. You didn't have the breast tissue on your slide; did you investigate how much of the injected dose goes to the breast? The comment is apropos Dr. Engel's remark, questioning whether small amounts, physiological amounts, also appear in the bile in large part. Many years ago (before the era of radioactive labeled compounds), we studied biliary excretion of estrogens and found we had to give large doses of estrogen in order to get any biological activity in the bile which we could measure. We were criticized as not dealing with a physiological mechanism when administering these huge amounts of estrogen. Consequently we gave gonadotropins and forced the ovary itself to put out estrogens; again there was a very high biliary excretion. I wouldn't be at all astonished if in Dr. Jensen's animals the estrogen were in the bile.

**E. V. Jensen:** In answer to your question about breast, this is a very interesting story which we hope to be able to say something about in time, but I am not prepared to do so at present. In regard to your comment, we would be very happy to be able to account for the rest of the radioactivity in the bile. From our standpoint, though, accounting for the total radioactivity is of secondary interest, because our primary objective is to determine what is happening to the steroid in the "target" tissue and, further, how this differs from its fate in "nontarget" tissues.

**M. M. Mason:** I was interested in your report of anti-uterotrophic activity. You showed the results with only one compound, and the order of inhibition was about 60 %. We have tested to date about 300 or 400 compounds and we have about 100 compounds that show anti-uterotropic effect over 50 %. We would like to know whether any of the nonsteroidal compounds show the same mechanism. It would be interesting in the investigation of anti-uterotropic activity to find out where this blocking takes place. With this very elegant system you have evolved, residual hormone might very well show where this blocking takes place, and whether the estrogen is still present in the target tissue despite the lack of growth.

**E. V. Jensen:** We have looked only at fluorohydroxyprogesterone in this experiment, since, in an investigation of estrogen inhibition that Dr. Huggins and I carried out and reported in 1955, this was found to be the most effective inhibitor studied. Obviously this is just a preliminary approach to the mechanism of hormone antagonism. One should measure not only how much radioactive estrogen reaches the uterus with and without the administration of inhibitor, but also whether differences exist in the nature of the radioactive material present in the tissue. But since it now appears that in the absence of inhibitor the active material in the uterus is unchanged estradiol, it would be rather unexpected if the inhibitor caused the uterus to convert the estradiol into something else. But we shall have to do more along this line, as you suggest.

**G. C. Mueller:** Dr. Jensen, you certainly have filled in a tremendous gap in the information that we have wanted for a long time; that is, the state of hormones in the tissue during response to hormone. This beautiful work is an example of experimentation executed with good command of organic chemistry and good knowledge of the biological picture. I was wondering, however, if you would care to disclose something of your techniques in radioactive counting. In our experience it can be very difficult with some of these tritiated substances.

**E. V. Jensen:** This presented quite a problem when we began, since there was no simple satisfactory method for the determination of tritium in biological material. The difficulty lies in the very low energy of the beta radiation from tritium which renders end-window or even gas-flow counters inadequate.

We have developed a procedure in which the tritium of the sample is converted to water, which is then counted in an automatic liquid scintillation counter. In this method, the dried tissue sample is heated at 650° C. with copper and copper oxide in a sealed tube of special glass, according to a procedure described by Wilzbach and Sykes some years ago for the determination of isotopic carbon in organic compounds. This treatment converts the carbon to carbon dioxide, the nitrogen to molecular nitrogen, and the tritium and hydrogen to water, which is easily condensed from the other gases in a vacuum manifold and transferred to a counting bottle. Although several manipulations are required for each sample, the fact that you can process a large number of samples simultaneously renders the method suitable for routine assay. Using this combustion technique, there is no interference in the scintillation counting from colored or quenching substances present in blood and tissues. So far as I know, this is the only method that we possibly could have used for the large number of determinations that we have carried out. Description of this method should appear in the *Archives of Biochemistry and Biophysics* before the end of the year.

**Y. J. Topper:** I should like to comment further on the question of steroid responsiveness of so-called "target" organs and "nontarget" organs. Some time ago we reported on observations indicating that progesterone had a considerable stimulatory effect on the oxidation of galactose by liver *in vitro*. The only other tissue in the mammalian system which we found responsive in this respect is gut. In order to see whether there was any physiological counterpart to this *in vitro* effect we made a study of three galactosemic children. Galactosemia is a disease characterized by an inability to metabolize galactose completely. This is a consequence, as was beautifully demonstrated by Kalckar and his associates, of an enzyme deficiency. The enzyme, galactose-1-phosphate uridyl transferase, is missing in these individuals. We were able to show that, whereas these children are essentially incapable of metabolizing galactose to carbon dioxide during a control period, after several days of progesterone administration their ability to metabolize a tracer dose of galactose approaches that of the normal subject. I might add that following progesterone treatment the blood cells derived from these individuals are still incapable of metabolizing galactose. It appears that the liver, an organ not usually considered to be a target organ for progesterone, has been able at least partially to circumvent the enzymatic block in response to this hormone.

**G. Pincus:** I would like to continue with this idea of a target organ. I think that there is scarcely any tissue in the body which is not responsive to estrogens. I had the opportunity of reviewing this some time ago, and as far as I recall the eyeballs are not affected by estrogens. Every other tissue has been recorded in one way or another to respond to estrogens, sometimes very surprisingly, other times rather superficially. So I am wondering whether it is quite correct to speak of the uterus and vagina as "the" target organs.

**E. V. Jensen:** The original reason for picking on uterus and vagina is because these are tissues which grow spectacularly in response to the estrogen stimulation. Growth response could be one basis of assigning the term "target organ." I have tried to point out that such an assignment could be based on two other criteria, namely, the shape of the steroid incorporation curve and the chemical nature of the radioactive material that is present in the tissue. In fact, according to the latter criterion, one might have to define a target organ as one which doesn't do anything to the steroid, since in uterus the radioactive material seems to be free estradiol, whereas in a tissue such as liver something does happen to the steroid. I certainly agree with Dr. Pincus that estrogens must affect most, if not all, the cells of the body. Yet, no matter what one calls the different types of organs, I think one should distinguish tissues such as uterus and vagina from others such as liver, kidney, and muscle. This is what I tried to bring out.

**S. Kushinsky:** I should like to ask Dr. Jensen (1) if he has examined fatty tissue for radioactivity content, (2) the location of the sample of muscle which was analyzed, and (3) the site of injection of the radioactive material.

**E. V. Jensen:** I'll answer your last question first. The material was injected subcutaneously in the back. The muscle was a thigh muscle, the M. *Quadriceps femoris*. In regard to the fatty tissue, we have no data on this as yet.

**V. P. Hollander:** Since the estrogen-stimulated rat uterus is hyperemic and has a high water content, I would like to know how much radioactivity is associated with the tissue fluid and how much with solid residue.

**E. V. Jensen:** The uteri in our experiments are wet but not bloody. These are rather atrophic uteri from castrate or immature rats. The uteri taken 2–6 hours after estrogen administration have grown a little; they are slightly bigger than the controls on both the dry and wet weight basis, but they are not bloody. There is a little bit of luminal fluid present, and of course, in the 7-day experiments, there is a lot of luminal fluid. In one 7-day experiment we measured the radioactivity in the luminal fluid and, somewhat to our surprise, found it to be very low. In the tissue water, obtained on drying the uteri for assay, there is definitely a little radioactivity, but this volatile material is very small compared to the nonvolatile.

**U. Kim:** It is interesting to note that Dr. Jensen's work included the anterior pituitary gland as one of the target organs of estrogens. It is our belief that estrogens stimulate mammotropes of the anterior pituitary to produce hormone or hormones which, in turn, stimulate the mammary gland. In other words, estrogens are mediated by pituitary to act on mammary tissue. We think this concept can be substantiated by the classical experiments of pituitary tumor induction by chronic administration of estrogens in rats. Dr. Furth and his associates have demonstrated the function of such tumors. We also observed that, in absence of pituitary, estrogens failed to give mammary gland stimulation. This phenomenon was also observed in hormone-responsive mammary tumors. By grafting functional mammosomatotropic tumors we have been able to revive mammary tumors which had regressed following various endocrine ablative therapies.

**E. V. Jensen:** I agree with you that the question of the breast is very important, and it is one that we are studying. However, one is limited in how much he can do at a time, and as yet I don't have a story to tell about this.

**C. A. Villee:** I was struck by the fact that when you inject estradiol you recover essentially only estradiol. However, when you inject estrone you recover quite a mixture of things. This seems very curious to me. I wonder if you would like to comment on that?

**E. V. Jensen:** This is in the uterus. I would like to be able to say more about estrone because it is a very interesting question. Whereas most of the other experiments reported have been repeated and confirmed, this one with estrone represents a single experiment which needs repeating. The various radioactive fractions must be rechromatographed and positively identified. What presumably is the estradiol fraction is somewhat larger than any other fraction, but there certainly appears to be a variety of substances present. At this time, we can say only that this gives a preliminary indication that estrone is different from estradiol, and it may be that the biologically active agent is estradiol into which part of the estrone is metabolically converted. We shall just have to look further into this phenomenon.

# The Prostate As a Target Organ for Steroids

WILLIAM WALLACE SCOTT

*The James Buchanan Brady Urological Institute, The Johns Hopkins Hospital,
Baltimore, Maryland*

The prostate gland is of great interest to the physician, especially the urologist, for a number of important reasons: its normal growth and development is certainly dependent on hormones; its remarkable secretion almost certainly is important in fertility; nodular hyperplasia of the gland is incontestably the most common symptomatic new growth in the male; and prostatic cancer is the most common cancer in the male in terms of incidence and prevalence, although not in terms of mortality.

During the normal course of events, placental mammals are born with prostate glands. During the last trimester of fetal life and for a short time after birth, distinct histological changes can be seen in the prostate which include squamous metaplasia and focal hyperplasia of fully differentiated prostatic epithelium. The prostate gland of the newborn male is distinctly palpable on digital examination through the rectum. These changes occur at a time when changes also occur in the breast, uterus, and vagina of females, and it has been suggested that they are caused by gonadal hormones, derived either from the mother or from the fetal gonads. Sections of the testis of the premature infant or newborn, when stained for lipid, show that the interstitial cells of Leydig accept the stain as in the adult, and suggest that these cells are producing a hormone or hormones (15). Shortly after birth retrogressive changes occur in the prostate and the interstitial cells of Leydig disappear. It is not until the testes again begin to elaborate their hormones at puberty that we again note changes in the size, histology, and function of the prostate gland. Shortly after puberty the prostate gland attains adult size and histologic appearance and begins to secrete its fluid. Whereas the exact function of the gland is not known, its secretion, which constitutes approximately one-half of the volume of ejaculate, serves as a carrier for spermatozoa and probably provides nourishment for them. Barring the occurrence of inflammation and calculi, few changes are observed during the next thirty to forty years. Thereafter benign nodular hyperplasia develops in most glands, and carcinoma in many.

Dependence of the normal adult prostate gland upon androgenic substances derived from the testis seems incontestable. Thus, it has been shown that castration in the young adult animal invariably results in atrophy of the prostate gland and profound alteration in its secretion. Such atrophy can be prevented by administration of appropriate amounts of testosterone or the gland can be "restored" to "normal" with testosterone if atrophy is allowed to occur. "Maintained" or "restored" glands are normal as far as we know at present. Thus, maintenance or restorative doses of testosterone administered to a castrate result in a gland which is of normal size, weight and histology and one which behaves normally in terms of respiration (2, 3), succinic oxidase and cytochrome oxidase activities (5), lipogenesis (19), etc. Its content of certain free amino acids and peptides (1, 18), citric acid (13, 16) and acid phosphatase (7, 12) are normal.

Dependence of the normal adult prostate gland upon the pituitary also seems to be well established. Thus, hypophysectomy in animals such as the dog (12) and rat (6) results in prostatic atrophy which is even more profound than that observed after castration. Chorionic gonadotropin in adequate dosage will restore the prostate weight of the hypophysectomized rat to normal. Almost surely, this occurs as the result of androgen production by the Leydig cells of the testis under stimulation by the luteinizing hormone.

In 1955, we (6) reported that in rats which have been both hypophysectomized and castrated, the response of the prostate to testosterone is not as great as that of the prostate of the castrate rat with an intact pituitary gland. Simultaneous administration of prolactin in the form of Squibb's Luteotrophin®, ACTH, thyroxine, or chorionic gonadotropin, and testosterone propionate was carried out in hypophysectomized castrate rats. Prolactin administration always resulted in an augmentation of the effect of testosterone propionate under these circumstances, but had no demonstrable effect when given alone. Thyroxine administration had similar but less striking effect. Also in 1955, Huggins et al. (11) found that the administration of pituitary growth hormone with testosterone resulted in greater growth of the preputial glands, seminal vesicles, and ventral prostates of hypophysectomized castrate male rats than did the administration of testosterone alone. In our own experiments, it is possible that the synergism noted may have been due to contamination of the prolactin used with pituitary growth hormone. These experiments should be repeated with purer materials. At any rate, it appears as if certain tropic hormones of the pituitary may synergize the action of testosterone.

Segaloff and his associates (23) have reported that prolactin may sensitize the hypophysectomized rat ventral prostate to the action of androgen produced by the administration of luteinizing hormone. They suggest that the enhancement effected by growth hormone preparations can probably be attributed to the lactogenic contaminant present in the preparations. However, Lostroh et al. (14) believe that the results they have obtained cannot be interpreted in this way, because "growth hormone was in every instance more effective than lactogenic hormone in enhancing the prostatic response to ICSH." Finally in this regard, others, including Paesi *et al.* (20), have reported on the ability of pituitary extracts to potentiate androgenic action in the hypophysectomized castrate.

The role of the adrenal in prostatic growth and function remains obscure. However, it seems clear that the prostatic atrophy that invariably follows castration is irreversible unless androgenic substances are given, even though adrenal function remains undisturbed. In the author's experience, the human adult castrate's prostate remains atrophic and seminal secretions are reduced to almost nothing. The administration of testosterone propionate to such patients results in prompt restoration of the normal volume of seminal plasma and the gland becomes palpable digitally.

As a clinician who sees patients each day with some form of prostatic disease or malfunction, I am much more interested in such than the normal growth and development of the prostate gland of the animal, except as such studies of the normal gland bear on prostatic disease or malfunction.

In the sections that follow, I shall discuss briefly the question of endocrine regulation of abnormal prostatic growth—specifically benign nodular hyperplasia and prostatic cancer—and conclude with a resume of a search for steroids having antiandrogenic action.

## BENIGN NODULAR HYPERPLASIA

Numerous theories have been advanced concerning the etiology of nodular hyperplasia, but none has been accepted in the sense that generally recognized preventative or therapeutic measures have been based on it. However, at present most investigators in the field believe that the condition results from an imbalance of androgenic and estrogenic hormones. As nearly as can be determined with histologic methods, the primary lesion in nodular hyperplasia consists of multicentric aglandular nodules arising in estrogen-sensitive periurethral fibromuscular tissues located between the vesical neck and the colliculus seminalis with secondary invasion by epithelium which forms glands. As these benign spheroids increase in size, the normal prostatic tissue is gradually pushed to the periphery and is compressed between the expanding adenomata and the relatively inelastic true capsule of the gland. Urologists refer to the nodular hyperplastic mass as the "inner prostate" and the compressed subcapsular layer as the "outer prostate," and yet the inner prostate probably is not prostate at all. From what is known, it appears that the "inner prostate" or benign nodular hyperplasic tissue is estrogen sensitive, whereas the outer true prostate is androgen sensitive.

A number of endocrine preparations have been used in the past twenty years in an attempt to replace surgery, but to date such studies are inconclusive. As Clarke (4) has noted, "Conclusions as to the efficacy of endocrine or other new methods of treatment are only valid if cases are followed up for a considerable period of time." Based on a series of 93 cases of prostatic obstruction, treated by neither prostatectomy nor endocrines, he suggests a minimum of five years for evaluation of therapy. In his untreated patients, followed for an average period of over four years, a large number showed a sustained improvement after instrumentation alone.

In concluding this phase, I submit, because of the commonness of benign nodular hyperplasia, the incapacity which it may cause, and the possibility that it may be controlled by endocrine therapy, that a cooperative effort to study the effects of steroids in this condition should be instituted, as it has in prostatic cancer. One cannot but wonder how effective known antiestrogenic steroids might be.

## Prostatic Cancer

Prostatic cancer appears to arise always, or almost always, in the true prostate gland, which if compressed by the development of nodular hyperplasia becomes known as the "outer prostate." And, as far as we can tell now, prostatic cancer, like normal adult prostatic tissue, is androgen sensitive and often responds favorably to treatment directed toward removing androgens by castration or by inhibiting androgen production and/or action by estrogen administration. Dr. Herbert Brendler, in the chapter below on prostatic cancer, indicates that to date the best forms of therapy for disseminated prostatic cancer are castration and/or estrogen therapy. However, not all patients are responsive to such therapy and all eventually relapse on such therapy. Because of these responses, it is imperative that further search be made for chemical inhibitors of prostate growth stimulators.

## A Search for Inhibitors

During the past five years a part of our research has been the testing of steroids for possible antiandrogenic action. The method used initially was published in 1957 (21), and recent modifications constitute the subject of a paper now in preparation. Briefly, the index of antiandrogenic action is expressed in terms of the ability of the compound tested to inhibit prostatic growth in the normal rat when the compound is given alone, or in the castrate when the compound is administered with a known stimulator such as testosterone. Thus it seems possible to detect antagonism of both *endogenous* and *exogenous* androgenic action.

To date we have tested between 60 and 70 steroids, among which are steroids with androgenic, estrogenic, and progestational action of varying degree. Each compound was tested in dosages of 2.0, 1.0, and 0.5 mg. subcutaneously every other day for 14 days in castrates whose prostate glands were maintained with 0.4 mg. testosterone propionate subcutaneously administered at the same intervals and for the same length of time. I will not enumerate every steroid tested, but rather will present a few generalizations relating antiandrogenic action with androgenic, estrogenic, and progestational activity: (a) Regardless of their hormonal activity, none of the compounds tested showed significant inhibition of prostatic growth in the castrate young adult rat maintained on testosterone propionate. Slight synergism was noted in a few instances. Species differences must occur, because Huggins and Clark (9) and we (17) have demonstrated repeatedly that estrogenic steroids will effectively inhibit the prostate-stimulating action of testosterone propionate in the castrate dog. Others have demonstrated estrogen-androgen antagonism in the capon. (b) Only steroids with estrogenic action were found to inhibit prostatic growth to a significant degree in the intact rat. In the dosages tested, several progestational compounds were inactive. The data for the estrogenic steroids tested are shown in Table I. It is possible that there are a few exceptions to this generalization, but we don't think so. A compound such as 17α-ethynyl-19-nortestosterone inhibited prostatic growth in the intact rat, but all samples tested contained some of the 3-methyl ether of ethynylestradiol, and the purer the compound was said to be, the less the inhibition noted.

The results that we have obtained with our test are similar in several respects to those obtained by Huggins et al. (11), using the growth of the preputial glands of the hypophysectomized female rat as an indicator of activity. Of the steroids which they tested, only compounds in the androstane series were highly effective in promoting growth of the preputial glands. Growth was not induced by any of several steroids with a phenolic ring A, and administration of these steroids had no effect on the promotion of preputial growth by testosterone.

A number of the compounds tested in the rat were also tested in the dog, using the Huggins (10) prostatic fistula preparation in which the effect of the steroid is measured in terms of alteration in the volume of pilocarpine-induced prostatic secretion. In such it was noted that only estrogenic steroids were effective in causing a reduction in secretion in the intact dog or the castrate maintained on testosterone propionate. Such inhibition was also noted in the hypophysectomized castrate dog, an observation heretofore not recorded (Fig. 1).

Of considerable interest to us and of possible importance to those using androgenic steroids in cancer chemotherapy is the observation that two closely related compounds, 4,4-dimethyl-5-androsten-17β-ol-3-one and 4,4-dimethyl-5-androstene-3β,17β-diol, appear to have a remarkable capacity to potentiate prostatic secretion in the testosterone-maintained castrate

TABLE I

INHIBITION OF PROSTATIC GROWTH IN THE INTACT AND CASTRATE RAT BY ESTROGENIC STEROIDS

| Test compound (T.C.) | Intact | | | | Castrate | | | | |
|---|---|---|---|---|---|---|---|---|---|
| | T.C. (mg.) | Total prostate weight (mg.) | Ratio PW:BW | Index | T.P. (mg.) | T.C. (mg.) | Total prostate weight (mg.) | Ratio PW:BW | Index |
| 2,3-bis-$p$-Hydroxyphenyl-valeronitrile | 2 | 187 | 0.59 | 30 | 0.5 | 2.0 | 286 | 1.04 | 104 |
| Estrone, glycolic acid ether | 2 | 273 | 0.98 | 58 | 0.5 | 2.0 | 459 | 1.64 | 123 |
| 1,3,5(10)-Estratriene-3,16α-diol | 2 | 251 | 0.66 | 35 | 0.5 | 2.0 | 527 | 1.40 | 95 |
| 1,3,5,(10)-Estratriene-3,16α-diol-3-methyl ether | 2 | 499 | 1.19 | 64 | 0.5 | 2.0 | 520 | 1.34 | 91 |
| α-Estradiol | 2 | 104 | 0.43 | 22 | 0.4 | 2.0 | 353 | 1.54 | 131 |

fistula preparation (Fig. 2). Such an action has never been observed before in our laboratory. Additional testosterone propionate will not do it, nor will these compounds exert an androgenic action in the castrate dog which receives no testosterone. It is my understanding that Dr. Edward Lewison of the Breast Cancer Group is comparing the effects of this compound when given with testosterone to testosterone alone in women with disseminated breast cancer.

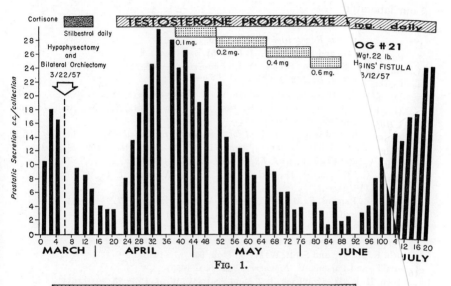

Fig. 1.

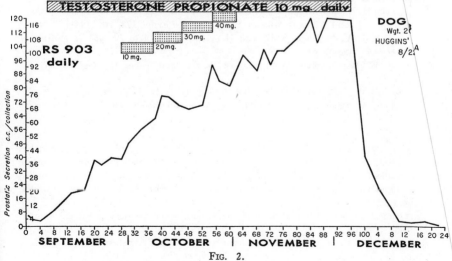

Fig. 2.

In conclusion, I believe that, if we are to continue to screen compounds in animals for trial in patients with disseminated prostatic cancer who have relapsed on castration-estrogen therapy, we must develop new methods of screening. If it is possible to induce rapidly an adenocarcinoma of the prostate gland of the animal which is hormone dependent, as Huggins and his associates (8) have developed a mammary carcinoma in female rats, we might well have a better tool. Such efforts in the dog and rat are in progress in our laboratory (22).

REFERENCES

1. Awapara, Texas Repts. Biol. and Med. 10, 22 (1952).
2. Barron, E. S. G., and Huggins, C. J. Urol. 51, 630 (1944).
3. Butler, W. S., III, and Schade, A. L. Endocrinology 63, 271 (1958).
4. Clarke, Brit. J. Urol. 9, 254 (1937).
5. Davis, S., Meyer, R. K., and McShan, W. H. Endocrinology 44, 1 (1949).
6. Grayhack, J. T., Bunce, P. L., Kearns, J. W., and Scott, W. W. Bull. Johns Hopkins Hosp. 96, 154 (1955).
7. Gutman, A. B., and Gutman, E. B. Proc. Soc. Exptl. Biol. Med. 41, 277 (1939).
8. Huggins, C., Briziarelli, G., and Sutton, H., Jr. J. Exptl. Med. 109, 25 (1959).
9. Huggins, C., and Clark, P. J. J. Exptl. Med. 72, 747 (1940).
10. Huggins, C., Masina, M. H., Eichelberger, L., and Wharton, J. D. J. Exptl. Med. , 543 (1939).
11. Huggins, C., Parsons, F. M., and Jensen, E. V. Endocrinology 57, 25 (1955).
12. Huggins, C., and Russell, P. S. Endocrinology 39, 1 (1946).
13. Humphrey, G. F., and Mann, T. Biochem. J. 44, 97 (1949).
14. Kostroh, A. J., Squire, P. G., and Li, C. H. Endocrinology 62, 833 (1958).
1 Lynch, K. M., Jr., and Scott, W. W. J. Urol. 64, 767 (1950).
Mann, T., and Parsons, V. Biochem. J. 46, 440 (1950).
Marden, H. E., Jr., Grayhack, J. T., and Scott, W. W. J. Urol. 73, 703 (1955).
Marvin, H. N., and Awapara, J. Proc. Soc. Exptl. Biol. Med. 72, 93 (1949).
Nyden, S. J., and Williams-Ashman, H. G. Am. J. Physiol. 172, 588 (1953).
Paesi, F. J. A., DeJongh, S. E., and Hoogstra, M. J. Acta Physiol. et Pharmacol. Neerl. 4, 445 (1956).
1. Scott, W. W., Hopkins, W. J., Lucas, W. M., and Tesar, C. J. Urol. 77, 652 (1957).
22. Scott, W. W., Schirmer, H. K. M., and Bradley, H. J., Jr. In preparation.
23. Segaloff, A., Steelman, S. L., and Flores, A. Endocrinology 59, 233 (1956).

DISCUSSION

R. Grinberg: The relationship between steroid hormones and the prostate gland has been studied in rats and human beings by our group. The relationship of the prostate gland of the rat with the testicle, the ovary, and the adrenal gland has been studied with intraprostatic grafts [Brachetto-Brian, D., and Grinberg, R. Rev. soc. arg. biol. 27, 199-204 (1951)].

Our clinical studies with patients suffering from benign prostatic adenoma showed that some patients are relieved of their symptoms by estrogen and progesterone, injected together in the muscle, in a proportion of 1/100 mg. [Grinberg, R., Jaroslavsky, M., and Cupesock, M. Rev. arg. endocrinol. & metabolism 3, 167-184 (1957)].

**W. W. Scott:** The indexes which we have observed for all progestational compounds in the castrate rat maintained on testosterone, as described, have never been less than 85, compared to a control index of 100. Certainly the degree of inhibition is very slight; and the same holds true in the prostatic fistula dog, either the intact or the castrate maintained on testosterone.

**G. Pincus:** When you test competitive inhibitors, the effect is proportional to some mysterious partition coefficient. For example, if the estrogens have a very high affinity for a tissue, and you try to displace them, you sometimes have to use very large quantities of the displacer. To give you an example, if you try to overcome the effects of estrogen with progesterone in the rabbit, the ratio usually has to be at least 10:1, usually 20:1 or higher. I noticed the highest ratio you mentioned was 5:1. Have you any data indicating whether, if you did use a larger ratio, you might see some effect?

**W. W. Scott:** For the 60 to 70 compounds we screened, we do not.

**R. Hertz:** May I ask Dr. Scott to discuss the adrenal factor in relation to the prostate and his present view of the place of adrenalectomy in the control of prostatic disease?

**W. W. Scott:** I am not sure just what role the adrenal plays in prostatic growth. As I said earlier, it is certain that in the adult human male, castration leads to profound atrophy of the prostate. This atrophy persists throughout the life of the individual unless androgenic substances are given. In the early 1940's, Dr. Huggins and I performed the first adrenalectomies for relapsing prostatic cancer, because we felt that the adrenal was an extragonadal source of androgens. In part, this belief was based on measurements of total 17-ketosteroids, a considerable rise in these values being noted after a transient postcastration fall. No bioassays were done on these urines.

One patient lived for 4 months after bilateral adrenalectomy. Cortisone was not available then. After removal of both adrenals of a patient, we observed a profound fall of the urinary 17-ketosteroids to very low levels, and yet he died of prostatic cancer. More recently in our own laboratory, we have measured the urinary steroids in a series of patients with widespread prostatic cancer before and after several forms of endocrine therapy. The method used was that developed by the late Dr. Conrad Dobriner and Dr. Tom Gallagher, which permits measurement of the 11-deoxy and 11-oxy urinary 17-ketosteroids. We have found that androsterone and etiocholanolone fall after castration, only to rise to rather high levels.

Estrogen administration may cause these levels to fall and may be associated with clinical improvement. Cortisone, in amounts of 100 mg. per day will do the same thing, but 50 mg. per day will not.

My indication for bilateral adrenalectomy in the relapsing patient with prostatic cancer would be failure to improve on castration therapy, estrogen therapy in low and high dosage, and following cortisone therapy in a dosage of at least 100 mg. per day. Actually, relatively few adrenalectomies have been carried out for prostatic cancer, many fewer than in disseminated breast cancer in the female.

**H. Spencer:** I would like to ask Dr. Scott whether a patient with metastatic carcinoma of the prostate, who is not responsive to a certain dose of estrogen used in the treatment of prostatic cancer, such as 15 mg. of diethylstilbestrol per day, would respond to a larger dose? The next question is: what are the pathologic changes in the normal prostate when cortisone is administered to dogs?

**W. W. Scott:** In such an individual, I would advise castration before trying larger doses of estrogen. At present, the Prostate Study Group is comparing the effectiveness of large and small doses of estrogen. The results of these studies are not yet available.

In answer to your second question, I do not know the effect of cortisone on the prostate gland of the dog.

**G. E. Block:** I would like to ask Dr. Scott about his experience with hypophysectomy in patients with disseminated carcinoma of the prostate who have relapsed after successful orchiectomy, or have continued with unabated disease after an unsuccessful orchiectomy.

**W. W. Scott:** The first hypophysectomy for prostatic cancer was carried out in our institution in 1948 by Dr. A. Earl Walker, our Professor of Neurosurgery. This was done before cortisone was available. The patient died on the eleventh postoperative day in profound hypoglycemia with no apparent effect on his cancer. We have since attempted hypophysectomy in ten additional patients with widespread prostatic cancer. In our experience, it is extremely difficult to secure total removal. Often enough, following presumably total hypophysectomy, there is little clinical evidence of panhypopituitarism, and at postmortem examination, a sizable amount of pituitary remains. I am convinced that when hypophysectomy is complete, it is effective in providing considerable relief in those patients who have previously responded to other forms of endocrine therapy. Admittedly, evaluation of such treatment is difficult.

At present we have under observation a man subjected to hypophysectomy in November, 1958. This man had been castrated, had received estrogen in both low and high dosage and cortisone. He was in profound relapse at the time of hypophysectomy, exhibiting marked weight loss, lymphedema of both lower extremities, pain requiring opiates, etc. Very recently he has had mild back pain thought to be secondary to osteoarthritis. His lymphedema is gone. He has regained all the weight he lost.

I think that more work should be done on hypophysectomy in the treatment of prostatic cancer. I for one believe that the results following hypophysectomy in breast cancer are superior to those following bilateral adrenalectomy.

# Effect of Steroids on Calcium Dynamics

Eugene Eisenberg

*Department of Medicine, University of California School of Medicine,
San Francisco, California*

The effects of steroid hormones on calcium metabolism have been observed in many species of animals. The spectacularly rapid bone deposition and resorption in the spongiosa of birds during the period of egg laying were first reported in 1934 (18). The subsequent investigations relating these changes to estrogen have been extensively reviewed (9, 14). Large doses of estrogen also affect the endosteal bone of mice (10, 23) and rats (25) but differently than in birds. The roughly analogous effects of androgen on bone growth may be seen in the growth and calcification of buck antlers (26).

Such observations led Albright and his co-workers (1-3) to examine the effects of these agents on calcium balance in man. The calcium retention described by them has subsequently been reported by others. In a recent review of published balance studies, Henneman and Wallach (16) concluded that estrogens given to postmenopausal women with osteoporosis do induce calcium retention; androgens given to senile men induce a more modest degree of calcium retention. In most studies the positive balance was a reflection of decrease in urinary excretion with no significant change in fecal calcium excretion. How gonadal steroids effect this retention of calcium is not known.

The loss of skeletal structure and the negative calcium balance associated with an excess of adrenocortical hormones are also well documented (3). The knowledge of whether these effects are secondary to an inhibition of bone growth or to an increase in bone resorption would be of considerable importance.

The internal movement of calcium in man has recently been studied by means of radioactive tracers (4, 6–8, 12, 13, 15, 17). Although the procedures and methods of calculation vary somewhat, recalculation of the data by the same methods gives comparable results. Several studies have shown that bone does not discriminate between calcium and strontium (19, 22). Bauer *et al.* (5) showed that after simultaneous intravenous injection of radiocalcium and radiostrontium, the two elements moved into the skeleton at the same rate. *Stable* strontium has been used as a tracer for calcium in our studies because it permits tests on young people and repeated tests on the same subjects.

The basis and methods for this test will be reported in detail elsewhere (12) but may be reviewed here briefly. There are two main pools of calcium in the body: a rapidly exchangeable pool which includes the calcium in blood, extracellular fluid, and surface crystal of bone, and a second reservoir, the less accessible calcium in deeper layers of bone. Calcium is removed from the exchangeable pool by urinary excretion and by incorporation into bone and is returned to the pool by bone resorption and gastrointestinal absorption of dietary calcium (Fig. 1). After injecting 10 meq. of strontium

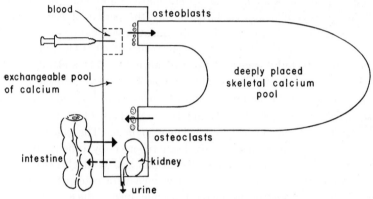

FIG. 1.  Model for analysis of calcium movement.

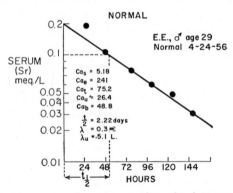

FIG. 2.  Plot of serum strontium concentrations after intravenous injection.

into the exchangeable pool, we can measure the half-time of tracer in the miscible pool by periodic sampling of the pool for 4–6 days. The serum specific activities are plotted on semilogarithm paper, and the half-time is measured (Fig. 2). The fractional rate constant is derived from Formula I, Table I. The size of the exchangeable calcium pool ($Ca_e$) may be calculated from the dilution of tracer (Formula II); the product of pool size and fractional rate of turnover gives total calcium turnover rate ($Ca_t$) (Formula III).

The portion accounted for by urinary excretion ($Ca_u$) is derived from an integration of urinary and serum specific activities (Formula IV). The estimated rate of osteogenesis ($Ca_b$) is the difference between total turnover rate and urinary excretion rate (Formula V). In the absence of diarrhea and steatorrhea, fecal excretion accounts for a negligible proportion of intra-venously injected calcium and strontium (7, 13, 24). Since the rate of osteo-genesis is computed from $Ca_t$—$Ca_u$, any other loss, e.g., through feces or sweat, would result in overestimation of the figure for osteogenesis.

TABLE I

FORMULAS

| | | |
|---|---|---|
| **(I)** $k = 0.693/t_{\frac{1}{2}}$ | $k$ | = fractional rate constant |
| | $t_{\frac{1}{2}}$ | = "half-time" derived by plotting serum specific activities |
| **(II)** $Ca_e = d/s_0$ | $Ca_e$ | = exchangeable calcium pool size |
| | $d$ | = dose of tracer |
| | $s_0$ | = serum specific activity at time zero |
| **(III)** $Ca_t = kCa_e$ | $Ca_t$ | = total turnover rate |
| **(IV)** $Ca_u = \int_{t_1}^{t_2} dU \bigg/ s_0 \int_{t_1}^{t_2} e^{-kt}dt$ | $Ca_u$ | = urinary excretion rate |
| | $U_{t_2-t_1}$ | = urinary content of tracer between time one and time two |
| $= (U_{t_2-t_1})k\big/(s_{t_1}-s_{t_2})$ | $s_{t_1},\ s_{t_2}$ | = serum strontium concentration at time one and time two |
| **(V)** $Ca_b = Ca_t - Ca_u$ | $Ca_b$ | = rate of osteogenesis |

We have studied the effects of sex steroids by comparing rates of osteo-genesis in normal control subjects with those in postmenopausal and senile osteoporotic patients and by noting the changes induced by the administra-tion of androgen or estrogen (Table II) to the subjects for 6–8 weeks. The effects of catabolic adrenal steroids were studied by observing changes induced by giving these agents to normal subjects (Table III) and by measuring calcium dynamics in two patients with far-advanced Cushing's disease and osteoporosis. Three sets of subjects without bone disease were used as controls: one group of young adults of average physical activity, another group of older women matched to the osteoporotic patients for age, height and weight, and a third group of athletes.

The normal exchangeable pool is about 225 meq. or 4.5 gm. of calcium, and the rate of osteogenesis is about 50 meq. or 1000 mg. per 24 hours

(Table III). These coincide with the figures derived for normal subjects by Bauer *et al.* (4) and by Bauer and Ray (6) from studies with radioactive calcium and strontium, respectively. The rate of osteogenesis in our normal subjects at routine activity differs from that reported by Heaney and Whedon (15), perhaps because their one control subject was a 65-year-old man at bed rest. The skeletal dynamics of older women free of radiographic osteoporosis did not differ from those of the normally active control group of both sexes. The dramatic effect on the skeleton of vigorous exercise can be seen in the data for members of the San Quentin Prison football team. In this group of athletes the exchangeable pool was greatly expanded and the rate of osteogenesis was 46 % greater than that of healthy persons at normal activity.

TABLE II

COMPOUNDS USED TO STUDY EFFECTS OF STEROID HORMONES ON CALCIUM DYNAMICS

| Compounds | Dose |
| --- | --- |
| Androgens | |
|     Fluoxymesterone | 10 mg./day |
|     Testosterone enanthate | 200 mg./14 days |
| Estrogens | |
|     Conjugated equine estrogens | 2.5 mg./day |
|     Methallenestril | 6 mg./day |
| Corticoids | |
|     Cortisol | 200 mg./day |
|     Triamcinolone | 20 mg./day |
|     Prednisone | 20 mg./day |
|     Dexamethasone | 3 mg./day |

The postmenopausal osteoporotics had small miscible pools and reduced rates of osteogenesis. These figures are the same as those reported for osteoporotic patients by Heaney and Whedon (15), who used $Ca^{45}$ as a tracer. It is noteworthy that in both normal and osteoporotic subjects about 20 % of the total exchangeable pool is going to bone each day. Therefore, if the rate of osteogenesis in osteoporotics is reported as a proportion of the pool, as Fraser *et al.* have done (13), the subnormal rate of osteoporosis is no longer apparent.

Cushing's disease is also characterized by reduction in the exchangeable pool. This small pool is turning over rapidly because of the greatly increased rate of urinary excretion despite a drastically reduced rate of osteogenesis. Again, the proportion of total pool being used for bone formation is about 20 %.

Administration of androgens and estrogens resulted in no alteration in the exchangeable pool size (Table IV), but decreased the rate of turnover.

TABLE III

CALCIUM DYNAMICS IN VARIOUS CONDITIONS

| Subjects | Number | Exchangeable calcium pool (meq.) | Total calcium turnover rate (meq./24 hr.) | Urinary excretion rate (meq./24 hr.) | Rate of osteogenesis (meq./24 hr.) |
|---|---|---|---|---|---|
| Healthy at normal activity | 24 | 228 ± 7[a] | 73.3 ± 3.6[a] | 21.0 ± 1.6[a] | 52.4 ± 2.4[a] |
| Normal, matched to osteoporotic | 8 | 215 ± 13 | 72.0 ± 5.7 | 21.9 ± 3.5 | 49.3 ± 3.2 |
| Athletes | 14 | 299 ± 13 | 105.7 ± 3.9 | 30.4 ± 1.3 | 76.1 ± 3.6 |
| Postmenopausal osteoporotic | 37 | 162 ± 5 | 44.7 ± 2.0 | 12.3 ± 1.1 | 32.3 ± 1.4 |
| Cushing's disease | 2 | 106,141 | 43.7,75.8 | 30.9,43.0 | 12.8,32.2 |

[a] Mean ± standard error for all groups except Cushing's disease.

Androgens effected this decrease solely by reducing the rate of urinary excretion, whereas estrogen reduced the rate of osteogenesis as well. Surprisingly, no increase in osteogenesis was found after administration of either of these calcium-retaining agents. Administration of large amounts of corticoids to normal subjects for 4 weeks increased the pool turnover. The increase was associated with an accelerated rate of urinary loss, as in spontaneous Cushing's disease. In this short period of time the rate of osteogenesis also increased, instead of dwindling as it does in Cushing's disease.

TABLE IV

CHANGES OF CALCIUM DYNAMICS FROM PRETREATMENT VALUES AFTER ADMINISTRATION OF VARIOUS CLASSES OF STEROIDS

| Number of subjects | Steroid | Exchange-able calcium pool (meq.) | Total calcium turnover rate (meq./ 24 hr.) | Urinary excretion rate (meq./ 24 hr.) | Rate of osteo-genesis (meq./ 24 hr.) |
|---|---|---|---|---|---|
| 12 | Androgens | 0 | —12% | —25% | 0 |
| 15 | Estrogens | 0 | —18% | —20% | —18% |
| 15 | Corticoids | +10% | +30% | +77% | +15% |

Since the bone mass in hypercorticism is reduced and osteoblastic activity is not primarily inhibited, it is apparent that osteolysis must be accelerated. Clark and his associates (11) have found that cortisone accelerates release of radioactive calcium previously incorporated in the skeleton of the rat. Such mobilization of calcium over a long period of time would lead to the loss of skeleton found clinically. Since part of the exchangeable pool of calcium consists of skeletal surface crystals, reduction in bone surface area could lead to the small exchangeable pool found in Cushing's disease. To test this hypothesis, serial studies are being done in patients who require long-term corticosteroid therapy.

In view of the marked decrease in skeletal mass characteristic of post-menopausal osteoporosis, it is not surprising that the exchangeable pool is small and the rate of osteogenesis reduced. Further suppression of the sub-normal rate of osteogenesis by estrogen is an unexpected finding. It has been postulated that the beneficial effects of estrogen in postmenopausal osteoporosis result from stimulation of osteoblastic activity. Treatment of senile and postmenopausal osteoporosis with androgens and estrogens has stopped the progressive vertebral collapse seen in this disease (16, 21). However, serum alkaline phosphatase does not increase, as would be expected if osteoblastic stimulation were indeed the mechanism. Also, bone density is not changed in serial roentgenograms (21), and serial bone biopsies on patients receiving long-term estrogen therapy in our clinic have shown no alterations in histologic appearance. It thus appears that osteoporosis can only be arrested, and not reversed. To explain the prolonged calcium retention induced by estrogens one must postulate that these agents reduce the rate of bone resorption. Unfortunately, quantitation of osteolysis in man is not possible by present techniques. In the rapidly growing rat, however, large doses of estrogens prevent resorption of endosteal bone (25). The degree of bone resorption induced by injecting adult rats with parathyroid hormone is decreased by estrogen therapy (20). Our data suggest a similar effect on the human skeleton. Whether this is a primary effect on the skeleton or is secondary to calcium retention mediated by the kidney cannot be ascertained from existing data.

## Summary

The actions of estrogen and androgen on the human skeleton were measured using nonradioactive strontium as a tracer for calcium in postmenopausal osteoporotic patients. These compounds caused calcium retention without stimulation of osteoblastic activity. Hence, one must assume that they decreased osteolysis. Administration of large doses of corticoids to normal human subjects increased the urinary excretion rate of calcium. The early and slight increase in bone accretion rate is probably compensatory, since it is succeeded in long-standing hypercorticism by a great decrease. It remains to be determined whether these effects are exerted directly on bone or are secondary to effects on other organ systems.

### Acknowledgments

These studies were initiated under the guidance of Professor T. R. Fraser, University of London Postgraduate Medical School, and are being continued with Dr. G. S. Gordan, University of California School of Medicine, San Francisco. We gratefully acknowledge the assistance of Dr. H. F. Loken and Mr. Warren Lubich.

Strontium gluconate was generously supplied by Dr. A. Cerletti and Mr. H. Althouse of Sandoz, Inc.; fluoxymesterone (Halotestin) and cortisol (Cortef) by Dr. H. Upjohn of The Upjohn Co.; testosterone enanthate (Delatestryl) and triamcinolone (Kenacort) by Drs. E. C. Reifenstein, Jr., and Dr. H. Rudel of E. R. Squibb & Sons; methallenestril (Vallestril) by Dr. I. C. Winter of G. D. Searle & Co.; conjugated equine estrogens (Premarin) by Dr. J. Jewell of Ayerst Laboratories; prednisone (Deltra) and dexamethasone (Decadron) by Dr. E. Alpert of Merck Sharp & Dohme.

This work was supported in part by grants allocated by the Committee on Research, University of California School of Medicine, San Francisco; and from the American Medical Association; Ayerst Laboratories; G. D. Searle & Co.; Merck Sharp & Dohme; E. R. Squibb & Sons; and The Upjohn Co.

### References

1. Albright, F. *Recent Progr. in Hormone Research* **1**, 293 (1947).
2. Albright, F., Bloomberg, E., and Smith, P. H. *Trans. Assoc. Am. Physicians* **55**, 298 (1940).

3. Albright, F., and Reifenstein, E. C., Jr. "Parathyroid Glands and Metabolic Bone Disease." Williams & Wilkins, Baltimore, Maryland, 1948.
4. Bauer, G. C. H., Carlsson, A., and Lindquist, B. In "Radioaktive Isotope in Klinik und Forschung" (K. Fellinger and H. Vetter, eds.), Vol. 3, p. 25. Urban and Schwarzenberg, Munich, 1958.
5. Bauer, G. C. H., Carlsson, A., and Lindquist, B. Acta Physiol. Scand. 35, 56 (1955).
6. Bauer, G. C. H., and Ray, R. D. J. Bone and Joint Surg. 40A, 171 (1958).
7. Bellin, J., and Laszlo, D. Science 117, 331 (1953).
8. Bronner, F., Harris, R. S., Maletskos, C. J., and Benda, C. E. J. Clin. Invest. 35, 78 (1956).
9. Budy, A. M. Ann. N. Y. Acad. Sci. 64, 428 (1956).
10. Budy, A. M., Urist, M. R., and McLean, F. C. Am. J. Pathol. 28, 1143 (1952).
11. Clark, I., Geoffroy, R. F., and Bowers, W. Endocrinology 64, 849 (1959).
12. Eisenberg, E., and Gordan, G. S. In preparation.
13. Fraser, R., Harrison, M., and Ibertson, K. Quart. J. Med. 29, 85 (1960).
14. Gardner, W. U., and Pfeiffer, C. A. Physiol. Revs. 23, 139 (1943).
15. Heaney, R. P., and Whedon, G. D. J. Clin. Endocrinol. and Metabolism 18, 1246 (1958).
16. Henneman, P., and Wallach, S. A.M.A. Arch. Internal Med. 100, 715 (1957).
17. Krane, S. M., Brownell, O. L., Stanbury, J. B., and Corrigan, H. J. Clin. Invest. 35, 874 (1956).
18. Kyes, P., and Potter, T. S. Anat. Record 60, 377 (1934).
19. Lengemann, F. W. Proc. Soc. Exptl. Biol. Med. 94, 64 (1957).
20. Manunta, G., Saroff, D., and Turner, C. W. Proc. Soc. Exptl. Biol. Med. 94, 785 (1957).
21. Moldawer, M. A.M.A. Arch. Internal Med. 96, 202 (1955).
22. Palmer, R. F., Thompson, R. C., and Kornberg, H. A. Science 127, 1505 (1958).
23. Segaloff, A., and Cahill, W. M. Proc. Soc. Exptl. Biol. Med. 54, 162 (1943).
24. Spencer, H., Brothers, M., Berger, E., Hart, H. E., and Laszlo, D. Proc. Soc. Exptl. Biol. Med. 91, 155 (1956).
25. Urist, M. R., Budy, A. M., and McLean, F. C. J. Bone and Joint Surg. 32A, 143 (1950).
26. Wislocki, G. B., Aub, J. C., and Waldo, C. M. Endocrinology 40, 202 (1947).

## DISCUSSION

**H. Spencer:** We found, in our studies carried out in man with $Ca^{45}$ and $Sr^{85}$, given simultaneously, by intravenous injection or oral ingestion of these tracer doses, that strontium is only a qualitative indicator of calcium metabolism, since there are considerable quantitative differences in urinary excretion, in intestinal absorption, and in retention of the two radioisotopes in the body. Preferential excretion of strontium by the kidney, higher absorption of calcium than of strontium via the intestinal tract, and the higher retention of $Ca^{45}$ indicate the body's preference for calcium rather than for strontium. The analysis of bone samples of patients who have received simultaneous injections of $Sr^{85}$ and $Ca^{45}$ intravenously, at varying time intervals before death (2 hours to 8 months) revealed that the concentration of the $Ca^{45}$ is much higher than of $Sr^{85}$. Dr. Eisenberg mentioned that the stool excretion of $Sr^{85}$ is negligible. In our observations, the fecal excretion of $Sr^{85}$ is as high as 15–20 % of the dose after the intravenous injection of this tracer, and the fecal radiostrontium excretion may vary with the calcium metabolism of the individual. For instance, if the urinary radio-strontium excretion is very low, the fecal $Sr^{85}$ excretion may be as high or even higher than the urinary radiostrontium excretion.

It is very interesting to learn that Dr. Eisenberg's calculations show that the rate of osteogenesis is decreased when estrogen is administered. One would not expect this. However, we have found that, although the urinary calcium excretion decreases when estrogens are given, the retention of infused calcium does not increase during estrogen therapy in certain types of patients. This would be in agreement with Dr. Eisenberg's theory that osteogenesis is not increased, but that the decrease of urinary calcium may be due rather to decreased resorption of calcium from bone. Also, estrogens may act on the kidney as well, since the $Sr^{85}$ plasma levels are higher in the phase of estrogen administration than in the control study, which may indicate increased tubular resorption of strontium and possibly also of calcium.

**A. White:**   Dr. Spencer, would you indicate what quantity of strontium you used, and in what form the strontium was administered?

**H. Spencer:**   Strontium as the chloride was administered carrier free in doses ranging from 0.1 to 0.4 microcurie per kilogram body weight.

**E. Eisenberg:**   We are aware of the many differences between calcium and strontium as they are handled by the human body. The problem of absorption in the gut is circumvented in this method by injecting the strontium directly into the exchangeable pool. Bauer, Carlsson, and Lindquist showed that the total retention of strontium by the body was lower than total retention of calcium because of the preferential urinary excretion rate of strontium. But the strontium retained in the body did move into the skeleton at the same rate as the calcium. We find strontium clearance by the kidney to be between three and five times that of calcium. You noticed perhaps that the figures for the rate of calcium excretion were in the order of some 20 meq. per day. These figures of calcium excretion are as determined by strontium. The ratio of strontium clearance to calcium clearance is the factor by which we would have to multiply the actual urinary calcium to get the figure for the rate of calcium excretion measured by this technique. The difference which the kidney causes in the total turnover of strontium is accounted for in this method because the urinary excretion rate is measured directly and subtracted from the total turnover; the remaining difference which is going to bone is assumed to be the same for the two elements on the basis of the work quoted. We found that, after infusing doses varying from 2 up to 12 meq. of strontium, the fecal excretion, over the period of time in which serum levels were measured, in most cases was less than 6–8 % in the absence of diarrhea or steatorrhea.

**T. C. Hall:**   I am curious about the effect on buck antlers' calcification because of the work that Dr. Aub and I did over a long period of time. We were not exactly able to pin it down as an androgenic effect, and I'd like to hear a little comment on that point.

**E. Eisenberg:**   The apparent difference in antler development between the buck and the doe is what I was referring to. I have no data to support this other than the common observation.

**M. J. Brennan:**   Did you do any studies to determine whether or not any of the steroids which you used, has an effect on the ratio of protein-bound to free calcium in serum?

**E. Eisenberg:**   Dr. Hans Loken has been investigating this particular aspect in our laboratory and to date has not uncovered any difference in the ratio of free to protein-bound calcium or strontium.

# The Effect of Estrogen Therapy on Incorporation of Formate-C$^{14}$ into Human Breast Cancer *in Vitro*

RICHARD J. WINZLER, HOWARD H. SKY-PECK, S. G. TAYLOR, III, AND
SYDNEY KOFMAN

*University of Illinois College of Medicine, and Department of Medicine, Presbyterian-St.
Luke's Hospital, Chicago, Illinois*

The beneficial effects of estrogens on the clinical course of metastatic breast cancer in some patients has been observed by many investigators (1, 3, 5, 7). It is well known, however, that many patients do not respond, and in some cases a more rapid progression of the disease appears to result from estrogen administration.

It has not been clear what, if any, metabolic changes are induced in the breast cancer by estrogen therapy, nor is their any information on the relation of such possible metabolic effects to the subsequent course of the disease. The studies that I should like to discuss were initiated in the hope of clarifying some of the metabolic actions underlying effects of estrogens on the growth and metabolism of breast cancer.

During the course of this work it has become evident that estrogens may have early stimulating or inhibiting effects on certain metabolic processes in breast cancers and that these effects are reflected in the subsequent course of the disease. Consequently some effort has been expended in determining whether early objective procedures can be developed which might have predictive value assessing the effectiveness of estrogen therapy in individual patients.

The work was initiated by studying the *in vitro* incorporation of radioactive formate into the proteins and nucleic acids of slices of normal and neoplastic breast tissue. The tissues were taken by surgical biopsy from patients with metastatic carcinoma of the breast before and during a course of therapy with 17β-estradiol. The patients selected for these studies had disseminated cancer of the breast and were previously untreated or showed no clinical evidence of effect from previous therapy. The selection of radioactive formate for these studies was made because its distribution in the components of protein and nucleic acid is relatively limited and the pathways for its incorporation into these components have been extensively studied.

The major components into which formate-$C^{14}$ is incorporated in animal tissues are the C-2 and C-8 positions of purines, the ureido carbon of histidine, the beta carbon of serine, the methyl group of thymine, and the methyl groups of methionine, choline, etc.

Neoplastic tissues weighing 0.5–2 gm. were obtained by biopsy, and normal tissues were taken from the same individual from the contralateral uninvolved breast. The tissues were placed in cold Krebs-Ringer-bicarbonate medium and within 15 minutes were sliced into thin slices. Alternate slices were used for metabolic studies or were fixed in formalin and stained with hematoxylin and eosin for histological examination.

The slices used for metabolic studies were incubated at 38° C. with Krebs-Ringer-bicarbonate-glucose medium in an atmosphere of 5 % $CO_2$-95 % $O_2$ in the presence of 1 μc. of formate-$C^{14}$ for periods up to 5 hours.

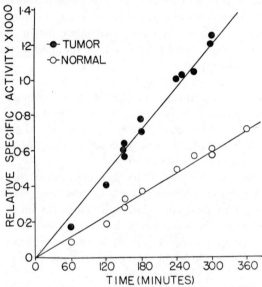

Fig. 1. Time course of formate incorporation into the proteins of normal and cancerous tissue. About 100 mg. of sliced tissue incubated in Krebs-Ringer-bicarbonate-glucose medium containing 1 mg. (1 μM) $C^{14}$-formate and lipid-free, nucleic acid-free "protein fraction" isolated. Specific activities expressed as (c.p.m./mg. protein) /(c.p.m./mg. formate) × 1000.

After incubation, the lipid-free nucleic acid-free "protein fraction" was isolated by precipitation of the incubation medium with cold trichloroacetic acid (TCA) and extraction with lipid solvents and with hot trichloroacetic acid. The amount and radioactivity of the residual protein was then determined. Ribonucleic acid (RNA) and deoxyribonucleic acid (DNA) were determined in the hot trichloroacetic acid extracts by their reactions with orcinol and with diphenylamine. In some experiments RNA and DNA were separated from the cold TCA extract by the method of Elson et al. (2). Separations of serine from the protein and of thymine and the purines from nucleic acid were made by standard chromatographic methods after appropriate hydrolysis (6).

Formate incorporation into protein fraction proceeds at a linear rate for at least 6 hours in both normal and cancerous tissue. This is shown in Fig. 1, which gives the relative specific activities [(cpm/mg. protein)/ (cpm $\mu M$ formate) $\times$ 1000] of the protein fractions as a function of time.

The heterogeneity of breast tissue is well known, and one of the misgivings we had in initiating these studies was the fear that this heterogeneity would introduce sampling problems that would lead to wide variability in results obtained. Although this is no doubt a complicating factor, we found that the rate of formate incorporation into normal breast tissue was sur-

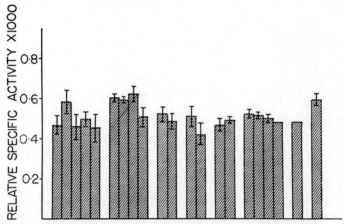

FIG. 2. Incorporation of formate-$C^{14}$ into the protein fraction of normal breast tissue. Incubation time 5 hours; other conditions as in Fig. 1. From Sky-Peck *et al.* (6).

prisingly constant when the same individual was studied at different times or when different individuals were compared. This is shown in Fig. 2. Here the average formate incorporation in 5-hour incubation periods with 45 patients yielded a relative activity of 0.47 $\pm$ 0.12 $\times$ $10^{-3}$.

The situation with breast cancer tissue was quite different, formate incorporation varying widely between tissues from different patients. This is shown on Fig. 3 for tissues from untreated patients. It is evident that formate uptake ranges from values considerably higher than the normal (shown by the crosshatched area) to values appreciably lower than normal. Attempts were made to correlate these uptake rates with differences in cellularity of the tissues, with differences in DNA and RNA content, and with differences in the relative proportion of stromal and carcinomatous cells. However, no clear-cut correlation of formate uptake with any of these measurements was evident. In general, the tissues having the highest rate of formate uptake came from patients whose tumors had been showing the most rapid growth rates. Tissues from slowly growing or static tumors had the lowest rates of formate incorporation into the "protein fraction." This is shown for a series of cases in Table I (4).

The results obtained in biopsies taken 1 week after initiation of estrogen therapy were somewhat surprising. In no case was formate incorporation into the "gross protein fraction" of the noncancerous breast tissue significantly altered. In most cases, however, there was a significant increase or a significant decrease in the extent to which formate was incorporated into protein of the cancer tissues in comparison with the pretreatment period.

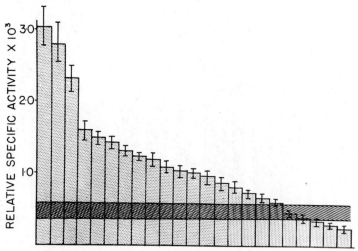

FIG. 3.   Incorporation of formate-$C^{14}$ into the protein fraction of neoplastic breast tissue.  Incubation time 5 hours.  Other conditions as in Fig. 1.  From Sky-Peck *et al.* (6).

This is apparent in Fig. 4, which shows the pretreatment formate uptake into normal and cancer tissue and the uptake after 7 days of therapy in 16 patients. On the right are the patients whose tumors were stimulated to take up more formate, and on the left those whose tumors were inhibited by therapy. In this series, attempts were made to correlate the effects of the therapy on formate incorporation with the subsequent response of the patient to continued therapy. This is shown by means of letters, *P* (progressing), *R* (regressing), and *S* (static), under each patient's number. It is seen that those patients whose breast tumors showed an increased *in vitro* formate uptake following initiation of therapy continued to progress, whereas those showing decreased formate uptake became static or showed regression. These observations could not be correlated with any change in appearance, cellularity, or DNA or RNA content of the tissue. We have as yet no data which permit us to do more than speculate as to the biochemical significance of the observations. It was not always possible to place a patient cleanly into one of these categories, since occasionally tumors in one area regressed while those in other areas progressed under the influence of therapy. Usually, however, this presented no problem.

TABLE I

THE RELATION BETWEEN FORMATE-$C^{14}$ INCORPORATION AND STATUS OF DISEASE[a]

| Patient | RSA of tumor[b] | Status of tumor |
|---|---|---|
| 1 | 3.78 | Rapid progression |
| 2 | 2.91 | Rapid progression |
| 3 | 2.85 | Rapid progression |
| 4 | 2.83 | Rapid progression |
| 5 | 1.92 | Rapid progression |
| 6 | 1.82 | Rapid progression |
| 7 | 1.61 | Rapid progression |
| 8 | 1.58 | Rapid progression |
| 9 | 1.45 | Rapid progression |
| 10 | 1.45 | Rapid progression |
| 11 | 1.42 | Rapid progression |
| 12 | 1.29 | Rapid progression |
| 13 | 1.26 | Rapid progression |
| 14 | 1.21 | Moderate progression |
| 15 | 1.19 | Moderate progression |
| 16 | 1.16 | Rapid progression |
| 17 | 1.15 | Moderate progression |
| 18 | 1.11 | Moderate progression |
| 19 | 1.04 | Moderate progression |
| 20 | 0.92 | Moderate progression |
| 21 | 0.91 | Moderate progression |
| 22 | 0.83 | Slow progression |
| 23 | 0.81 | Moderate progression |
| 24 | 0.81 | Moderate progression |
| 25 | 0.75 | Slow progression |
| 26 | 0.70 | Moderate progression |
| 27 | 0.59 | Slow progression |
| 28 | 0.56 | Regression |
| 29 | 0.44 | Static |
| 30 | 0.42 | Static |
| 31 | 0.38 | Static |
| 32 | 0.37 | Static |
| 33 | 0.33 | Static |
| 34 | 0.12 | Static |
| 35 | 0.11 | Static |

[a] From Kofman et al. (4).
[b] RSA, relative specific activity.

Thus far we have considered results obtained only with the "protein fraction" freed of lipids and nucleic acids. For any real insight into the influence of estrogen therapy on formate incorporation, it is necessary to go beyond the "protein fraction" and to study the individual components of the proteins, nucleic acids and their acid-soluble precursors. This we have be-

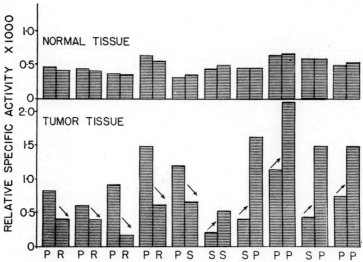

Fig. 4. Effect of 1 week of estrogen therapy on formate-$C^{14}$ incorporation into normal and cancerous breast tissue. Incubation time 5 hours. Other conditions as in Fig. 1.

gun to do, and, although we are in the early stages of this work, certain information is beginning to accumulate. Table II shows that, of the radioactivity in the TCA-insoluble fraction, about 90 % remains with the protein residue and 10 % is extracted with the nucleic acids by hot trichloroacetic acid. This relation is not affected by estrogen therapy in this patient, although an increase of formate incorporation into both fractions was in-

TABLE II

DISTRIBUTION OF $C^{14}$ FROM FORMATE IN THE FRACTIONS OF A BREAST TUMOR BEFORE
AND AFTER INITIATION OF ESTRADIOL THERAPY

|  | Before therapy | After 7 days of therapy |
|---|---|---|
| Protein fraction RSA | 1.19 | 2.34 |
| Bound $C^{14}$ in protein (%) | 89.9 | 89.1 |
| Bound $C^{14}$ in nucleic acid (%) | 10.1 | 10.9 |
| Protein $C^{14}$ in β-carbon of serine (%) | 87 | 86 |
| CPM/μM serine | 760 | 1470 |

duced. Thus, incorporation into both nucleic acid and protein was stimulated by estrogen therapy. The radioactivity in the residual protein fraction was primarily present as serine. This was shown by hydrolyzing the protein, separating the amino acids on ion exchange columns, oxidizing these with periodate, and collecting, as the dimedon derivative, the formaldehyde released from the beta carbon of serine. Serine was also isolated from the hydrolyzate by paper chromatographic methods, and its specific activity determined. The results of these two types of experiment on a patient before and after initiation of estrogen therapy are also shown in Table II. It is seen that close to 90 % of the radioactivity in the "protein fraction" is in the beta carbon of serine, and that the increase in formate uptake into the protein fraction noted in the tumor of this patient was associated with an increase in the specific activity of serine. Therefore, one of the effects of estrogen therapy in this patient was to increase the over-all rate of formation of serine from formate and/or the incorporation of serine into proteins. An attempt to assay this latter possibility is being made with labeled serine and other amino acids in place of formate.

In addition to its incorporation into protein-bound serine, formate is converted into nucleic acid purines and thymine and into their free nucleotide precursors. As has already been indicated, about 10 % of the TCA-insoluble radioactivity is taken up into the nucleic acids extracted with hot trichloroacetic acid. This radioactivity is primarily located in the adenine and guanine of RNA and in the thymine of DNA. The purines of DNA had very low specific activity. These observations are illustrated in Table III and were obtained with tissue from a postmenopausal patient with meta-

TABLE III

EFFECT OF ESTRADIOL THERAPY ON INCORPORATION OF FORMATE-$C^{14}$ INTO THE NUCLEIC ACID PURINES AND PYRIMIDINES OF NORMAL AND NEOPLASTIC BREAST TISSUE[a]

|  | Normal breast | | Tumor breast | |
| --- | --- | --- | --- | --- |
|  | Before therapy | 7 Days after initiation of therapy | Before therapy | 7 Days after initiation of therapy |
| RNA adenine | 153 ± 14[b] | 258 ± 16 | 280 ± 18 | 450 ± 17 |
| RNA guanine | 93 ± 8 | 144 ± 17 | 137 ± 19 | 193 ± 11 |
| DNA thymine | 53 ± 3 | 52 ± 3 | 46 ± 6 | 110 ± 9 |
| DNA purines and other pyrimidines | † | † | † | † |
| Protein fraction | 0.55 ± .15[c] | 0.56 ± .16 | 1.19 ± .1 | 2.34 ± .1 |

[a] From Sky-Peck et al. (6).
[b] Specific activity, counts per minute per micromole; average of four determinations.
[c] Relative specific activity.
† Insignificant.

static carcinoma of the breast who showed, clinically, a marked "estrogen flare" following estradiol therapy.

Estradiol therapy for 7 days caused an increased uptake of formate-$C^{14}$ into the purine bases of RNA in both normal and tumor tissue and into the DNA thymine of the tumor. It, therefore, appears that, in addition to affecting formate incorporation into protein-bound serine, estradiol therapy also may affect formate incorporation into the nucleic acid bases. In this case, however, it appears that the turnover of RNA of normal tissue may be influenced. Corresponding studies on formate incorporation into the nucleic acids of tumor whose formate uptake into protein-bound serine is inhibited have not yet been carried out.

The most striking observation of these studies is the fact that estradiol therapy does not significantly affect formate incorporation into the protein of normal breast tissue but may stimulate or may inhibit its incorporation into breast cancer tissue. We are, however, a long way from being able to interpret this observation. We do not know whether we are dealing with a net synthesis of new protein and nucleic acid, or with a metabolic turnover, or with exchange reactions with pre-existing protein and nucleic acid. We do not know whether estrogen therapy directly or indirectly affects formate activation and incorporation into acid-soluble serine, purine, and thymine, or whether the effect is on the incorporation of these into protein and nucleic acid. We may perhaps be dealing with an effect of estrogen therapy on the pool sizes of these precursors. Studies to solve some of these problems are planned or are under way.

We can say that any net synthesis that does occur is very small—less than 1 % of the protein-bound serine being derived from the added radioformate during the incubation period of 5 hours.

The appearance of formate in the DNA thymine makes us feel that some synthesis of new DNA does occur during the experiment. The activity of the DNA thymine, however, is only 0.1 % that of the added formate, and we see this only because the thymine pool is very small and its equilibration with added formate is very rapid. Addition of 100 µg. of thymidine completely inhibits formate incorporation into DNA-thymine.

In spite of our limited knowledge, the sensitivity of formate incorporation into breast cancer to stimulation or inhibition by a short term of estradiol therapy seems clear. Further exploration of the biochemical bases of these effects may provide clues concerning the theraputic effectiveness of estrogens and perhaps may yield information of predictive value for assessing the potential effectiveness of estradiol therapy in individual patients.

### REFERENCES

1. Adair, F. E., Mellors, R. C., Farrow, J. H., Escher, G. C., and Urban, J. A. *J. Am. Med. Assoc.* **140**, 1193 (1949).
2. Elson, D., Gustafson, T., and Chargaff, E. *J. Biol. Chem.* **209**, 285 (1954).
3. Huggins, C. B. *J. Natl. Cancer Inst.* **15**, 1 (1954).
4. Kofman, S., Sky-Peck, H. H., Perlia, C. P., Economou, S. G., Winzler, R. J., and Taylor, S. G., III. *Cancer* **13**, 425 (1960).
5. Pearson, O. H., Li, M. C., MacLean, J. P., Lipsett, M. B., and West, C. D. *J. Am. Med. Assoc.* **159**, 1701 (1955).
6. Sky-Peck, H. H., Kofman, S., Taylor, S. G., and Winzler, R. J. *Cancer Research* **20**, 125-132 (1960).
7. Taylor, S. G. *Am. J. Med.* **21**, 688 (1956).

### DISCUSSION

**T. L. Dao:** I would like to ask Dr. Winzler about the incorporation of $C^{14}$-formate in the protein of cancerous breast tissue. Half of the patients showed a decrease of $C^{14}$-formate intake and the other half had an increase of incorporation of $C^{14}$-formate in the protein during estrogen therapy. Did you have any cases which showed no change of the $C^{14}$-formate uptake (besides the normal breast tissues) and, if so, what were the clinical courses of these patients?

**R. J. Winzler:** About 30 patients have now been studied. Of the 30 patients, about 10 have shown a stimulation, about 15 an inhibition, and the remaining 5 showed no effect that we can be sure of. In the 25 that do show either stimulation or inhibition of their very specific activities, the correlation with the subsequent course of the disease was very good. I do not recall what the clinical course was with the patients whose formate incorporation was neither stimulated nor inhibited by therapy.

**A. Segaloff:** Two questions. First, have you tried the effect of androgens? Secondly, if I understand your figures, there was essentially no change in formate incorporation in the serial biopsies. I presume that the patients were bearing breast cancer elsewhere and these were biopsies from the normal breast; but I was troubled by finding that when you gave large doses of estrogen there wasn't a substantial increase in formate incorporation from the estrogenic stimulation of the normal breast. Have I misconstrued what was done?

**R. J. Winzler:** No. This is exactly what was done. Most of these patients were postmenopausal patients and there was no increase in formate incorporation under these conditions in the normal breast tissues, even though therapy was continued for some time. In answer to the second question, we have tried the effects of prednisolone and testosterone on a few patients. The data, however, are too sparse for comment.

**R. Huseby:** My question also relates to the age and the status of endocrine stimulation of the control breast tissue. Certainly 1 week of estradiol therapy does not bring about much stimulation of the postmenopausal breast, whereas 1–4 months of such stimulation will. I wonder, therefore, if you have studied the incorporation of formate in normal breast tissues after longer periods of estrogen stimulation?

**S. G. Taylor, III:** We've got some data on repeated biopsies on the contralateral breast of individual patients, but we don't have enough data on the long-term effect of estrogen in the normal breast. There does appear to be a slight stimulation of the normal breast with estrogens, but only within the standard deviation. The interesting thing about these biochemical observations is that we have seen this drop in the specific activity of the biopsy specimen within 1 week after starting therapy, but we have not seen regression of the tumor clinically for up to 3 months.

**R. Huseby:** The question that I had in mind was whether or not you had followed patients that were on estrogen therapy over a period of months, and taken several breast biopsies? After about 1 month of therapy and progressing on to 7 or more months, an extensive proliferation and over-all increase in breast epithelium and fibrous connective tissue occurs in most, but not all, patients. This conversion of a postmenopausal breast, composed mainly of fat with relatively little fibrous connective tissue and epithelium, to one that is highly lobular and contains much more epithelium and fibrous connective tissue, certainly must represent a considerable formation of new protein. Is this reflected in formate uptake?

**R. J. Winzler:** One of the patients shown in Fig. 3 was one repeatedly studied over the course of several months. I don't know whether the breast showed the morphologic changes that you spoke of, but at least there was no change in the rate of formate uptake. I don't know the histological data on this particular patient.

**M. J. Brennan:** If the breast had been under the influence of fairly large amounts of estrogen at the time that the estradiol was given, it might well be that the rate of incorporation from a small dose of estradiol would not change appreciably. However, if it had not been under previous estrogenic influence a marked change in a positive direction might have been looked for, at least in some instances. This would be true in respect to both the breast and the tumor if they were positively responsive to the hormone. Is there any correlation, therefore, between an increase in uptake in these studies and measurements of pretreatment urinary estrogen excretion, vaginal smears, or gonadotropins, which might give us an indication whether the patient showing increased uptake has been more or less estrogen free in the pretreatment period?

**S. G. Taylor, III:** We have no information on the urinary estrogens. We have been doing some studies on vaginal smears but have not correlated that with other information to date. I think it should be done. There also was some minor variation in the incorporation of $C^{14}$ in normal breast tissue, that is, tissue from the contralateral breast of patients with cancer of the breast. Perhaps we should not call it *normal* breast tissue, but it showed no sign of tumor on biopsy. Does that answer the question?

**H. J. Greene:** Do the antifolic agents effect the incorporation of formate?

**R. J. Winzler:** Yes. The incorporation into serine, purine, and thymine is inhibited by very low concentrations of amethopterin.

**G. Gordan:** Regardless of any of our *a priori* ideas, it seems to me that these important data merit congratulations. If, at the end of 1 week, you can predict from formate incorporation which cases are going to progress and which regress, you really have something. It would be helpful to have a few more details about what you mean by "regression" and "progression." I ask this because, if you are using the terms as defined in protocol studies, a case in which most lesions are regressing, while some new ones are developing, is classified as "progressing." In such patients, by chance, you may have hit a progressing lesion when other lesions were regressing. In other words, the tissue you used may not have represented what was going on in all the cancer, throughout the body.

**S. G. Taylor, III:** That is an extremely important point. We have taken a biopsy from a lesion that seems to be static clinically and another lesion in the same patient that is clinically progressing. There is a difference in the incorporation of formate in these two lesions; so we have to be extremely careful in interpreting a finding, whether it is a reflection of what is going on in the body or only in one individual lesion. In general, the tissue which is most active clinically and biochemically, usually reflects what is going on.

**A. Segaloff:** Can you shorten the interval still further by putting the estrogen in the incubation mixture instead of into the patient?

**R. J. Winzler:** Estradiol added to the incubation medium has no effect. We have shortened the interval to 3 days in a few instances, and found essentially the same effect—either stimulation or inhibition. We have very few of these cases so far but hope to use even shorter intervals than this.

**A. White:** I wish to ask what seems to be an odd question, which requires some explanation. Have you looked at the effects of estrogen treatment on the utilization of other substrates by mammary tissue *in vitro,* specifically the glucose of the medium? I ask this question because, using the transplantable lymphosarcoma in the rat, we have demonstrated that estradiol, while not being one of the potent steroids studied, does have a marked inhibitory effect on the incorporation of glycine into the total proteins and the total nucleic acids of the tissue. It subsequently developed that all the steroid inhibitory effects could be explained on the basis of their effects on glucose utilization and on the supply of adenosine triphosphate in the system. If glucose utilization were the basis of the effects you observed, it would save a great deal of experimental effort.

**R. J. Winzler:** We have done a few incubations using other amino acids, none using glucose, and none measuring oxygen consumption or glycolysis rates. These are now being set up, along with ATP analysis in the tissues, using the firefly lantern technique. In the course of time we will have information on other substrates to see whether this is a specific effect on formate metabolism or a generalized effect.

**F. C. Greenwood:** I would like to return to the discussion on the expected increase in incorporation by treating a normal breast with estrogen. Dr. Huseby has shown the dramatic histological effect in the normal postmenopausal breast treated with estrogen, but I don't think this is biochemically a dramatic site of protein synthesis. If you take enzyme assays on the rat breast during pregnancy, for example, these have always shown a rather dull increase. I would not expect a rapid rate of incorporation under these conditions. Lactation is the condition in which one obtains a rapid synthesis of protein, probably comparable to that induced in the uterus by estrogen.

**R. J. Winzler:** I should have pointed out that the incorporation of formate in this system is actually much less than it is in other tissues that we have studied— animal tumors particularly, and also leucocytes. The incorporation into the tumor as well as the normal breast tissues is really very low, about one-sixth that into liver, for example. I don't think we have adequately answered the question raised about the prolonged effect of estrogen on normal breast tissue. This will take more work, but we will certainly do it.

**G. E. Block:** This is in amplification of Dr. Brennan's question: Do these patients represent a homogeneous clinical group? In other words were they all postmenopausal or were they all premenopausal; had they all been castrated, or what was their glandular status?

**S. G. Taylor, III:** They were a very heterogenous group. Some studies were made on premenopausal, some on postmenopausal patients. Observations were made before, during, and following estrogen therapy, and before and after various ablative procedures.

# IV. STEROIDS AND EXPERIMENTAL TUMORS

## Studies of Hormone Dependency Employing Interstitial Cell Testicular Tumors of Mice[1]

ROBERT A. HUSEBY

*Department of Surgery, University of Colorado Medical Center, Denver, Colorado*[2]

The study of the characteristics of hormone dependency of a group of transplantable testicular interstitial cell tumors originally induced in BALB/c mice has proved most interesting and, we believe, rather enlightening. Although in most strains of mice, as in man, the spontaneous occurrence of this tumor type is infrequent, it has been shown by several investigators that chronic treatment of male mice of several inbred strains with large doses of estrogenically active substances, either steroidal or nonsteroidal, is associated with the development of a high incidence of tumors of interstitial cell origin. Cytologically, these tumors appear to be malignant, and biologically they may invade the tunica albuginea and occasionally other surrounding structures and metastasize to the periaortic and left suprarenal lymph nodes. In spite of these manifestations of malignancy, it was found that many of the tumors would not grow progressively when isografted into intact male animals unless the recipients were also estrogenized (for reviews see 1, 7). It is of interest, however, that Gardner (6) was able to show that the nongrowing isografts in untreated males, though dormant for many months, remained viable, for they would begin to grow progressively soon after estrogen administration was instituted.

Since the early observations were made before the hormone dependency of certain truly malignant neoplasms was well established, many investigators regarded the behavior of these induced tumors in the mouse as curious but of only passing interest, while others raised the question whether they were really malignant neoplasms or merely hormonally induced atypical hyperplasias. However, as more examples of hormone-dependent malignant neoplasms were recorded and studied both in human subjects and in experimental animals, it became evident that the induced interstitial cell tumors of the mouse testis were, in fact, of such a nature. They appear to have several features to recommend their intensive investigation. They can be

---

[1] Aided by grants from the Damon Runyon Memorial Fund for Cancer Research Inc., and by grant No. C-3950 of the National Institutes of Health.

[2] *Present address:* Eleanor Roosevelt Institute for Cancer Research, American Medical Center, Denver, Colorado.

induced readily in several available inbred strains of mice so that the stimuli found to be necessary to support growth of isografts can be compared with those that influence their induction. They are sufficiently distinctive morphologically, and their genesis can be followed closely enough, to avoid any confusion with neoplasms that might be thought to arise from "rests" of other endocrine tissues within the substance of the testis. Their ability to remain dormant but viable for relatively long periods of time is reminiscent of the situation seen in certain malignancies of the human population. And, finally, since they frequently produce significant amounts of hormones, one can study the biosynthesis of these hormones in essentially pure cultures of abnormal interstitial cells (3).

## STUDIES OF TUMORIGENESIS

The first problem was to determine as many factors as possible that might influence the genesis of these tumors. In this regard, we (10, 11) were able to show that excessive estrogen stimulation was not essential for the development of a high incidence of tumors in BALB/c mice when the testes were maintained within the abdominal cavity. The intra-abdominal position not only enhanced tumorigenesis in association with estrogen stimulation, but also after many months by itself produced changes in the interstitial cells suggestive of early neoplasia. It was also found that with mild estrogen stimulation of the intra-abdominal testis, the striking changes noted in the interstitial cells prior to tumor development in heavily estrogenized mice (8) did not occur; so that the precursors of the neoplastic cells apparently were rather normal-appearing interstitial cells. Finally it was demonstated that 2 to 4 months after estrogen administration was instituted a change occurred in the interstitial cells that greatly increased the frequency with which they would become neoplastic when transplanted subcutaneously into castrate mice that were heavily estrogenized. Since this change occurred before any morphologic evidence of neoplasia appeared, it might well represent the initial step in interstitial cell tumorigenesis and, we believe, deserves considerable further investigation.

In none of our studies have we obtained evidence to support the thesis that excessive stimulation by pituitary tropic hormones represents the primary impetus to interstitial cell tumorigenesis (5). Though the mild dose of exogenous estrogen used in the studies employing intra-abdominally placed testes was found not to influence the response of seminal vesicles of castrate male mice to the administration of graded doses of testosterone propionate, the seminal vesicles of intact males ingesting this stilbestrol-containing diet are routinely slightly smaller than are those of males ingesting no estrogen. It is possible, of course, that stilbestrol acting directly on the interstitial cells could reduce their responsiveness to gonadotropins. Preliminary observations in our laboratory with hypophysectomized mice treated with human chorionic gonadotropin (HCG)[3] in graded doses suggest that this may be true to a certain degree; however, when an amount of HCG sufficient to maintain seminal vesicular weights at a near-normal level is administered daily for 2 weeks, the differences noted in the seminal vesicles of estrogenized and nonestrogenized animals are of the same magnitude as those seen in intact animals. All these observations seem to be consistent with the thesis that with this degree of estrogenization the level of circulating gonadotropins is not abnormally high. Nevertheless, since it has not yet been determined whether or not estrogen in the total absence of gonadotropic stimulation is capable of inducing tumors, it certainly is possible that gonadotropic stimulation at normal, or even at lower than normal, levels plays an essential role, along with estrogen, in the induction of this type of neoplasm.

### EARLIER STUDIES OF HORMONE DEPENDENCY

Our initial studies (10, 11) were designed to investigate under what endocrinological conditions isografts of several tumor lines would grow to macroscopic size within a reasonable period of time. For these studies, seven transfer lines were serially transplanted until their growth rate was such that explants when placed in estrogenized hosts would reach an average size of approximately 0.5 gm. within a four-month period. Throughout these studies, all animals in any one experiment were sacrificed at the time when the more rapidly growing tumors had reached this desired size, so that it is possible that had the experiments been allowed to continue longer, additional animals would have developed macroscopic tumors. However, this experimental design seemed to us to afford the best quantitation of relative growth rates.

It should also be mentioned that on morphologic and biologic grounds the primary tumors most usually appear to be composed of a heterogeneous population of neoplastic cells. With serial transplantation this obvious heterogeneity decreased rather rapidly, but recently evidence has been obtained that would indicate that even after as many as twenty-two transfer generations in one tumor line and nineteen generations in another the resultant tumors contained at least two populations of cells whose response to endocrine alterations were distinctly different. This heterogeneity of cell population may indeed contribute to the complexity of the results obtained in these studies.

---

[3] Human chorionic gonadotropin (Follutein) was kindly supplied by Dr. Edward C. Reifenstein, Jr., of the Squibb Institute for Medical Research.

The most striking fact that became evident early was that the tumor lines under investigation possessed very different characteristics of dependency with the only common factor that growth was always at its height in estrogenized animals. Beyond this, however, no consistent pattern evidenced itself. Thus, the 4092 tumor was found to grow essentially as well in castrate animals of either sex as in estrogenized animals and yet did not grow in intact females or in intact males. On the other hand, tumors 166189, 4061, and 157220 Line A grew distinctly better in intact females than in those that had been ovariectomized. Tumor 4061 by the third transfer generation was found to grow well in intact male mice, in fact better than in either castrate males or females, yet the administration of large doses of testosterone propionate to castrate males tended to slow the growth rate and reduced the number of individuals growing the tumor. The administration of this same dose of testosterone propionate to intact male mice bearing the 157220 Line A tumor, on the other hand, augmented tumor growth whereas similar treatment of animals bearing three other tumor lines was ineffectual in this regard.

Although tumor line 157220 Line B appeared to retain completely its marked degree of dependency throughout fifteen transfer generations over a period of more than five years, on the basis of observations made during the first transfer generations, it is fairly evident that the other lines had lost some degree of dependency during the early transfers when we were deliberately selecting toward more rapidly growing tumors. The results of these initial studies of dependency, therefore, are consistent with the interpretation that, when multiple changes are required for tumorigenesis and for the conversion of dependent tumors to autonomous ones, such alterations may occur in a rather random fashion, so that tumors of the same cell type evolve that have very different characteristics of dependency. It should be remembered, however, that changes might also be induced in the tumor cells during serial transfer in an unusual endocrine environment so that tumors might evolve that are dependent for continued growth upon stimuli that they did not originally require. In this regard, it might be mentioned that although the usual course of events was for tumor lines to become less dependent the more they were transplanted, in one instance a tumor apparently progressively increased in its dependency after the seventh serial transfer suggesting either that the tumor cells changed or that the more dependent cells outgrew the less dependent ones, an explanation that is difficult to reconcile with the fact that the growth rate of the tumors declined during this period.

Three additional factors were investigated in some detail. The first of these was the effect of the intra-abdominal position. During the course of other experiments, it was noted with two different tumor lines that transplants in the spleen of untreated intact males grew to macroscopic size more often than did explants in the subcutaneous tissues of the same animals. Experiments were then set up employing the 157220 Line B tumor, a tumor that had developed in a cryptorchid testis of a mouse ingesting the mildly estrogenizing diet, and had retained through many transplants a high degree of dependency. When explants were placed both in the spleen and in the subcutaneous tissues of recipients consuming this diet, the intrasplenic explants grew to macroscopic size in 15 of the 21 animals while in none were macroscopically evident tumors found in the subcutaneous tissues. It seems evident, then, that one of the factors, other than estrogen per se, that was found to enhance tumorigenesis also facilitated the growth of the explants.

Secondly, we wished to determine if estrogenic substances might stimulate the growth of tumors directly without the mediation of other organs such as the pituitary. This seemed possible to test by placing bits of tumor in the subcutaneous tissues and in the spleen of the same animal and then inserting an estrone-cholesterol pellet in juxtaposition to the intrasplenic transplant. If the concentration of estrone in the pellet was properly adjusted, it should be possible to bathe the intrasplenic explant in estrone while the subcutaneous one would be deprived of this stimulation because of hepatic inactivation of estrone as it drained from the spleen over the portal circulation. Experiments with the two tumor lines that would not grow in the intra-abdominal position in the absence of estrogenic stimulation were carried out, and in both instances small areas of growing tumor were found rather frequently next to the intrasplenic estrone-cholesterol pellets whereas the subcutaneous explants routinely were composed only of ceroid-filled cells and a few atypical tumor cells—the histological pattern we have become accustomed to seeing in explants that are not growing. Pure cholesterol pellets when placed next to the explants in the spleen exerted no growth-promoting effect. Because of the tendency of several of the tumor lines to grow when placed in the spleen without the addition of estrone, we have not been able to extend these observations to other lines; but, at least, in the two different lines that could be investigated it would appear that estrone exerted a growth-stimulating effect directly upon the tumor cells, an effect that was not mediated through other organs such as the pituitary. This, of course, does not imply that in the absence of other stimulatory factors estrone could maintain tumor growth by itself.

Finally the effect of the administration of a purified sheep pituitary LH preparation[4] was investigated. This preparation was well suited for our

[4] Purified sheep pituitary LH No. 227-80 was generously supplied by Doctors Sanford L. Steelman and James B. Lesh of the Armour Laboratories.

purpose since even after 4 months of continuous daily administration it was found to be effectively stimulating normal interstitial cells, as evidenced by their hyperplasia and hyperfunction. The results obtained in these studies were perplexing. Although such treatment was ineffective in promoting growth of the completely dependent 157220 Line B tumor, it did allow some tumor growth in intact males bearing grafts of three tumor lines of intermediate dependency (157220 Line A, 166189, and 4658). However, employing two lines that grew only inconsistently in castrate males (166189 and 4061), it was found that treatment of such animals with this LH preparation resulted in no growth stimulation. This would suggest that the growth-promoting effect noted in the intact males was mediated via the testes, possibly as a result of an increased production of estrogen by the hyperstimulated interstitial cells. Even more perplexing were the observations that the growth of the 157220 Line A tumor in either estrogenized males or in castrate females, of 166189 in estrogenized males and intact females, and of 4092 in castrate females was either distinctly slowed or completely inhibited by the administration of this hormone preparation. This latter observation seems more enigmatic in view of the fact that as a result of the combined estrogen-sheep LH treatment normal interstitial cells underwent extensive hyperplasia, so much so in fact that after 4 months of such treatment the testes often were composed almost entirely of interstitial cells with but few tubular elements remaining. This then represents another instance (9, 12, 13) of an endocrine manipulation inducing an extensive proliferation of the normal cells of origin while inhibiting the growth of their malignant counterpart, a situation that is difficult to explain by invoking the current ideas relative to the genesis of dependent neoplasms.

## The Effects of Hypophysectomy

From the preceding studies, it was impossible to get any idea of the role the pituitary might play in either the formation or the continued growth of these interstitial cell testicular tumors. Therefore, a study of the effects of hypophysectomy alone and in combination with certain substitutive therapies was undertaken (14). For the purpose of these investigations, five tumor lines that, at the time the studies were initiated, exhibited lesser degrees of dependency were selected with the hope that fewer factors would be required to maintain the growth of such tumors. In fact, two of the tumor lines, 4658 and 164041, by this time showed no response to hormonal alterations less drastic than hypophysectomy, and both of these were found to grow consistently in hypophysectomized hosts though their growth rate was somewhat slowed. Though one of these lines was apparently producing no hormones, the other, 164041, was an active androgen producer, and it was found that this tumor continued to produce androgens in as great quantities in hypophysectomized animals as in those with functioning pituitaries. Therefore, it would appear that these two tumor lines during the course of multiple serial transplantations had become "growth independent" and in the one case also "function independent."

On the other hand, the three tumor lines that had continued to exhibit some degree of hormone responsiveness, not only would not grow when transplanted into hypophysectomized hosts, but if allowed to grow to a measurable size in nonhypophysectomized animals would show definite regressive changes when the pituitary of the host was removed. These tumors, therefore, were definitely dependent for their continued growth upon one or more pituitary factors. Initial attempts at substitutive therapy using the purified sheep pituitary LH preparation were largely unsuccessful, for the diminution in size was not prevented. However, function was preserved to some extent and in two of the tumor lines (166189 and 4061) cellular morphology was maintained to a degree for a few days. Recent experiments employing human chorionic gonadotropin (HCG) have yielded more encouraging results. Here it was found that the growth and morphology of the 4092 tumor, though unaffected by sheep pituitary LH, were completely maintained by this latter less purified preparation. Contrariwise, treatment of hypophysectomized animals with HCG had no effect upon either the maintenance of growth or the morphology of 4061 tumors. Although the responsiveness of the 4092 tumor to large doses of HCG would seem to indicate that these tumor cells were dependent for their continued growth upon gonadotropic hormones, this does not necessarily mean that excessive stimulation with such hormones was a responsible factor in tumorigenesis. Certainly the effectiveness of smaller, more "physiological," doses of HCG will have to be studied; and the possibility always exists that during the seventeen serial transfers in castrate female animals alterations in the tumor cells occurred rendering them dependent upon a stimulus upon which they were not originally dependent.

The functional dependence of these three growth-dependent tumors is of some interest since, as far as could be determined, tumors of the 166189 line continued to produce hormones for at least 2 weeks after hypophysectomy of the host even though during this period they decreased markedly in size and showed significant morphological alterations. Thus it appears that in this instance a dissociation between growth dependency and function dependency had occurred. Tumor 4092, on the other hand, apparently ceased producing hormones as soon as pituitary stimulation was interrupted.

It is also of interest that in the five tumor lines studied, there was no correlation between growth dependency and morphology. Actually, on purely cytologic grounds, the 164041 tumor would have been considered the least malignant and the 4658 tumor the most malignant, yet both were apparently growth independent. It would appear from this small series that function was more related to morphology, since both of the tumors that produced goodly amounts of androgenically active hormones were composed of cells bearing the most resemblance to normal interstitial cells, whereas the tumors that were producing estrogenic and/or progestational hormones or were nonfunctional were composed of the more abnormal-appearing cells.

## POSSIBLE USEFULNESS OF ORGAN CULTURE TO PREDICT HORMONE DEPENDENCY

The use of organ culture techniques has yielded interesting results in the study of the relationship of certain normal tissues to hormone stimulation. For example, when tissue from prelactational mouse mammary glands was cultured in the commercially available 199 medium (15) using the Chen technique (2), it was noted that the alveolar structures disintegrated unless certain specific hormones, namely cortisol and lactogenic hormone, were added to the medium (4). On the other hand, tissues not under such intimate hormonal control were maintained well in this media and hormone-independent mouse mammary carcinomas would also be maintained. This suggested to Dr. Joel Elias that this might represent a useful technique to distinguish between hormone-dependent and hormone-independent neoplasms.

As an initial step, we sent Dr. Elias as "unknowns" representatives of six different tumor lines varying widely in their degree of dependence. Multiple organ cultures of two tumors from each line were set up and histological observations were made after 5 and 10 days of culture. The behavior of the tumors in this *in vitro* system correlated very well with the known behavior of the tumors *in vivo*. The fragments of tumor from the two lines that were autonomous, i.e., would grow in hypophysectomized mice, were well maintained for the duration of the experiment in the unfortified 199 medium. On the other hand, fragments of tumors from the four lines that had retained some hormone dependency showed evidence of disintegration after 5 days of culture, and many of the still obviously viable cells appeared cytologically similar to those seen in tumors that were regressing following hypophysectomy. By the tenth culture day, the explants had disintegrated to a much greater degree, and the extent of this disintegration appeared roughly parallel to the degree of hormone dependency exhibited *in vivo*. Thus fragments from the one tumor that could be grown consistently only in estrogenized mice had completely disintegrated and largely disappeared, while in those from the less dependent tumors there were still some viable appearing, though cytologically altered, cells.

Although these initial results are suggestive, in order to establish for certainty the validity of this technique we will have to find a hormone or combination of hormones that when added to the 199 medium will maintain the cellular integrity of hormone-dependent tumor. Preliminary experiments in our laboratory using the 4092 tumor and adding human chorionic gonadotropin to the medium have yielded encouraging, but as yet not conclusive, results. The addition of this hormone to the media definitely seems to alter the morphology of the surviving cells, but as yet we have not perfected our technique of culture to the point that we can be certain that it also increases the degree of cell survival.

However, since this is a relatively simple culture technique, should this line of investigation prove fruitful, it would seem that this might well be useful also in determining which cancers in the human patient are hormone dependent and thereby to predict with accuracy which patients might benefit from one or more of the various endocrine procedures now known to be useful in the palliative treatment of human cancer.

## SUMMARY

Although we have collected a considerable volume of data and have established certain basic facts relating to the nature of hormone dependency in these experimentally induced testicular interstitial cell tumors, many of the most fundamental questions remain unanswered. Certainly we need to determine all the principle factors influencing tumorigenesis in order to establish what influence they might have in sustaining the growth of isografts. With this information it might then be possible to maintain explants of a number of dependent tumors in organ culture and to investigate their *in vitro* versus their *in vivo* hormone requirements. As a corollary to this line of investigation, we must determine if, while growing in an unusual endocrine environment, tumor cells can be induced to become dependent for their continued growth upon stimuli on which they were not originally dependent. In another vein, it will be important to establish whether the ultimate behavior of a group of tumor cells is at all dependent upon the number of tumor cells present. In other words, in altered endocrine situations does the failure of isografts to grow progressively always parallel regression of established tumors? Also, in chronic experiments will dependent tumors that have regressed following hypophysectomy remain in this inactive state indefinitely as apparently do the small isografts, or will some of the cells in the larger tumor mass become autonomous and begin again to proliferate even in the absence of pituitary stimulation?

Although one is never justified in applying information obtained in one type of tumor in a certain species to other tumor types in other species, one would hope that answering these questions in this particular material might be helpful in interpreting similar phenomena of tumor dependency in other species, such as man, in which rigid control of conditions is not possible.

I feel that our text, in contrast to that cited by a previous speaker, must be "complexity, longevity, tenacity," for nature seldom is simple; and as Augustus Caesar has reminded us: "Hasten slowly. Do not let impetuosity betray you into imprudence."

REFERENCES

1. Andervont, H. B., Shimkin, M. B., and Canter, H. Y. *J. Natl. Cancer Inst.* **18**, 1 (1957).
2. Chen, J. M. *Exptl. Cell Research* **7**, 518 (1954).
3. Dominguez, O. V., Samuels, L. T., and Huseby, R. A. *Ciba Foundation Colloq. on Endocrinol.* **12**, 231 (1958).
4. Elias, J. J., and Rivera, E. *Cancer Research* **19**, 505 (1959).
5. Gardner, W. U. *Anat. Record* **68**, 339 (1937).
6. Gardner, W. U. *Cancer Research* **5**, 497 (1945).
7. Gardner, W. U. *Ciba Foundation Colloq. on Endocrinol.* **12**, 239 (1958).
8. Hooker, C. W., and Pfeiffer, C. A. *Cancer Research* **2**, 759 (1942).
9. Huggins, C., and Mainzer, K. *J. Exptl. Med.* **105**, 485 (1957).
10. Huseby, R. A. *Ciba Foundation Colloq. on Endocrinol.* **12**, 216 (1958).
11. Huseby, R. A. Unpublished data.
12. Huseby, R. A., and Thomas, L. B. *Cancer* **7**, 54 (1954).
13. Jacobs, B. B., and Huseby, R. A. *J. Natl. Cancer Inst.* **23**, 1107 (1959).
14. Jacobs, B. B., and Huseby, R. A. Unpublished data.
15. Morgan, J. F., Morton, H. J., and Parker, R. C. *Proc. Soc. Exptl. Biol. Med.* **73**, 1 (1950).

DISCUSSION

**G. S. Gordan:** I would like to express admiration for Dr. Huseby's willingness to oppose Dr. Huggins' admonition and his reminding us that these extremely complex matters do require time. This prompts me to ask the following question. Dr. Huseby has shown what hormonal dependency means in animal tumors; he has also had a great deal of experience with human breast cancer. Can we say on the basis of present information that certain breast tumors are, or are not, hormone dependent? I stress the word "dependent" in contrast to "sensitive."

**R. A. Huseby:** Although this may seem a matter of semantics, it is important. Some human tumors, both of the prostate and of the breast, regress following a variety of endocrine alterations of the host. This, in fact, was the origin of the concept of hormonal dependency of tumors. Certainly in the case of regressions that follow ablative procedures, it seems safe to assume that the continuing growth of a tumor at that particular time was, in fact, dependent upon some hormonal factor. Whether or not the same can be said of regressions in response to additive therapies is much less certain. The term "responsive," on the other hand, seems to have different connotations to different people, but usually suggests that a tumor responds either functionally or growthwise to some hormonal manipulation. In the testicular tumors that we have discussed, the three tumors that showed any hormonal responsiveness to lesser hormonal alterations regressed following hypophysectomy and, therefore, seemed to me to represent truly hormone-dependent tumors as well as hormone-responsive tumors.

What causes the regrowth of a tumor that has regressed in response to a hormone therapy is far from understood. One possibility is that the tumor cells during their dormancy change and no longer need the same stimulation for their continued growth that they did originally. In other words, the tumor has become autonomous. It is also probable that in some instances the hormonal milieu of the host may again change so that the necessary stimulant is again provided to the cells. This latter explanation is a bit difficult to understand in the case of hypophysectomy, and we hope that with this experimental material we will be able to investigate these problems further.

**R. L. Noble:** One part of Dr. Huseby's description which caught my attention particularly was a tumor that, I understood, showed increasing hormonal dependency. I would like to ask if there is any reason why this tumor, in its course of development, should develop an increasing dependency. As you are aware, we know fairly well how to reduce hormone dependency, but I think anything to give any insight as to how one could increase hormone dependency might lead to something practical. One other question: I presume that the various estrogens are interchangeable for tumors that are dependent on estrogens. Can one substitute the natural and the synthetic estrogens?

**R. A. Huseby:** To answer the last question first, as far as we know the estrogens, whether they are steroidal or nonsteroidal, are essentially interchangeable both in tumor production and in maintenance of growth. There are slight differences, however, as Dr. Gardner has shown. Certain strains of mice are more susceptible to one type of estrogen than to another as far as tumor production is concerned, but in general it appears that estrogen stimulation is the most important thing.

Now concerning increasing dependency: This was a tumor that was growing rather uniformly. During the seventh transfer generation it took about 4 months to attain an average size of 0.5 gm. in intact female animals, but only about 10 weeks to grow to the same size in castrate males ingesting our stilbestrol-containing diet. However, five transfers later, although it was growing slightly more rapidly in intact female animals, it now took 5 months to grow to the 0.5-gm. size in estrogenized castrate male recipients, even though in estrogenized castrate females it grew at the same rate as it did in the intact females. Since that time it has continued to be more difficult to handle, and by the twentieth transfer generation it grew only very inconsistently in male animals, no matter how much estrogen they were given. In addition, its growth rate had slowed down perceptibly in intact female animals, but it has grown better in these than in castrate female animals ingesting stilbestrol. There seem to be two possible explanations for such a phenomenon: either the tumor cells had changed as a result of their abnormal endocrine milieu and had become dependent upon some factor upon which they were not originally dependent, or the more dependent tumor cells had outgrown the more independent ones. The latter explanation seems difficult to accept since throughout much of the period of change the growth rate of the tumor had slowed rather than increased. However, how one can intentionally increase the dependency of these tumors is not known.

**R. Grinberg:** I would like to ask Dr. Huseby for further information on the relation between the so-called "dormant" cells and the hormones.

**R. A. Huseby:** The question relates to the dormancy, but retained viability, of transplanted tumor cells when they are put into an endocrine milieu that will not sustain growth. This was first described by Dr. Gardner, and we have repeated it in our material. For example, a dependent tumor is inoculated into an intact male animal, and no growth results. If one examines the area of the graft microscopically one finds small atypical cells that we have come to recognize as abnormal tumor cells, and some ceroid-filled macrophagic-appearing cells. This situation can be maintained for many months, but if the animal is then given estrogen in quantities that would have allowed growth of the isograft initially, within a month or so these areas of dormant tumor will begin to grow and become palpable. At this time they will look, microscopically, essentially the same as if they had started to grow immediately after transplantation into estrogenized hosts. This to me is very reminiscent of the situation seen in certain human cancers such as breast cancer, where the patient may go ten, fifteen, or even twenty years after radical mastectomy without showing evidence of metastatic disease, and then may come into the clinic one day with extensive disease that has apparently developed very rapidly.

**G. C. Mueller:**  Dr. Huseby, have you carried out experiments looking for this sort of steroid dependency in tissue culture systems?

**R. A. Huseby:**  We have just started doing the organ culture work discussed in the presentation. There is a big difference between organ culture as we are attempting to use it and the conventional tissue culture, as I am sure you are well aware. Our goal in the organ culture studies is to maintain survival of the cells without an outgrowth. Thus we use a medium which is not particularly rich in nutrients and to which such magical things as embryo extract have not been added. We have not conducted any true tissue culture studies. It is obvious, I think, that one matter that should be explored is the use of the clone technique to get cultures from single cells, in order to study the responsiveness of such tumors transplanted back into mice. We have not done this because of the large number of animals necessary for such studies if any significant number of clones were to be investigated. There is also always the possibility that the tissue culture passage might alter the characteristics of the tumor cell.

**U. Kim:**  We have appreciated Dr. Huseby's beautiful work very much and in many points agree with him. However, we use the terms "dependency" and "autonomy" in a slightly different manner. To us the dependent tumor is the one that does not grow in untreated host; for example, estrogen-induced rat pituitary tumors do not grow in untreated (nonestrogenized) rats; thyrotropic mouse pituitary tumors induced by radiothyroidectomy grow only in athyroid animals; and some of the hydrocarbon-induced tumors grow only in hosts treated with the same carcinogen. However, after repeated transplantations these dependent tumors become independent of the conditioning, and then we call them autonomous. Though these autonomous tumors may be independent of carcinogenic condition they still can be responsive to hormonal treatments. This we call autonomous but responsive. Many spontaneous and most of the methylcholanthrene-induced mammary carcinomas belong to this category. Finally, this responsiveness disappears and the tumors grow in any host and are indifferent to any kind of treatment. We classify them as autonomous-nonresponsive tumors; many radiation-induced tumors and mouse mammary carcinomas are of this type. Therefore, in treating a given tumor by various endocrine ablations, their effectiveness seemed to depend on the degree of dependency or autonomy at the time the treatments were initiated.

**R. A. Huseby:**  Different terms can be used, but I think it is time that we try to standardize our nomenclature a bit. If one can demonstrate that a tumor regresses significantly in size after an ablative procedure such as hypophysectomy, this tumor must be considered as being dependent: dependent for its continued growth on something other than circulating nutritional elements, etc. However, whether or not regressions of established tumors following administrative hormonal therapies reflect the same phenomenon is still an open question. In one mouse mammary tumor that Dr. Jacobs and I studied, we were able to show that the tumor responded nicely to several hormonal situations and yet would grow in hypophysectomized animals. In other words, we could augment or depress its growth by endocrine manipulations, but never could prevent its growth. This, according to Dr. Furth's definition, would be a growth-autonomous yet a growth-responsive tumor. However, in the case of three of the interstitial cell tumors studied, even though they would grow in many types of animals, they would regress following the removal of the pituitary. Therefore, I think we must put them in the growth-dependent group.

Growth rate and function do not necessarily go hand in hand. One of our most rapidly growing tumors, 164041, was also our best androgen-producing tumor. One of our slowest growing tumors produced no hormones as far as we could detect. Again there is no good correlation between dependency and autonomy of these tumors and their histological appearance. The 164041 tumor is composed of cells that are rather similar to normal interstitial cells, and yet it is hormone-independent whereas some of the other tumors that are hormone dependent are much more abnormal in their histological appearance. Actually there is a better correlation in this material between function and histology. Those tumors that produce androgens in significant amounts tend to have larger cells, with eosinophilic-staining cytoplasm more reminiscent of normal interstitial cells, than do those that are producing estrogen or are hormonally nonfunctional.

**W. H. Daughaday:**  I was very much interested on the effect of cryptorchidism on the induction of the tumors. Is this a temperature effect or do you have other speculations about the mechanism? Would you be willing to extrapolate this to the clinical situation?

**R. A. Huseby:**  I would not like to extrapolate the results we reported to the clinical situation, since the tumors that are purported to be influenced by the cryptorchid position in the human population are not of interstitial cell origin. The influence of the cryptorchid testis in tumorigenesis in our material has interested us greatly. One might guess that it is temperature, for certainly it has been shown that the tubular elements are greatly influenced by temperature changes and, of course, the tubules in our material have atrophied essentially down to the Sertoli cells. We tried to conduct one experiment, a year or so ago, in which we put just one of the testes up into the abdomen and then placed the mice on the stilbestrol-containing diet. But it would appear that testes like to be in the scrotum, for without exception when we autopsied the animals the intra-abdominally placed testis had migrated to the opposite side and down into the scrotal sac on that side. We will have to repeat this experiment using more forceful means of keeping the wanderers where we want them.

# Steroid-Responsive Neoplasms in Rats and Mice[1]

## W. F. Dunning

*Cancer Research Laboratory, University of Miami, Coral Gables, Florida*

A recent report (1) on the responsiveness of seven isologously transplanted rat neoplasms to a group of steroid compounds showed that cortisol was the most effective inhibitor of tumor growth. A transplantable lymphosarcoma R 2788 and acute leukemia IRC 741 proved to be the most responsive of the neoplasms. Further exploration of the responsiveness of these neoplasms to related adrenal cortical compounds and the results of testing a group of related neoplasms in rats and mice will be reported. The search for more responsive transplantable neoplasms has continued, and the results of testing three recently transplanted rat neoplasms will also be reported.

## Material and Methods

The neoplasms were inoculated subcutaneously on the right side or bilaterally by trocar in adult rats or mice of the same inbred strain as the bearer of the primary tumor. All the neoplasms grew progressively in 100 % of the untreated inoculated animals of the line of the bearer of the primary tumor or in $F_1$ hybrids derived from the same line. Groups of 10 were assigned randomly as controls or to the chemicals to be tested. The injection schedule was initiated 24 hours after inoculation and maintained until death of one of the group appeared imminent.

The chemicals were suspended in a methylcellulose solution SPF 17874 (Upjohn Company) and injected daily or on some other prearranged schedule in 0.2-ml. doses in the subcutaneous tissues alternately in the right or left flank at a distance from the site of inoculation of the neoplasm.

The rats and mice were weighed and inspected for tumors weekly. As soon as the tumors were palpable they were measured. In each case the three largest diameters were recorded in centimeters and an average diameter was obtained for each tumor at weekly intervals until death of the host. Postmortem examination included inspection for gross metastases and preservation of representative sections of the neoplasm, auxiliary and mediastinal lymph nodes, lungs, liver, spleen, kidney and endocrine glands.

## Results

Table I summarizes the response obtained in Fischer line 344 rats inoculated with acute leukemia IRC 741 following treatment with four adrenal

[1] The work reported in this paper was supported by contract SA-43-ph-1681 with the Cancer Chemotherapy National Service Center, National Institutes of Health, United States Public Health Service.

## TABLE I

RESPONSE OF TRANSPLANTED ACUTE LEUKEMIA IRC 741 IN FISCHER LINE 344 RATS TO HORMONAL AGENTS WHEN TREATMENT WAS INITIATED 24 HOURS AFTER TRANSPLANTATION

| Compound | Total dose (mg./kg.) | No. of inj. | Inj. inter. (days) | Number treated | | At end $R_x$ period | | | | Difference in W.B.C. |
|---|---|---|---|---|---|---|---|---|---|---|
| | | | | Rats | Tumors | % Change body wt. | Tumor diameter $R_x$/cont. | % Change, survival | % Toxic deaths | |
| Cortisol | 194 | 14 | 1 | 10 | 10 | −18 | 0.53 | 19 | 0 | −127,000 |
| Prednisone | 65 | 5 | 1 | 10 | 10 | 40 | 0.96 | 0 | 0 | − 27,000 |
| 9α-Fluorocortisol | 65 | 5 | 1 | 10 | 10 | −18 | 0.60 | −5 | 0 | −110,000 |
| Decadron | 60 | 3 | 2 | 10 | 0 | — | 0.00 | — | 100 | — |
| Decadron | 12 | 6 | 2 | 10 | 6 | −18 | 0.53 | 0 | 40 | − 86,000 |
| Decadron | 12 | 12 | 1 | 10 | 8 | −11 | 0.53 | 5 | 20 | − 88,000 |
| Decadron | 6 | 6 | 2 | 10 | 10 | 4 | 0.77 | 3 | 0 | − 75,000 |
| Decadron | 6 | 12 | 1 | 10 | 10 | −15 | 0.63 | 5 | 0 | − 63,000 |

cortical compounds. It shows that none of the compounds prevented the development of the disease. Decadron, 9α-fluorocortisol, and cortisol effectively reduced the growth of the subcutaneous tumor and significantly reduced the white blood count (WBC). Cortisol was the only compound that increased the average survival of the rats. It was tolerated for a longer period than any of the other compounds. Daily injections of 15 mg./kg. of all the compounds except prednisone proved to be toxic to these rats. Decadron was toxic at 1 mg./kg.

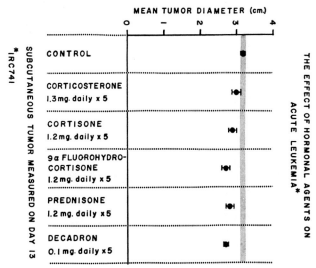

FIG. 1. A comparison of the mean tumor diameter of IRC 741 in each treated group with the mean ± P.E. of the control group after the fourth daily injection.

Figure 1 shows the comparative reduction in size of established subcutaneous tumors in rats that were treated for 5 consecutive days starting on the tenth day after inoculation with IRC 741. The rats weighed approximately 100 gm. at the beginning of treatment. These tumor measurements were made after the fourth injection of approximately 12 mg./kg. for all the compounds except Decadron. The dose for the latter compound was 1 mg./kg. The tumors were consistently smaller in the treated rats, and the small differences in average diameter were statistically significant except in the case of corticosterone.

Table II summarizes the results obtained with cortisol, 9α-fluorocortisol, and Decadron on R 2788 lymphosarcoma in adult A × C line 9935 piebald rats and with cortisol on R 3251 lymphosarcoma (Fig. 2) in Fischer line 344 rats. Daily injections of 10 mg./kg. of cortisol were toxic but this dose

## TABLE II

RESPONSE OF TRANSPLANTED LYMPHOSARCOMA R 2788 IN A × C LINE 9935 RATS AND LYMPHOSARCOMA R 3251 IN FISCHER LINE 344 RATS TO HORMONAL AGENTS WHEN TREATMENT WAS INITIATED 24 HOURS AFTER TRANSPLANTATION

| Tumor no. compound | Total dose (mg./kg.) | No. of inj. | Inj. inter. (days) | Number treated | | At end $R_x$ period | | | % Toxic deaths | % Cures |
| --- | --- | --- | --- | --- | --- | --- | --- | --- | --- | --- |
| | | | | Rats | Tumors | % Change body wt. | Tumor diameter $R_x$/cont. | % Change survival | | |
| R 2788 Lymphosarcoma | | | | | | | | | | |
| Cortisol | 172 | 17 | 1–2 | 10 | 20 | −7 | 0.93 | 4 | 0 | 0 |
| 9α-Fluorocortisol | 27 | 4 | 1 | 10 | 18 | −16 | 0.74 | 5 | 10 | 0 |
| 9α-Fluorocortisol | 50 | 5 | 2 | 10 | 14 | −27 | 0.00 | 42 | 40 | 0 |
| Decadron | 40 | 4 | 2 | 10 | 0 | −29 | 0.00 | — | 100 | 0 |
| R 3251 Lymphosarcoma | | | | | | | | | | |
| Cortisol | 198 | 22 | 2 | 10 | 15 | −10 | 0.83 | −8 | 0 | 0 |

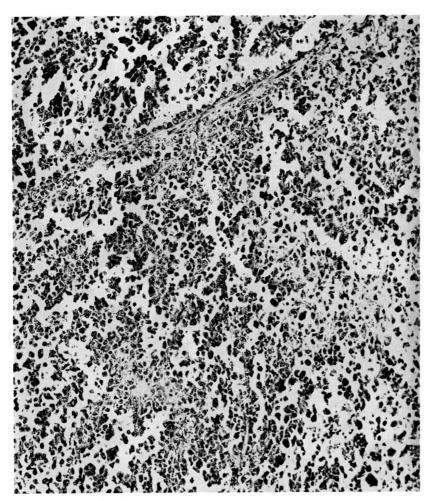

Fig. 2. Section of R 3251, a primary lymphosarcoma of the mesenteric lymph nodes in a 452-day-old Fischer line 344 male rat (magnification × 105).

was tolerated on an every other day schedule. Cortisol was better tolerated than the other compounds but was less effective in controlling the growth of the tumor. The best response was obtained with 9α-fluorocortisol administered at 10 mg./kg. every other day for five injections. Four of 10 rats died from the toxicity of the drug (3 with no evidence of neoplasia). No tumors were discernible in the surviving 6 at the end of the treatment period, but these rats died with tumors an average of 11 days after the untreated tumor rats. The average survival of the tumor bearers was increased 42 %.

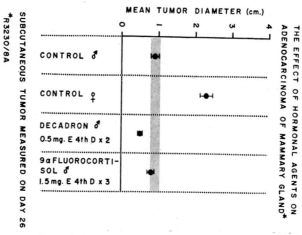

Fig. 3.  A comparison of the mean tumor diameter ± P.E. of R 3230 in males and females and males treated with Decadron and 9α-fluorocortisol.

Table III shows that these compounds were equally toxic to Yoshida rats and were ineffective in controlling the growth of the Yoshida lymphoma. This homologously transplated lymphoma proved (2) to be more responsive to other carcinostatic agents than R 2788 but was relatively unresponsive to maximum tolerated doses of cortisol, prednisone, or 9α-fluorocortisol.

Likewise, maximum tolerated doses of 9α-fluorocortisol (Table IV) proved to be ineffective in controlling the growth of transplanted squamous cell carcinomas of the prostate (M-C 972 and M-C 961) in A × C line 9935 Irish rats, spindle cell sarcoma IRS 4337 in Copenhagen line 2331 rats, or R 3230 adenocarcinoma of the mammary gland in Fischer line 344 rats. Figure 3 shows graphically for the latter tumor, the difference observed in diameter of the tumors in males and females and the comparative inhibition obtained in males treated with Decadron and 9α-fluorocortisol.

Lampkin and Potter (3) described a transplantable lymphosarcoma in

## TABLE III

RESPONSE OF SUBCUTANEOUSLY TRANSPLANTED YOSHIDA LYMPHOMA IN YOSHIDA RATS TO HORMONAL AGENTS WHEN TREATMENT WAS INITIATED 24 HOURS AFTER TRANSPLANTATION

| Compound | Total dose (mg./kg) | No. of inj. | Inj. inter. (days) | Number treated | | At end $R_x$ period | | | | |
|---|---|---|---|---|---|---|---|---|---|---|
| | | | | Rats | Tumors | % Change body wt. | Tumor diameter $R_x$/cont. | % Change survival | % Toxic deaths | % Cures |
| Cortisol | 18 | 3 | 4 | 8 | 8 | — 3 | 1.03 | —24 | 0 | 0 |
| Prednisone | 30 | 4 | 1 | 8 | 8 | —12 | .92 | —43 | 0 | 0 |
| 9α-Fluorocortisol | 18 | 3 | 4 | 8 | 8 | —25 | .85 | —35 | 0 | 0 |
| 9α-Fluorocortisol | 30 | 4 | 1 | 8 | 8 | —28 | .74 | —47 | 25 | 0 |
| 9α-Fluorocortisol | 50 | 5 | 2 | 8 | 7 | —30 | .51 | —50 | 100 | 0 |
| Decadron | 6 | 3 | 2 | 8 | 0 | —25 | .00 | | 100 | 0 |
| Decadron | 11 | 2 | 4 | 8 | 0 | —30 | .00 | | 100 | 0 |

TABLE IV

RESPONSE OF SEVERAL ISOLOGOUSLY TRANSPLANTED SOLID NEOPLASMS IN RATS TO 9α-FLUOROCORTISOL AND DECADRON WHEN TREATMENT WAS INITIATED 24 HOURS AFTER TRANSPLANTATION

| Compound and tumor no. | Total dose (mg./kg) | No. of inj. | Inj. inter. (days) | Number treated | | At end $R_x$ period | | | | % Cures |
| --- | --- | --- | --- | --- | --- | --- | --- | --- | --- | --- |
| | | | | Rats | Tumors | % Change body wt. | Tumor diameter $R_x$/cont. | % Change survival | % Toxic deaths | |
| 9α-Fluorocortisol | | | | | | | | | | |
| *Squamous cell carcinoma of prostate* | | | | | | | | | | |
| M-C 972 | 56 | 7 | 1 | 9 | 4 | −20 | 0.85 | −8 | 77 | 0 |
| M-C 961 | 31 | 5 | 4 | 10 | 20 | −22 | 1.00 | −7 | 0 | 0 |
| *Spindle cell sarcoma* | | | | | | | | | | |
| IRS 4337 | 20 | 3 | 2 | 10 | 10 | −15 | 0.88 | 0 | 0 | 0 |
| *Adenocarcinoma of mammary gland* | | | | | | | | | | |
| R 3230 | 19 | 3 | 2 | 10 | 20 | −10 | 0.89 | 0 | 0 | 0 |
| Decadron | | | | | | | | | | |
| M-C 961 | 22 | 3 | 2 | 10 | 0 | −33 | | | 100 | 0 |
| IRS 4337 | 20 | 3 | 2 | 10 | 8 | −25 | | | 100 | 0 |
| R 3230 | 5 | 2 | 2 | 10 | 20 | −14 | 0.55 | | 40 | 0 |

TABLE V

RESPONSE OF SEVERAL SUBCUTANEOUSLY TRANSPLANTED MALIGNANT LYMPHOMAS IN MICE TO CORTISOL AND CORTISONE WHEN TREATMENT WAS INITIATED 24 HOURS AFTER TRANSPLANTATION

| Compound and tumor no. | Total dose (mg./kg.) | No. of inj. | Inj. inter. (days) | Number treated | | At end $R_x$ period | | | | |
|---|---|---|---|---|---|---|---|---|---|---|
| | | | | Mice | Tumors | % Change body wt. | Tumor diameter $R_x$/cont. | % Change survival | % Toxic deaths | % Cures |
| Cortisol | | | | | | | | | | |
| M 3713 | 145 | 6 | 1 | 10 | 8 | −3 | 0.50 | 7 | 0 | 20?[a] |
| M 3509 | 425 | 20 | 1 | 10 | 10 | −7 | 1.13 | 22 | 0 | 0 |
| M 3445 | 168 | 6 | 1 | 10 | 10 | 7 | 0.87 | 11 | 0 | 0 |
| M 3445 | 238 | 12 | 1 | 10 | 10 | −16 | 0.31 | −12 | 0 | 0 |
| Cortisone | | | | | | | | | | |
| M 3509 | 125 | 5 | 1 | 10 | 7 | −6 | 0.18 | 21 | 0 | 30?[a] |
| M 3713 | 125 | 5 | 1 | 10 | 10 | 0 | 0.33 | 49 | 0 | 0 |
| P 1798 | 250 | 12 | 1 | 10 | 10 | −18 | 0.33 | 45 | 10 | 0 |
| P 1798 | 125 | 5 | 1 | 11 | 11 | −2 | 0.25 | 31 | 0 | 0 |

[a] Cures (?) because tumors failed to grow progressively after reinoculation.

## TABLE VI

RESPONSE OF SEVERAL SUBCUTANEOUSLY TRANSPLANTED MALIGNANT LYMPHOMAS IN MICE TO 9α-FLUOROCORTISOL WHEN TREATMENT WAS INITIATED 24 HOURS AFTER TRANSPLANTATION

| Tumor no. | Total dose (mg./kg.) | No. of inj. | Inj. inter. (days) | Number treated | | At end $R_x$ period | | | | |
|---|---|---|---|---|---|---|---|---|---|---|
| | | | | Mice | Tumors | % Change body wt. | Tumor diameter $R_x$/cont. | % Change survival | % Toxic deaths | % Cures |
| M 3713 | 150 | 6 | 1 | 9 | 2 | 4 | 0.00 | 28 | 11 | 66 |
| M 3713 | 125 | 5 | 1 | 10 | 2 | −25 | 0.00 | 193 | 80 | 0 |
| P 1798 | 125 | 5 | 1 | 11 | 5 | −2 | 0.00 | 70 | 18 | 45 |
| P 1798 | 125 | 5 | 1 | 10 | 7 | −13 | 0.00 | 50 | 0 | 30 |
| P 1798 | 100 | 10 | 1 | 10 | 9 | −13 | 0.00 | 90 | 0 | 10 |
| M 3509 | 125 | 5 | 1 | 10 | 6 | −7 | 0.00 | 0 | 40 | 0 |
| M 3445 | 162 | 6 | 1 | 10 | 10 | −10 | 0.56 | 17 | 20 | 0 |
| M 3307[a] | 125 | 5 | 1 | 8 | 8 | −4 | — | 20 | 0 | 0 |

[a] Acute lymphatic leukemia.

TABLE VII

RESPONSE OF SEVERAL SUBCUTANEOUSLY TRANSPLANTED MALIGNANT LYMPHOMAS IN MICE TO DECADRON WHEN TREATMENT WAS INITIATED 24 HOURS AFTER TRANSPLANTATION

| Tumor no. | Total dose (mg./kg.) | No. of inj. | Inj. inter. (days) | Number treated | | At end $R_x$ period | | | | |
| | | | | Mice | Tumors | % Change body wt. | Tumor diameter $R_x$/cont. | % Change survival | % Toxic deaths | % Cures |
|---|---|---|---|---|---|---|---|---|---|---|
| P 1798 | 125 | 5 | 1 | 9 | 5 | −17 | 0.00 | 110 | 0 | 44 |
| P 1798 | 100 | 10 | 1 | 9 | 1 | −18 | 0.01 | 141 | 10 | 77 |
| M 3713 | 125 | 5 | 1 | 10 | 9 | − 8 | 0.11 | 50 | 10 | 0 |
| M 3713 | 125 | 5 | 2 | 10 | 3 | −15 | 0.00 | 75 | 70 | 0 |
| M 3445 | 125 | 5 | 1 | 10 | 5 | 4 | 0.58 | 30 | 50 | 0 |
| M 3445 | 50 | 5 | 1 | 10 | 6 | 3 | 0.79 | 15 | 40 | 0 |
| M 3509 | 125 | 5 | 1 | 9 | 8 | − 6 | 0.09 | 25 | 11 | 0 |

Balb/C mice that was more responsive to cortisone than any of the rat neoplasms that have been tested thus far. Table V shows the relative responsiveness of this neoplasm and three other transplantable mouse lymphomas to cortisone or cortisol. AKR or AKR $F_1$ hybrid mice inoculated with M 3509 and M 3713 and Balb/C mice inoculated with P 1798 tolerated five daily injections of 24 mg./kg. of cortisone with very little loss of body weight, showed a significant inhibition (0.18 to 0.33 of the diameters of the tumors in controls) in growth of the subcutaneous tumors, and showed an increase of 21–49 % in average survival. A total dose of 250 mg./kg in twelve daily injections was somewhat more toxic to the Balb/C mice inoculated with P 1798. M 3509 seemed to be the most responsive to cortisone. Three of 10 mice survived for 90 or more days with no evidence of neoplasia. M 3713 responded well to six daily injections of 25 mg./kg. of cortisol. In this case the average diameter of the tumors was reduced to 50 % of the average diameter of the tumors in the controls. The treated mice sustained a loss of only 3 % in body weight. Twenty per cent appeared to be cured, but the tumors failed to grow progressively in these mice after reinoculation. M 3509 did not respond as well to a total dose of 425 mg./kg. of cortisol when it was administered in twenty daily injections as it did to five daily injections of cortisone administered at a slightly higher dosage level. M 3445 in C3H mice was less responsive to cortisol than the other lymphomas.

Unpublished data from Lampkin-Hibbard (Tables VI and VII) show that all five mouse lymphomas responded well to five or six daily injections of 25 mg./kg. of 9α-fluorocortisol. Except for M 3445 no tumors were discernible in the treated mice after the completion of the treatment and at the time that the tumors in the untreated control mice were measured. The average diameter of M 3445 subcutaneous tumors in mice treated with 9α-fluorocortisol was reduced to 56 % of the average diameters of the tumors in untreated control mice. Complete cures, i.e., mice that survived for 90 or more days without evidence of neoplasia and succumbed in the expected time to a second challenge with the tumor, were obtained in 66 % of treated mice inoculated with M 3713, and in 30–45 % of the mice inoculated with P 1798. For the latter tumor one cure out of ten and a 90 % increase in average survival time of the mice that died with tumors resulted from treatment with ten daily injections of 9α-fluorocortisol at 10 mg./kg.

P 1798 proved to be the most responsive of the mouse lymphomas tested with Decadron, as shown in Table VII. Cures were obtained in 44 and 77 % of the mice treated, respectively, with five daily injections of 25 mg./kg. and ten daily injections at 10 mg./kg. No cures were obtained in similarly treated mice inoculated with the other three lymphomas. Mice inoculated with M 3445 were less tolerant of the drug, and these tumors were less

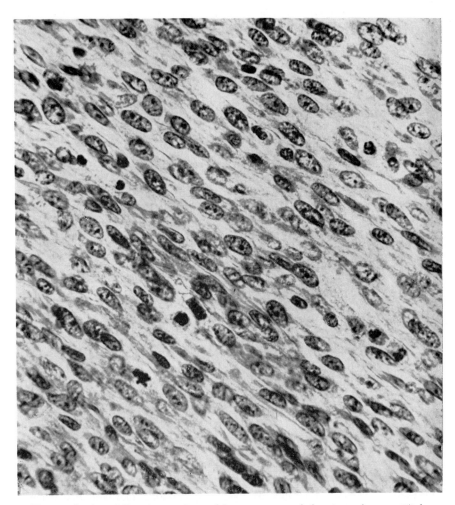

FIG. 4.   Section of R 3234, a primary leiomyosarcoma of the uterus from a 407-day-old A × C line 9935 Irish rat (magnification × 600).

responsive than the other lymphomas. After five daily injections at 25 mg./kg. and 10 mg./kg., 50 and 40 % succumbed, respectively, and the subcutaneous tumors in the survivors were reduced to only 58 and 79 % of the tumors in the controls. The dose of Decadron tolerated by these mice, however, was at least ten times that tolerated by any of the rats thus far tested.

## New Transplantable Rat Neoplasms

Three of the recently transplanted rat neoplasms were sufficiently responsive to some of the steroid compounds to be of interest. The first of these, R 3234 (Fig. 4), a leiomyosarcoma of the uterus, was observed as a spon-

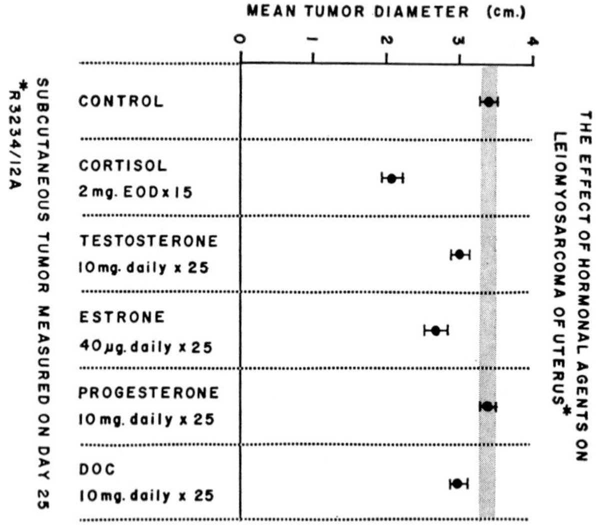

Fig. 5. A comparison of the mean tumor diameter of R 3234 in each treated group with the mean ± P.E. of the control group in A × C line 9935 Irish male rats.

taneous neoplasm in a retired A × C line 9935 Irish breeder rat 407 days old. It grew rapidly in 100 % of the inoculated rats of both sexes of this inbred line. Rats with bilateral transplanted tumors succumbed in an average of 30 days in a range of 25–35 days. Table VIII and Fig. 5 show the response of this neoplasm to daily injection of 40 μg. of estrone, 10 mg. of deoxycorticosterone, testosterone, and progesterone, and injections every other day of 2 mg. of cortisol. Figure 5 shows the comparative average diameters of the tumors in control and treated rats 25 days after inoculation. The tumor growth appeared to be unaffected by daily injections of 10 mg. of progesterone and significantly inhibited by the other compounds. Testosterone increased the average survival period from $29 \pm 0.91$ to $36 \pm 0.42$

TABLE VIII

RESPONSE OF SUBCUTANEOUSLY TRANSPLANTED R 3234 LEIOMYOSARCOMA OF THE UTERUS IN A ×C LINE 9935 IRISH RATS TO VARIOUS HORMONAL AGENTS WHEN TREATMENT WAS INITIATED 24 HOURS AFTER TRANSPLANTATION

| Compound | Dose per inj. | Total | No. of inj. | Number | | Initial body wt. (gm.) | Days to death (Mean ± P.E.) | 25 Days | |
| --- | --- | --- | --- | --- | --- | --- | --- | --- | --- |
| | | | | Rats | Tumors | | | Tumor diameter (Mean ± P.E.) | Body wt. (gm.) |
| SPF 17874 | 0.2 cc. | 5 cc. | 25 | 9 | 18 | 171 | 29 ± .91 | 3.4 ± .07 | 152 |
| Cortisol | 2 mg. | 30 mg. | 15 | 8 | 16 | 235 | 36 ± 1.9 | 2.1 ± .11 | 171 |
| Estrone | 40 μg. | 1 mg. | 25 | 8 | 16 | 220 | 30 ± .84 | 2.7 ± .11 | 166 |
| Deoxycorticosterone | 10 mg. | 250 mg. | 25 | 8 | 16 | 200 | 30 ± .59 | 3.0 ± .06 | 163 |
| Testosterone | 10 mg. | 250 mg. | 25 | 8 | 16 | 216 | 36 ± .42 | 3.0 ± .03 | 193 |
| Progesterone | 10 mg. | 250 mg. | 25 | 8 | 16 | 216 | 31 ± .42 | 3.4 ± .05 | 194 |

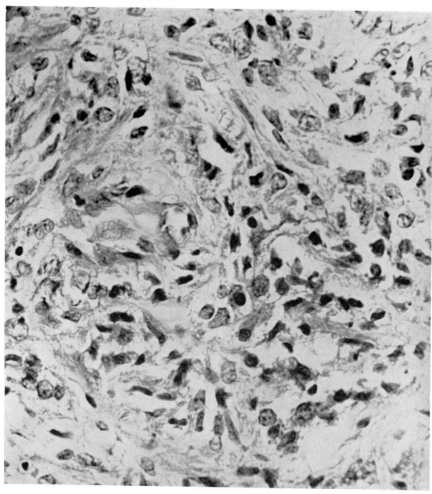

FIG. 6.  Section of R 3244 primary fibrosarcoma of mammary gland from a 509-day-old Fischer line 344 rat (magnification × 600).

days. The other compounds caused sufficient weight loss and evidence of toxicity to increase the variability or limit the survival period to approximately that of the untreated rats.

The second tumor R 3244, a relatively acellular fibrosarcoma of the mammary gland (Fig. 6), was observed as a spontaneous neoplasm in a breeding Fischer line 344 female rat 509 days old. The transplanted tumors grew more slowly than the previously described neoplasm and killed the host in an average of 65 days. Table IX and Fig. 7 show that this tumor

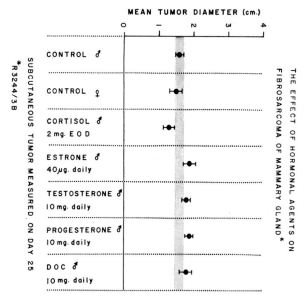

Fig. 7. A comparison of the mean tumor diameter of R 3244 in each treated group with the mean ± P.E. of the control group in Fischer line 344 male rats.

grew equally well in males and females, and after 25 daily injections the tumors were slightly larger in rats treated with all the steroid compounds except cortisol. The differences were somewhat greater at 32 days. Data on the average survival of the rats are not yet available.

The most interesting of the newly transplated neoplasms is R 3230, an adenocarcinoma of the mammary gland. This tumor (Figs. 8 and 9) was observed in a 332-day-old Fischer line 344 breeding female. It grows more rapidly when transplanted in intact females than when transplanted in males. The average survival of rats with bilateral tumors is 60 days for females and 90 days for males. Table X and Figs. 3, 10, and 11 show the response of this neoplasm to several steroid compounds. It appears to be slightly

TABLE IX

Response of Subcutaneously Transplanted R 3244 Fibrosarcoma of the Mammary Gland in Fischer Line 344 Rats to Various Hormonal Agents When Treatment Was Initiated 24 Hours after Transplantation

| Compound | Sex | Dose per inj. | Total (mg.) | No. of inj. | Number | | Average initial body wt. | 25 Days | |
|---|---|---|---|---|---|---|---|---|---|
| | | | | | Rats | Tumors | | Tumor diameter (Mean P.E.) | Body wt. (gm.) |
| SPF 17874 | M | 0.2 cc. | — | 25 | 10 | 20 | 207 | $1.6 \pm 0.08$ | 204 |
| SPF 17874 | F | 0.2 cc. | — | 25 | 10 | 20 | 134 | $1.5 \pm 0.09$ | 138 |
| Cortisol | M | 2 mg. | 50 | 25 | 10 | 20 | 174 | $1.3 \pm 0.08$ | 169 |
| Estrone | M | 40 μg. | 1 | 25 | 10 | 20 | 180 | $1.9 \pm 0.09$ | 165 |
| Deoxycorticosterone | M | 10 mg. | 250 | 25 | 10 | 20 | 163 | $1.8 \pm 0.10$ | 179 |
| Testosterone | M | 10 mg. | 250 | 25 | 10 | 20 | 171 | $1.8 \pm 0.08$ | 181 |
| Progesterone | M | 10 mg. | 250 | 25 | 10 | 20 | 154 | $1.9 \pm 0.06$ | 177 |

TABLE X

RESPONSE OF SUBCUTANEOUSLY TRANSPLANTED R 3230 ADENOCARCINOMA OF THE MAMMARY GLAND IN FISCHER LINE 344 RATS TO VARIOUS HORMONAL AGENTS WHEN TREATMENT WAS INITIATED 24 HOURS AFTER TRANSPLANTATION

| Tumor no. and compound | Sex | Dose per inj. | Total | No. of inj. | Number Rats | Number Tumors | Initial body wt. (gm.) | Days to death (mean ± P.E.) | Tumor diameter (mean ± P.E.) | Body wt. (gm.) |
|---|---|---|---|---|---|---|---|---|---|---|
| R 3230/6A | | Daily | | | | | | | 35 Days | |
| SPF 17874 | M | 0.2 cc. | 6.0 | 30 | 10 | 20 | 200 | 83 ± 2.6 | 1.6 ± .09 | 208 |
| SPF 17874 | F | 0.2 cc. | 6.0 | 30 | 9 | 18 | 144 | 57 ± 1.7 | 3.6 ± .06 | 179 |
| Cortisol | M | 4.2 mg. | 44 | 17 | 10 | 18 | 216 | 86 ± 2.5 | 1.2 ± .06 | 194 |
| Estrone | M | 40 µg. | 1.2 | 30 | 11 | 22 | 208 | 62 ± 3.4 | 2.2 ± .09 | 181 |
| Deoxycorticosterone | M | 10 mg. | 300 | 30 | 10 | 20 | 203 | 46 ± 2.4 | 3.5 ± .07 | 215 |
| Testosterone | M | 10 mg. | 300 | 30 | 10 | 20 | 202 | 58 ± 3.1 | 3.4 ± .08 | 217 |
| Progesterone | M | 10 mg. | 250 | 25 | 10 | 20 | 189 | 45 ± 2.5 | 4.1 ± .04 | 230 |
| R 3230/8A | | E.O.D.[a] | | | | | | | 54 Days | |
| SPF 17874 | M | 0.2 cc. | 6.0 | 30 | 10 | 20 | 222 | 94 ± 3.8 | 3.2 ± .13 | 233 |
| Control | F | — | — | — | 11 | 22 | 157 | 54 ± 2.0 | 4.7 ± .15 | 207 |
| Estriol | M | 400–200 µg. | 7.2 | 30 | 10 | 20 | 208 | 64 ± 3.1 | 4.2 ± .21 | 210 |
| Hexestrol | M | 120–60 µg. | 2.1 | 30 | 10 | 20 | 201 | 77 ± 2.5 | 3.6 ± .09 | 204 |
| R 3230/9A | | E.O.D. | | | | | | | 26 Days | |
| SPF 17874 | M | 0.2 cc. | 0.6 | 3 | 10 | 20 | 195 | 79 ± 4.0 | 0.9 ± .06 | 202 |
| Control | F | — | — | — | 10 | 20 | 164 | 67 ± 2.1 | 2.3 ± .11 | 165 |
| Decadron | M | 0.5 mg. | 1.0 | 2 | 10[b] | 20 | 205 | — | 0.5 ± .02 | 176 |
| 9α-Fluorocortisone | M | 1.5 mg. | 4.5 | 3 | 10 | 20 | 230 | — | 0.8 ± .05 | 206 |

a Every other day.
b Five died from toxicity with small tumors.

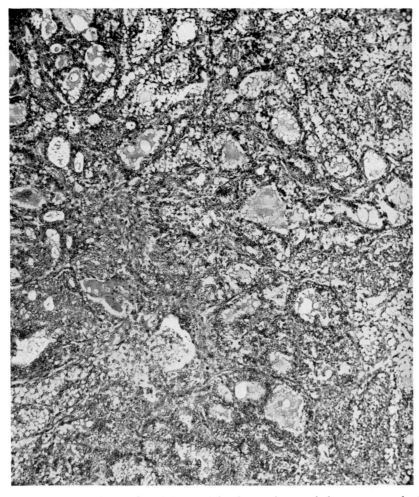

Fig. 8. Section of transplanted R 3230/1A adenocarcinoma of the mammary gland in Fischer line 344 female rat (magnification × 105).

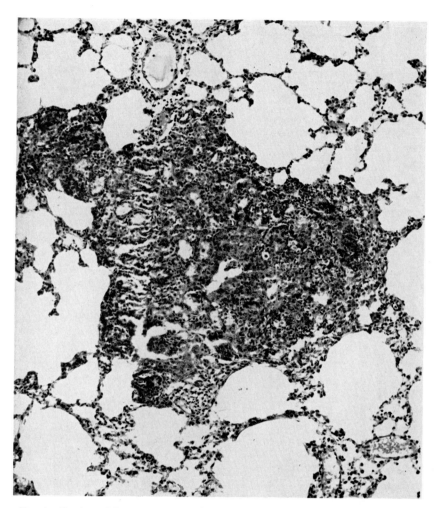

FIG. 9. Section of lung metastases of R 3230/1A from Fischer line 344 female rat 92 days after transplantation (magnification × 105).

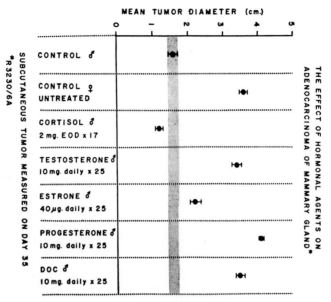

Fig. 10. A comparison of the mean tumor diameter of R 3230 in each treated group with the mean ± P.E. of the control group in Fischer line 344 male rats.

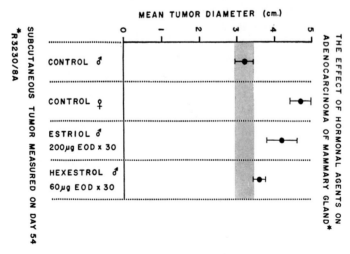

Fig. 11. A comparison of the mean tumor diameter of R 3230 in normal females and estrogen-treated males with the mean ± P.E. of the control in intact Fischer line 344 male rats.

inhibited by the adrenal cortical compounds and stimulated by all the other steroids that have been tested. The tumors in males treated with progesterone were larger than those in normal females. Tumors in males treated with estrogens, testosterone, and deoxycorticosterone were almost as large as in the females and the average survival time of the hosts was correspondingly reduced.

The morphological changes that were observed in tumors from hosts that were treated with some of these compounds are of special interest. In intact adult females the tumor appears to be a papillary cyst adenocarcinoma as shown in Fig. 8. In intact males areas of metaplastic squamous epithelium are characteristically found as shown in Fig. 12. Treatment with estrone stimulated secretory activity as shown in Fig. 13. Treatment with testosterone appeared to stimulate the growth of the stroma and reduce the glands to relatively benign-appearing single-layered structures, as shown in Fig. 14. Progesterone likewise stimulated the stroma but also preserved the glandular structures, giving the appearance of a mixed tumor as shown in Fig. 15. Figure 16 shows definite squamous epithelium with pearl formation in a tumor from a rat that died 50 days after the completion of the course of treatment with 10 mg. of testosterone.

Decadron and 9α-fluorocortisol proved to be toxic to these rats. After two injections of 2.5 mg./kg. of the former, 40 % of the rats died. The tumors were significantly reduced in the survivors that lived to be measured 26 days after transplantation of the tumor.

The estrogenic compounds estriol and hexestrol were effective in stimulating the growth and secretory activity of this neoplasm. Larger doses were required to attain the increased average diameter of the tumors and reduced average survival period than was observed to result from treatment with 40 µg. of estrone. About twice the dose of hexestrol and six times the dose of estriol gave comparable results.

These estrogens were also compared for effectiveness with estrone on several other neoplasms. Figure 17 shows that 40 µg. of estrone, 60 µg. of hexestrol, and 200 µg of estriol injected every other day for twenty injections significantly stimulated the growth of transplanted squamous cell carcinoma of the prostate (M-C 972). Figures 18 and 19 show that all three of these compounds slightly inhibited the subcutaneous growths of IRC 741 in Fischer line 344 rats and a previously described adenocarcinoma of the mammary gland R 2426 transplanted in August line 7322 rats. The latter tumor is similar in morphology to R 3230 that was stimulated by these compounds.

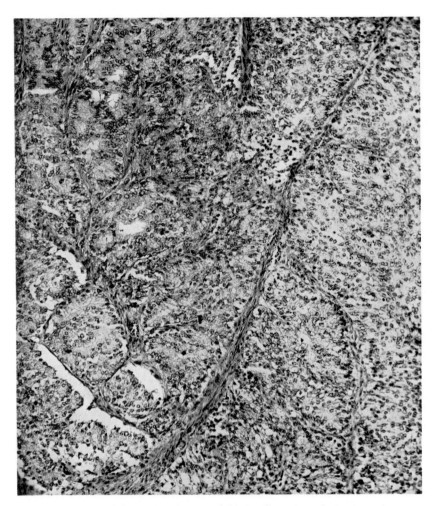

FIG. 12. Section of R 3230/5A in normal Fischer line 344 male 77 days after transplantation (magnification × 105).

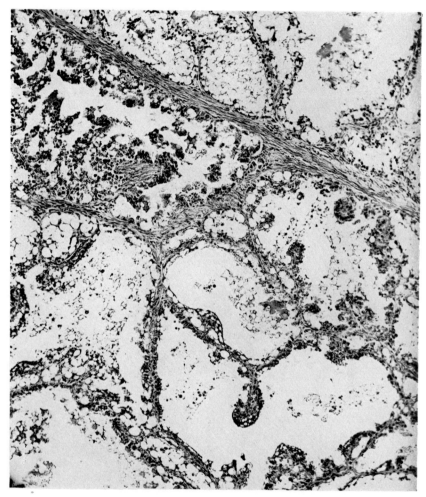

FIG. 13. Section of R 3230/6A in Fischer line 344 male rat treated for 34 days with 40 μg. estrone (magnification × 105).

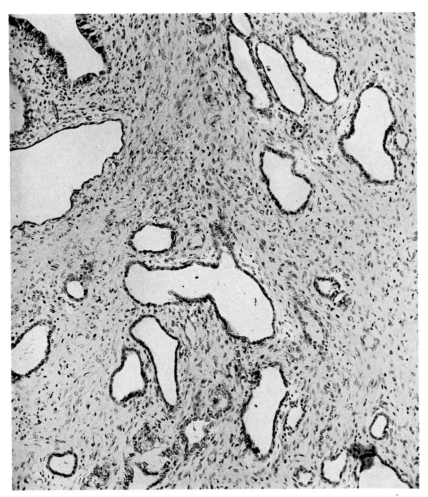

FIG. 14. Section of R 3230/6A in Fischer line 344 male rat after 30 daily injections of 10 mg. of testosterone (magnification × 105).

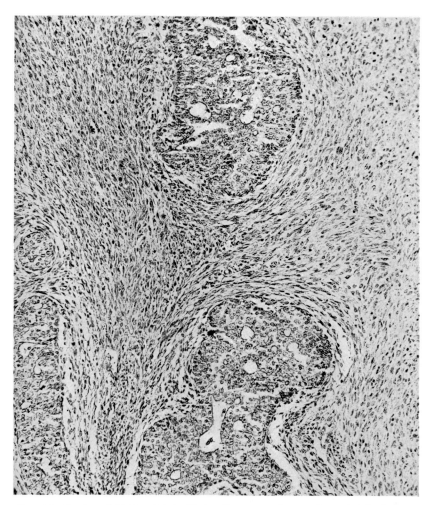

Fig. 15.   Section of R 3230/6A in Fischer line 344 male rat after 25 daily injections of 10 mg. of progesterone (magnification × 105).

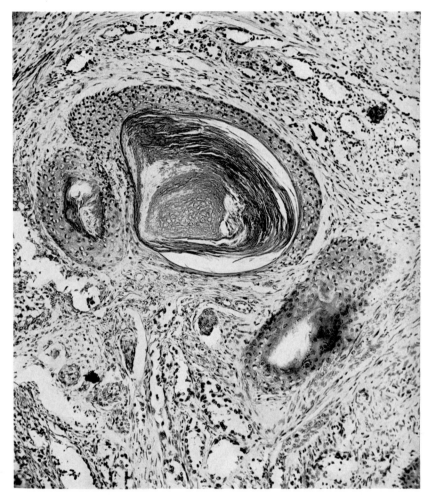

Fig. 16. Section of R 3230/6A in Fischer line 344 male rat 50 days after completion of course of 30 daily injections of 10 mg. of testosterone showing epithelial pearl formation (magnification × 105).

## SUMMARY

1. Three subcutaneously transplanted rat neoplasms, acute leukemia IRC 741, lymphosarcoma R 2788, and the Yoshida lymphoma, were shown to be less responsive to maximum tolerated doses of a group of adrenal cortical compounds than a group (P 1798, M 3445, M 3509, and M 3713) of subcutaneously transplanted mouse lymphomas.

2. The tumor-bearing mice were able to tolerate twice the dose of cortisol and 9α-fluorocortisol and ten times more Decadron than was tolerated by the rats.

3. Three newly transplanted rat neoplasms were tested for responsiveness to a group of steroid compounds. They were as follows: R 3234, a leiomyo-

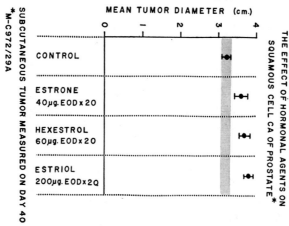

Fig. 17. A comparison of the mean tumor diameter of MC 972 in normal and estrogen-treated A × C line 9935 Irish male rats.

sarcoma of the uterus in A × C line 9935 Irish rats; R 3244, a fibrosarcoma of the mammary gland in Fischer line 344 rats; R 3230, an adenocarcinoma of the mammary gland in Fischer line 344 rats.

4. R 3234 was found to be inhibited by cortisol, testosterone, and deoxycorticosterone and unaffected by treatment with progesterone.

5. R 3244 was inhibited by cortisol and slightly stimulated by estrone, testosterone, progesterone, and deoxycorticosterone.

6. R 3230 was inhibited by cortisol and Decadron and stimulated by progesterone, testosterone, deoxycorticosterone, and estrone, estriol and hexestrol. Characteristic changes in morphology resulted from treatment with some of these compounds.

7. The growth of a previously described adenocarcinoma of the mammary

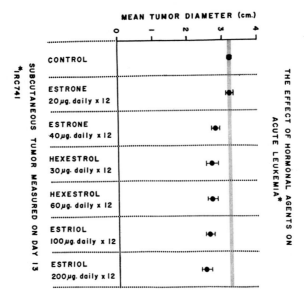

FIG. 18. A comparison of the mean tumor diameter of subcutaneous growths of IRC 741 in control and estrogen-treated immature Fischer line 344 rats.

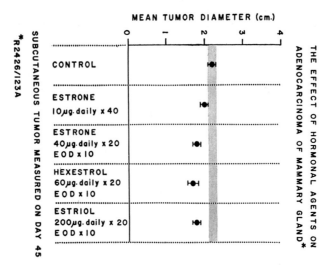

FIG. 19. A comparison of the mean tumor diameter of R 2426 in control and estrogen-treated August line 7322 male rats.

gland R 2426 and acute leukemia IRC 741 was slightly inhibited by estrone, estriol, and hexestrol.

8. A subcutaneously transplanted squamous cell carcinoma of the prostate (M-C 972) was stimulated by similar treatment with estrone, estriol, and hexestrol.

### REFERENCES

1. Dunning, W. F. *Ann. N. Y. Acad. Sci.* **76**, 696 (1958).
2. Dunning, W. F. *Ann. N. Y. Acad. Sci.* **76**, 643 (1958).
3. Lampkin, J. M., and Potter, M. *J. Natl. Cancer Inst.* **20**, 1091 (1958).

### DISCUSSION

**J. Lampkin-Hibbard:** I would like to add a few facts about the P 1798 lymphosarcoma. First, regarding the change in its response to cortisone: mice treated with 15–25 mg./kg. for 5–7 days survived on the average over 300 days in the second transfer generation (untreated controls lived 48 days), whereas similarly treated animals survived only 45 days in the 49th transfer generation (untreated controls, 29 days). Tumor size was also affected, most by 9α-fluorohydrocortisone, less by prednisone and prednisolone, still less by hydrocortisone and cortisone, and not at all by corticosterone and 11-dehydrocorticosterone. A subline of this lymphosarcoma, resistant to 9α-fluorohydrocortisone, has been developed [Lampkin-Hibbard, J. McC. *J. Natl. Cancer Inst.* **24**, 1353 (1960)].

When this subline is implanted into one side of a mouse while the sensitive tumor is implanted contralaterally, differential effects of a treatment may be observed. During treatment with 9α-fluorohydrocortisone the resistant tumor grew at a rate similar to that of controls, even when the dosage was maximal (25 mg./kg.). This occurred regardless of the time treatment was initiated. When 5 days of treatment at maximal dosage was initiated 24 hours after tumor implantation, the sensitive line was completely suppressed, but the resistant line grew continuously. The same thing happened when treatment with 9α-fluorohydrocortisone, for 5 days, was begun 14 days after tumor implantation.

**Charles Harris:** I may have missed this on the slides that were shown, but I wonder whether Dr. Dunning's tumors, which were inhibited by estrogen, were tumors that had been transplanted to male or female rats. I ask this question because, in the induced tumor, when the hormones are introduced at the start of methylcholanthrene therapy before the tumor develops, estrogen promotes the growth of tumor in the male but inhibits it in the female. In other words, are the properties in your tumor inherently the property of the tumor or could they be related to the sex of the recipient?

**W. F. Dunning:** Both the one which I showed that was inhibited with the estrogenic compounds and the one that was stimulated with the estrogenic compounds had been transplanted into adult intact males.

**R. L. Noble:** The last remarks of Dr. Dunning concerning the difficulties in transplanting an estrogen-induced tumor were of considerable interest. We also have had difficulty in attempting to transplant this type of tumor. Admittedly we do not have the elegant inbred strains of rats, but in our ill-bred strains the transplants apparently remain dormant and will not grow. However, with these tumors I believe there is a strong possibility that the hormone dependency may also be related to pituitary hormones. I would ask Dr. Dunning if she has attempted to stimulate these transplants, perhaps by growth hormone or lactogenic hormone, as well as estrone.

**W. F. Dunning:** No, we haven't tried any other hormones, but we have noted that palpable tumors appear only after time enough has intervened for the pituitary in the recipient host to have increased in size. The transplanted tumors grow better in the hosts that are more responsive in the growth of the pituitary—that is in the Fischer rat or the August rat—than in some of the rats in which the pituitary responds more slowly to estrogen.

**U. Kim:** I would like to comment on Dr. Dunning's last remark about this tumor. If you give it time, it will become autonomous. We have observed similar estrogen dependency in other tumors; for instance, estrogen-induced pituitary tumors grew only in estrogen-treated animals for the first several subpassage generations. However, as passage was repeated, they eventually became autonomous and grew well in untreated hosts.

**W. F. Dunning:** I can only comment that I am still waiting.

**R. Hilf:** It appeared to me that wherever you had a decrease in the tumor size, you also had a concomitant loss in body weight. Do you have any indication or data concerning the effect of nutrition on tumor growth?

**W. F. Dunning:** There were some in which we had considerable decrease in size of the tumor without loss in body weight. Loss in fluid is a major fact, or perhaps also the reduction in size of the subcutaneous mass in the acute leukemia treated with adrenal cortical compounds. The animals become almost dehydrated.

**J. H. Bryant:** In our work on cortisone-sensitive and cortisone-resistant transplantable mouse lymphosarcomas, developed after the method of Potter and Lampkin-Hibbard, we tried to ascertain the effects of steroids on the metabolism of these tumors. Our results indicate that certain steroids inhibit the utilization of glucose in these tumors, perhaps at the level of glucose phosphorylation as described by Dr. White. Our particular interest was to compare the metabolism of the cortisone-resistant tumor with that of the cortisone-sensitive tumor. We were hoping to describe a mechanism of resistance. In *in vitro* experiments some steroids showed the same inhibitory effect on the conversion of glucose to $CO_2$ in both types of tumors. However, the effect of hydrocortisone was distinctive in that it inhibited the conversion of glucose to $CO_2$ in the sensitive tumor but not in the resistant tumor. It may be that this is an *in vitro* expression of the cortisone resistance seen *in vivo*. This was a tumor, P 2450, that Dr. Michael Potter developed for use in these studies.

I would like to make a point which might apply to some experiments described here and elsewhere on the effects of steroids in normal and abnormal tissues. Assumptions are made that the steroid that is added to an experimental preparation *in vivo* or *in vitro* is in fact the compound which accomplishes the observed effect in the experimental preparation. This assumption is not always warranted. In our experiments we found that these lymphomatous tissues extensively transformed hydrocortisone into as many as ten chromatographically distinct metabolites. Thus, at this time we cannot say that hydrocortisone is indeed the compound which accomplishes the experimental effect that we observe.

# Steroids and Experimental Mammary Cancer

E. Myles Glenn, S. Lee Richardson, Barbara J. Bowman,
and Stanley C. Lyster

*Department of Endocrinology, The Upjohn Company, Kalamazoo, Michigan*

## Introduction

Until recently, knowledge concerning the influence of hormones on mammary cancer had been largely derived from studies in man. A major drawback to this area of research has been a lack of suitable methods for study in experimental animals. Within the past four years, Huggins (1, 2) and Glenn *et al.* (3, 4) have demonstrated that the mammary fibroadenoma of the rat closely resembles the steroid-dependent mammary tumors in man.

The limited success of steroid therapy in mammary carcinoma and in certain forms of leukemia calls for an evaluation of the effects of many new steroids in these and other types of neoplasms in both man and experimental animals. Although the naturally occurring steroids have limited effectiveness against mammary carcinoma, the occasional objective remission of this disease warrants the belief that when the chemotherapeutic control of mammary cancer is discovered, the steroid hormones or their congeners will be found to be near the center of the problem (5).

The historical development of the mammary fibroadenoma as an assay tool has been discussed previously (1–4) and need not be repeated here. The mammary fibroadenoma of the rat is unique in that it has certain functional traits of its tissue of origin. It responds to the administration or withdrawal of the appropriate hormones. In this regard it resembles its human counterpart—within certain reasonable limits. Since the mammary fibroadenoma of the rat responds to hormonal therapy and to the removal of the ovaries, adrenals, and pituitary, several important questions were considered before we initiated a program of research in this area. Does the mammary fibroadenoma of the rat respond only to steroids having known biologic effects? If so, what are the benefits to be derived from the use of a technique which is more time consuming and laborious than the standard techniques used to analyze the known biologic activities of steroids? In addition, does the mammary fibroadenoma of the rat merely represent an end point which detects only those compounds that are effective pituitary inhibitors? If so, the use of this relatively complicated bioassay procedure adds nothing new or original to the wealth of data that are available, or that can be more readily obtained, in this area. If these primary questions can be answered in the affirmative, the assay methods for the analysis of antitumor effects, described by both Huggins (1, 2) and Glenn (3, 4). become of minor and questionable significance. These were among the most important considerations which motivated the research to be described in the following sections.

Huggins has shown that the dihydrotestosterone-responsive mammary fibroadenoma of the rat eventually loses its responsiveness to this hormone. Does this mean that the tumor has become refractory to all other $C_{19}$ steroids? Detailed evidence to be presented later indicates quite the contrary. A so-called "testosterone-resistant" tumor is not necessarily a "$C_{19}$ steroid-resistant" tumor; it is also not necessarily a "hormonally-insensitive" tumor.

This investigation was also concerned with the relative antitumor effects of $C_{21}$ steroids on the transplanted mammary adenocarcinoma of C3H mice. Others (6, 7) have shown previously that the C3H adenocarcinoma is inhibited by prednisolone and hydrocortisone. The following results are merely an extension of these more original contributions. Since the C3H tumor has lost its responsiveness to gonadal hormones, the most important question was: Will it be possible to discover a steroid that will inhibit both the C3H mammary adenocarcinoma and the rat mammary fibroadenoma? The following investigations show that it is indeed possible to discover a steroid that will inhibit both types of tumor. Another question relating to studies with the C3H mammary adenocarcinoma was: since C3H mammary tumor growth is inhibited by $C_{21}$ steroids, will it be possible to discover closely related synthetic steroids which, having none of the other well-known metabolic effects of adrenocortical steroids (e.g., glycogenic and anti-inflammatory activity) will nevertheless have antitumor activity? Results to date suggest that the antitumor effects of the adrenal hormones and their synthetic derivatives are intimately related to their other metabolic effects. In our experience, a so-called "inactive" glycogenic or anti-inflammatory steroid has not yet been discovered which also has significant antitumor activity in C3H mice.

The most important and critical, and as yet unanswered, question arising from these studies is: Can the results obtained in rats and mice be readily extrapolated to studies in man? Although correlations have been found for the known steroids, i.e., estradiol, progesterone, testosterone, and others, the more recent observations reported in the following sections have not been adequately examined in the female with breast cancer.

## METHODS

### Rat Mammary Fibroadenoma, Responsive Tumor

Since the percentage of animals in which transplanted tumors grow varies from one series of experimental animals to another, and since the number of "takes" per rat varies when multiple transplants are employed, procedures described by Huggins *et al.* (1, 2) have been slightly modified in the interest of greater assay reproducibility.

Original tumors were obtained from Dr. Huggins' laboratory in February, 1957. They were transplanted to a large number of female Sprague-Dawley rats and have subsequently produced a tumor strain used successfully in our laboratories for the last two years.

Female Sprague-Dawley rats (45–50 days old, 140–160 gm.) are anesthetized with 1.0 cc. of 1.0 % Na Cyclopal by intraperitoneal injection. Incisions are made into the back of each animal, and channels in the subcutaneous connective tissue made with surgical forceps to about ½ inch caudal to each front leg on both sides. One operator removes "seed" tumors (one "seed" tumor-bearing animal sacrificed for each 100 recipients) and prepares them for implantation by cutting slices of uniform thickness and punching uniform pieces of tumor (70 ± 20 mg.) with nasal cutting forceps. Transplants, one on each side, are quickly inserted into previously made channels and the incisions closed with surgical clips. The animals are housed in cages in constant temperature, constant humidity, animal quarters. Animals are allowed tap water and Purina laboratory chow ad libitum. Two operators can carry out the entire operation described above on two to three hundred rats in 1½–2 hours.

Tumors are allowed to grow for 35 days; animals are then palpated for actively growing tumors. Those with extremely small or no tumors are discarded; those with very large tumors are set aside for subsequent "seed" tumors. The remaining animals are randomized in "haphazard" fashion by placing in large carrying cages, removing animals, and dividing into dosage groups of eight to ten animals. Test compounds are administered, orally or subcutaneously, as finely dispersed suspensions in 0.5 or 0.2 ml. of carboxymethyl cellulose vehicle. Treatment is continued for 30 days, after which animals are sacrificed and autopsied. The eight to ten animals used for each experimental group usually provide sixteen to eighteen tumors of rather uniform size. Three groups of controls are used in every experiment: an *initial control*, ten tumor-bearing animals sacrificed at the end of the 35-day growth period; a *final control*, consisting of untreated animals in which tumors have grown for 65 days; and a *hormone control*, consisting of ten animals to which 1.0 mg. per day of testosterone propionate has been administered subcutaneously for 30 days (day 35–day 65). The last control is to insure that tumors in the experimental rats are hormone sensitive and have not mutated to the Huggins "Class II" (2), "hormone-insensitive" mammary fibroadenoma.

### Rat Mammary Fibroadenoma, Testosterone Propionate-resistant Tumor

Methods employed in this assay were essentially the same as those described for the responsive tumor, except that only one tumor was implanted into each animal. "Seed" tumors were removed from tumor-bearing animals which had shown complete resistance to testosterone propionate administration for at least four successive transplant generations. In this assay, the hormone control group received testosterone propionate (1.0 mg. per day) to insure continued resistance of the tumor.

### C3H Mammary Adenocarcinoma

This tumor grows equally well in both male and female C3H mice; it was originally obtained from Dr. Morris K. Barrett of the National Institutes of Health. Lack of sufficient supplies of females necessitated the use of 10–12-week-old male mice throughout. Fifty per cent suspensions in 0.9 % NaCl of the tumor were prepared in a tissue press under aseptic conditions. Of this suspension 0.2 ml. was injected subcutaneously into the back of the recipient. Compounds were administered subcutaneously in 0.2 ml. of carboxymethyl cellulose vehicle, starting on the day following tumor implantation and continuing for 18 days.

Before being used for tumor implantation, C3H mice were adequately housed in our animal quarters for at least 2 weeks before initiation of experiments. They were allowed a 0.7 mg./cc. solution of Panmycin[1] in their drinking fluid ad libitum. On the day of implantation animals were removed from this regimen and placed on tap water, on which they were continued thereafter.

Prednisolone, standard for this assay, was administered at the 300-µg. per day per mouse level to at least twenty animals during every assay or experimental investigation. Tumors and animals were weighed at the end of each experiment. Both control and treated specimens of this tumor, as well as the two experimental fibroadenomas, were routinely examined for histological differences.

Anti-inflammatory, glycogenic, androgenic, progestational, estrogenic, and "myotropic" activities of $C_{21}$ and $C_{19}$ steroids were determined by standard assay procedures. These assay methods have been described previously and will not be repeated here.

### RESULTS

### Testosterone Propionate-responsive Tumor

A characteristic growth rate curve for the testosterone propionate-sensitive mammary fibroadenoma is shown in Fig. 1. Tumors grow slowly, if at all,

---

[1] Panmycin: tetracycline hydrochloride, The Upjohn Co., Kalamazoo, Michigan.

during the first 20 days after tumor implantation. Subsequent growth rate proceeds in a somewhat logarithmic fashion. The 35-day period was selected for procurement of established tumors since they were readily inspected both visually and manually at this time. In several experimental series of animals (250–300 animals per series), the mammary fibroadenoma implants completely failed to "take." When such animals were implanted again, 35 days after the initial implantation, tumors grew as successfully as in other series.

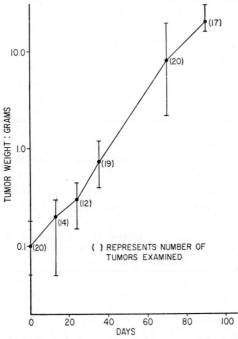

Fig. 1. Growth rate of the testosterone propionate-responsive mammary fibroadenoma of the rat (3).

Explanations for these obvious failures are unavailable. Either the endocrine status of the host or the viability of the initially transplanted tumors may be responsible for these failures.

Variations in size of both the 35-day and 65-day tumors (Table I) necessitated the use of adequate numbers of controls for assay purposes. Consistency in tumor size was obtained within each experimental series of animals, but not from one series to another. Therefore, when comparative results were desired, they were derived from the same group of tumor-inoculated animals. In short, although the effects of steroid hormones on tumor growth were qualitatively the same, the quantitative determinations of effects on tumor growth had to be derived with great care and selection of tumors.

TABLE I

VARIATION IN SIZE OF TP-RESPONSIVE MAMMARY FIBROADENOMAS 35 AND 65 DAYS AFTER TRANSPLANTATION (3)

| Experiment number | 35-Day tumors | | | 65-Day tumors | | |
|---|---|---|---|---|---|---|
| | Number of rats | Number of tumors | Mean tumor weight (gm.) | Number of rats | Number of tumors | Mean tumor weight (gm.) |
| 1040 | 10 | 19 | 0.697 | 10 | 16 | 8.400 |
| 1037 | 10 | 19 | 0.605 | 10 | 17 | 11.400 |
| 1035 | 10 | 16 | 0.879 | 10 | 14 | 11.203 |
| 1034 | 10 | 17 | 0.977 | 10 | 18 | 10.210 |
| 1032 | 10 | 17 | 0.459 | 10 | 19 | 4.430 |
| 1028 | 10 | 19 | 0.436 | 10 | 16 | 7.960 |

The variation in the number of transplants that grew successfully (47–77 %) from one series of experimental animals to another also necessitated the use of well-established tumors for assay purposes (Table II). It is evident that, with such variation in the number of transplant successes, the initiation of steroid treatment beginning on day 1 of tumor implantation

TABLE II

VARIATION IN NUMBER OF TUMOR "TAKES" AFTER TRANSPLANTATION OF TP-RESPONSIVE MAMMARY FIBROADENOMA (3)

| Experiment number | Number of animals | Number of tumors transplanted | Number of animals with tumors after 35 days | % |
|---|---|---|---|---|
| 1040 | 200 | 400 | 130 | 65 |
| 1037 | 200 | 400 | 90 | 45 |
| 1035 | 200 | 400 | 120 | 60 |
| 1034 | 200 | 400 | 102 | 51 |
| 1032 | 200 | 400 | 128 | 64 |
| 1029 | 200 | 400 | 135 | 67 |
| 1028 | 200 | 400 | 150 | 75 |
| 1026 | 200 | 400 | 95 | 47 |
| 1024 | 200 | 400 | 150 | 75 |
| 1020 | 156 | 312 | 107 | 68 |
| 1017 | 202 | 404 | 134 | 66 |
| 1015 | 200 | 400 | 155 | 77 |
| 1018 | 200 | 400 | 130 | 65 |
| | 2558 | 5116 | 1626 | Avg. 64 |

might have led to erroneous conclusions. Attempts were made to increase the number of successful implants in female rats by means of prior treatment with various steroids, i.e., estradiol and/or progesterone, without apparent success. Attempts were also made to grow tumors in ovariectomized females treated with various amounts of both progesterone and estradiol for varying periods. These experiments also did not lead to greater incidence of tumor "takes."

Testosterone propionate (TP) was chosen as reference standard for this assay. A sufficient number of animals was treated with this steroid in every

TABLE III

EFFECT OF TESTOSTERONE PROPIONATE ON GROWTH RATE OF TP-RESPONSIVE MAMMARY FIBROADENOMA[a] (3)

| Treatment | Number of animals with tumors (35 Days) | Number of takes | | Mean tumor weight (gm.) | % |
|---|---|---|---|---|---|
| | | 35 Days | 65 Days | | |
| Initial Control | 10 | 18 | — | 0.602 | — |
| Final Control | 10 | — | 16 | 8.950 | — |
| TP[b] | 10 | — | 17 | 1.030 | 95 |
| Initial Control | 10 | 19 | — | 0.356 | — |
| Final Control | 10 | — | 17 | 4.420 | — |
| TP | 10 | — | 20 | 0.568 | 95 |
| Initial Control | 10 | 19 | — | 0.913 | — |
| Final Control | 10 | — | 17 | 6.070 | — |
| TP | 10 | — | 18 | 1.040 | 98 |
| Initial Control | 10 | 16 | — | 0.950 | — |
| Final Control | 10 | — | 15 | 10.210 | — |
| TP | 10 | — | 14 | 1.130 | 99 |
| Initial Control | 10 | 15 | — | 1.062 | — |
| Final Control | 10 | — | 14 | 17.880 | — |
| TP | 10 | — | 11 | 1.250 | 99 |
| Initial Control | 10 | 17 | — | 0.977 | — |
| Final Control | 10 | — | 13 | 10.200 | — |
| TP | 10 | — | 20 | 1.180 | 98 |

[a] Selected at random from series of controls for period of 6 months.
[b] 1.0 Mg. per day for 30 days, subcutaneously (approximately 5 mg./kg.).

assay. In Table III the consistent inhibitory effects of TP on the responsive tumor are shown. The administration of 1 mg. per day of this steroid caused tumor inhibition in the range of 95–99 %. Administration of TP neither induced regression of tumor growth nor caused markedly discernible histological differences between tumors from control and treated animals.

Later, an experiment was designed to determine if steroid withdrawal following the marked inhibitory effects produced by testosterone propionate would result in resumption of tumor growth. Data shown in Fig. 2 indicate that, if sufficient time is allowed, the initially inhibited tumor will resume its original growth pattern. These results suggest that testosterone merely halts the further progression of mammary fibroadenoma growth; it does not bring about death of tumor cells.

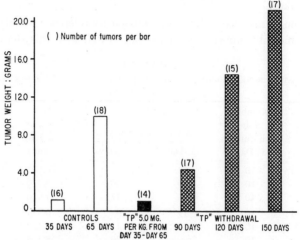

FIG. 2.   Effect of testosterone propionate withdrawal on subsequent tumor growth of the responsive mammary fibroadenoma.

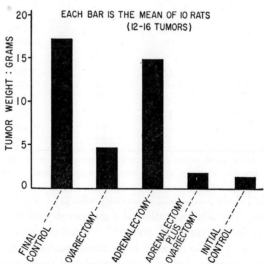

FIG. 3.   Effect of ovariectomy, adrenalectomy, and the combined procedure on growth of the responsive mammary fibroadenoma (3).

TABLE IV

EFFECT OF HYDROCORTISONE ON TP-RESPONSIVE MAMMARY FIBROADENOMA GROWTH, ENDOCRINE GLANDS, AND TARGET ORGANS OF THE FEMALE RAT[a] (10)

| Number of rats | Dose (mg./kg./ day) | Body weight gain (gm.) | Number of tumors | Average tumor weight (gm.) | Uterus (mg.) | Ovaries (mg.) | Preputial gland (mg.) | Adrenals (mg.) |
|---|---|---|---|---|---|---|---|---|
| 10 | — | +23 | 15 | 9.01 | 464 | 100 | 91 | 63 |
| 8 | 0.5 | + 7 | 12 | 7.63 | 478 | 98 | 70 | 74 |
| 8 | 1.0 | +13 | 14 | 7.54 | 450 | 88 | 75 | 60 |
| 8 | 2.0 | + 2 | 11 | 9.17 | 447 | 91 | 75 | 64 |
| 8 | 4.0 | − 7 | 12 | 9.71 | 395 | 102 | 88 | 49 |
| 8 | 8.0 | −25 | 13 | 8.85 | 401 | 112 | — | 41 |

[a] Conditions: Hydrocortisone administered daily, starting 35 days after initial implantation of tumor and continued for 30 days. Animals autopsied on 66th day after initial implantation.

The effect of removal of various endocrine sources is shown in Fig. 3. Adrenalectomized rats were maintained on 0.9 % NaCl and 0.2 mg. of hydrocortisone per day. It is apparent that combined removal of both the adrenals and ovaries results in greater inhibition of tumor growth than that produced by either procedure alone. These latter procedures also fail to induce death of tumor cells, since the inhibited tumors were subsequently transplanted successfully to normal female recipients.

Hydrocortisone, when administered at varying dose levels, had little effect on tumor growth (Table IV), despite the marked "catabolic" effects which it produced in the host. These results are emphasized because they have direct bearing on later developments in the research with mammary tumors.

The above results are in contrast to those following the administration of estradiol which, at low doses stimulates, at higher doses begins to inhibit, tumor growth (Table V). Injection of estradiol at higher dose levels than

TABLE V

EFFECT OF ESTRADIOL ON TP-RESPONSIVE MAMMARY FIBROADENOMA DEVELOPMENT AND VARIOUS ENDOCRINE ORGANS OF THE FEMALE RAT[a] (10)

| Group | Number of tumors | Body weight gain (gm.) | Uterus (mg.) | Ovaries (mg.) | Preputial gland (mg.) | Adrenal (mg.) | Tumor weight (gm.) |
|---|---|---|---|---|---|---|---|
| Initial Controls | 19 | | | | | | 0.559 |
| Final Controls | 17 | +16 | 443 | 109 | 77 | 58 | 7.460 |
| Estradiol (μg./kg.) | | | | | | | |
| 0.05 | 12 | +24 | 467 | 110 | 108 | 68 | 7.980 |
| 0.10 | 12 | +20 | 474 | 102 | 88 | 68 | 9.900 |
| 0.20 | 12 | +19 | 478 | 118 | 69 | 64 | 15.570 |
| 0.50 | 12 | +22 | 529 | 100 | 120 | 69 | 15.780 |
| 1.50 | 12 | +26 | 440 | 93 | 86 | 62 | 15.040 |
| 3.00 | 15 | +15 | 418 | 90 | 77 | 67 | 13.870 |
| 6.00 | 11 | + 7 | 441 | 86 | 83 | 64 | 14.120 |
| 12.00 | 14 | + 9 | 446 | 87 | 88 | 71 | 7.830 |
| 24.00 | 15 | +13 | 623 | 73 | 99 | 74 | 10.020 |
| 48.00 | 13 | 0 | 759 | 63 | 81 | 67 | 9.090 |
| 80.00 | 14 | − 4 | 688 | 56 | 97 | 68 | 6.340 |

[a] Conditions: Estradiol administered daily, starting 35 days following initial implantation of tumor; continued for 30 days. Final autopsy: 66 days after initial implantation.

those shown in Table V caused marked inhibition of tumor growth. These are extremely interesting results, similar to those obtained by Huggins (1, 2), but definitive explanations regarding the biphasic effects of this ovarian steroid on tumor growth are not available. On the other hand, the administration of progesterone has little, if any, effect on established tumor growth

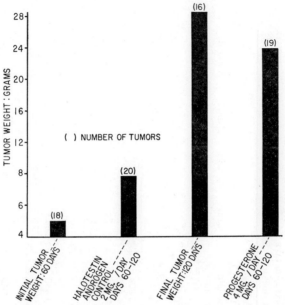

FIG. 4. Effect of progesterone administration on growth rate of responsive mammary fibroadenoma (3).

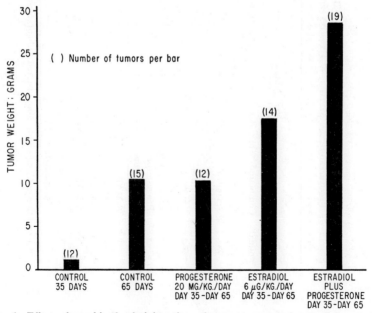

FIG. 5. Effect of combined administration of progesterone and estradiol on growth rate of benign mammary fibroadenoma.

## TABLE Va

EFFECT OF PROGESTERONE, 6α-METHYL-17-HYDROXYPROGESTERONE ACETATE (6-MAP), AND TESTOSTERONE PROPIONATE ON GROWTH RATE OF TP-RESPONSIVE MAMMARY FIBROADENOMA AND VARIOUS ENDOCRINE ORGANS[a] (10)

| Number of animals | Compound | Amount (mg./day) | Number of tumors | Body weight gain (gm.) | Average tumor weight (gm.) | Uterus (mg.) | Ovaries (mg.) | Preputial gland (mg.) | Adrenals (mg.) |
|---|---|---|---|---|---|---|---|---|---|
| 10 | Original control | 0 | 18 | — | 0.528 | — | — | — | — |
| 10 | Final control | 0 | 16 | +12 | 4.550 | 450 | 91 | 95 | 64 ± 4 |
| 8 | Progesterone | 1 | 15 | +13 | 6.800 | 271 | 70 | 84 | 55 ± 6 |
| 8 | Progesterone | 2 | 12 | +26 | 6.020 | 244 | 64 | 89 | 59 ± 7 |
| 8 | Progesterone | 4 | 12 | +20 | 4.890 | 224 | 48 | 93 | 58 ± 2 |
| 8 | Progesterone | 8 | 13 | +29 | 5.040 | 221 | 43 | 86 | 45 ± 4 |
| 8 | 6-MAP | 1 | 11 | +18 | 2.520 | 233 | 42 | 98 | 22 ± 2 |
| 8 | 6-MAP | 2 | 13 | +15 | 0.950 | 234 | 38 | 90 | 19 ± 3 |
| 8 | 6-MAP | 4 | 16 | +14 | 1.850 | 263 | 36 | 87 | 21 ± 5 |
| 8 | 6-MAP | 8 | 15 | + 8 | 0.880 | 272 | 40 | 87 | 20 ± 3 |
| 8 | Testosterone propionate | 1 | 14 | +42 | 1.530 | 746 | 63 | 277 | 44 ± 6 |

[a] Conditions: Compounds administered subcutaneously for 30 days.

(Fig. 4). However, when combined with estradiol, the stimulatory effects of this steroid become markedly enhanced (Fig. 5).

When compared to progesterone, 6α-methyl-17α-acetoxyprogesterone Provera,[2] or 6-MAP), a progestational agent which is twenty to forty times as potent as progesterone on endometrial proliferation (9), inhibits subsequent tumor growth. These effects may be related to the marked pituitary inhibition which this steroid produces in female rats (Table Va). It should be

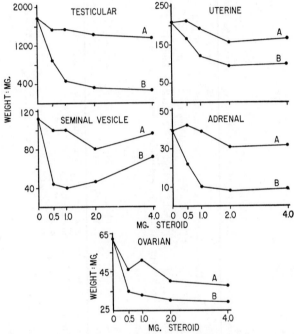

Fig. 6. Effect of 6α-methyl-17-hydroxyprogesterone acetate (6-MAP) and progesterone on testicular, seminal vesicle, uterine, adrenal, and ovarian weights of male and female 21-day-old weanling rats. Steroids administered for 20 days (10). A, progesterone; B, 6-MAP.

emphasized that the larger amounts of 6α-methyl-17α-acetoxyprogesterone administered here are, at least, equivalent to the administration of 160–320 mg. of progesterone. Administration of such amounts of the latter have not been attempted. That this progestational agent (6-MAP) is a patent pituitary inhibitor in male and female weanling rats is shown in Fig. 6 (10). It is evident that Provera produces inhibitory effects on the adrenals and testes of weanling rats which cannot be duplicated by larger amount of progesterone.

---

[2] Provera: 6α-methyl-17-acetoxyprogesterone, The Upjohn Co., Kalamazoo, Michigan.

## TABLE Vb

Duration of Effect of Hydrocortisone and 6-MAP (Provera) on Adrenal and Other Organ Weights[a] (10)

| Compound | Dose (mg./day) | Cumulative body weight gain (gm.) | | Uterus weight (mg.) | | Ovarian weight (mg.) | | Preputial gland weight (mg.) | | Adrenal weight (mg.) | |
|---|---|---|---|---|---|---|---|---|---|---|---|
| | | End of treatment | 2 Weeks later | End of treatment | 2 Weeks later | End of treatment | 2 Weeks later | End of treatment | 2 Weeks later | End of treatment | 2 Weeks later |
| None | — | 45 | 87 | 261 | 172 | 72 | 61 | 95 | 72 | 49 | 52 |
| Hydro-cortisone | 3 | —20 | 2 | 205 | 145 | 74 | 52 | 65 | 60 | 17 | 39 |
| 6-MAP | 4 | 37 | 79 | 147 | 121 | 51 | 34 | 84 | 84 | 20 | 20 |

[a] Conditions: Five intact rats per group. Injected subcutaneously once daily for 2 weeks, half the animals sacrificed; kept untreated for two additional weeks, remaining animals sacrificed.

Part of this inhibitory activity may be related to the prolonged duration of action of this steroid, since its adrenal inhibitory effects persist for at least 2 weeks following complete cessation of administration to female rats (Table Vb). Conversely, equal inhibitory doses of hydrocortisone produce the expected response, but adrenals resume their growth rate toward normal during the 2 week withdrawal period. These results are emphasized because they, too, bear on the later developments of research in this area.

TABLE VI

EFFECT OF TESTOSTERONE PROPIONATE ON TUMOR AND HORMONAL TARGETS OF FEMALE RATS (3)

| Testosterone propionate[a] (mg./kg./day, 30 days) | Tumor weight (gm.) | Uterus weight (mg.) | Preputial glands (mg.) | Adrenal (mg.) | Ovary (mg.) |
|---|---|---|---|---|---|
| 0 | 8.210 | 582 | 99 | 62 | 90 |
| 0.5 | 5.420 | 280 | 152 | 62 | 49 |
| 1.0 | 4.890 | 339 | 161 | 51 | 38 |
| 2.5 | 0.850 | 820 | 229 | 48 | 44 |
| 5.0 | 0.620 | 901 | 321 | 48 | 56 |

[a] Ten rats per dose, 12–13 tumors per group of rats. Pretreatment tumor weight 0.621 gm. Testosterone propionate administered subcutaneously between days 35 and 65 after tumor implantation.

TABLE VIa

EFFECT OF TESTOSTERONE PROPIONATE ON GROWTH OF SEMINAL VESICLES AND LEVATOR ANI MUSCLES OF CASTRATE MALE RATS[a] (3)

| Testosterone propionate (mg./kg./day, 20 days) | Number of rats | Seminal vesicle (mg.) | Levator ani (mg.) |
|---|---|---|---|
| 0 | 10 | 10 | 49 |
| 0.25 | 10 | 74 | 79 |
| 0.50 | 10 | 141 | 116 |
| 1.00 | 10 | 212 | 159 |
| 2.00 | 10 | 280 | 171 |
| 4.00 | 10 | 331 | 189 |
| 8.00 | 10 | 349 | 179 |

[a] These data were obtained following subcutaneous administration of testosterone propionate for 20 days to 27-day-old castrate male rats.

In Tables VI and VIa, the effects of equivalent doses of testosterone propionate on the various end organs of the female tumor-bearing rat and the castrate male rat are shown. It is apparent that, at dose levels which cause significant tumor inhibition in female rats, significant androgenic effects are produced in both sexes. For practical purposes, the response of the preputial gland of the female rat has been selected as a measure of "androgenicity."

This gland invariably responds to $C_{19}$ steroids with known androgenic activity in male rats (8).

When the basic parameters shown above were fairly well substantiated by experiments repeated several times, we were in a position to begin assaying compounds for antitumor activity. Selection of compounds presented a problem, since all so-called biologically active $C_{19}$ steroids (androgens) would be expected to produce tumor inhibition. To make the problem more interesting, both relatively "inactive" and active $C_{19}$ steroid androgens which had been tested in castrate male rats were selected—with emphasis on the former.

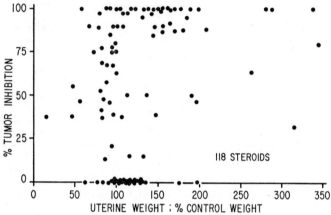

Fig. 7.  Tumor inhibition by $C_{19}$ steroids and effect on uterine weight.

The selection of the appropriate dose levels to employ for studies in the mammary fibroadenoma assay also presented a problem. Since mammary cancer, either its transplanted or naturally occurring prototypes, is non-physiological, we selected "nonphysiological" doses of steroids. In most instances, 3.0 mg. of steroid per rat (180–220 gm) were administered daily for a period of 30 days. When compounds appeared to be interesting in these preliminary studies, they were subsequently assayed orally and sub-cutaneously at many dose levels.

A primary consideration emphasized in the introduction was: are all $C_{19}$ steroids that inhibit tumor growth necessarily androgenic? For analysis of this latter response, the preputial gland was chosen as the end point in female rats. Other indexes, such as changes in body weight and in ovarian, adrenal, and uterine weights, were also used to gain an approximate insight into the character of the steroids being tested. In Figs. 7, 8, and 9 attempted correlations between $C_{19}$ steroid antitumor effects and other end organ responses (uterus, ovaries, and preputial glands) are illustrated. In Fig. 10

are shown the attempted correlations for $C_{19}$ steroid antitumor effects in female rats and androgenic effects in castrate male rats. It is apparent, from the 80–118 steroids selected at random from our files, that positive correlations cannot be made between these parameters. The original question was:

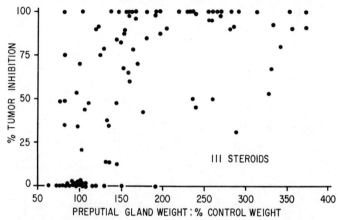

FIG. 8. Tumor inhibition by $C_{19}$ steroids and effects on preputial gland weight.

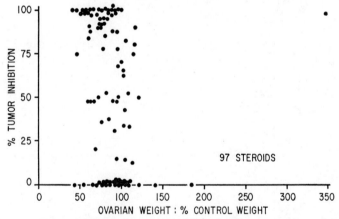

FIG. 9. Tumor inhibition by $C_{19}$ steroids and effect on ovarian weight.

Can tumor inhibition be predicted from an analysis of other well-known biologic activities of $C_{19}$ steroids? On the basis of these data, we believe that such positive predictions cannot be made.

Examination of some of the $C_{19}$ steroids which produced significant tumor inhibition, with little or no effect on preputial gland development, led to a number of interesting observations. In Fig. 11 the effects of subcutaneous

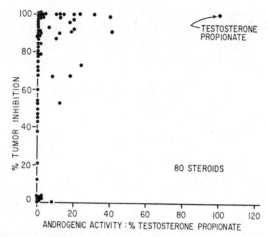

FIG. 10. Correlation between androgenic activity and tumor inhibitory activity of $C_{19}$ steroids.

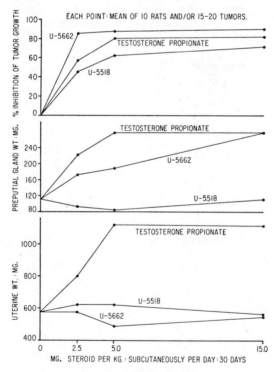

FIG. 11. Tumor inhibitory effects of subcutaneously administered 9β,11β-epoxy-17-methyltestosterone (U-5518) and 11α-hydroxy-17-methyltestosterone (U-5662) (4).

administration of 11α-hydroxy-17-methyltestosterone (U-5662) and 9β,11β-epoxy-17-methyltestosterone (U-5518) on tumor growth and other end organs are illustrated. It is evident that both agents are as effective as testosterone propionate as antitumor agents, yet exert different effects on both the uterus and preputial glands. In Fig. 12 the results of oral administration of the same compounds are shown. For these latter studies, the two

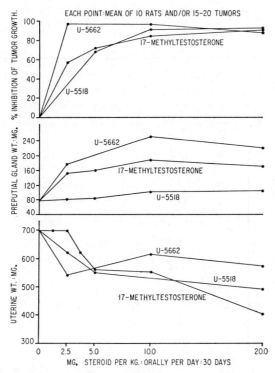

Fig. 12. Tumor inhibitory effects of orally administered U-5518 and U-5662 on established mammary fibroadenoma (4).

derivatives were compared to 17-methyltestosterone. It is evident that, at dose levels which produced marked tumor inhibition, U-5518 did not stimulate the preputial glands as did 17-methyltestosterone and U-5662.

When administered to castrate male rats, neither U-5518 nor U-5662 were found to be androgenic (Fig. 13). These steroids were also found to be devoid of estrogenic activity (Table VII). In addition, these two interesting derivatives of 17-methyltestosterone did not modify the response of the uteri of female castrate rats to estradiol.

A rather interesting result was obtained when the comparative antitumor

TABLE VII

Uterotropic and Anti-uterotropic Activity of 11α-Hydroxy-17-Methyltestosterone
(U-5662) and 9,11-Epoxy-17-Methyl-testosterone (U-5518) (4)

| Preparation | Number of rats | Dose per day (20 days) | Uterus (mg.) |
|---|---|---|---|
| A  CMC Vehicle | 10 | 0.2 cc. | 22 |
| B  Estradiol | 10 | 0.8 µg./kg. | 143 |
| C  U-5518 | 10 | 15.0 mg./kg. | 23 |
| D  U-5662 | 10 | 15.0 mg./kg. | 19 |
| B + C | 10 | — | 143 |
| B + D | 10 | — | 164 |

effects of 19-nortestosterone and 2-methyl-19-nortestosterone (U-5520) were
compared in female rats. Whereas 19-nortestosterone is an effective antitumor agent as well as a potent preputial gland stimulator, 2-methyl-19-
nortestosterone has essentially the same antitumor activity but does not

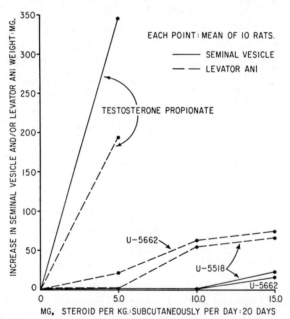

Fig. 13. Androgenic activity of testosterone propionate, U-5662, and U-5518 (4).

stimulate the preputial glands (Table VIII). These preliminary results led
to further analysis of 2-methyl-19-nortestosterone and, as results in Fig. 14
illustrate, 2-methyl-19-nortestosterone inhibits the mammary fibroadenoma
without producing effects on the preputial glands. In contrast to the oral
effectiveness of 11α-hydroxy-17-methyltestosterone and 9β,11β-epoxy-17-

TABLE VIII

EFFECT OF 19-NORTESTOSTERONE, 2-METHYL-19-NORTESTOSTERONE, AND TESTOSTERONE
PROPIONATE ON GROWTH OF TP-RESPONSIVE MAMMARY FIBROADENOMA (4)

| Preparation | Dose (mg./kg.) | Number of animals | Number of tumors | Preputial glands (mg.) | Tumor weight (gm.) | % Inhibition |
|---|---|---|---|---|---|---|
| Final controls | — | 8 | 11 | 99 | 8.375 | — |
| 19-Nortestosterone | 15 | 8 | 15 | 317 | .980 | 100 |
| 2-Methyl-19-nor-testosterone | 15 | 8 | 11 | 103 | .820 | 100+ |
| Testosterone propionate | 5 | 8 | 11 | 279 | 1.130 | 98 |
| Initial controls | — | 10 | 16 | — | .950 | — |

methyltestosterone, 2-methyl-19-nortestosterone is inactive by this route of administration.

When the pituitary inhibitory effects of U-5662, U-5520, and U-5518 were compared, it was discovered that only 2-methyl-19-nortestosterone (U-5520) inhibited testicular development in the male rat (Table IX). That the

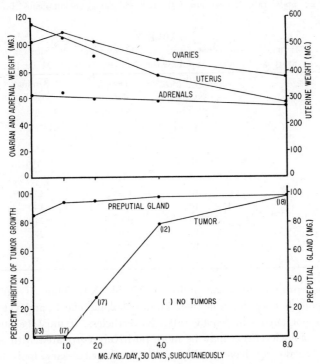

FIG. 14. Tumor inhibitory effects of 2-methyl-19-nortestosterone (U-5520) (4).

latter compound is probably an effective pituitary inhibitor is reflected by changes in uterine, ovarian, and adrenal weights following its administration to female rats (Fig. 14). As in the findings with U-5662 and U-5518, 2-methyl-19-nortestosterone was found to be less than 1 % as effective as

TABLE IX

EFFECT OF 2-METHYL-19-NORTESTOSTERONE, 9-11-EPOXY-17-METHYLTESTOSTERONE, AND 11α-HYDROXY-17-METHYLTESTOSTERONE ON GROWTH RATE OF TESTES[a] (4)

| Number of animals | Compound | Testes (mg.) | Seminal vesicles (mg.) | Adrenals (mg.) | Body weight gain (gm.) |
|---|---|---|---|---|---|
| 10 | Controls | 2274 | 269 | 33 | 113 |
| 10 | 9,11-Epoxy-17-methyl-testosterone | 2192 | 200 | 33 | 100 |
| 10 | 11α-Hydroxy-17-methyl-testosterone | 2187 | 201 | 30 | 117 |
| 10 | 2-Methyl-19-nor-testosterone | 1130 | 132 | 29 | 106 |

[a] Weanling male rats, 70–80 gm.; treated 40 days, subcutaneous injections, 15 mg./kg./day.

TABLE X

EFFECT OF 2-METHYL-19-NORTESTOSTERONE AND TESTOSTERONE PROPIONATE ON GROWTH RATE OF SEMINAL VESICLES AND LEVATOR ANI OF CASTRATE MALE RATS (4)

| Compound | Number of rats | Dose, S.C. (mg./kg.) | Seminal vesicle (mg.) | Levator ani (mg.) |
|---|---|---|---|---|
| Vehicle | 10 | 0.1 cc. | 6 | 41 |
| 2-Methyl-19-nor-testosterone | 10 | 15.0 | 34 | 97 |
| Testosterone propionate | 10 | 0.25 | 74 | 80 |
| | 10 | 0.50 | 140 | 118 |
| | 10 | 1.00 | 210 | 150 |
| | 10 | 2.00 | 277 | 170 |
| | 10 | 4.00 | 320 | 185 |
| | 10 | 8.00 | 351 | 161 |

testosterone propionate as an androgen (Table X). Thus, it can be seen that compounds may differ in their known biologic effects and yet be effective antitumor agents in female rats. Nevertheless, it must be emphasized that other biologic effects may be more positively correlated with antitumor activity. We do not have readily available the necessary tools for determining the ability of these steroid derivatives to modify the secretion or activity of, for example, growth hormone and lactogenic hormone which have been shown by Huggins (1) to increase the growth rate of the benign mammary fibroadenoma.

That a steroid can exist which exerts maximum antitumor effects and at the same time minimum effects on the preputial glands is fairly well demonstrated in Fig. 15. These data resulted from the administration of the potent androgen 9α-fluoro-11β-hydroxy-17-methyltestosterone (Halotestin).[3] When compared to previous figures and tables and Fig. 17, it is apparent that this compound produces antitumor effects at subcutaneous dose levels that

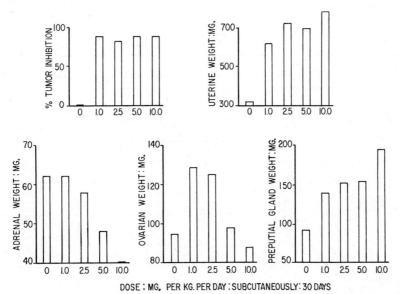

FIG. 15.   Effect of 9α-fluoro-11β-hydroxy-17-methyltestosterone on uterus, ovaries, preputial glands, adrenals, and benign fibroadenoma (4).

produce less "androgenic" activity in female rats than testosterone propionate or 17-methyltestosterone.

A few of the structural requirements for mammary tumor inhibition are illustrated in Table XI. Compounds shown here represent only a small number of those which have been studied. However, it can be seen that a large number of structural modifications on the $C_{19}$ steroid molecule can be made without bringing about loss of antitumor activity. The presence of a double bond between C-4 and C-5 on the steroid molecule is not a necessary requirement for the production of antitumor effects. The presence of a

---

[3] Halotestin: 9α-fluoro-11β-hydroxy-17-methyltestosterone, The Upjohn Co., Kalamazoo, Michigan.

ketone configuration at C-3 is also not absolutely necessary for antitumor activity. The presence of a ketone or hydroxyl grouping at C-17 appears to be essential, since substitution with an oxime or methyl group leads to complete loss of antitumor activity. Introduction of substituents at C-2, C-9, and C-11 modifies the ratio of antitumor activity to preputial gland-stimulat-

TABLE XI. RELATION BETWEEN STEROID STRUCTURE AND TUMOR INHIBITION (TP RESPONSIVE TUMOR)

| | | | | | | | |
|---|---|---|---|---|---|---|---|
| ANTI TUMOR ACTIVITY % INHIBITION | 100 | 90 | 95 | 53 | 100 | 50 | 83 |
| PREPUTIAL GLAND WEIGHT % CONTROLS | 352 | 284 | 255 | 327 | 163 | 260 | 150 |
| ANDROGENIC ACTIVITY ORALLY (% MT) | 31 | 0 | TRACE | 115 | 0 | 55 | 20 |
| PARENTERALLY (% TP) | 100 | 0 | TRACE | 12 | 0 | 0 | — |

| | | | | | | | |
|---|---|---|---|---|---|---|---|
| ANTI TUMOR ACTIVITY % INHIBITION | 79 | 98 | 75 | 0 | 0 | 87 | 97 |
| PREPUTIAL GLAND WEIGHT % CONTROLS | — | 269 | 125 | 101 | — | 198 | — |
| ANDROGENIC ACTIVITY ORALLY (% MT) | TRACE | TRACE | 0 | 0 | 0 | 2000 | 260 |
| PARENTERALLY (% TP) | 0 | 0 | 0 | 0 | 0 | 10 | TRACE |

| | | | | | | | | |
|---|---|---|---|---|---|---|---|---|
| ANTI TUMOR ACTIVITY % INHIBITION | 88 | 90 | 100 | 90 | 91 | 100 | 99 | 100 |
| PREPUTIAL GLAND WEIGHT % CONTROLS | 153 | 333 | 104 | — | 123 | 199 | 196 | 162 |
| ANDROGENIC ACTIVITY ORALLY (% MT) | 0 | 40 | 0 | 0 | 31 | 25 | TRACE | TRACE |
| PARENTERALLY (% TP) | 0 | 20 | 0 | 12 | 0 | 10 | 0 | 0 |

Note: All 2-methyl substituents are in the alpha position.

ing activity in female rats as well as androgenic activity in male rats. It may be summarily stated that a potent androgenic steroid in male rats will be an effective antitumor agent in female rats. It cannot be stated that an inactive steroid androgen in male rats will be an inactive antitumor agent in female rats.

### Testosterone Propionate-Resistant Tumor

It was observed, after many successive transplant generations, that some of the mammary fibroadenomas became resistant to the tumor inhibitory effects of testosterone propionate. One of the resistant tumors was selected for further investigation and transplanted; the transplanted tumors tested for resistance to testosterone propionate were used for subsequent studies. A control group, to which 5.0 mg./kg. of testosterone propionate had been administered, was included in each of the following series of experiments to assure continued resistance.

Figure 16 illustrates that, although the mammary fibroadenoma is resistant to increasing amounts of testosterone propionate, it is not resistant to the administration of $9\alpha$-fluoro-$11\beta$-hydroxy-$17$-methyltestosterone (Halotestin). These results are more interesting when one considers the observations which

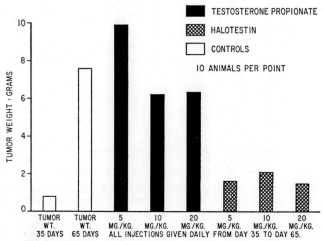

FIG. 16. Effect of Halotestin and testosterone propionate on growth rate of testosterone-resistant mammary fibroadenoma.

show that, when injected subcutaneously, this steroid is less "androgenic" in ovariectomized female rats than testosterone propionate (Fig. 17). The studies recorded in Fig. 16 have been repeated many times with essentially the same results. These results are interpreted to mean that a "testosterone propionate-resistant" tumor is not necessarily a "$C_{19}$ steroid resistant" tumor.

In many series of "testosterone propionate-resistant" tumors it was noted that the growth rate far exceeded the growth rates previously obtained with the "testosterone propionate-responsive" tumor. Perhaps the rapid proliferation of some of these tumors was sufficient to outweigh the influence of testosterone propionate on their subsequent rate of growth. This idea gains further encouragement when data shown in Fig. 18 are analyzed. This figure illustrates that the testosterone propionate resistant tumor is still markedly depressed by the combined process of adrenalectomy-ovariectomy. Neither procedure alone produces a marked inhibitory effect. Note that this resistant tumor appears to be somewhat similar to that reported by Huggins (2). However, the Huggins' Class II tumor is only slightly affected by hypophysectomy. It should be emphasized that Huggins did not employ

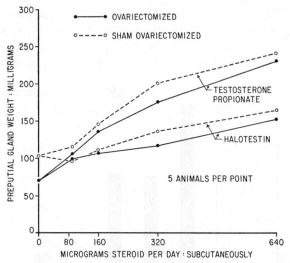

FIG. 17.  Comparative potencies of Halotestin and testosterone propionate on growth rate of preputial glands in ovariectomized and sham-ovariectomized female rats.

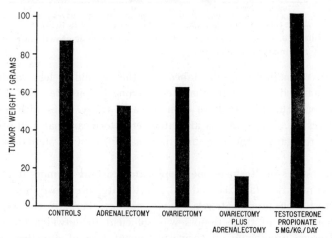

FIG. 18.  Effect of ovariectomy, adrenalectomy, and the combined procedures on growth of testosterone-resistant tumor. Conditions: 20 rats per group; operation performed 35 days after initial implantation; autopsy on day 65.

well-established growing tumors for assay purposes. We have shown in previous publications (3, 4) that differences in response exist between well-established growing tumors and tumors treated from day 1 of tumor implantation. It is our belief that the dihydrotestosterone-resistant tumor which Huggins described was still androgen sensitive for the following reason. He showed that the sensitive tumor finally became refractory to dihydrotestosterone. However, if the 3-methylcholanthrene were administered orally along with dihydrotestosterone, to animals bearing the resistant tumor, marked tumor inhibition occurred. Glenn et al. (11), later showed that orally administered 3-methylcholanthrene merely potentiated the biologic activity of administered androgens. If the amounts of dihydrotestosterone administered had been increased to rather high pharmacologic levels, the Huggins' Class II tumor may still have responded to the androgen.

We have attempted to determine why the mammary fibroadenoma becomes resistant to testosterone propionate and not to the potent androgen 9α-fluoro-11β-hydroxy-17-methyltestosterone (Halotestin). Preliminary results, which are not complete, suggest that the sensitive tumor does not metabolize testosterone; the resistant tumor does. Neither the resistant nor responsive tumors are capable of metabolizing Halotestin. The conclusions to be inferred from these data are that the continued synthesis of androgen-metabolizing enzymes in the tumor inactivates the hormone, and antitumor effects are depressed. In fact, Halotestin is not the only derivative of testosterone that will inhibit the testosterone-resistant tumor. A brief summary of results in Table XII shows that other $C_{19}$ steroids exist that are capable of depressing the growth rate of a testosterone propionate-resistant mammary fibroadenoma.

TABLE XII

$C_{19}$ STEROIDS THAT INHIBIT TESTOSTERONE PROPIONATE-RESISTANT TUMOR

| Compound | Mg./kg./day | Androgenic activity (% of TP) | Preputial gland (% of Control) | % Tumor inhibition |
|---|---|---|---|---|
| 11-Keto-17-methyltestosterone | 15.0 | Negative | 254.0 | 100.0 |
| 9α-Fluoro-11β-hydroxy-17-methyltestosterone | 5.0 | 12.0 | 205.0 | 85.0 |
| 6α-17-Dimethyltestosterone | 15.0 | 14.0 | 200.0 | 95.0 |
| Testosterone propionate | 15.0 | 100.0 | 405.0 | 10.0 |
| 6α-Fluoro-17β-hydroxy-5α-androstan-3-one | 15.0 | Negative | 409.0 | 91.0 |
| 6α-Methyl-9α-fluoro-21-deoxy-17-acetoxy-prednisolone (U-17323) | 5.0 | Negative | —40.0 | 73.0 |

Androgenic activity determined in castrate male rats at 100-μg. per rat dose levels (approximately 1.0 mg./kg.).

High dose levels of estradiol produce a slight inhibitory effect on the TP-resistant mammary fibroadenoma; progesterone administration results in a significant increase in tumor size (Fig. 19); when combined, a greater increment in growth rate occurs (Fig. 20). In the latter figure it is shown that the antitumor agent, 5-fluorouracil, has only a slight inhibitory influence on

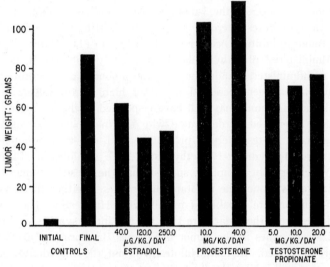

FIG. 19. Effect of estradiol, progesterone, and testosterone propionate on growth of TP-resistant mammary fibroadenoma. Conditions: steroids administered daily for 30 days; 10 rats per group.

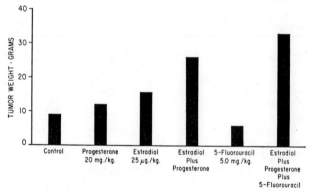

FIG. 20. Effect of combined administration of estradiol and progesterone on growth rate of the testosterone-resistant mammary fibroadenoma. Conditions: 10 rats per group; compounds administered daily for 30 days, steroids subcutaneously, 5-fluorouracil intraperitoneally.

tumor growth; it is unable to prevent the increase in growth resulting from combined administration of progesterone and estradiol.

As was indicated previously, hydrocortisone administration fails to alter growth of the responsive neoplasm; in addition, prednisolone is also ineffective. The administration of prednisolone to animals bearing the resistant tumor also fails to alter tumor growth (Fig. 21). These latter experiments were primarily performed to determine if the combined administration of prednisolone and Halotestin would cause regression of tumor growth since the former is a potent "catabolic" agent in female rats. Combination of the

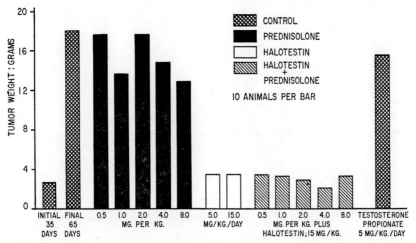

Fig. 21. Effect of Halotestin, prednisolone, and their combination on growth of testosterone-resistant mammary fibroadenoma. Prednisolone administered every other day with and without Halotestin.

two steroids does not produce greater inhibitory effects than can be produced with Halotestin alone. These results are shown because they, too, bear on the future developments of research in this area—to be described in a later section.

Correlations between steroids that inhibit the testosterone propionate-resistant tumor and androgenic activities in male and female rats also failed to lead to convincing evidence that one process is necessarily related to the other (Figs. 22 and 23). It has also been found that the compounds described in preceding sections, $11\alpha$-hydroxy-17-methyltestosterone and $9\beta$,-$11\beta$-epoxy-17-methyltestosterone, which had been shown to inhibit the responsive tumor, failed to inhibit the testosterone propionate-resistant tumor. On the other hand, 2-methyl-19-nortestosterone, which inhibited the responsive tumor, also effectively inhibited the resistant tumor.

## C3H Mammary Adenocarcinoma

It was necessary, first, to determine the known hormonal parameters which are important to the development of this tumor in mice.

Examination of Fig. 24 shows that ACTH administration causes retardation of tumor growth—a dose-related phenomenon. In the same illustration

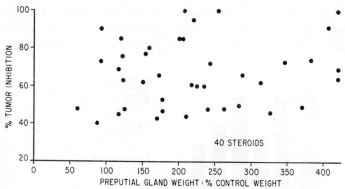

FIG. 22. Relationship between preputial gland stimulation and tumor inhibition (testosterone-resistant mammary fibroadenoma).

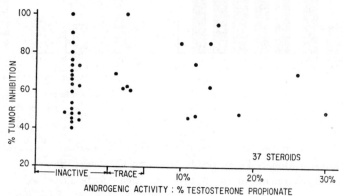

FIG. 23. Relationship between androgenic activity and tumor inhibition (testosterone-resistant mammary fibroadenoma).

it is shown that pregnant mare's serum gonadotropin (Gonadogen[4]) has a slight but significant inhibitory influence on tumor growth.

Luteotropin, growth hormone, and estradiol have little influence on growth rate of the C3H mammary tumor (Figs. 25 and 26). Testosterone and progesterone (5–20 mg./kg.) also fail to alter growth rates of the C3H mammary adenocarcinoma.

---

[4] Gonadogen: The Upjohn Co., Kalamazoo, Michigan.

It may be concluded from the above results that ACTH, probably via its effects on adrenal hormone synthesis or release, causes retardation of mammary tumor growth in the C3H mouse. This conclusion is valid since both prednisolone and hydrocortisone also produce inhibitory effects on growth rate of the mammary adenocarcinoma of C3H mice (6, 7). It is evident that prednisolone is about 2.5 times as potent as hydrocortisone with regard to its ability to inhibit mammary adenocarcinoma development (Fig. 27). This is an interesting observation, since the glycogenic potency

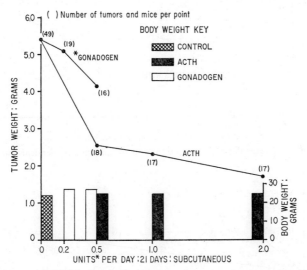

FIG. 24. Effect of ACTH and Gonadogen on growth rate of mammary adenocarcinoma of C3H mice. Gonadogen: 1 Cartland-Nelson unit* is equivalent to 20 international units.

of the synthetic steroid is of the same order of magnitude (5.8 times) in this species (Fig. 28).

In Fig. 29 the comparative effectiveness of prednisolone and deoxycorticosterone are shown. It is evident that deoxycorticosterone, a potent sodium-retaining steroid in adrenalectomized animals and man, is without effect on tumor growth. Halotestin, although having the ability to inhibit the mammary adenocarcinoma of mice (Fig. 30) fails to cause tumor inhibition beyond the 50 % range—a result that is not too exciting. Conversely, prednisolone causes increasing decrements in tumor growth rate to the 95 % level.

To define the parameters of effectiveness of prednisolone on tumor growth, the following experiments were performed. Groups of 20 animals were transplanted with tumors in the usual fashion. Some animals were pretreated with prednisolone; others were treated at various times after tumor implantation. Results of these experiments are shown in Fig. 31. It is evident that prednisolone merely retards tumor growth; it fails to alter subsequent tumor growth when administered before tumor implantation; it fails to

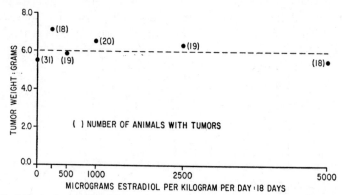

Fig. 25. Effect of estradiol-17β on growth rate of mammary adenocarcinoma of C3H mice.

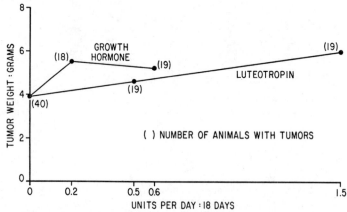

Fig. 26. Effect of growth hormone and luteotropin on growth rate of mammary adenocarcinoma of C3H mice.

alter subsequent growth following its withdrawal; it also fails to cause regression, but retards tumor growth after tumors are established and growing autonomously. The conclusions to be drawn from these studies are: (1) Prednisolone does not bring about the death of mammary adenocarcinoma cells. (2) Prednisolone merely slows the growth rate of mammary tumor cells in C3H mice. (3) Prednisolone effects may be related primarily to those produced in the host. This latter idea led to the development of the following experiments.

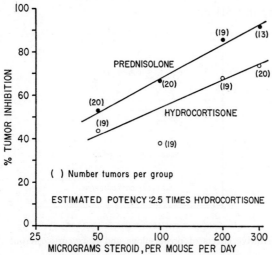

FIG. 27. Comparative effects of hydrocortisone and prednisolone on tumor inhibition in C3H mice.

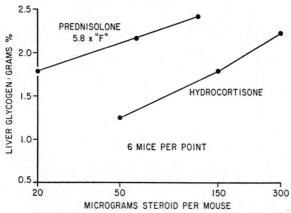

FIG. 28. Glycogenic potency of hydrocortisone and prednisolone in C3H mice.

It may be that the tumor-inhibitory effects that were being observed for the adrenocortical steroids were merely a reflection of other metabolic effects of these compounds. Data illustrated in Fig. 32 show that only those $C_{21}$ steroids that are effective glycogenic agents in adrenalectomized rats are also effective antitumor agents in C3H mice. Inactive glycogenic steroids are either completely inactive or produce less than 60 % inhibition of tumor growth. It is also of interest that the more potent glycogenic agents in rats do not show the same potency correlations when examined for tumor inhibitory activity in C3H mice.

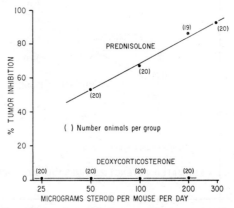

FIG. 29. Comparative effects of prednisolone and deoxycorticosterone on C3H mouse tumor growth.

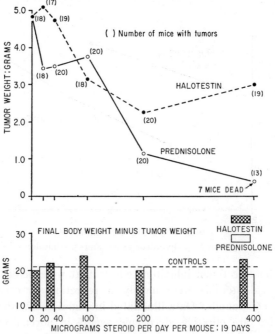

FIG. 30. Comparative effectiveness of Halotestin and prednisolone on C3H mammary tumor growth.

These latter observations prompted an examination of the glycogenic potencies of some $C_{21}$ steroids in C3H mice. When compared to glycogenic potencies in rats, these $C_{21}$ steroids are, with the exception of prednisolone, less active glycogenic and antitumor agents in the mouse (Table XIII). It

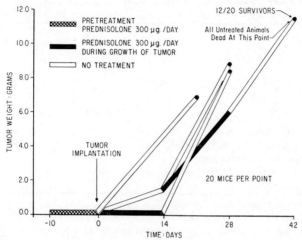

FIG. 31. Effect of prednisolone on mammary tumor growth in the C3H mouse.

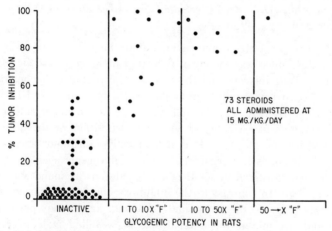

FIG. 32. Relationship between glycogenic activity of $C_{21}$ steroids and anti-tumor activity in C3H mice.

has also been found that the rate of metabolism of $C_{21}$ steroids in the liver of the mouse is markedly different than that observed for the rat. These observations, with their theoretical and practical implications and their relation to studies in man, will be the subject of another communication and will not be described in further detail. It is sufficient at this juncture merely to indicate that studies with the C3H mammary tumor led to developments in other areas which may ultimately be equally important to those reported herein.

TABLE XIII

GLYCOGENIC POTENCIES OF VARIOUS $C_{21}$ STEROIDS IN RATS AND MICE[a]

| Compound | Glycogenic Potency | | C3H Tumor potency, mouse | Anti-inflammatory potency, rat |
|---|---|---|---|---|
| | Rat | Mouse | | |
| Hydrocortisone | 1 | 1 | 1 | 1 |
| Prednisolone | 3 | 6 | 3 | 3 |
| 9α-Fluoroprednisolone | 42 | 15 | 9–10 | 14 |
| 6α-Methyl-9α-fluoroprednisolone | 126 | 3 | 4 | 24 |
| 6α-Methyl-21-deoxy-9α-fluoroprednisolone | 25 | 1 | 4 | 135 |
| 9α-Fluoro-16α-hydroxyprednisolone | 33 | 19 | 3 | 7 |
| 6α,9α-Difluoroprednisolone acetate | 442 | 24 | 3 | 66 |
| 6α-Methylprednisolone | 9 | —[b] | 2 | 6 |

[a] Conditions: Adrenalectomized fasted male rats and intact fasted male mice were used for glycogen assays in the two species: 6–10 animals per group for glycogen assays; four dose levels of each steroid analyzed simultaneously with four dose levels of hydrocortisone. At least four dose levels (20 mice per point) used to compare antitumor potencies in C3H mice. Numbers shown in table have been calculated to nearest digit.

[b] Equal to prednisolone. Results obtained from two separate assays in both C3H and Rockland male mice (20–25 gm.).

At this point, we were of the opinion that the assessment of antitumor activity in C3H mice was merely a reflection of other metabolic effects of $C_{21}$ steroids. That this may be the case can be partially demonstrated by the use of the extremely potent progestational agent, 6α-methyl-17-acetoxy-progesterone (Provera). This steroid had been found, under rather special circumstances, to cause significant glycogen deposition in the adrenalecto-mized fasted female rat (10). It is not an active antitumor agent in C3H mice (Fig. 33), nor is it a particularly active glycogenic agent in the same species when administered under the same conditions as found successful in the rat (Fig. 34). In contrast to the inhibitory effects it produced in wean-ling male rats (Fig. 6), this compound (2–40 mg./kg. per day per mouse for 2 weeks) did not inhibit the adrenal size of weanling male mice. These latter results emphasize that the mouse is not only quantitatively but quali-tatively different from the rat insofar as $C_{21}$ steroid effects are concerned.

In summary, it is pertinent to emphasize that steroids and their deriva-tives of different glandular origins have the ability to inhibit mammary tumor development in two different species of animals bearing two and possibly three different types of mammary cancer. Steroids active against the TP-responsive mammary fibroadenoma of rats, testosterone, 9β,11β-epoxy-17-methyltestosterone, and 11α-hydroxy-17-methyltestosterone, are not active against the C3H tumor; steroids that are effective in the C3H

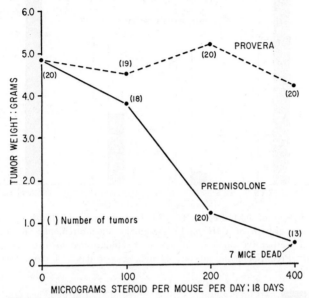

Fig. 33. Effect of 6α-methyl-17-acetoxyprogesterone (Provera) on growth rate of mammary adenocarcinoma of C3H mice.

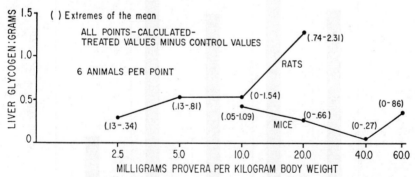

Fig. 34. Comparative glycogenic activity of 6α-methyl-17-acetoxyprogesterone (Provera) in rats and C3H mice (10).

tumor, i.e., hydrocortisone and/or prednisolone, are not effective against the mammary fibroadenoma (Fig. 35). This being the case, it would be ideal to discover a steroid that effectively inhibits both the C3H tumor in mice and preferably the "testosterone propionate-resistant" tumor in rats.

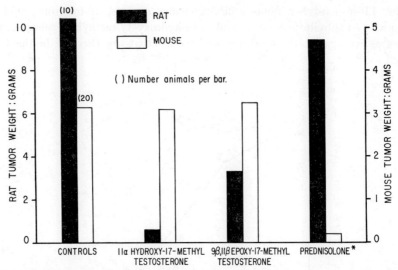

Fig. 35. Effects of 9β,11β-epoxy-17-methyltestosterone and 11α-hydroxy-17-methyl-testosterone on growth of C3H mouse mammary adenocarcinoma and rat mammary fibroadenoma (responsive tumor). All steroids* administered at 15.0 mg. per kilogram body weight. Prednisolone in rats at 5.0 mg./kg. per day: 14 days, treatment withdrawn 14 days.

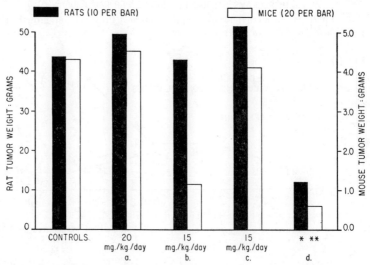

Fig. 36. Tumor-inhibiting effect of progesterone (a.), hydrocortisone (b.), testosterone propionate (c.), and 6α-methyl-9α-fluoro-21-deoxy-17-acetoxyprednisolone (U-17323) (d.). Solid bar (*): rats, 5 mg./kg. per day for 14 days; no treatment for 14 days. Open bar (**): mice, 15 mg./kg. per day.

Figure 36 illustrates the tumor inhibitory effects of 6α-methyl-9α-fluoro-17-acetoxy-21-deoxyprednisolone (U-17323) in C3H mice as well as in rats bearing the TP-resistant mammary fibroadenoma. This steroid has been found to be a potent progestational as well as glycogenic agent (Table XIV). This is the only steroid we have examined to date that effectively inhibits both the C3H adenocarcinoma of mice and the TP-resistant mammary fibroadenoma of rats.

TABLE XIV

EFFECT OF 9α-FLUORO-11β,17-HYDROXY-6α-METHYL-1,4-PREGNADIENE-3,20-DIONE-17-ACETATE (U-17323) ON VARIOUS ENDOCRINE PARAMETERS

| Compound | Glycogenic activity | Progestational activity |
|---|---|---|
| Hydrocortisone | 1.0 | 0 |
| Progesterone | 0 | 1.0 |
| Prednisolone | 3.0 | 0 |
| 6α-Methyl-17-acetoxyprogesterone (Provera) | 0.2[a] | 20–40[b] |
| U-17323 | 7.3 | 8–16[c] |

[a] Results derived from previous published reports (10). Glycogenic activity determined in adrenalectomized fasting rats; progestational activity in rabbits.

[b] Subcutaneous injection.

[c] Results derived from preliminary data, subcutaneous injection.

A few of the steroids, their antitumor activities and related effects, are shown in Table XV. These compounds represent only a few of those which have outstanding antitumor and other biologic effects in experimental animals.

## DISCUSSION AND CONCLUSIONS

It is evident from an examination of the data referred to in the preceding sections that hormonal therapy of experimental breast cancer in animals is a highly effective procedure. However, it is equally evident that, in the rat and mouse, the steroids studied are not "cures" for experimental mammary cancer. Tumors resume normal growth rate patterns when steroid therapy is withdrawn. Prior treatment of animals before tumor implantation is also without effect on subsequent tumor growth. These results are interpreted to mean that the steroid hormones thus far examined in experimental mammary cancer are merely palliative measures. However, knowledge gained in this specialized field may mean that the ultimate control of mammary cancer can be expedited in this and related areas of tumor research.

It is interesting to note that the $C_{19}$ steroids are "anabolic," i.e., they cause animals to gain considerably more weight than nontreated animals; yet they have antitumor activity in female rats. On the other hand, the

## TABLE XV

SUMMARY OF ANTITUMOR AND RELATED BIOLOGIC EFFECTS OF SOME $C_{19}$ AND $C_{21}$ STEROIDS IN EXPERIMENTAL ANIMALS

| Compound | Hormonal properties[a] | | | | | | | Tumor effectiveness | | |
|---|---|---|---|---|---|---|---|---|---|---|
| | Andro. | Utero. | Prog. | Glyc. | Anti-in. | Gon. In. | ACTH In. | TP-Responsive | TP-Resistant | Mouse adenocarcinoma |
| 9β,11β-Epoxy-17-methyl testosterone | < 1% of TP | 0 | + | 0 | 0 | 0 | 0 | +++ | 0 | 0 |
| 11α-Hydroxy-17-methyl-testosterone | < 1% of TP | 0 | − | 0 | 0 | 0 | 0 | +++ | 0 | 0 |
| 17α-Hydroxy-6α-methyl progesterone acetate | 0 | 0 | +++ | +,− | +,− | +++ | +++ | ++ | 0 | 0 |
| 2α-Methyl-19-nor-testosterone | < 1% of TP | 0 | − | 0 | 0 | ++ | 0 | +++ | +++ | 0 |
| 9α-Fluoro-11β,17α-dihydroxy-6α-methyl-1,4-pregnadiene-3,20-dione 17-acetate | 0 | 0 | +++ | +++ | +++ | ++ | +++ | − | ++ | +++ |
| 9α-Fluoro-11β-hydroxy-17-methyltestosterone | ++ | ++ | − | 0 | 0 | + | 0 | +++ | +++ | + |
| 1-Dehydrohydrocortisone | 0 | 0 | 0 | +++ | +++ | − | +++ | 0 | 0 | +++ |
| Testosterone propionate | + | +++ | − | 0 | 0 | ++ | 0 | +++ | 0 | 0 |
| Progesterone | 0 | 0 | + | 0 | 0 | + | 0 | 0 | 0 | 0 |
| Hydrocortisone | 0 | 0 | 0 | + | + | 0 | + | 0 | 0 | ++ |

[a] Andro. = androgenic; Utero. = uterotropic; Prog. = progestational; Glyc. = glycogenic; Anti-in. = anti-inflammatory; Gon. In. = gonadotropin inhibitor; ACTH In. = ACTH inhibitor.

biologically active $C_{21}$ steroids studied here are, for the most part, effective "catabolic" agents, i.e., they are thymolytic and cause loss in body weight; yet they also inhibit a tumor in a different species of animal. With regard to the rat mammary fibroadenoma, tumor inhibition may be related for the most part to effective inhibition of pituitary function. With regard to the mammary adenocarcinoma of C3H mice, tumor inhibition may be related primarily to effects on the host as well as to direct effects on the tumor. Huggins has shown fairly conclusively that the $C_{19}$ steroids that inhibit mammary fibroadenoma development cause stimulation of normal mammary gland tissue. It is almost unnecessary to emphasize, then, that the factors which cause growth of the normal gland, as well as factors which affect body growth in general, may not necessarily reflect the factors involved in the growth of the neoplastic gland.

The benign mammary fibroadenoma represents an autonomous growth that is rather remarkable. This tumor grows in the period of 4–6 months to sizes which are, for the most part, larger than the rat which bears the tumor. It is not unusual to have a 250-gm. rat with a 350-gm. tumor. One of the primary reasons why this tumor causes death is related to the inability of the host to gain access to food. However, in the case of the testosterone propionate-resistant tumor, we have noted earlier deaths of animals which are unrelated to tumor size. The explanations for these differences await further experiments. Gross pathological examination reveals that neither tumor has metastasized to adjacent or distant sites. Aside from its possible usefulness in the study of mammary carcinoma, the mammary fibroadenoma represents a possible tool for a prolonged study of factors that modify or alter growth of neoplastic or normal tissue. However, such studies would necessarily be accomplished in the hypophysectomized rat bearing a rapidly growing tumor, since this tumor is predominantly under hormonal control via the pituitary.

Before starting a program in this area, one could speculate that all $C_{19}$ steroid androgens are antitumor agents and that all related nonandrogens are ineffective. In the experimental animal, at least, this is not a true generalization. We have made a generalization in the work presented in the foregoing sections. Studies with the C3H mammary adenocarcinoma reveal that only those $C_{21}$ steroids that are metabolically active are effective antitumor agents in the mouse. These statements must be interpreted solely on the basis of the number of compounds examined and the species in which they are examined. In this area, not only do we have the problem of tumor differences in response to steroids, but we also have the additional problem of species differences. With the testosterone-responsive mammary fibroadenoma, we have some justification for believing that it represents a somewhat analogous situation to that occurring in man. The C3H mammary adenocarcinoma is a species-specific tumor that may have little relation to the development of mammary cancer in man. Conversely, the fact that correlations can be made between known steroid antitumor effects in animals and those in man does not necessarily imply that unknown steroids discovered in animals will show the same degree of positive correlation between the two species.

Huggins has emphasized in the past (5), and we should like to re-emphasize in the present, that the study of mammary cancer in both man and experimental animals represents a unique situation. First, here is a neoplasm that is promoted, and inhibited, in all probability, by hormones. Both the promoting and inhibiting hormones are natural products of the physiological environment. Growth and development of prostatic carcinomata are also influenced by known physiological controlling mechanisms. Is it too much to envisage that other neoplasms may be dominated by similar types of controlling forces? If so, future developments in this area must await the discovery and investigation of numerous other endocrine mechanisms.

In the studies that we have presented it would have been ideal to show investigations at the enzyme level demonstrating the defect in metabolism of the benign fibroadenoma compared to normal mammary gland tissue. The relative deficiency in blood supply of the benign fibroadenoma and its rapid rate of growth, suggest that it is dependent upon an anaerobic type of energy metabolism. The acquisition of data of this type, were they available, would do little toward increasing our understanding regarding the discovery of agents useful in the treatment of mammary cancer. In addition, enzyme studies concerning the mechanism whereby some steroids stimulate and others inhibit the mammary fibroadenoma would presumably do little toward advancing our knowledge regarding the types of agents to use for treatment of mammary cancer in experimental animals. It is perhaps too early in the development of biochemistry to apply basic knowledge from this area to the treatment of mammary cancer. This is an unfortunate state of affairs and relegates research in this area to the hit-or-miss type of endeavor. Nevertheless, the knowledge that one group of steroids causes increased growth rate of mammary tumors and another group causes depression of growth rate, should be sufficient to prompt the synthesis and development of analogs or derivatives of these and related steroids that will essentially "fool" the tumor—thereby bringing about the possible death of mammary tumor cells. Thus far, it appears that the steroids investigated in this communication merely prevent cellular proliferation or division but do not induce actual death of cancer cells. The latter objective is the desired one.

Although it is possible to demonstrate in the experimental animal the existence of steroids that have antitumor effects without other so-called "undesirable" qualities, i.e., androgenicity or estrogenicity, the search for better and more improved types of antimammary tumor therapy must proceed in other directions. If such research is to be fruitful, it must be based upon the acquisition in the laboratory of tumors which simulate those occurring in man. The endocrine-dependent tumors represent a somewhat analogous situation to that observed in man, but in these areas, too, experimental tools are inadequate. Mammary tumors in animals that simulate the hormonally resistant tumors in man have not been discovered. It is the latter type that causes the greatest concern.

The observations which show that a tumor becomes resistant to one type of $C_{19}$ steroid and remains responsive to analogs of the same steroid represents an observation that may, or may not, have its counterpart in humans with breast cancer. However, such basic information should be applied to studies in man to determine whether this relationship exists. This may mean the difference between 5-month and 10-month survival of the patient with mammary cancer. Such possibilities remain to be determined.

It is possible to find steroids that will inhibit both mammary cancer in rats (a benign fibroadenoma) and mammary cancer in mice (a more malignant adenocarcinoma). However, it must be emphasized that, in the mouse, the levels of $C_{21}$ steroids necessary to induce 90–100 % depression of tumor growth are verging on the near-toxic levels for these substances. It is necessary to emphasize that many $C_{21}$ steroids that cause 100 % inhibition of tumors in mice also produce sick hosts. The steroid that produces tumor inhibition in both rats and mice (U-17323) has a pronounced "catabolic" effect in rats. Nevertheless, prednisolone also has the same action in rats but does not produce antitumor effects. One cannot satisfactorily ascribe the antitumor activity of this agent to a so-called "antianabolic" effect on the host. With the $C_{19}$ steroids, it is gratifying to note that antitumor effects are produced in animals which gain more weight and appear healthier than their nontreated controls. Generally, the story of antitumor agents is a story of host toxicity, but in this instance the opposite situation exists.

Initiation of a program of research in this area was approached with limited objectives. These limited objectives have been partially attained and a few were outlined in the preceding sections. It is the belief of these investigators that further knowledge in this area awaits the development and acquisition of knowledge in the more basic areas of endocrinology. In fact, all the limited experiments and results presented here have had as their foundation the tremendous store of basic knowledge that has been acquired in the fields of adrenal, pituitary, and reproductive physiology. Many approaches to this problem are being used in other areas; this research represents an extremely small facet of the entire problem. It is unfortunate that further insight into the mammary cancer problem has not been forthcoming, but the primary reason for this has arisen from our complete lack of knowledge in the more fundamental areas of research which are not directly related to the cancer problem.

### ACKNOWLEDGMENTS

The original tumor for the mammary fibroadenoma studies, as well as much helpful advice, was supplied by Dr. Charles Huggins. Numerous members of the Chemistry Department of The Upjohn Company contributed to these studies; without their help, suggestions, and supplies of compounds these studies would not have been possible.

### REFERENCES

1. Huggins, C., Torralba, Y., and Mainzer, K. *J. Exptl. Med.* **104**, 525 (1956).
2. Huggins, C., and Mainzer, K. *J. Exptl. Med.* **105**, 485 (1957).
3. Glenn, E. M., Richardson, S. L., and Bowman, B. J. *Endocrinology* **64**, 379 (1959).
4. Glenn, E. M., Richardson, S. L., Lyster, S. C., and Bowman, B. J. *Endocrinology* **64**, 390 (1959.)
5. Huggins, C. *J. Natl. Cancer Inst.* **15**, 1 (1954).
6. Sparks, L. L., Daane, T. A., Hayashida, T., Cole, R. D., Lyons, W. R., and Li, C. H. *Cancer*, **8**, 271 (1955).
7. MacAlpin, R. N., Blair, S., Gillies, D., Lyons, W., and Li, C. H. *Cancer* **11**, 731 (1958).
8. Glenn, E. M. Unpublished data.
9. Barnes, L. E., Schmidt, F. L., and Dulin, W. E. *Proc. Soc. Exptl. Biol. Med.* **100**, 820 (1959).
10. Glenn, E. M., Richardson, S. L., and Bowman, B. J. *Metabolism Clin. and Exptl.* **8**, 265 (1959).
11. Glenn, E. M., Lyster, S. C., Bowman, B. J., and Richardson, S. L. *Endocrinology* **64**, 419 (1959).

### DISCUSSION

**R. L. Noble:** I must congratulate Dr. Glenn on the tremendous amount of work which he has done with these tumors. I would like, however, to express a word of caution about the use of the preputial glands to indicate androgenic activity. While it is true that androgen stimulates these glands in the rat, many years ago Dr. Collip and I showed that they are under a direct control of the anterior pituitary. Following hypophysectomy, the preputial glands atrophy and can be restored by fractions which we then thought contained growth hormone. It is conceivable therefore that in attempting to assay for androgens you might be affecting the pituitary and so, indirectly, the preputial glands.

The opening remarks of the speaker rather interested me; following his thanks to Dr. Huggins for interesting him in the problem, he congratulated himself for having the determination now to get out of the problem. Yet, listening to the presentation one was struck by the fact that this approach to the screening of steroids seemed reasonable. Dr. Glenn and his associates have demonstrated that there was activity against a tumor which did not parallel other biological activity; this seems to be very informative. Historically, we were faced with a tremendous enthusiasm for the use of the fibroadenoma, perhaps justifiable, although I think there were a few small dissenting voices. The enthusiasm for the use of this tumor seems now to have waned—particularly if Dr. Glenn is giving it up. We seem to be faced with a resurgence of interest in the use of carcinogen-induced mammary adenocarcinoma. Perhaps it's time to take stock before plunging ahead with this new mammary adenocarcinoma, and to review the pitfalls that have been exposed using the fibroadenoma.

**M. Glenn:** I agree with Dr. Noble with regard to the use of the preputial glands as a measure of the androgenic activities of $C_{19}$ steroids in female rats. However, it is a convenient end point in the same animal in which we are also measuring tumor inhibition. When we find steroids that fail to produce stimulation of the preputial glands, yet still inhibit tumor growth, we then examine these steroids more critically in castrate male rats to determine if, at the same dose levels, the steroids are indeed androgenic or completely lacking in this property.

Insofar as my comment congratulating myself on getting out of the problem is concerned, I'd like to emphasize that I did most of the work shown here—a rather boring situation when one has many other interesting problems. Secondly, since we have turned up so many steroids which affect the mammary fibroadenoma, but which apparently do not possess androgenic activity, we would prefer to wait and see whether any clinical correlations exist between these observations in rats and the observations that may be made in man. If such correlations actually exist there may be, as you say, a resurgence of interest in this particular tumor.

Dr. Noble pointed out the extreme variabilities in tumor growth rates and I also mentioned this in the beginning of the manuscript. This is an extremely difficult tumor with which to work.

Lastly, the comments regarding the 3-methylcholanthrene-induced tumor: We have not attempted to get into this area of research because the initial results with these induced tumors appear to correlate fairly well with the results that we obtained with the mammary fibroadenoma—that is, the steroids which are effective there are also effective here; —the ablative procedures are also effective against both preparations. Unless we can be convinced that we are not actually duplicating everything that we have already done, I think we will just leave it alone.

**A. White:** In view of the discrepancy or divergence between the data obtained for glycogenic activity of certain steroids in rats as compared to mice, have you found similar divergences in possible comparisons of anti-inflammatory activities in the two species? There might be a correlation between antitumorigenic activity and anti-inflammatory activity. Secondly, in describing the search for a relationship between the antitumorigenic activity of $C_{21}$ steroids and/or the anti-inflammatory, you spoke also of their glycogenic and/or anti-inflammatory activity. This suggests that you have in mind a steroid in which you have dissociated the anti-inflammatory and the glycogenic activity.

**M. Glenn:** In answer to your last question first. We have not obtained such steroids —that is, steroids which have glycogenic activity without anti-inflammatory activity. I apologize for using the terminology "and/or." It wasn't in the manuscript. You ask if there was a correlation between antitumor activity in C3H mice and anti-inflammatory activity. We are now investigating this problem, and there is some difficulty in setting up the proper assays for anti-inflammatory activity in C3H mice.

**C. Harris:** I would like to go back to the question of the methylcholanthrene-induced tumors versus the fibroadenomas, and raise the question about the criteria for malignancy. There was a saying that once a tumor is transferrable it is malignant, and in this case the fibroadenoma possibly would fit this classification. However, histologically a fibroadenoma is a benign tumor. The methylcholanthrene-induced tumor in the female rat is a glandular tumor which histologically appears malignant and sometimes fulfills the criteria for malignancy, in that it metatasizes and invades adjacent tissues. The female rat treated with methylcholanthrene and testosterone propionate during pubescence will develop a tumor that is fibroadenomatous, and sometimes if enough testosterone is given the tumor will become just a fibrous mass in which no glands can be seen at all. This fibrous mass is completely benign, histologically and behaviorally. In the middle group depending upon the balance between the estrogen and androgen at the time the methylcholanthrene is given, one gets a tumor that is like a cystosarcomaphyllodes—it is almost, histologically, as if the cells themselves can't make up their minds which way to go—whether to form glands or to form stroma. The question of malignancy here is more difficult to assess because people feel there is a tendency to local recurrence; certainly in the human problem with regard to this tumor, the cystosarcomaphyllodes has always been a problem. In methylcholanthrene induction we see a spectrum going from a complete histological malignancy to benignity as well as including a middle form of tumor, which is in a sense indeterminate. If indeed there is no difference in the response of these tumors to the various treatments, it speaks possibly for some relationship between the stroma and glandular components in the metabolic response to these drugs. Heretofore we have always thought of stroma as something independent of the glandular elements, possibly having a completely different metabolic makeup. I would like to know if Dr. Glenn has gone into this problem at all and whether, in this treatment, when there is retardation of growth it is distinctive of one or the other element.

**M. Glenn:** With regard to the question whether the retardation is related to one or another histological element in the tumor: I'm not a pathologist. However, every tumor which was shown here has been examined by a competent pathologist and it appears that one cannot distinguish a treated tumor from a control. Therefore, we have disregarded the pathological picture in the analysis of the results which we have presented here.

Next you ask whether the mammary fibroadenoma is malignant. There is disagreement about this among experts, and I don't feel competent to take sides. With regard to the studies with 3-methylcholanthrene and testosterone, these are very interesting, but we have no data in this area and cannot speak positively. However, I should like to say that Dr. Huggins reported that, when the TP-responsive tumor became resistant to dihydrotestosterone, it was subsequently inhibited, if 3-methylcholanthrene were administered orally with the dihydrotestosterone. We became interested in this problem and began administering 3-methylcholanthrene, as well as other related carcinogenic hydrocarbons, to castrate male rats given 17-methyltestosterone orally. We found that by this route of administration 3-methylcholanthrene produces marked potentiation of the biologic effects of 17-methyltestosterone. We have completed about sixteen carcinogenic hydrocarbons, some of which are and some of which are not carcinogenic. The reported relationship holds up with these compounds; that is, those that have been shown to be carcinogenic potentiated 17-methyltestosterone, those that have been shown to be noncarcinogenic in small animals, did not show the potentiation.

**A. Segaloff:** I would like to ask whether you feel that this last compound is going to be "the answer." Secondly, I wonder if you have tried some dosage response curves aimed at getting preputial gland stimulation like that of an optimal dose of testosterone, in order to see whether relatively ineffective or weak androgens work on the tumor at high dosage?

**M. Glenn:** As to whether we believe that the last compound is the answer—no, we do not. We have no feelings in this regard except to say that it was pleasing to find a steroid that possessed these activities, since we hadn't observed them before. As to your last question regarding stimulation of the preputial gland and differences in the response, we do not have this information.

**D. Holtkamp:** We discussed the anti-inflammatory, the immunologic, and the glycolytic aspects of $C_{21}$ steroid therapy, but nobody has mentioned the metastatic aspects of this type of therapy. I think it is well known that a number of the tumors will respond to the $C_{21}$ steroids with a regression of the tumor but with an increase in the number of metastases. The increased number of metastases has not been taken into account in the work discussed here today.

Secondly, I'd like to propose a possible screening procedure or a transplant procedure, based on some work I did years ago with Dr. Robert M. Hill. This might relate to the glycolytic and nonglycolytic aspects of tumor metabolism and growth. We induced tumors in thigh muscles of rats by injection of methylcholanthrene, and then studied the tumor itself and the "normal" tissue which was adjacent to this tumor [*Federation Proc.* **9**, 184 (1950); *Cancer Research* **15**, 354 (1955)]. This was studied *in vitro* for succinate utilization and oxalacetate utilization, using them as indexes of oxygenating mechanisms [*Arch. Biochem. Biophys.* **34**, 216 (1951)]. The tissue which was adjacent to the tumor had decreased efficiency in succinate and oxalacetate utilization. The control for these experiments was tissue from the contralateral side of the animal. Next, we implanted marbles into these same areas of the leg [*Federation Proc.* **10**, 197 1951)] and again there was a reduction in the oxidative mechanisms. Implanted paraffin had the same effect. Cutting the insertion or cutting the origin of the muscle produced the same effect. Denervation, likewise, had the same effect. Finally, we denervated the muscle and then exercised this muscle by regular, electrical, stimulation and brought the oxidative mechanism back up toward normal. All in all, I'm wondering if the denervated muscle, or the site in which a marble had been implanted the previous week, could possibly be used to expedite screening procedures or to cause a higher percentage of "takes" in tumors that are difficult to transplant. Is there possibly an increase in the glycolytic system in such a preparation? Would tumors planted into this preparation expedite the initial growth of those tumors? I know of no further work on this line of investigation.

**M. Glenn:** I think these are extremely interesting comments. As to the increased metastates following the administration of $C_{21}$ steroids, we haven't observed this phenomenon in the C3H mice. This does not preclude that it may act in this fashion in other species.

**H. M. Lemon:** We have been interested for some years in the therapeutic effects of corticoids given to women who have breast cancer and whose ovaries have been removed. I wanted to ask Dr. Glenn in relation to the lack of effect which he found with corticoids in the fibroadenoma animals, whether he tried the combination of oophorectomy and cortisone therapy?

**M. Glenn:** No, we didn't try a combination of oophorectomy and $C_{21}$ steroid administration. We did try prednisolone administration in increasing amounts with 9α fluoro 11β 17 methyltestosterone. We were unable to produce greater inhibitory effects with the combination than we could produce with the $C_{19}$ steroid alone.

**J. Fried:** On the assumption that this compound that Dr. Glenn put on the board is, so to speak, the essence of his trying work, I think it becomes of extreme interest what the complete endocrine spectrum of this compound is. I do not recall whether it had glucocorticoid activity. Looking at the structure, one would predict quite potent progestational activity.

**M. Glenn:** This steroid is about seven to eight times as potent as hydrocortisone as a glycogenic agent in rats and, in preliminary studies, it is equal to 6α-methyl-17-acetoxyprogesterone as a progestational agent; so it has a combination of very interesting biologic effects. The compound, so far as I know, is not androgenic; but this is a preliminary statement.

**E. Jensen:** I would like to make a philosophical comment concerning Dr. Noble's statement about restraint on our enthusiasm for either the mammary fibroadenoma or the methylcholanthrene-induced tumor as aids in screening. I agree with Dr. Noble that there are certain difficulties in the use of these tumors, and I think that the search should continue for better animal tumors in the endocrine area. The presentation of Dr. Dunning this morning gives an example of how work is going forth in this direction. However, I think that it would be a mistake to wait for perfection, unless we just intend to bequeath the whole problem of cancer chemotherapy to our grandchildren. So, I would like to congratulate Myles Glenn for taking these imperfect tools and using them to obtain information which I believe will prove valuable in the cancer chemotherapy program.

Now I would like to ask Dr. Glenn about the testosterone-resistant tumor which I believe he said was not affected very much by either ovariectomy or adrenalectomy alone, but was markedly inhibited by both together. I wondered what is the effect of hypophysectomy in comparison to the removal of steroidogenic organs.

**M. Glenn:** We haven't hypophysectomized animals having the TP-resistant tumor because of the extreme difficulty that we have had in keeping these animals alive with the rapidly growing tumors.

**E. Jensen:** It seems to me that Dr. Huggins has made the rather interesting observation that hypophysectomy was not nearly so effective in inhibiting the tumor as was the combination of ovariectomy and adrenalectomy, indicating that there must be some factor independent of pituitary control but yet involving the gonads or the adrenal.

**M. Glenn:** That's true; Dr. Huggins says that his dihydrotestosterone-resistant tumor is no longer inhibited by removal of the pituitary. We have pointed out before that marked differences exist in response of tumors which are treated from day 1 and day 35 of tumor implantation. I don't know if this is a possible explanation, and I would be most unwilling to say that our TP-resistant tumor is the same as Dr. Huggins' dihydrotestosterone-resistant tumor. They were derived under entirely different circumstances.

**G. Pincus:** If you look at the formula of this compound that is active against all tumors tested it is obvious that the side chain might be removed and you would get a $C_{19}$ steroid, which would be a 6-methyl-$\Delta^1$-9α-fluoro-11-hydroxytestosterone—and I wonder if such a compound has been tested. Secondly, have you tested related androgens, if not that particular compound, in the C3H adenocarcinoma?

**M. Glenn:** We have tested a number of $C_{19}$ steroids in the mammary adenocarcinoma and found them ineffective. However, with 9α-fluoro-11β-hydroxy-17-methyltestosterone, we can produce rather consistent inhibition, but never greater than, say, 40%. I can't recall that we have determined the activities of a compound related to this one which is a $C_{19}$ steroid. Dr. Babcock may be able to answer this question.

**J. Babcock:** We have not assayed the particular 9-fluoro derivative you mentioned, Dr. Pincus, but the same compound without the 9-fluorine has been tested and is an active compound in the mammary fibroadenoma, both the TP-resistant and the TP-sensitive strains. It has probably not been tested in the C3H tumor.

**K. L. Sydnor:** I have examined a number of biologically active and inactive androgens in the hypophysectomized female rat. I have not found an inactive biological androgen that would make the preputial glands in a hypophysectomized female rat grow. I have not yet examined a biologically active androgen that did not fail to make the preputial gland grow in the hypophysectomized female rat. I think this might answer Dr. Noble's comment.

**U. Kim:** Dr. Glenn should be re-encouraged by the rapid mammary tumor induction method with methylcholanthrene, which was initiated by Dr. Shay and improved by Dr. Huggins. As stated by Dr. Huggins, a high percentage of these methylcholanthrene-induced mammary carcinomas are hormone responsive, as in humans. Since we consider mammary fibroadenomas as benign neoplasias, and they are readily curable by simple excision, I do not think it is advisable to use fibroadenomas for screening of various competitive compounds for therapeutic evaluation. After Dr. Huggins' and Dr. Noble's extensive studies on this tumor, it is now of purely academic interest to use mammary fibroadenomas in steroid screening. One may want to do a comparative study between fibroadenomas and carcinomas in their hormone responsiveness, or pathogenesis.

In regard to the hormone-responsive tumors, it is our concept that the progression of hormone dependence to autonomy is a one-way track: it is irreversible. Therefore, we think one should look for some way to detect hormone-responsive tumors, and treat them while they are still responsive and controllable.

# Steroid Effects on Heterologously-Transplanted Human Tumors[1]

George W. Woolley, John J. Harris, Philip C. Merker, Joy E. Palm,[2] and Morris N. Teller

*Division of Human Tumor Experimental Chemotherapy, Sloan-Kettering Institute for Cancer Research, and Sloan-Kettering Division Cornell University Medical College, New York, New York*

## I. Introduction

Reports of the use of transplantable human tumors for experimental chemotherapy in the rat (26), hamster (7), mouse (18), and on the chorio-allantoic membrane of the chick embryo (10), have appeared. Recently, it was desired to know whether experimental human tumors could be used, and possibly uniquely, for hormonal anticancer evaluations.

Steroids have been of special interest in cancer for a number of reasons: (1) The secondary sex sites of man and of several experimental animals are sites having high incidence of cancer. (2) Substances structurally related to steroids (3-methylcholanthrene is an example) are cancer-producing chemicals. (3) Hormonal imbalance, produced both by the absence of hormones through glandular ablation, and the pharmacological use of steroid materials may lead to (a) the unexpected occurrence or increased incidence of cancer, and in other instances to (b) the prevention of cancer. And finally (4) steroids and related hormones have been found to be useful in modifying and aiding in the control of cancer of man. The latter influence has been effected through both glandular ablation (ovariectomy, adrenalectomy, and hypophysectomy) and direct hormone administration.

Four systems are being utilized at present in our studies for growth of the human tumors: rat, mouse, egg, and hamster. Each host system presents unique differences and, therefore, will be considered separately both in regard to methodology and to hormone anticancer evaluation. Four human tumors have been selected for major study: a sarcoma H.S.#1, an epidermoid carcinoma H.Ep.#3, an intestinal adenocarcinoma, H.Ad.#1, and a bronchiogenic carcinoma A-42 (Fig. 1). Because these studies are still in progress and also because of the breadth and extent of the work, only a few examples can be presented at this time—and these not in a comparative manner. It

[1] This study was supported in part by Contracts SA-43-ph-1923 and SA-43-ph-2445 from the Cancer Chemotherapy National Service Center, Research Grant CY-3784 from the National Cancer Institute, National Institutes of Health, and Grant T-47 from the American Cancer Society.

[2] At present: Research Associate, Wistar Institute of Anatomy and Biology, Philadelphia, Pennsylvania.

is anticipated that eventually there will be enough points in common in the system outlined so that the results may be considered as a whole.

## II. Studies of Human Tumors Grown in the Egg

The chick embryo has been used in cancer research by various investigators since the classic studies of Murphy of 1912 (19). Time and space will not permit a complete review of the literature. Following studies involving growth of animal tumors on the chorioallantoic membrane (CAM) of the chick embryo, (23, 24), reports have appeared in the literature regarding the use of transplantable human tumors in the egg for chemotherapy studies (3, 4, 8, 9, 10). Preliminary chemotherapy studies (12) using

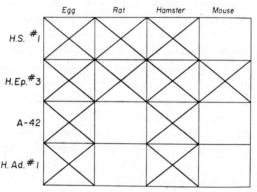

Fig. 1. Anticancer evaluation against experimental human tumors. X = test developed.

hormones and related substances as test agents against human tumors grown on the CAM of chick embryos have indicated that such tumors can evaluate potential antitumor agents in the endocrine category.

Previous reports have indicated that the various types of human tumors differed from each other in their response to chemotherapy agents of other categories (8, 9, 10, 11). The studies reported here indicate similar tumor differences in response to hormones and related substances.

### 1. Procedures

Each egg received a single tumor fragment at 9 days of incubation. Observation for tumor growth occurred 4 days after implantation, and, at this time, tumor-bearing eggs were selected for the tests and single-dose injections of the test agents were made in the yolk sac. Evaluations were made 6 days after the beginning of therapy. The dose of the agent to be treated was suspended in 0.5 ml. of sesame oil. The four types of human tumors mentioned above were used in these studies: Toolan's epidermoid carcinoma

(H.Ep.#3), sarcoma (H.S.#1), and adenocarcinoma (H.Ad.#1), and Skiff's bronchogenic carcinoma (A-42).

## 2. *Experimental*

In Tables I and II, where the number of eggs in the treated group equal six or less, the results are based on single tests. In all other instances, the number of eggs in the treated group exceeds six and this represents pooled data of two or more tests or replications. Pooled results were obtained by combining individual test results for a given tumor at a given dose level and treated as values of a large sample. In other words, the individual tests or replications are considered as subsamples taken from the same population. In Fig. 2, many of the agents used as a basis for the summary are still in

| TUMOR | CORTICOIDS | PROGESTOGENS | ANDROGENS | ESTROGENS |
|---|---|---|---|---|
| A – 42 | ± +   8/9 | ±   4/6 | ± +   13/19 | ± +   6/7 |
| HAD NO. 1 | ± −   1/4 | ± −   2/5 | ±   5/9 | ± −   1/5 |
| HEP NO. 3 | ±   4/9 | ± −   2/6 | ± −   10/19 | −   0/7 |
| HS NO. 1 | ±   7/9 | ±   4/6 | +   17/19 | ± +   5/7 |

FIG. 2. Response of human tumors to steroids and related agents. Fractions indicate number of activities per number tested. Symbols indicate response of tumor to class of agent tested.

the restricted or confidential category; thus, the actual results and references by name could not be presented.

*a. Progesterone.* The results of testing progesterone (4-pregnene-3,20-dione) are indicated in Table I. A comparison among the tumor types clearly indicates that the tumors respond differently to identical doses of the same

### TABLE I
#### EFFECT OF PROGESTERONE[a] ON HUMAN TUMORS IN EGGS

| Tumor | Number of eggs | | % Inhibition | |
|---|---|---|---|---|
| | Treated | Control | Embryo | Tumor |
| A-42 | 10 | 13 | 32 | 64 |
| H.Ep.#3 | 14 | 23 | 17 | 47 |
| H.Ad.#1 | 5 | 7 | 38 | 21 |
| H.S.#1 | 11 | 17 | 21 | 78 |

[a] At 4 mg. per egg.

agent, with H.S.#1 having the best response, i.e., 21 % difference in weight between treated and control embryos and 78 % difference between treated and control tumors. Only one test was made against H.Ad.#1, but the results indicate that this tumor was more resistant to progesterone than was the embryo (38 % difference between treated and control embryos and 21 % difference between treated and control tumors). Although A-42 tumors were inhibited 64 %, the embryo effects (32 % inhibition) were sufficiently high to reduce the significance of the tumor inhibition.

*b. Hydrocortisone.* H.Ad.#1 did not respond to hydrocortisone (11β,-17α,21-trihydroxy-4-pregnene-3,20-dione) at 0.1 mg. per egg (Table II),

TABLE II

EFFECT OF HYDROCORTISONE ON HUMAN TUMORS IN EGGS

| Tumor | Dose (mg.) | Number of eggs | | % Inhibition | |
|---|---|---|---|---|---|
| | | Treated | Control | Embryo | Tumor |
| A-42 | 0.1 | 26 | 27 | 19 | 63 |
| H.Ep.#3 | 0.1 | 3 | 6 | 50 | 57 |
| | 0.05 | 16 | 18 | 10 | 5 |
| H.S.#1 | 0.1 | 5 | 7 | 37 | 66 |
| | 0.05 | 6 | 11 | 10 | — |
| H.Ad.#1 | 0.1 | 11 | 15 | 29 | 27 |
| | 0.05 | 6 | 6 | 10 | 12 |

although this dose was somewhat toxic to the embryos. At the same dose level, A-42, H.Ep.#3, and H.S.#1 were moderately inhibited; however, the embryos bearing H.Ep.#3 and H.S.#1 showed signs of considerable toxicity, thus reducing the significance of the inhibition of these tumor types. A-42 was the only type of tumor to exhibit significant reduction without undue embryo toxicity. When the dose of hydrocortisone was dropped to tolerated dose levels (0.05 mg) for embryos bearing H.Ep.#3 and H.S.#1, tumor inhibition was lost.

*c. Testosterone Propionate.* The results of testing testosterone propionate at 20 mg. per egg against the four types of human tumors are summarized in Table III. The response of H.Ep.#3, A-42, and H.S.#1 are similar with respect to degree of tumor inhibition. Inhibition of H.S.#1 was slightly greater than that of the other tumor types. H.Ad.#1 failed to respond at this dose level.

*d. Androsterone.* Summarized in Table IV are the results of testing androsterone at 10 mg. per egg against the four human tumor types. Here is a striking example of how the degree of sensitivity to a particular agent may vary with tumor types. The order of sensitivity among the tumor types to androsterone placed H.S.#1 as the most sensitive (81 % inhibition), followed by A-42, H.Ep.#3, with H.Ad.#1 (35 % inhibition) the least sensitive.

### TABLE III
EFFECT OF TESTOSTERONE[a] PROPIONATE ON HUMAN TUMORS IN EGGS

| Tumor | Number of eggs | | % Inhibition | |
|---|---|---|---|---|
| | Treated | Control | Embryo | Tumor |
| H.Ep.#3 | 12 | 16 | 4 | 41 |
| A-42 | 9 | 12 | — | 43 |
| H.S.#1 | 9 | 13 | 5 | 51 |
| H.Ad.#1 | 15 | 22 | 5 | 19 |

[a] At 20 mg. per egg.

### TABLE IV
EFFECT OF ANDROSTERONE[a] ON HUMAN TUMORS IN EGGS

| Tumor | Number of eggs | | % Inhibition | |
|---|---|---|---|---|
| | Treated | Control | Embryo | Tumor |
| A-42 | 10 | 16 | — | 63 |
| H.Ep.#3 | 10 | 12 | 14 | 42 |
| H.S.#1 | 9 | 14 | — | 81 |
| H.Ad.#1 | 22 | 31 | — | 35 |

[a] 3α-hydroxyandrostan-17-one at 10 mg. per egg.

### TABLE V
EFFECT OF ESTRONE[a] ON HUMAN TUMORS IN EGGS

| Tumor | Number of eggs | | % Inhibition | |
|---|---|---|---|---|
| | Treated | Control | Embryo | Tumor |
| A-42 | 16 | 21 | — | 62 |
| H.Ep.#3 | 11 | 16 | — | 15 |
| H.S.#1 | 16 | 22 | — | 63 |
| H.Ad.#1 | 9 | 13 | 6 | 8 |

[a] 3β-Hydroxy-1,3,5(10)-estratrien-17-one at 20 mg. per egg.

*e. Estrone.* The results of testing estrone at 20 mg. per egg are summarized in Table V. A-42 and H.S.#1 show similar degrees of inhibition, 62% and 63 %, respectively, and H.Ep.#3 and H.Ad.#1 failed to respond at this dose level. There were no signs of toxicity to the embryo in either case.

An attempt has been made to group the endocrine materials tested into general categories, i.e., corticoids, progestogens, androgens, and estrogens, and to summarize (Fig. 2) the responses of the four types of tumor to materials in the various categories. The fractions in each square represent the number of active agents in a particular group over the number tested for a given tumor type. The symbols (—, ±, +, etc.) occurring within a square represent the ranking of a particular group of endocrine materials in terms of its effectiveness against a particular type of tumor.

For example, H.Ep.#3 did not respond to any of the seven estrogens tested: thus, the ranking of estrogen against H.Ep.#3 is "—." H.S.#1 responded to seventeen out of nineteen androgens tested and the level of activity of these androgens against H.S.#1 was high: thus, the ranking of androgens against H.S.#1 is "+." Another example is to be found among the corticoids, where H.Ad.#1 responded to only one of the four corticoids tested, and though this one agent gave moderate inhibition, the ranking of corticoid against H.Ad.#1 is "± −." Following this procedure, one could rank these four types of human tumors growing in the egg according to their sensitivity, in general, to endocrine materials, as follows: rank 1—H.S.#1; rank 2—A-42; rank 3—H.Ad.#1; rank 4—H.Ep.#3.

A study (Fig. 2) indicates that there is little margin between ranks 1 and 2 and between ranks 3 and 4. Because of this, one could rank the response of these tumors to endocrine materials in another way. Rank 1 could very well include H.S.#1 and A-42, and rank 2 would include H.Ad#1 and H. Ep.#3. When using the latter scheme of ranking, there is a much greater margin of sensitivity between the ranks.

### 3. Discussion

In view of the results presented here, it is difficult to think in terms of effectiveness of a potential antitumor agent without indicating its target. An agent may be negative against one type while destroying another type of tumor.

Another consideration borne out by the evidence is that one agent within a particular group of compounds may be quite effective in inhibiting tumor growth whereas another agent within the same group, even closely related, may be totally ineffective against the same type of tumor. This raises the question regarding the necessity of considering individuality of potential chemotherapeutic agents, as well as the individuality of a particular tumor type. It may be inferred from this that the success achieved in chemotherapy may well depend upon the closeness of fit of the individual agent to the individual tumor type.

### 4. Summary

The results of testing corticoids, progesterones, androgens, and estrogens against four types of transplantable human tumors (H.Ep.#3, H.Ad.#1,

A-42, and H.S.#1) growing on the CAM of chick embryos have been presented.

Comparative testing, i.e., testing the same agent against the four types of tumors, clearly demonstrates differences among the tumor types in their sensitivity to certain antitumor agents. The results indicate that transplantable human tumors growing on the CAM of the chick embryo may be used to evaluate potential antitumor activity of endocrine materials. Comparisons among the tumor types of their sensitivity to the various classes of endocrine materials tested indicate that H.S.#1 and A-42 are considerably more sensitive to endocrine materials than are H.Ad#1 and H.Ep.#3.

### III. Studies of a Human Tumor Grown in the Swiss Mouse

#### 1. Method

A detailed description of the transplantation, conditioning, and chemotherapy procedures for the Swiss mouse-H.Ep.#3 tumor-testing program has been published (17). However, a brief description of the method is presented for purposes of orientation.

Female Swiss Webster mice (Taconic Farms) each weighing 15–22 gm. are used as hosts. Since three tumors, each weighing a minimum of 2.0 gm., are required in the transplant procedure and because of the difficulty of maintaining a continuous transplant line of H.Ep.#3 in Swiss mice, 7–14-day-old H.Ep.#3 tumors grown in X-irradiated and cortisone-treated rats are used. The tumor is first separated from the muscle and bone of the donor rat; it is minced with scalpels, and then diluted in the ratio 1 part tumor:1 part saline fortified with potassium penicillin G (1000 units/ml.) and streptomycin sulfate (2 mg./ml.). Minced suspensions are injected through a 16-gauge needle fitted to a 2-ml. Luer Lok syringe. All transplantations are made intramuscularly into the right thigh. Immediately thereafter, each mouse receives a single dose of cortisone acetate (150 mg./kg.) subcutaneously in the nape of the neck. No further conditioning is required.

Chemotherapy trials are conducted against three tumor-bearing mice. Control groups also contain three mice. In general, one set of control mice services three test groups. Therapy is usually started 24 hours after transplantation and continued for 7 days. Animals are sacrificed 9 days after transplantation, and net tumor weights are determined by subtracting the weight of the opposite uninjected thigh from the weight of the tumor-bearing thigh. The average net tumor weights of the treated and control groups are then compared.

Test data are evaluated on the basis of "per cent inhibition" computed from the average net tumor weight of the local control group for that day, or in relation to the lower limits (95 % confidence) of the historical grand average.

In general, the grading system has been adopted as shown in the Tabulation.

| General effect | % Inhibition | Average weight of 3 treated tumors |
|:---:|:---:|:---:|
| — | 0–35 | > 1.4 gm. |
| ± | 36–58 | 1.4–1.0 gm. |
| + | > 58 | < 1.0 gm. |

As in other chemotherapy programs, final decisions as to the disposition of a compound take into account reproducibility of test results: a compound, in order to "pass," must be effective (+ or ± grade) in two out of the first three preliminary trials; otherwise it is classified "reject." A passed compound is given a complete dose titration and tested orally.

The grading system given above is re-examined approximately every six months on the basis of the performance of the system as a whole. To date, and after one and a half years of operation, shifts of several percentage points have taken place, but these have had no particular bearing on final decisions. The entire H.Ep.#3 testing program, therefore, has been essentially stable and very satisfactory from the laboratory standpoint.

## 2. Results

a. $C_{21}$ Steroids: In preliminary tests, it was found that the conditioning agent cortisone, in doses of 500 mg./kg., inhibited the growth of H.Ep.#3 and that hydrocortisone, at 250–125 mg./kg. also acted as an antitumor agent. Therefore, it was not unexpected to observe that analogs of these two steroids were also inhibitory to tumor growth. Five steroids in this class, other than cortisone or hydrocortisone, were significantly inhibitory: Decadron, 9α-fluorohydrocortisone, 9α-fluoroprednisolone, prednisolone, and prednisone, (Table VI).

In some cases, such as with 9α-fluorohydrocortisone, the effects were produced at doses close to an $LD_{50}$. In other cases, lower toxicity was associated with the antitumor effects as demonstrated by Decadron at 62 mg./kg. and prednisolone at 250 mg./kg. The nonfluorinated steroids, prednisolone, prednisone, and hydrocortisone acetate, produced their effects at higher doses (250–125 mg./kg.) than the fluorinated steroids (62–31 mg./kg.).

In the case of 9α-fluorohydrocortisone, antitumor activity and toxicity were spread over a broad range: 125–16 mg./kg. (Table VII). At doses lower than 16 mg./kg., toxicity to the host and antitumor activity are not present. Liver lesions resembling fatty degenerative changes were observed

TABLE VI

EFFECT OF A SERIES OF $C_{21}$ STEROIDS ON H.EP.#3 GROWING IN THE CONDITIONED SWISS MOUSE

| Compound[a] | Dose | Number of trials | Mortality | Average tumor weight (gm.) | Effect |
|---|---|---|---|---|---|
| Decadron | 62 | 4 | 3/12 | 1.0(0.9–1.1) | ± |
| | 31 | 2 | 0/6 | 1.5(1.1–1.8) | |
| 9α-Fluoro-hydrocortisone | 62 | 7 | 11/21 | 1.2(1.0–1.4) | ± |
| | 31 | 3 | 2/9 | 1.5(1.3–1.6) | |
| 9α-Fluoro-prednisolone | 62 | 2 | 4/6 | | |
| | 31 | 2 | 1/6 | 0.8(0.7–0.9) | + |
| | 16 | 2 | 0/6 | 1.7(1.5–1.8) | |
| Prednisolone | 250 | 6 | 6/18 | 1.0(0.8–1.1) | + |
| | 125 | 3 | 0/9 | 1.5(1.3–1.8) | |
| Prednisone | 250 | 5 | 2/15 | 1.1(0.8–1.4) | ± |
| | 125 | 2 | 1/6 | 1.1(0.7–1.6) | ± |
| | 31 | 2 | 2/6 | 1.6 | |
| Hydrocortisone acetate | 250 | 5 | 1/15 | 1.2(0.9–1.7) | ± |
| | 125 | 3 | 2/9 | 1.2(0.8–1.5) | ± |
| Control (historical) | | | 7/153 | 2.2(1.4–3.0) | |

[a] Administered subcutaneously.

TABLE VII

EFFECT OF 9α-FLUOROHYDROCORTISONE ON H.EP.#3 GROWING IN THE CONDITIONED[a] SWISS MOUSE

| Dose (mg./kg. × 7, S.C.) | Number of trials | Mortality | Host body weight change (gm.) | Average tumor weight (gm.) | Effect |
|---|---|---|---|---|---|
| 500 | 2 | 5/8 | | | |
| 125 | 5 | 6/14 | —1.1 | 0.8(0.7–1.0) | + |
| 62 | 7 | 11/21 | —0.3 | 1.2(1.0–1.4) | ± |
| | 4[b] | 4/12 | —0.2 | 1.1(1.0–1.2) | ± |
| 31 | 3 | 2/9 | —0.2 | 1.5(1.3–1.6) | ± |
| | 3[b] | 1/9 | —0.2 | 1.4(1.2–1.6) | ± |
| 16 | 2[b] | 1/6 | —2.2 | 1.1(0.9–1.4) | ± |
| Controls | 17 | 0/54 | +1.6 | 2.2(1.4–3.2) | |
| | 9[b] | 0/27 | +1.3 | 2.6(1.7–3.4) | |

[a] X-Irradiation 100r, total body; cortisone acetate four doses (1.5, 1.0, 1.0, 1.0, mg. per mouse).

[b] No X-irradiation; cortisone acetate 1 dose 3 mg. per mouse (150 mg./kg.).

at 125, but not at 62, mg./kg. Severe liver pathology was noted for hydro-cortisone acetate at 500, 250, and 125 mg./kg.; prednisone at 250 and 62 mg./kg.; and prednisolone at 500, 250, and 125 mg./kg. Liver damage was not necessarily confined to these steroids because it was also associated with at least one relatively ineffective $C_{19}$ steroid, 1-dehydrotestololactone. With the exception of 9$\alpha$-fluoroprednisolone, the tumor-inhibitory activity and host toxicity were displayed by these steroids when the oral route was used. Only Decadron and prednisolone were active when tested against the 4-day-old established tumor transplants (Table VIII).

TABLE VIII

Effects of Oral and Post 4-Day Therapy With $C_{21}$ Steroids on H.Ep.#3 Growing in the Conditioned Swiss Mouse

| Compound | Oral | | Therapy started after 4 days | |
|---|---|---|---|---|
| | Dose (mg./kg.x7) | Effect | Dose (mg./kg.) | Effect |
| Decadron | 62 | ± | 62 | — |
| | | | 31 | ± |
| 9$\alpha$-Fluorohydrocortisone | 125 | ± | 250 | — |
| | 62 | — | 62 | — |
| 9$\alpha$-Fluoroprednisolone | 31 | — | 31 | — |
| | 250 | ± | 125 | ± |
| Prednisolone | 125 | ± | 125 | — |
| | | | 62 | — |
| Prednisone | 250 | ± | 125 | — |
| | 500 | — | 250 | — |
| Hydrocortisone acetate | 500 | ± | 125 | — |
| | 250 | ± | | |

*b. $C_{19}$ Steroids.* Steroids of this class were without significant antitumor activity. Of thirty-eight compounds, thirty-five were rated ineffective and three gave "suggestive" evidence of antitumor effects. Data on these three compounds are presented in the form of a graph (Fig. 3) in which individual tests are plotted relative to their local controls and the historical grand mean tumor weight. For testosterone propionate, results were negative; for 1-dehydrotestololactone, one test was inhibitory but other trials showed no effect. In the case of the three "suggestive" $C_{19}$ steroids, average treated tumor weights tended to be close to, if not below, the lower limit of 1.4 gm., and inhibitions using local controls ranged from 38 to 50 %. It is possible that compounds closely related to these three steroids may be more active.

*c. $C_{18}$ Steroids.* Like the $C_{19}$ class, the $C_{18}$ steroids did not produce consistent, major antitumor effects in the mouse-H.Ep.#3 system (Fig. 4). When test data are examined against historical control limits (Table IX,) it is seen that estrone (in three tests), hexestrol and diethylstilbestrol (in one test each) produced average treated tumor weights (Fig. 4, open circles) of

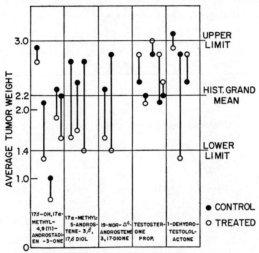

FIG. 3. $C_{19}$-Steroids H.Ep.#3 (IM) in conditioned Swiss mouse. All compounds tested at 500 mg./kg. times 7 by subcutaneous route.

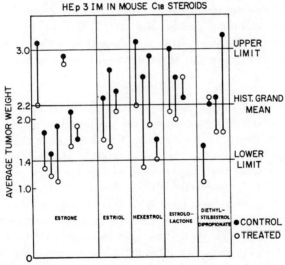

FIG. 4. H.Ep.#3 (IM) in mouse $C_{18}$ steroids. All compounds tested at 500 mg./kg. times 7 by subcutaneous route.

less than 1.4 gm. In several tests, estrone, estriol, hexestrol, and diethyl-stilbestrol produced inhibitions ranging from 41 to 50 % based on comparisons of treated (open circles) and local control (solid circles) tumor weights. Estrone, estrololactone, and diethylstilbestrol also produced, in at least one trial, average treated tumor weights that were *larger* than the local controls for that test. On the average, these five $C_{18}$ steroids did not

TABLE IX

EFFECT OF A SERIES OF $C_{18}$ STEROIDS ON H.EP.#3 GROWING IN THE CONDITIONED SWISS MOUSE

| Compound | Dose (mg./kg.) | Route | Number of trials | Mor-tality | Average tumor weight (gm.) | Effect |
|---|---|---|---|---|---|---|
| Estrone | 500 | S.C. | 7 | 1/21 | 1.8(1.1–2.8) | — |
| | 500 | P.O. | 1 | 0/3 | 1.6 | — |
| | 500 | S.C. | 4 | 3/12 | 1.5(1.1–2.2) | — |
| Hexestrol | 500 | P.O. | 1 | 3/3 | | |
| | 250 | P.O. | 1 | 0/3 | 1.5 | |
| Diethylstilbestrol | 500 | S.C. | 4 | 2/12 | 1.7(1.1–2.3) | — |
| Estrololactone | 500 | S.C. | 4 | 2/12 | 2.2(2.0–2.6) | — |
| Estriol | 500 | S.C. | 4 | 0/12 | 1.8(1.6–2.1) | — |
| Control (historical) | | | | 7/153 | 2.2(1.4–3.0) | |

produce remarkable antitumor effects; that is, treated tumor weights of less than 0.9 gm. or inhibitions greater than 60 %. At most, like the three $C_{19}$ steroids previously discussed, data are suggestive. Other steroids of this class did not even produce this slight degree of antitumor activity.

## 3. Discussion

A recent study of human epidermoid carcinoma (H.Ep.#3) growing in conditioned Swiss mice demonstrated the applicability of this system to chemotherapy studies (17). In an attempt to define more closely the limits of usefulness of this system to the special problem of steroid chemotherapy, approximately seventy-five steroids representing the three major chemical groups, $C_{18}$, $C_{19}$, $C_{21}$, were tested. It was found that consistent and clearly defined antitumor effects associated with host toxicity were present in the following steroids: hydrocortisone acetate, 9α-fluorohydrocortisone, 9α-fluoro-prednisolone, prednisolone, prednisone, and Decadron. Of these six agents, only Decadron and prednisolone inhibited tumor growth when therapy was started 4 days after transplantation. No well-defined antitumor activity could be demonstrated within the $C_{18}$ and $C_{19}$ categories. Several compounds within the $C_{19}$ group have been suggestive, namely: 17β-hydroxy-17α-methyl-4,9(11)-androstadien-3-one, 17α-methyl-5-androstene-3β,17β-diol, and 19-nor-4-androstene-3,17-dione. Because of the small numbers of steroids tested within each class (27 for $C_{21}$, 38 for $C_{19}$, and 11 for $C_{18}$) no definite conclusion can be made at this time about the over-all sensitivity of this human-tumor-mouse host system to steroids. However, from the existing data it is clear that the corticoid compounds are the most potent with respect to host toxicity and antitumor activity. Whether the antitumor effects are real, i.e., mediated through direct action on the tumor cell, or whether the inhibitory activity is due to an alteration in the nutritional relationship of host and tumor due to metabolic imbalances produced in the host by the steroids, cannot be defined at this time. These agents have had profound effects against some types of transplantable animal tumors (5, 20, 21, 25) and have been shown to be useful in some types of human cancer (6, 13, 14). In this respect, therefore, the transplantable H.Ep.#3 growing in the conditioned rat and mouse has not been unique in its behavior toward treatment with these corticoids.

The lack of sensitivity of the transplantable human tumor growing in conditioned mice or rats to $C_{18}$ and $C_{19}$ compounds has also been noted for transplantable animal tumors. In this respect, it is quite possible that the metabolic background of the host, i.e., mouse or rat, is not suitable to unmask significant antitumor activities in these classes of steroids. In our laboratories, the transplantable C3HBA tumor growing in C3H/JAX or $C_3D_2F_1$ hybrids responds to only a few of the $C_{18}$ and $C_{19}$ steroids in comparison to the larger number of $C_{21}$ compounds that are potent antitumor agents.

## IV. Studies of Human Tumors Grown in The Hamster

### 1. Introduction

Experimental chemotherapy of transplantable human tumors has become feasible in laboratory animals as a result of procedures for reducing the resistance of the host species to the heterologous grafts. These procedures consist primarily of the use of conditioning agents such as cortisone or X-irradiation (Toolan), which reduce the immunological competence of the animal to respond to foreign antigenic material.

The cheek pouch of the golden hamster (*Mesocritus auratus*) as a site for tissue implantation has been discussed by several investigators (2, 15, 22, 29), and the advantages of this site for establishing and maintaining human tumors in conditioned hosts have been described (29). In particular it has been reported that less conditioning of the host is required for the growth of many transplantable human tumors and that cortisone alone, without X-irradiation, is frequently sufficient for tumor growth. For these reasons the

cheek pouch of the hamster may have interest particularly to those investigators without the means for X-irradiation readily available.

The following is a report of a study on the effects of a series of steroid
compounds on two different tumors growing in the cheek pouch of the
hamster.

## 2. Materials and Methods

The hamsters used in this study were females each weighing 55–65 gm.
The tumors were H.S.#1, a sarcoma, and H.Ep.#3, a carcinoma, the human
origin of which has been described (29).

For maintenance of these tumors in the hamster, the tumors were transplanted intramuscularly because large amounts of material could be harvested
from this site. For therapy studies, the cheek pouch was used as the site of
implantation. The H.S.#1 sarcoma was implanted as a small fragment by
means of a 16-gauge trocar. The H.Ep.#3 tumor was implanted by 0.1 cc.
of a homogenized 50% suspension (60–70 mg.). Implantation of the tumor
material was performed in the following manner. With a large, blunt forceps
the many-folded membrane of the cheek of the anesthetized host was pulled
out through the mouth opening and grasped with the thumb and forefinger
of the left hand, thereby forming a pouch. The membrane was wiped with a
dry sterile gauze to remove any moisture or food particles. The trocar or
syringe needle was inserted near the host cheek wall and run backward
between the thumb and forefinger so that the material could be inserted at
the tip of the "pouch." Upon ejection of the tumor material the needle was
withdrawn and pressure exerted by the thumb and forefinger in order to
prevent leakage of tumor material. The pouch was then eased back into the
cheek area where the tissue re-assumed its multifold state, keeping the tumor
in place. Aseptic procedures were followed and the tumor transplantation
performed under a glass hood to reduce the possibility of contamination of
the tumor tissue.

The tumor-bearing hamsters were conditioned with three injections of
cortisone acetate on alternate days (60 mg./kg. per injection) starting on
the day of transplant. Therapy was initiated either 24 hours or 5 days post
transplantation. Groups of twenty-four animals receiving the same inoculum
composed a transplant group. This was divided at random into four groups
of six animals each. One such group served as a control and received the
agent used as compound vehicle. The other three groups of six each received
either the same chemical at different dosage or several chemicals. Steroids
were suspended in sesame oil. Compounds were prepared so that the amount
for a 60-gm. average group weight was in a volume of 0.5 cc. Injections were
given intraperitoneally once daily (excluding Sunday) unless otherwise

noted. For evaluation of compound effects, the animals were sacrificed and the tumors removed from the cheek pouch, cleaned of interior liquid or necrosis, and weighed on a Roller-Smith torsion balance. Histological samples were routinely taken. Detailed descriptions of the performance of these tumors with respect to percentage take, average weight, and other population characteristics are being presented elsewhere.

In brief, over the 5-month period from which the chemotherapy results to be reported below have been taken, the percentage take was high for both tumors: 96 % and 95 % for H.Ep.#3 and H.S.#1, respectively. The average weight of the control H.Ep.#3 tumors was 503.8 gm. with a coefficient of variation of 43 %, whereas the H.S.#1 sarcoma averaged 899.4 mg. with a coefficient of variation of 60 %. Mortality of tumor-bearing hosts during the experiments was negligible. Weight loss will be considered with compound effect. Experiments were terminated while the tumors were still in an active phase of growth but before they became large enough to erode the cheek pouch. H.Ep.#3 animals were autopsied on the tenth day post transplantation and H.S.#1 animals on the twelfth day.

Initial tests against H.Ep#3 and H.S.#1 were with doses of 750 mg./kg. of steroid. Compounds demonstrating any activity (arbitrarily considered to be 30 % or more inhibition on the initial test) were repeated, usually at several doses, and histology samples were taken.

The chemotherapy results reported here represent treatment on established tumors, i.e., therapy initiated 5 days after implantation of tumor. This procedure has been investigated primarily because the shorter test period represents a saving of both time and compound, a factor of some importance, providing that the test is not so conservative that potentially useful compounds are missed. In addition, in the unique case of the hamster among laboratory mammals, the use of the cheek pouch as a transplantation site provides a means of observing tumor growth very easily *before* therapy is initiated. Consequently compounds which are costly and/or of limited availability need not be wasted on experimental groups in which the original inoculum is growing poorly.

### 3. Results

The effects of a variety of steroids on each of the two tumors have been studied. Twenty-seven steroids tested against both tumors have been considered with respect to the steroid classification. Reactions from "no effect" to relatively high inhibitions have been obtained.

*a. Corticoids.* Eight corticoids tested include: corticosterone, prednisone, prednisolone, 9α-fluorocortisol, hydrocortisone (free form and acetate), 9α-fluoroprednisolone, and 11-deoxycorticosterone. Of these eight compounds, seven inhibited H.S.#1 extensively and only one, 11-deoxycorticosterone failed to inhibit this tumor.

The growth of H.Ep.#3 was inhibited by four of the eight corticoids: prednisone, prednisolone, hydrocortisone, and 9α-fluoroprednisolone. The inhibitions of H.Ep.#3 caused by these four corticoids represent the most marked effect against this tumor by any steroids in the hamster when therapy was initiated on the fifth day, although nonsteroid compounds as inhibitory have been found.

b. *Androgens.* Both tumors were moderately affected by one of the thirteen $C_{19}$ compounds tested: 4-androstene-3,17-dione. In addition, H.Ep.#3 was moderately affected by 19-nortestosterone and the growth of H.S.#1 was moderately inhibited by 17α-methyltestosterone and markedly inhibited by 9α-fluoro-11-keto-17-methyltestosterone. In view of the general inactivity of this class of compounds against the tumors (nine had no effect against either tumor) the considerable, consistent responses of H.S.#1 to this compound are interesting and will be studied further.

c. *Estrogens.* The results of testing only two estrogens, hexestrol and estrone, are included. Both of these failed to exert a consistent inhibitory effect on either tumor.

d. *Progestogens.* Of the four progestogens included—progesterone, pregnenolone, 17α-hydroxyprogesterone 17-acetate; and 11α-hydroxyprogesterone—only one, the first mentioned, had a slight effect on H.S.#1. None inhibited the tumor H.Ep.#3.

### 4. Summary

The results of testing a series of twenty-seven steroids against two human tumors in the hamster have been presented with emphasis on the comparative responses of the different tumors, one a sarcoma, H.S.#1, and the other a carcinoma, H.Ep.#3, and the relative activity of different classes of steroids (Table X).

TABLE X

EFFECT OF STEROIDS ON HUMAN TUMORS IN HAMSTERS

| Effect | Corticoid | | Androgen | | Estrogen | | Progestogen | |
|---|---|---|---|---|---|---|---|---|
| | H.Ep.#3 | H.S.#1 | H.Ep.#3 | H.S.#1 | H.Ep.#3 | H.S.#1 | H.Ep.#3 | H.S.#1 |
| ± and + | 5 | 7 | 2 | 3 | 0 | 0 | 0 | 1 |
| — | 3 | 1 | 11 | 10 | 2 | 2 | 4 | 3 |

The sarcoma H.S.#1 responded to a greater percentage of the steroids under test than did the carcinoma. However, one compound was reported which acted against the carcinoma and had no observable effect on the sarcoma. Presumably in routine testing of many steroids, other compounds with similar selective effect on H.Ep.#3 will be found. These should be exhaustively studied since their activity against the more "resistant" of the two tumors may reflect basic metabolic effects of importance in chemotherapy.

Of the various classes of steroids, the corticoids exhibited the greatest effect on tumor growth. Whether this is due to an actual effect on the tumor or is a result of a cumulative effect of the test steroid and cortisone used for conditioning is impossible to say at this time, but it is a point worthy of further study.

Of the noncorticoid steroids inhibiting H.S.#1, the greatest inhibition of tumor growth was caused by 9α-fluoro-11-keto-17-methyltestosterone. Although only a few estrogens (two) and progestogens (four) are included, these compounds seem noticeably lacking in inhibitory activity against the present tumors.

From these data it appears that the H.S.#1 tumor responds more frequently to the steroid compounds (11/27 or 40 % positive compounds) than does the carcinoma, H.Ep.#3 (7/27 or 26 % positive compounds). Only one compound, 19-nortestosterone, was observed to have an effect against H.Ep.#3 and not against H.S.#1. The effect, though moderate, was consistent in two trials at the 750-mg/kg. dose with no toxicity. Further study of this compound will be made.

## V. Studies of Human Tumors Grown in the Rat

### 1. Introduction

Transplantable human tumors growing subcutaneously in the rat have been established as an experimental chemotherapy tool (1, 16, 18, 26, 27, 28). The two human tumors used in previous, as well as present, experiments were the epidermoid carcinoma H.Ep.#3 and the sarcoma H.S.#1, described elsewhere by Toolan (29). Previous results (30) have indicated that these tumors growing in other hosts (mouse, chick embryo, hamster) may be responsive to certain steroids. This investigation was undertaken to determine whether H.S.#1 and H.Ep.#3, growing subcutaneously in the rat, would be affected by steroid or steroidlike substances and thus would become useful in detecting such compounds of possible therapeutic value. The material presented here is only preliminary and is offered solely for possible comparison with other tumor systems presented elsewhere in this series of papers.

The test procedure has been described elsewhere (26). For experimental chemotherapy, 0.5 ml. of tumor suspension containing approximately 350 mg. tissue was injected subcutaneously in the right flank of X-irradiated rats. Immediately after transplantation, the rats were injected subcutaneously near the nape of the neck with 60 mg./kg. cortisone acetate in saline suspension. Rats bearing H.S.#1 tumors were injected again with cortisone on alternate days for a total of four doses; those bearing H.Ep.#3 were injected at 3–4-day intervals for a total of three doses.

TABLE XI

Effects of a Series of Compounds on the Subcutaneous Growth of H.S.#1 in the Rat

| Compound | Dose (mg./kg.) | Toxicity | | | | Average tumor weight (gm.) | | % Inhibition[b] |
| | | Average weight Δ (gm.) | | Mortality | | | | |
| | | T[a] | C[a] | T | C | T | C | |
|---|---|---|---|---|---|---|---|---|
| Testosterone propionate | 50 | +1 | —3 | 0/6 | 2/10 | 6.9 | 5.4 | 0[c] |
| | 100 | +3 | —4 | 0/11 | 3/15 | 5.8 | 4.2 | 0[c] |
| | 200 | —5 | —3 | 1/5 | 1/5 | 3.0 | 3.0 | 0 |
| | 500 | +9 | +6 | 0/6 | 0/6 | 7.5 | 2.4 | 0 |
| 4-Pregnene-3,11,20-trione (11-ketoprogesterone) | 25 | +6 | +7 | 0/6 | 0/6 | 4.4 | 5.6 | 0 |
| | 500 | +1 | +7 | 0/6 | 0/6 | 4.4 | 5.6 | 0 |
| 11α-Hydroxy-4-pregnene-3,20-dione (11α-hydroxyprogesterone) | 25 | +16 | +12 | 0/12 | 1/12 | 3.9 | 2.3 | 0[c] |
| | 500 | +12 | +12 | 1/12 | 1/12 | 4.5 | 2.3 | 0[c] |
| Hexestrol | 25 | +1 | +8 | 0/6 | 0/6 | 5.4 | 4.2 | 0 |
| | 500 | +3 | +8 | 0/6 | 0/6 | 2.6 | 4.2 | 38 |
| 1-Dehydrotestololactone | 25 | +15 | +23 | 1/6 | 3/6 | 9.0 | 8.3 | 0 |
| | 87.5 | +14 | +23 | 0/6 | 3/6 | 8.4 | 8.3 | 0 |
| | 350[d] | +11 | +14 | 0/6 | 0/6 | 5.9 | 3.9 | 0 |
| | 700 | +21 | +19 | 0/6 | 1/6 | 6.8 | 6.1 | 0 |
| 9α-Fluoro-17β-hydroxy-17-methyl-4-androstene-3,11-dione | 750 | +17 | +13 | 0/6 | 0/6 | 3.7 | 4.1 | 10 |
| 4-Chloro-17β-hydroxy-17α-methyl-4-androsten-3-one (4-Chloro-17α-methyltestosterone) | 25 | +25 | +7 | 0/6 | 0/6 | 3.6 | 5.6 | 36 |
| | 500 | +11 | +7 | 0/6 | 0/6 | 5.9 | 5.6 | 0 |
| 17β-Propionoxy-2α-methylandrostan-3-one | 500 | +7 | +12 | 1/12 | 1/12 | 4.2 | 3.7 | 0[c] |
| 17α-Methylandrostane-3β,11β,17β-triol | 25 | +9 | +8 | 0/6 | 1/6 | 4.4 | 3.8 | 0 |
| | 500 | +6 | +8 | 1/6 | 1/6 | 4.5 | 3.8 | 0 |
| 17β-Hydroxy-17-Methyl-androstane-3,11-dione | 25 | +9 | +8 | 1/6 | 1/6 | 5.3 | 3.8 | 0 |
| | 500 | +6 | +8 | 0/6 | 1/6 | 4.2 | 3.8 | 0 |

[a] T = Treated; C = control.

[b] H.S.#1 tumor inhibitions of less than 40% are considered negative.

[c] Results of two or more tests were pooled.

[d] Prepared in saline.

An experimental chemotherapy group was composed of thirty-six rats, with five treated subgroups and one control subgroup of six rats each. Three single tumors were used as the source of tumor tissue inoculum, each transplanted into twelve rats, two of which were placed into each of the six subgroups. The compounds were prepared in sesame or peanut oil in con-

TABLE XII

EFFECTS OF A SERIES OF COMPOUNDS ON THE SUBCUTANEOUS GROWTH OF H.EP.#3
IN THE RAT

| Compound | Dose (mg.kg.) | Toxicity | | | | Average tumor weight (gm.) | | % Inhibition[b] |
|---|---|---|---|---|---|---|---|---|
| | | Average weight $\Delta$ (gm.) | | Mortality | | | | |
| | | T[a] | C[a] | T | C | T | C | |
| Testosterone propionate | 50 | +7 | +2 | 0/3 | 0/6 | 3.8 | 3.1 | 0 |
| | 100 | 0 | +6 | 2/13 | 1/16 | 3.1 | 4.0 | 22[c] |
| | 500 | +11 | +10 | 0/18 | 0/18 | 3.3 | 3.4 | 3[c] |
| Δ4-Pregnene-3,11,20-trione (11-ketoprogesterone) | 1000 | +1 | +8 | 0/6 | 0/6 | 1.8 | 1.0 | 0 |
| 4,4'-(1,2-diethylene) di-phenol (hexestrol) | 500 | +3 | +8 | 0/6 | 0/6 | 2.4 | 1.0 | 0 |
| 1-Dehydrotestololactone | 25 | +18 | +15 | 1/6 | 0/6 | 3.0 | 3.5 | 0 |
| | 87.5[d] | +15 | +9 | 1/12 | 1/12 | 3.1 | 3.4 | 9[c] |
| | 700 | +23 | +18 | 0/12 | 0/12 | 3.3 | 5.5 | 40[c] |
| 4-Chloro-17β-hydroxy-17α-methyl-4-andros-ten-3-one (4-Chloro-17α-methyl-testosterone) | 1000 | +7 | +8 | 0/6 | 0/6 | 2.6 | 1.0 | 0 |

[a] T = Treated; C = control.

[b] H. Ep. #3 tumor inhibitions of less than 25% are considered negative.

[c] Results of two or more tests were pooled.

[d] Prepared in saline.

centrations such that one-half of the dose was injected subcutaneously in 0.1 ml. twice daily (except Sunday). Therapy was started 24 hours post transplantation and continued for 9 days for H.S.#1 and 7–8 days for H.Ep.#3. Test animals were sacrificed on the eleventh to twelfth day for H.S.#1 and ninth to eleventh day for H.E.p.#3 tumors, 24–48 hours after the last injection had been given. The tumors were excised, opened, and the debris removed before weighing. Only those tumors weighing 0.3 gm. or more were considered takes.

All instruments, glassware, and solutions were sterilized, and aseptic conditions were maintained throughout by the use of glass-enclosed chambers.

Purina Lab Chow, supplemented with rolled oats and sunflower seeds, and water were fed ad libitum. The animal room was maintained at approximately 74° F.

## 2. Results

The effects of the compounds on the subcutaneous growth of H.S.#1 and H.Ep.#3 are given in Tables XI and XII, respectively. Most of the results reported here are of single tests and are thus preliminary in nature. Included in the compounds tested against one or both tumors are one estrogen, two progestogens, and seven androgens. None of these at the doses used had any effect against H.S.#1, and only one, 1-dehydrotestololactone, had a small effect against H.Ep.#3. None of the compounds was toxic at the levels used, as measured by host weight change and mortality.

## 3. Summary and Conclusions

An initial, preliminary study was made of the effects of several steroids and steroidlike compounds on the subcutaneous growth of human tumors H.S.#1 and H.Ep.#3 in the rat. None of these compounds affected H.S.#1, and only one, 1-dehydrotestololactone, had a small effect against H.Ep.#3. Most of the compounds tested were androgens or androgenlike, and were necessarily representative of the class. Only further testing with representative compounds in the androgen, estrogen, progestogen, and corticoid classes can determine whether these tumors are responsive to such classes of compounds. This work is under way.

## VI.  DISCUSSION

It has been observed that experimental human tumors will yield anticancer evaluations for each of the four main biological types of steroids: androgens, estrogens, progestogens, and corticoids. The tumors A-42 and H.S.#1 appear to be modified in growth by all classes when grown in the egg even though the tumors are normally not considered to be hormone dependent. The intramuscularly grown H.Ep.#3 in the mouse appears to be sensitive only to certain $C_{21}$ steroids. Evidence has been presented that hamster-grown tumors may be unique and useful objects for evaluations with several classes of steroids. It is of interest that in the studies thus far a number of the materials affect H.S.#1 in the hamster and a few, only H.Ep.#3. These differences may be utilized in further studies. Subcutaneously grown tumors in the rat should be explored more extensively. In general, it may be interpreted that within the systems discussed changes of hormonal balance modified the tumor metabolism sufficiently so that one may evaluate the anticancer potential of endocrine materials. Human tumors as studied appear to be more versatile in their steroid anticancer evaluation qualities than a number of the animal tumors thus far employed (25).

The present studies may have special pertinence since human tumor tissue has been employed. Certainly the tissues are closely related to the species of origin—the clinical cancer patient. The observed differences following change of host and change of tumor can be exploited and be employed toward an understanding of the mechanisms involved.

## VII. SUMMARY

Methods have been developed for chemotherapy evaluations against the human tumors H.S.#1, H.Ep.#3, A-42, and H.Ad.#1. Insofar as the techniques are developed, tests may be conducted when the tumors are grown in the egg, rat, mouse, and hamster. Differences have been demonstrated in the ability of several steroid and hormonelike materials to inhibit the growth of these tumors under the experimental test techniques developed. Differences have also been observed when a given tumor has a change of host, i.e., both tumor type and tumor host background are of influence in the chemotherapeutic evaluations obtained.

### REFERENCES

1. Armaghan, V., and Bergstresser, D. *Proc. Am. Assoc. Cancer Research* **2**, 92 (1956).
2. Chute, R. N., Sommers, S. C., and Warren, S. *Cancer Research* **12**, 912 (1952).
3. Dagg, C. P., Karnofsky, D. A., Toolan, H. W., and Roddy, J. *Proc. Soc. Exptl. Biol. Med.* **87**, 223 (1954).
4. Dagg, C. P., Karnofsky, D. A., Stock, C. C., Lacon, C. R., and Roddy, J. *Proc. Soc. Exptl. Biol. Med.* **90**, 489 (1955).
5. Dunning, W. F. *Ann. N. Y. Acad. Sci.* **76**, 696 (1958).
6. Ellison, R. R. "The Medical Clinics of North America," p. 748. Saunders, Philadelphia, Pennsylvania. 1956.
7. Handler, A. H., Adams, R. A., and Farber, S. *Proc. Am. Assoc. Cancer Research* **2**, 210 (1957).
8. Harris, J. J. *Cancer* **9**, 756 (1956).
9. Harris, J. J. *Proc. Am. Assoc. Cancer Research* **2**(3), 211 (1956).
10. Harris, J. J. *Ann. N. Y. Acad. Sci.* **76**, 409 (1958).
11. Harris, J. J. *Proc. Am. Assoc. Cancer Research* **3**, 26 (1959).
12. Harris, J. J., and Woolley, G. W. *Ann. N. Y. Acad. Sci.* **76**, 729 (1958).
13. Hill, J. M., Marshall, G. J., and Falco, D. J. *J. Am. Geriat. Soc.* **4**, 627 (1956).
14. Hyman, C. B., and Sturgen, P. *Cancer* **9**, 965 (1956).
15. Lemon, H. M., Lutz, B. R., Pope, R., Parson, L., Handler, A. H., and Patt, D. I. *Science* **115**, 461 (1952).
16. Marsh, W. S., and Cullen, M. R. *Ann. N. Y. Acad. Sci.* **76**, 752 (1958).
17. Merker, P. C., and Woolley, G. W. *Cancer Research* **19**, 664 (1959).
18. Merker, P. C., Teller, M. N., Palm, J. E., and Woolley, G. W. *Antibiotics & Chemotherapy* **7**, 247 (1957).
19. Murphy, J. B. *J. Am. Med. Assoc.* **59**, 874 (1912).
20. Nandi, J., and Bern, H. A. *Cancer Research* **18**, 790 (1958).
21. Noble, R. L. *In* "The Hormones" (G. Pincus and K. V. Thimann, eds.), Vol. 3, p. 750. Academic Press, New York, 1955.

22. Patterson, W. B., Chute, R. N., and Sommers, S. C. *Cancer Research* **14**, 656 (1954).
23. Schrek, R., and Avery, R. C. *Am. J. Pathol.* **13**, 45 (1937).
24. Stevenson, H. N. *J. Cancer Research* **3**, 63 (1918).
25. Stock, C. C., and Sugiura, K. *Ann. N. Y. Acad. Sci.* **76**, 720 (1958).
26. Teller, M. N., Merker, P. C., Palm, J. E., and Woolley, G. W. *Ann. N. Y. Acad. Sci.* **76**, 742 (1958).
27. Teller, M. N., Palm, J. E., Merker, P. C., Harris, J. J., and Woolley, G. W. *Cancer Research* **18**, 522 (1958).
28. Teller, M. N., Palm, J. E., Merker, P. C., Harris, J. J., and Woolley, G. W. *Antibiotics Ann.* p. 518 (1959).
29. Toolan, H. W. *Cancer Research* **14**, 660 (1954).
30. Unpublished data. Division of Human Tumor Experimental Chemotherapy, Sloan-Kettering Institute.

### DISCUSSION

**G. Pincus:** Were any of these explants taken from patients who were actually treated with steroids?

**G. Woolley:** I have no knowledge concerning previous treatment, hormonal or otherwise, of the donor patients.

**K. B. Olson:** The patient from which A-42 came was not treated with cortisol or any of the estrogens. This was a tumor isolated from a patient who died about a month after excision of a lung cancer by Dr. John Skitt. It is being continuously grown at Albany Medical College.

I would like to add that we have an interest in the subject of steroid treatment of lung cancer. About two years ago we treated a small number of patients with estrogens and with androgens. At that time Dr. Kennedy very kindly gave me some data which he had from the Massachusetts General Hospital on castration and lung cancer, which I believe were entirely negative. We could not show any benefit to the patients. This was a small number of cases. Since then we have treated perhaps 15 or 20 cases of lung cancer with cortisone and prednisone. We have seen no beneficial effects. I should say that with cortisone over a short period of time some patients do get a little euphoria, but we saw no real tumor regression.

**H. M. Lemon:** In the Boston area we are quite troubled with the irregular growth of the transplants in the hamster's cheek pouch. I would like to ask Dr. Woolley whether he has had that problem too. Secondly, I would like to inquire what he has found on histological examination of the regressed transplants?

**G. Woolley:** As far as the tumors in the hamsters are concerned, we had the unfortunate experience of losing Dr. Joy E. Palm who had been working with these tumors and thus we have not been able to complete our studies concerning variability of growth up to this time. Dr. Merker might like to discuss variability of tumor growth in the mouse where work has progressed further than in the hamster.

**P. C. Merker:** With cooperation of Mr. Mantel, Head of the Experimental Statistics Section at the National Cancer Institute, analysis of tumor weights has revealed that the assay system is essentially stable. A recent compilation of data collected over a one-year period, revealed that the average tumor weight of three tumors is 2.3 gm. and, except for four instances in approximately 100 groups, average tumor weights ranged from 1.5 to 3.8 gm. Because of this stability, routine testing has been with as few as three tumor-bearing mice and a similar number of control animals. With such small groups, and employing repeated assays, it has been found that results obtained for test compounds have been relatively consistent.

**E. Schwenk:** I can confirm the observation made by Dr. Lemon about the variable growth rates of transplants of the hamster cheek pouch tumors. We usually take the tumor and transfer it into the cheek pouch of 12 hamsters. The first tumor that we used was the original as obtained by Professor Lutz and his co-workers in Boston when they developed the cheek pouch method in hamsters, supplied by him to us. This was a methylcholanthrene-induced sarcoma of the thigh and showed in our experiments quite variable rates of growth when it was measured at the fourth, seventh, and eleventh days after the transplant into the cheek pouch. In the last half year we were fortunate to get from Dr. Fortner of the Sloan-Kettering Institute, an adenosarcoma of the hamster which grows very much better than the first tumor and much faster to quite a large size in the cheek pouch and which also shows a more uniform rate of growth. We have shown that the cheek pouch technique can be successfully used in testing of compounds for tumorostatic properties [Stevens, D. F., and Schwenk, E., *Naturwissenschaften* **45**, 218 (1958)].

**G. Woolley:** We do practice two or three things that may help cut down variability. One is to wait until the tumor gets to be 5 days of age; at this time a uniform group is selected and then randomized between test and control groups. We have also learned that certain tumors can be transplanted most successfully by trocar as a mince and by means of a syringe and needle. This may also be of aid in reducing the amount of tumor growth variability.

**R. W. Talley:** I noticed that there seemed to be a difference in the response of various tumors in different species. Do you have any correlation at all between a specific tumor and the type of steroid to which it might have responded? Did the H.S.#1 respond better to corticoids in all species or was there any correlation?

**G. Woolley:** We have insufficient data to answer this question.

**R. W. Talley:** Would you think that these steroids, then, are affecting the host system more than the tumor itself?

**G. Woolley:** In some instances, as shown in the tables presented, the embryo was modified more than the tumor. In other instances the tumor was modified more than the embryo.

**J. J. Harris:** As I understand the question, it concerns the agreement in response of a given human tumor, grown in the several types of hosts, to a particular type of steroid. In other words, whether the response of a given tumor to a particular type of steroid depends upon the kind of host in which it is grown.

I think Dr. Woolley has already stated that we do not have at present the four types of human tumors growing in the four types of hosts. We are currently working toward that goal. Any attempt to make comparisons among the systems of their response to steroids before the denominators of tumors and test agents are common to all hosts would be premature.

**P. C. Merker:** I have also had the opportunity to study the effect of steroids on intramuscular transplants of H.Ep.#3 growing in the X-irradiated and cortisone-treated rat. When test data from the rat and mouse intramuscular H.Ep.#3 systems were compared, no essential significant differences were found. The $C_{18}$ and $C_{19}$ steroids were generally inactive, whereas the $C_{21}$ corticoids were toxic and active tumor inhibitory agents.

**H. M. Lemon:** May I ask whether anybody has a human breast or prostate adenomacarcinoma which is serially passing in the experimental animal? Perhaps the lack of obtaining at least many strains of these tumors indicates something about the necessity of endogenous steroids for support of growth of the tumors.

**G. Woolley:** I would like to say that I don't believe this problem is completely hopeless. We are searching and have found an alternate method of conditioning which eliminates the necessity of cortisone. This involves the use of Zymosan. Tumor growth, although excellent, is variable. Conditioning of this sort would be of possible aid in securing new tumor types for study.

**P. C. Merker:** Another fascinating area in this heterologous transplantation field, has been the use of newborn mice as hosts for the H.Ep.#3 tumor. It grows exceedingly well for at least 12–14 days before regressing, when transplanted into newborn mice less than 24 hours old. We hope to explore this system in terms of experimental chemotherapy, and since X-ray and cortisone are not required, it will be interesting eventually to correlate test results with data from the egg-H.Ep.#3 system.

**M. Shear:** The work of Rubin in Texas may provide another approach for those who are casting about for alternative procedures to affect the host. Rubin, among other aspects of his work, transplanted the Gardner lymphosarcoma of C3H mice into C3H mice and, as expected, found that it took in 100% of the cases and grew progressively with resultant death of all the mice. In DBA/2 mice this tumor took in some of the cases and then regressed after about 10 days. On the other hand, when he first painted the skin of the DBA mice with methylcholanthrene for brief periods, then the out-of-strain tumor took in 100% of the cases, grew at the same rate as it did in its own strain, and killed all the mice. Treatment with methylcholanthrene indeed is a simple method. However, even though the manipulative procedure is simple, it may well involve a whole series of extraordinarily complex phenomena.

**G. Woolley:** I certainly appreciate your suggestion, Dr. Shear, and I hope we have more of them.

**P. C. Merker:** We have attempted to grow H.Ep.#3 in C3H mice bearing methylcholanthrene-induced subcutaneous tumors and have not been successful.

Since I mentioned the induced methylcholanthrene tumor, I would like to add that the $C_{21}$ corticoids discussed by Dr. Woolley had no remarkable inhibiting effect on the growth of established induced tumors or on the survival of mice bearing the induced tumor.

**H. Brendler:** Although I have had no immediate experience working with human prostatic cancer transplants, I have had some information which may be of help to Dr. Lemon. During the course of our own work with a mouse prostatic cancer originally induced by Dr. W. E. Smith in Dr. Peyton Rous' laboratory, I recall some work done at the Memorial Center by Joseph Patti, using 24-hour-old mice. This work was reported by him in *Cancer Research* in two articles, as well as I can recollect.

**R. Hilf:** In one of the slides it appeared as though there were a few instances in which the treated animals had larger tumors than the controls. Was this just an artifact or did you possibly pursue this further to see if this was a real hormonal stimulation?

**G. Woolley:** I believe that this could be looked upon as variation well within the standard deviation.

**J. H. Leathem:** Dr. Woolley, do you see any relationship between the response of the host animal in terms of species sensitivity to steroids and the tumor response? In our experience, if one gives androgen the order of response would be rat, mouse, hamster. The hamster is the least responsive. Secondly, is there any correlation between corticoid effects on tumors and corticoid effects on liver glycogen deposition? Species differences may influence glycogen responses to corticoids and to tumors.

**G. Woolley:** This type of information is of real interest to us.

# Steroid-Induced Tumors in Animals

## O. MÜHLBOCK

*The Netherlands Cancer Institute, Amsterdam, The Netherlands*

Although the main object of this meeting is to consider the biological aspects of steroids in relation to cancer chemotherapy, it seems useful to deal also with the activity of steroids in relation to the genesis of cancer. First, further insight may be gained by the study of the carcinogenic action of certain steroids, which may be helpful in the elucidation of the effects on tumor growth. Secondly, prophylactic measures as a form of cancer therapy could be feasible, if the hormonal induction mechanism can be recognized. Thirdly, the carcinogenic action of certain steroids used in cancer therapy should be taken into account in certain cases. A review of the steroids with regard to their carcinogenic action reveals the surprising fact that as yet the only steroids by which tumors could be induced in animals are the estrogenic hormones. A carcinogen is hereby defined as a compound which, when appropriately applied to animals, gives rise to the appearance of cancers that would not have appeared otherwise.

The term estrogen, however, is not limited to steroid compounds, but broadly refers to all substances to which the animals respond in at least one common manner—vaginal epithelial proliferation and cornification. That would mean that a substance which causes this specific biological effect can be expected to be carcinogenic irrespective of the chemical structure.

Other steroid hormones to be considered as possible carcinogens are progesterone and testosterone. There is no convincing evidence that progesterone itself can cause cancer in animals, whereas it has been repeatedly shown that it can augment the effect of other carcinogens significantly. The same applies to testosterone or other androgenic steroids.

A survey of the tumors induced by estrogens is given in Table I. From this table it appears that the estrogens are potent carcinogens. Tumors have

TABLE I

TUMORS INDUCED BY ESTROGENS

| Site | Animal |
| --- | --- |
| Hypophysis | Mice, rats, hamsters |
| Testis | Mice |
| Mammary gland | Mice, rats |
| Uterus | Mice, rabbits, guinea pigs |
| Kidney | Hamsters |
| Epididymis | Hamsters |
| Bone | Mice |
| Lymphoid tissue | Mice |

331

been induced in a great variety of tissues and organs. For details see the review (1, 3, 5, 8, 11, 12, 14). The experiments have been done mostly with small rodents such as mice, rats, and hamsters.

The carcinogenic action of hormones and the mechanism involved have long been a matter for speculation and have repeatedly been discussed. For this review only a direct carcinogenic action of steroids shall be considered. Direct action means stimulation or inhibition of a target organ without intermediary steps. Indirect action would mean that, for example, an alteration of the endocrine balance could be caused by the steroids which then gives rise to the development of tumors. This is thought to be the case in the genesis of testicular tumors. Interstitial cell tumors can be induced by estrogens in certain inbred strains of mice. The probable effect of the estrogens is to stimulate secretion of interstitial cell stimulating hormone by the pituitary gland. This in its turn then induces the interstitial cell tumor.

In other cases it cannot yet be said whether estrogens have a direct or indirect carcinogenic effect, because we do not know anything about the mechanism. This is the case in lymphoid neoplasia, which in certain inbred strains of mice may be induced by administration of estrogens. Estrogens may be independently leukemogenic, but also they may augment other causative factors.

The most convincing direct carcinogenic effect of estrogens is the induction of cancer in the uterine cervix and vagina in mice. Gardner (6) has shown that the number of these cancers is larger and the induction time much shorter when estrogen is applied directly to these tissues. Large doses of estrogens given systematically had a much less carcinogenic effect.

Since the original experiment of Lacassagne (7), numerous experiments have been made on the influence of estrogenic hormones on the development of mammary tumors in mice. It may be stated, in general, that the administration of estrogens is followed by the occurrence of mammary cancer in gonadectomized mice of suitable strains when the mammary tumor agent, the Bittner factor, is present. Mice not carrying this factor, with only a few exceptions, develop no mammary tumors after treatment with estrogens. A complex hormonal mechanism is involved in the development of mammary cancer, but certainly estrogens can be considered as causative factors in the induction of these cancers.

The great experience with these mammary tumors and the relative ease with which they can be induced make it possible to design experiments to study the mechanism of this hormonal carcinogenesis. Our knowledge in this field is still minimal, but some points already have been definitely clarified.

Generally it may be stated that the carcinogenic effect of a hormone is related to the amount of the hormone acting on its target organ. An example may serve to illustrate this dose-response relationship. When a dose of estrogenic hormone which may represent the physiological level is given to agent-free C3H$_f$ mice, the animals have only a very few mammary tumors and only very late in life (Fig. 1). However, with a dose sixteen times higher nearly all animals develop mammary tumors very early in life (2). This clearly shows that the frequency of the tumors is dependent on the dose of hormones.

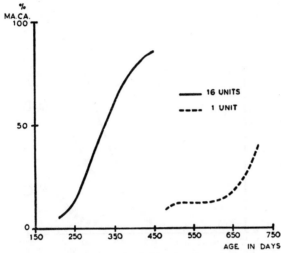

Fig. 1.  Mammary cancer frequency in C3H$_f$ mice dependent on the estrogen dosage.

In discussing the mechanism of steroid carcinogenesis, it has to be emphasized that a tumor will develop only if the organs are under continuous influence of the hormone. To prove this point, experiments were designed in which the total amount of the hormone administered in a given time was the same with continuous and with discontinuous treatment (13).

Three groups of castrated male mice were treated (Fig. 2). Group A: Estrone (100 µg. in 100 ml. in drinking water) was given continuously; 96 % of the mice developed mammary cancer. Group B: The double dose of estrone in drinking water was given, but the duration of the treatment was 2 months, then a pause of 2 months without estrone, again treatment for 2 months, and so on. The mammary tumor incidence in this group was 58 %. Group C: This group was treated with double the amount of estrone for 5 days, then left untreated for 5 days, and then treated again for 5 days with the double dose. The mammary tumor incidence was only 16 %.

These experiments show that only in the group with continuous treatment was there a high incidence of mammary cancer at an early age. The incidence was negligible in the group with intermittent treatment with pauses of 5 days, although at a given time the total hormone dose administered was the same in groups A and C. Apparently in group B, with a treatment of 2 months' duration there are already some changes toward malignancy in the cells, which by a renewal of the treatment lead to mammary cancer in a higher percentage.

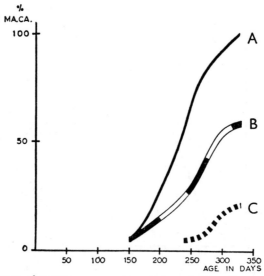

Fig. 2. Frequency of mammary cancer in castrate male mice after estrogen treatment: A, continuous treatment; B, discontinuous treatment, 2 months' interval; C, discontinuous treatment, 5 days' interval.

The same experiments have been done with the induction of tumors in the hypophysis after treatment with estrogenic hormones. After continuous treatment with estrone (100 µg. per 100 ml.) given in drinking water a tumor in the hypophysis was found after some time in 85 % of the animals. However, when the animals were treated with the double amount of estrone for 5 days, left untreated for 5 days, and then treated again for 5 days with the high dose of estrone, and so on, then only in 5 % of the animals was a tumor, usually small, observed, in spite of the fact that the total amount of estrone given was the same in both groups.

These results are of importance for the explanation of the mechanism of the hormonal carcinogenesis. Experiments with chemical carcinogenic substances, especially with certain remotely acting carcinogens, such as butter yellow or urethane, have shown that under certain circumstances a single dose is sufficient for the carcinogenic effect, although the carcinogenic substance is destroyed or excreted in a short time. Further conclusions are that the carcinogenic effect of butter yellow is irreversible and that a subthreshold dose does not exist (4). As the experiments with the steroid induction of mammary cancer show, all this is not necessarily the case in this type of carcinogenesis. It is not possible to induce cancer with one single large dose of hormone; neither is the tumor-inciting effect of hormone irreversible before tumor formation actually occurs. The conclusion must be that other mechanisms are instrumental in the hormonal induction of cancer, as compared with the so-called chemical carcinogenesis. A further conclusion is that no experimental evidence has been found for the often discussed assumption that estrogens are converted in the organism into true carcinogenic substances.

Although there is yet no direct evidence, it seems probable that estrogens themselves incite the neoplastic deviation in a cell or group of cells. It is evident that this can happen only if a growth-promoting effect by estrogens in the target organ is found. A long latency period is usually observed. It is likewise evident from our experimental experience that genetic and environmental factors play an important part in the genesis of the steroid-induced tumors.

The administration of estrogens to the animals is, of course, a highly artificial procedure. The question therefore arises if in the genesis of the spontaneous tumors the same principles are valid.

It is an old and well-confirmed observation that pregnancy promotes the development of mammary cancer in mice. It had therefore to be investigated if here too the number of pregnancies and the continuous or discontinuous state of pregnancy is of influence on the mammary tumor incidence.

TABLE II

MAMMARY TUMOR INCIDENCE IN FORCE-BRED DBA FEMALES

| Group | Number of animals | Mammary cancer (%) | Average tumor age (days) | Average age at death without tumors (days) |
|---|---|---|---|---|
| A (2 pregnancies) | 48 | 62 | 477 | 586 |
| B (7 pregnancies) | 69 | 97 | 382 | 533 |

The incidence of mammary tumors increases with the number of pregnancies. As an example of the investigations in our laboratory, only the results with the DBA strain (10) are given (Table II). Females of this strain with two pregnancies and with the litters discarded had a mammary tumor incidence of 62 % at an average age of 477 days, whereas females with seven litters, and with the litters discarded, had an incidence of 97 % at an average age of 382 days.

In this experiment as in others, the pregnancies followed in rapid succession. The next question then was, what is the influence of pregnancy on the tumor incidence when there are pauses between the pregnancies. In the experiments with estrogenic hormones the intermittent treatment resulted in a much lower incidence of mammary tumors than in those with continuous treatment.

TABLE III

THE INCIDENCE OF MAMMARY TUMORS IN MICE AFTER PREGNANCIES IN RAPID SUCCESSION (A) AND WITH PAUSES BETWEEN THE PREGNANCIES (B)

| Hybrid | Group | Number of animals | Tumor incidence (%) | Average tumor age (days) |
|---|---|---|---|---|
| $F_1$ (female WLL × male 020) | A | 35 | 87 | 321 |
| with mammary | B | 65 | 71 | 512 |
| tumor agent | | | | |
| $F_1$ (female C3H$_e$ × male CBA) | A | 41 | 54 | 537 |
| without mammary | B | 41 | 27 | 555 |
| tumor agent | | | | |

In Table III the incidence of mammary tumors in mice is compared after pregnancies in rapid succession and with pauses of 1–2 months between the pregnancies. Two $F_1$ hybrids were used, one with the mammary tumor agent (female WLL × male 020) and one without the agent (female C3H$_e$ × male CBA). In both experiments the number of pregnancies in the groups compared was the same and the young were discarded as soon as possible after birth. In both experiments the mammary tumor incidence was lower, and the average tumor age higher, in the group with pauses between the pregnancies.

The conclusion can be drawn that a continuous hormonal stimulation during pregnancy has a greater carcinogenic effect than a quantitatively equal but discontinuous stimulation. In this type of experiment one factor has to be taken into account in the evaluation of the results: the age of the animal when the hormonal stimulation takes place. In an experiment with six pregnancies in rapid succession, the hormonal stimulus ends after 6 months whereas in the experiment with a pause of 1 month between the pregnancies the hormonal stimulus ends only after 12 months. In the latter group the hormonal stimulus therefore acts on an older animal. Further experiments have to be done to prove whether this factor has an influence on the mammary tumor incidence.

How can we explain the genesis of spontaneous endocrine cancer on the basis of these facts? The carcinogenic effect of a hormone may be caused by the action of an increased amount of the hormone on the target organ as the consequence of increased production and secretion. Usually, however, we cannot find in the history of patients or in animals any signs of increased amounts of hormones. The hormonal balance seems normal.

That brings the possibility to the foreground that the susceptibility of the target organ to hormones may play a decisive part. That this possibility exists is illustrated in experiments with mice. The minimal effective dose of estrogenic hormone that causes vaginal estrus in an ovariectomized mouse is different in various inbred strains; e. g., if the minimal effective hormone dose in the $C_{57}BL$ strain is taken as unity, then this dose in the DBA strain is seven times higher (9). On the grounds of other observations also, it may be concluded that the ovaries of the mice of the DBA strain produce more estrogenic hormones than those in the $C_{57}BL$ strain. A normal estrous cycle is found in both strains. The higher production of estrogenic hormones is compensated by a lesser susceptibility of the vaginal epithelium—a normal cycle in the vagina occurs. But if we compare the susceptibility of the mammary gland in these two strains for estrogenic hormones, then it appears that both are equal in sensitivity. That would mean that throughout the life of the animal of the DBA strain, the mammary gland is under a stronger hormonal influence. It is conceivable that this stronger hormonal influence is instrumental in the development of mammary cancer in this strain. It may be that this principle plays a major role in the genesis of hormonal cancers.

TABLE IV

EFFECT OF PROGESTERONE AND TESTOSTERONE ON THE CARCINOGENIC ACTION OF ESTROGENS

| Tumors induced by estrogens | Effect on carcinogenic action | |
|---|---|---|
| | Progesterone | Testosterone |
| Hypophysis | Synergist | Antagonist |
| Testis | Antagonist | Antagonist |
| Uterus | Antagonist | Antagonist |
| Mammary gland | Synergist | Antagonist |
| Kidney | Synergist | Synergist |
| Lymphoid tissue | Antagonist | Antagonist |

As stated in the beginning, estrogens are the only steroid hormones that have so far proved to be carcinogenic. It is especially noteworthy that neither progesterone nor testosterone has any direct carcinogenic action. Nevertheless, they can profoundly alter the carcinogenic action of estrogens either acting as synergist or as antagonist. In Table IV experience in this field is summarized. The action of progesterone is synergistic in some cases and antagonistic in others. Testosterone in most cases has an antagonistic effect. The mechanism of the synergistic or antagonistic effects has to be studied in each case separately. In this respect much work still has to be done. There is no doubt that a further insight will help considerably in the elucidation of the carcinogenic effect of estrogens.

The corticosteroids have not been dealt with in this report. Whereas an influence of these steroids on the tumors has been found in many cases, the study on the influence in the genesis of the various tumors has given contradictory results.

REFERENCES

1. Bielschowsky, F., and Horning, E. S. *Brit. Med. Bull.* **14**, 106 (1958).
2. Boot, L. M., and Mühlbock, O. *Acta Unio Intern. Contra Cancrum* **12**, 569 (1956).
3. Burrows, H., and Horning, E. S. "Oestrogens and Neoplasia." Blackwell, Oxford, England, 1952.
4. Druckrey, H. *Oncologia* **7**, 155 (1954).
5. Gardner, W. U. *In* "Canadian Cancer Conference" (R. W. Begg, ed.), Vol. 2, p. 207. Academic Press, New York, 1957.
6. Gardner, W. U. *Cancer Research* **19**, 170 (1959).
7. Lacassagne, A. *Compt. rend. soc. biol.* **195**, 630 (1932).
8. Lipschütz, A. "Steroid Hormones and Tumors." Williams & Wilkins, Baltimore, Maryland, 1950.
9. Mühlbock, O. *Acta Brevia Neerl. Physiol. Pharmacol. Microbiol.* **16**, 22 (1948).
10. Mühlbock, O. *J. Natl. Cancer Inst.* **10**, 1259 (1950).
11. Mühlbock, O. *Advances in Cancer Research* **4**, 371 (1956).
12. Mühlbock, O. *Acta Unio Intern. Contra Cancrum* **15**, 62 (1959).
13. Mühlbock, O., and Boot, L. M. *Ciba Foundation Symposium on Carcinogenesis* p. 83 (1959).
14. Symposium of the American Cancer Society. *Cancer Research* **17**, 421 (1957).

## DISCUSSION

**U. Kim:** It is very interesting to note the reference made by Dr. Mühlbock to the possible relationship between the incidence of mammary tumors and the frequency of pregnancies in a certain strain of mice. Dr. Farquhar studied our mammosomatotropic pituitary tumor under the electron microscope and found that the size of cytoplasmic granules in tumor cells is the same as that of granules in the pituitary cells of lactating rats. We also observed in aging female breeding rats a high incidence of spontaneous, so-called chromophobe adenomas of pituitary that secreted mammosomatotropic hormone(s). This seems to us to indicate that repeated estrus, pregnancy, and lactation are conducive to the occurrence of tumors derived from these pituitary cells. These spontaneous pituitary tumors are essentially similar in function and morphology to those induced by chronic administration of estrogens.

**F. J. Agate, Jr.:** On the question of tumor induction by testosterone, I believe that malignant and metastasizing tumors of the hamster flank organ have been induced with testosterone by Kirkman[1] at Stanford, and I think by other people.

[1] Dr. Kirkman writes: "The benign, definitive flank organ tumor is induced by neither estrogen nor androgen alone, but by stilbestrol and testosterone propionate administered simultaneously. The respective role of each agent is yet to be clarified."

**O. Mühlbock:** I know that Dr. Kirkman has reported that testosterone may be carcinogenic in the hamster. According to a personal communication that action has to be investigated further.

**A. White:** I have two questions. One relates to the important concept that a continuous supply of estrogen must be present for the induction of tumors, in contrast to the single injection which has been described for some of the carcinogenic hydro-carbons. In view of your experiment in which you have provided the animals with an intermittent supply of estrogen at 5-day intervals, I wonder whether you have data on similar studies in which the period between injections is somewhat longer? I raise the question because of the experiments of Gardner, Dougherty, and Williams in which they showed that the induction of lymphatic leukemia in the CBA mouse as a result of a subcutaneously placed pellet of estrogen is related to a critical time during which the estrogen must be present in the animal. It was possible to demonstrate that if the estrogen pellet was withdrawn from the host at any time prior to 9 weeks following its implantation, the leukemia incidence was greatly reduced, or indeed was not likely to be significant as compared to the controls. However the 9-week period seemed to be a critical one in that the withdrawal of the pellet at any time after 9 weeks did lead subsequently to an incidence of leukemia as great as that seen in a similar group of animals in which the pellet remained continuously in place. The induction period was not altered and the incidence of leukemia was not altered. Thus, although for a period from 9 weeks of age to something considerably over a year estrogen was not present in the host, lymphatic leukemia did eventually appear. These experiments are intriguing in that they suggest that a specific period exists during which critical alterations are occurring. It might be possible to do certain metabolic studies with the view of studying fundamental biochemical changes that may occur at this critical period.

The other question relates to something which I may have inferred, and that was in the comparison of the relative amounts of estrogen required to produce stimulation of the vaginal epithelium in the mice of various strains. Did I understand you to intimate that in those strains in which a higher dose of estrogen was required experimentally, these animals must therefore be producing significantly more estrogen endogenously? Or could it be, in the absence of direct measurement, that all animals are producing, let us say, approximately the same levels of estrogen, but in the presence of a more responsive end organ, this particular strain of animal would then have a continuing excessive supply of estrogen which could lead to deleterious consequences? I was im-pressed by the fact that the CBA mouse, which is susceptible to the induction of lymphoma through estrogen treatment, had a low requirement for exogenous estrogen as measured by changes in the vaginal epithelium.

**O. Mühlbock:** With reference to your first question about longer intervals between treatments, maybe it is possible to show the slide (Fig. 2) again. In this experiment we gave estrone for 2 months and then paused for 2 months and again treated for 2 months with double the dose of estrone, and so on, so that at the end the same amount of hormone had been administered. The mammary tumor incidence is between those of both other groups; apparently there are some changes in the cells after treatment of long duration which gives a higher effect if the hormone is given again. I think you raised a very important question, which we hope to answer through experiments now under way.

With regard to your second question: we could show that in fact the ovaries of the DBA-strain produce more estrogens. We have done this by using the mammary tumor incidence as indicator. If you make $F_1$ hybrids between the DBA and C57 Black strains and transplant into them ovaries of the DBA strain or of the C57 Black strain, the mammary tumor incidence is much higher in the animals carrying DBA ovaries. I think that is a good argument for assuming that the production is higher. Elisabeth Fekete has come to the same conclusion after morphological investigations.

**G. W. Woolley:** I should like to call attention to evidence for the carcinogenic action of cortisone. In the study, cortisone acetate was administered to two strains of animals, C58 and AKR, and also to a group of hybrids between these two strains, at the level of 1 mg. per day for 3 successive days once each month throughout life. Some of each group of both males and females eventually presented an unexpected type of tumor for these strains—a parotid gland tumor. It was necessary in this case to administer the hormone periodically in order to minimize related infections. This type of study was later extended to two sublines of strain C3H mice. Interestingly, individuals of one sublime came down with this type of tumor and the other failed to do so. Since the tumor is known to be associated with a cell-free viruslike agent it is possible that cortisone facilitated its activity. The subline of C3H without tumors after cortisone treatment is known from other studies to be resistant to infection with the virus. This phenomenon perhaps forms a parallelism with estrogen and the milk factor association in breast cancer in mice.

**J. T. Velardo:** Coming back to the slide (Fig. 2) that Dr. Mühlbock just reprojected, I should like to ask what would happen if you hypophysectomized the animals during the 2-month interval between periods of treatment with estrone.

**O. Mühlbock:** We have done some experiments with hypophysectomy in various stages of the development of mammary cancer. The effect of hypophysectomy depends on the stage of the development of a tumor. If you do the hypophysectomy after even a very small carcinoma has developed it has no effect. But if the development is still in the stage of a hyperplastic nodule, then these disappear and no mammary cancer will develop later on.

**A. Segaloff:** Dr. Mühlbock, since all these carcinogens are phenolic steroids, is there a correlation with the estrogenicity, or do simple phenols which are of low estrogenic activity also induce these tumors? In other words is it a hormonal effect or is it possibly a phenolic effect? As I recall, Dr. Gardner pointed out some time ago that in some strains the less estrogenic estrogens are more effective in tumorigenesis.

**O. Mühlbock:** I have not tried different types of estrogen. In our experience the carcinogenic effect was always parallel to the estrogenic effect. As far as I know the Gardner experiment is the only exception.

**K. B. Olson:** There appears to me to be quite a conflict between clinical cancer as we see it and cancer as described by Dr. Mühlbock in the mouse, in that all the epidemiological studies of which I am aware would indicate that the fewer pregnancies the more likely a woman is to have cancer of the breast and the more pregnancies, the less likely. This is from world-wide studies, by Dr. Bogen and others. It is in marked contrast with what Dr. Mühlbock said about mouse breast cancer. Furthermore, we have a vast human experience in administering estrogens without any evidence that this produces cancer. There probably is a different age distribution, but certainly many estrogens have been given at least to the older age group of both sexes. Dr. Gray Twombly reviewed this human experience about five years ago, and he was unable to find any proof that exogenous estrogens had ever produced breast cancer in humans. I think there are some breast cancers reported after estrogen therapy for prostatic cancer, but I think pathologists would consider these metastatic from the prostate to the breast. There is evidence that increase of endogenous estrogens at an earlier age may produce breast tumors. I would like to have Dr. Mühlbock comment on the relation of his findings to human breast cancer because this is a very important clinical subject to many of us.

**O. Mühlbock:** Dr. Olson raised a very important point, to which of course we have given much attention and thought. Certainly statistics on human cancer on a world-wide basis reveal that mammary cancer is more frequent in unmarried women than in married women. But recent statistics confirm an old observation, made forty years ago in Holland, that this is not so in women with mammary cancer before the age of 45. That is one point. The second point is that if we compare the genesis of mammary cancer in mice with that in human beings, we must take into account the different hormonal status, disregarding pregnancy. A mouse has an estrous cycle every 4 or 5 days; there is ovulation and formation of a corpus luteum, but this corpus luteum doesn't produce hormone. In human beings, however, the corpus luteum formed produces progesterone, and the basic hormonal changes of pregnancy occur in the second half of every menstrual cycle. In the genesis of mammary tumor we have to take into account another factor that is very important—lactation. It was shown by English statistics many years ago that lactation has a retarding effect. With regard to the induction of mammary cancer by hormonal treatment: hormonal treatment with estrogens starts late in life. Usually menopausal syndromes necessitate this hormonal treatment. We know from experiments in mice also that treatment with estrogenic hormones in older mice does not lead to the development of mammary cancer.

**W. F. Dunning:** In reference to Dr. White's remark about the continuous versus the discontinuous treatment in the induction of breast cancer, we tried many years ago to produce breast cancer in rats with diethylstilbestrol pellets and found that 5 mg. in a cholesterol pellet from which the material was absorbed continuously produced practically 100% breast cancer. But if we put in 5 mg. of compressed diethylstilbestrol and allowed it to be absorbed (this took about 3 months) and if we waited until the testicles descended in the males and then implanted another 5-mg. pellet, with rest periods in between, there were no breast cancers. This was so, even if we made five consecutive implantations, in which case the rats had 25 mg. of diethylstilbestrol compared to less than 5 mg. absorbed from the cholesterol pellet.

**R. Grinberg:** One interesting way of studying the mechanism of action of hormones is to use intrasplenic grafts. We mixed intrasplenic grafts of uterus and ovary, and also of mammary gland and ovary [*Rev. soc. arg. biol.* **27**, 271-275 (1951)]. In the case of the mammary gland we saw that even big ovarian tumors grafted into the spleen could not produce similar changes in the mammary gland. But when the ovary was grafted with the adrenal gland we saw small adenomas in the mammary gland. The mechanism of action of the hormones in the human beings has also been studied, and we reported that in the Sheehan syndrome we couldn't induce changes in the mammary gland even with very large doses of estradiol benzoate [*Rev. asoc. med. arg.* **72**, 245-248 (1958)].

**J. Lampkin-Hibbard:** Can the lymphoid tumors induced by estrogens in your studies be transplanted from one generation to another? P1798 lymphosarcoma in BALB/C mice was induced by a diethylstilbestrol pellet and has grown for many transfer generations. Some other lymphoid tumors were induced in the same way and would not grow in inbred BALB/C mice.

**O. Mühlbock:** I have not tried any transplantation experiments with lymphoid tumors.

**T. L. Dao:** In a study of methylcholanthrene-induced mammary cancer, we found that pregnancy greatly increased the incidence, and shortened the latent period, or tumor formation. These observations are similar to those of Dr. Mühlbock. However, we found also that if female rats became pseudopregnant by mating with sterile males, the results in tumor induction were similar to those of our pregnancy experiments. Now, as I recall, you have done some experiments on pituitary isograft in certain strains of mice, I believe the 020 strain, and in these mice with pituitary isografts the mammary tumor incidence was high. I would like to ask you to comment on the tumor production by pituitary isograft. Is it due to occurrence of pseudopregnancy as a result of pituitary graft like those of our experiments?

**O. Mühlbock:** If you transplant pituitary into rats in the same manner as we did into mice, then you should get the same effect—continuous pseudopregnancy.

**K. E. Paschkis:** I would like to take up again what Dr. White said about the "critical period." Dr. White quoted the old experiments of Gardner and his associates. This phenomenon of a critical period in cancer induction is not limited to the estrogens. Such a critical period of exposure to the carcinogen—somewhat independent of total dose—has also been studied in the carcinogenic action of 2-acetylaminofluorene (AAF); Wilson and DeEds found that rats developed cancer if they ingested this carcinogen for 25–30 days. In our laboratories a high incidence of various cancers is observed in rats fed AAF for 90 days and then returned to stock diet. At this time no malignant changes are seen grossly or histologically, but certain metabolic alterations are already detectable, for instance, the utilization of an alternate pathway in the synthesis of ribonucleic acid (incorporation of uracil).

**M. M. Mason:** I would like to stress the importance of this problem of dose and time from an entirely different point of view. Workers in toxicology are very interested in the carcinogenic activities of many foodstuffs and food additives. The Food and Drug Administration is now urging that two-year trials be made on many substances. If it can be proved conclusively that carcinogenesis is initiated and determined in a period of two or three months, this would be of great importance.

# V. HORMONES AND HUMAN CANCER

## Evaluation of Endocrine Ablative Surgery in the Treatment of Mammary Carcinoma: A Preliminary Study on Survival

SAMUEL G. TAYLOR, III, AND CHARLES P. PERLIA

*Department of Medical Oncology of Presbyterian-St. Luke's Hospital and the Department of Medicine, University of Illinois College of Medicine, Chicago, Illinois*

The relative value of various treatments for primary breast cancer has been clarified by the simple study of survival rates. So has the natural history of breast cancer. The effectiveness of endocrine therapy in disseminated cancer of the breast has been based mainly on criteria for tumor regression (2–4, 7, 11). Because of the inherent difficulty in interpreting the evidence of objective regression, especially in retrospective studies, it would be helpful if other measurements of the effects of these procedures were investigated. If that therapy does produce an effect on the tumor and/or tumor host relationship in breast cancer, this should be reflected in changes in the survival rate. We have, therefore, collected material on survival as a method of measuring the efficacy of ablative procedures in disseminated breast cancer.

Because of the marked variation in the course of the disease, it is necessary to study a relatively large series for such an analysis to be meaningful. A project is under way under the auspices of the American College of Surgeons and the American College of Physicians[1] for the evaluation of endocrine ablative surgery in metastatic breast cancer. The Joint Committee of these two organizations has kindly made available to us the material collected to date. The present paper is in the form of a very preliminary report, as it will include only a small portion of the material to be analyzed. The completed final report of this study may well invalidate some of the apparent trends which appear here and will include other facets not to be brought out in our study.

### METHOD AND MATERIAL

One of the authors, (C. P.), an investigator for the Joint Committee, made site visits to the institutions listed below and with their cooperation obtained data by careful analysis of the charts on each patient who had undergone ablative surgery. The institutions from which data have been obtained to date are:

---

[1] These studies are supported by grants from the National Cancer Institute, United States Public Health Service. (CS-9576).

Iowa University Hospital, Iowa City, Iowa
Albany Hospital, Albany, New York
Presbyterian—St. Luke's, and Research and Educational Hospitals, Chicago, Illinois
Barnes Hospital, St. Louis, Missouri
Roswell Park Memorial Hospital, Buffalo, New York
Memorial Hospital, New York, New York
National Institutes of Health, Bethesda, Maryland
Medical College of Virginia, Richmond
Peter Bent Brigham Hospital, Boston, Massachusetts
Massachusetts General Hospital, Boston
M. D. Anderson Hospital, Houston, Texas

As this presentation is limited to survival, only cases closed by death are included. This necessarily excludes from our series patients with extraordinarily long survival following therapy and does not include some recent cases operated early in the course of disseminated disease. Cases with incomplete data and those dying within 30 days of the ablative procedure (classed as operative death) were excluded, as were patients with only local recurrence. All patients in this series had had a mastectomy for their primary disease. No attempt at evaluating these patients, in relationship to clinical evidence of tumor regression, has been made in this particular study.

Over 1200 cases of disseminated carcinoma of the breast who have undergone endocrine ablative surgery for metastatic disease have been processed from the above institutions to date; 555 have met the above criteria for the present survival study (to be referred to as the EAP series). These include 193 cases who had oophorectomy alone, 157 who had hypophysectomy, and 205 who had adrenalectomy. Of the total series of hypophysectomy and adrenalectomy cases from which the figures for patients who died were taken, 18.6 % and 17.0 %, respectively, are still living. All but a very few had had an oophorectomy preceding or in conjunction with adrenalectomy or hypophysectomy. Many patients in the EAP series were also treated with radiation in conjunction with, preceding, or following the ablative procedure. A few were given various chemotherapeutic agents late in their disease. Many had sex hormones or corticosteroid therapy preceding ablative therapy or when the disease was in clinical progression following an ablative procedure, but no cases were accepted when additive and ablative therapy were combined.

## RESULTS

It has been frequently pointed out (3, 6, 9) that the survival of patients following an ablative procedure is conspicuously longer if clinical regression is manifest than if it is not. So it is reasonable to assume that if an ablative procedure produces tumor regression in about one-third of the cases, the survival of the entire series should be longer than if no ablative procedure had been performed. We have, therefore, compared the survival of the various EAP groups with published series of patients who had had mastectomy and then developed recurrent disease. It had been impossible to find any series in the literature identical with the present one, but the similarity of Shimkin's series (10) (374 cases) and the androgen-estrogen series of the American Medical Association (1) (492 cases) seem adequate for some

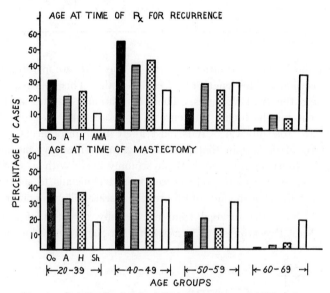

FIG. 1.   Age distribution in A.M.A., Shimkin, and EAP series.

comparisons. This has offered us an opportunity to compare a series completed before the general use of steroids for this disease and a series treated with sex steroids, with the EAP series.

Figure 1 shows the age distribution of the three series. For the A.M.A. series the age is given as the time of hormonal treatment of recurrence, whereas for Shimkin's series it is the age at mastectomy. For the EAP the age at both these times is available. This shows that the A.M.A. and Shimkin's series contain more patients in the older age group. Shimkin, however, found no appreciable difference in survival in his series in the different age groups. Therefore, this difference may not invalidate the comparisons to be presented.

The period between the primary treatment and the development of clinical evidence of disseminated disease, designated here as the "free interval," has been shown to influence survival (10) and is a rough measurement of the biological activity of the disease.

TABLE I
DISTRIBUTION OF CASES IN RELATION TO LENGTH OF FREE INTERVAL

| Group | < 24 Months[a] (%) | | > 24 Months (%) | |
|---|---|---|---|---|
| Shimkin | 58.8 | (217) | 42.0 | (157) |
| Oophorectomy | 69.0 | (113) | 31.0 | ( 60) |
| Adrenalectomy | 57.5 | (118) | 42.5 | ( 87) |
| Hypophysectomy | 59.8 | ( 94) | 40.2 | ( 63) |

[a] Figures in parentheses are the number of cases.

Table I shows the distribution of cases in the EAP groups and Shimkin's series in relation to the length of "free interval." This information is not available for the A.M.A. series. The distribution is quite similar in all groups except for the higher incidence of oophorectomy cases in the group having short "free interval." It is most likely that this reflects a more aggressive type of disease in that particular group. However, the lower percentage of adrenalectomy and hypophysectomy cases with a shorter "free interval" may be due to the reluctance of most clinicians to select patients for these procedures in the face of progressive disease following oophorectomy.

Figure 2 shows the survival from mastectomy to death of each group. The pooled ablative groups (555 cases) have a significantly longer survival

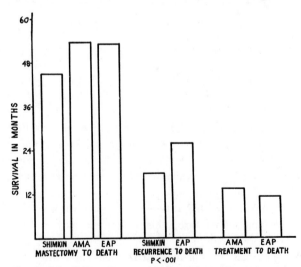

FIG. 2. Survival in EAP series compared with A.M.A. and Shimkin series

than Shimkin's series (374 cases), but there is no significant difference between the EAP and the A.M.A. series (492 cases).

Next the survival from recurrence to death of the ablative groups is compared with Shimkin's series. This information is not available in the A.M.A. series. Again, the survival of the former is significantly longer than in the untreated group ($P < 0.001$). There is no significant difference of survival from treatment when the pooled EAP is compared with the A.M.A. series.

The increased survival after recurrence in the EAP series compared with the untreated series of Shimkin is demonstrated in the survival curve in

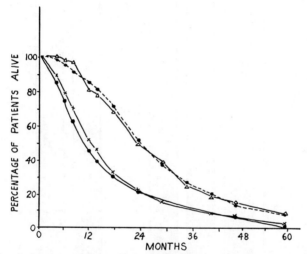

FIG. 3.  Survival after recurrence in EAP series compared with Shimkin series (●——●): adrenalectomy group, △——△; hypophysectomy group, ● - - - ●; oophorectomy group, X——X.

Fig. 3. More specifically it can be seen that the higher percentage of survival occurs in the adrenalectomy and hypophysectomy groups. The poorer showing of the oophorectomy group may partially be explained by the fact that this group includes a greater number of patients with a more aggressive tumor (a higher percentage with a short "free interval") and that many did not have further ablative surgery because their condition was rapidly deteriorating. The similarity of the adrenalectomy and hypophysectomy groups is obvious.

Figure 4 compares the survival of the three different types of ablative surgery from mastectomy, from recurrence, and from treatment, to death. It is apparent there is no difference between the adrenalectomy and hypophysectomy groups. It is also of interest that there is no significant difference between combined and sequential oophorectomy-adrenalectomy. There is, however, a significantly longer survival from mastectomy or recurrence to death for both the adrenalectomy and hypophysectomy groups as compared with the oophorectomy group ($P < 0.001$). Survival from treatment to death is similar for each type of surgery. It may be that the survival

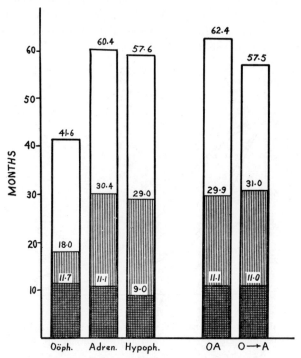

FIG. 4. Comparative survival of oophorectomized, adrenalectomized, and hypophysectomized groups from time of mastectomy (open bar), recurrence (vertical lines), and treatment (crosshatching) to death. OA = simultaneous oophorectomy-adrenalectomy; O→A = sequential oophorectomy-adrenalectomy.

from treatment to death in the oophorectomy group is lengthened by the fact that this ablative surgery was performed earlier in the course of disseminated disease.

That the survival from recurrence to death is greatly influenced by the biological activity of the tumor (8) is graphically demonstrated by Fig. 5. This shows that the survival from recurrence is directly related to the length of the "free interval." It also re-emphasizes the similarity of the adrenalectomy and hypophysectomy groups and the poorer survival for the oophorectomy group even when broken down into biologically similar groups.

Figure 6 separates the "free interval" into the two categories of $< 24$ months and $> 24$ months, and thus allows comparison with Shimkin's data. Again, there is a direct relation between the "free interval" and survival in the "untreated" group as well as the similarity between this group and the oophorectomy group.

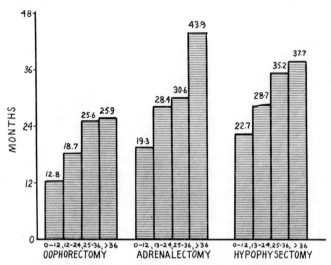

FIG. 5. Survival after recurrence in EAP groups related to length of "free interval."

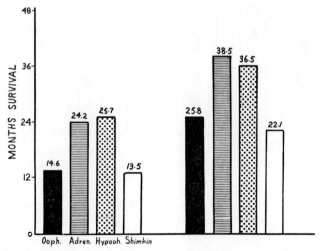

FIG. 6. Survival after recurrence in EAP and Shimkin groups. Bars at left, free interval less than 24 months; bars at right, more than 24 months.

A question in the minds of all clinicians in this field is whether an ablative procedure early in the course of disseminated disease is of greater value than if this treatment is delayed. With the figures available to date no correlation could be found between the interval from recurrence to treatment and survival in the oophorectomy or hypophysectomy group. In the adrenal-ectomy group there was a linear proportionality between these time intervals ($r = 0.1$). With the material available we have, therefore, been unable to demonstrate any increased survival by earlier ablative therapy.

TABLE II

DEFINITION OF STAGES

| | |
|---|---|
| Stage I: | Metastases to skin or subcutis, peripheral lymph nodes, or pleura |
| Stage II: | Metastases to bone with or without any to sites under Stage I |
| Stage III: | Metastases to viscera with or without any to sites under Stage I or II |

The three stages of disease as used in this paper are defined in Table II. This is an artificial classification and does not necessarily imply prognostic significance. However, it is useful for comparison of survival with Shimkin's figures. It should be pointed out that Shimkin's Stage I includes local

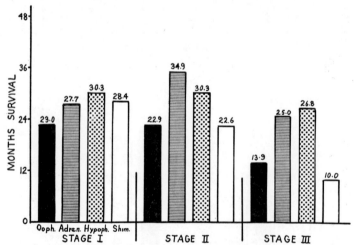

FIG. 7. Survival after recurrence in EAP and Shimkin groups: death by stage of recurrent disease.

recurrence whereas ours do not. Also pleural involvement is classed as Stage I in our figures, and Stage III in Shimkin's. In Figure 7 there is a significant difference between the oophorectomy versus hypophysectomy ($P < 0.001$) and oophorectomy versus adrenalectomy ($P < 0.001$) in Stage III. The same is true for Shimkin's series as compared to either adrenalectomy or hypophysectomy ($P < 0.1$). The same results are found for Stage II as for Stage III. However, for Stage I no significant difference could be demonstrated.

It is of interest that 48 % of the oophorectomy cases were in Stage III as compared with 39 % and 36 %, respectively, of the adrenalectomy and hypophysectomy cases. It must be emphasized that in the oophorectomy group evidence of intra-abdominal cancer is verified earlier because of laparotomy, whereas this may not be known, though frequently present, at the time of hypophysectomy or adrenalectomy. This may explain the slight difference in survival in the various stages in adrenalectomy and hypophysectomy cases.

Analyzing the survival for each group of cases in relation to the stage of the disease, we find a definitely lower figure in Stage III as compared to either Stage I or II for both the oophorectomy and Shimkin's group. This difference in survival is only minor for the adrenalectomy and hypophysectomy groups in the various stages. The reason for this is not readily apparent. The longer survival from recurrence of Stage II (most marked in the adrenalectomy and hypophysectomy groups) may be partially explained by the fact that the diagnosis of painful osseous metastases is made at an earlier date than would an asymptomatic nodule in the liver. However, the survival from mastectomy is also longer.

## DISCUSSION

Any set of these figures suggests improved survival in the adrenalectomy and hypophysectomy series. However, the multiplicity of factors other than the therapy influencing these figures must be taken into consideration in order to determine their validity. Shimkin's series includes many cases treated in the years preceding modern antibiotic therapy. It also includes cases with local recurrence only, which the A.M.A. and EAP series do not. The A.M.A. cases were treated before the days of more aggressive therapy for pleural effusion and the use of corticosteroids for the treatment of hypercalcemia and other complications. Furthermore, the possibility that ablative procedures may produce a worsening in the course of the disease (5, 13) may falsely decrease the survival figures of the total EAP group. In most institutions, ablative procedures, especially hypophysectomy or adrenalectomy, have until recently been used only in far advanced cases. All these factors influence survival one way or another. Furthermore, it has been shown that the stage of the disease at the time of mastectomy influenced the survival of those dying with disseminated disease (10). This has not been taken into consideration in this study. Certainly, though adrenalectomy and hypophysectomy appear to prolong life, it may be questioned by some whether six to twelve months of increased survival is adequate compensation for the physiological, psychological, and economic trauma produced by these procedures.

These figures do not tell the whole story. Though the total life span is increased by a relatively small figure, these additional months in a substantial number of patients were made more bearable. Furthermore, we are all aware that at the present time there is no systemic therapy that will produce as good a palliation. Only the British can say it better than we uneducated colonials, so I quote from a paper by Wade (12), "We may, therefore, describe them [the treated group] as 'enjoying' a survival period of so many months, whereas the untreated group might more accurately to be said to 'endure' a survival period of so many months."

### SUMMARY AND CONCLUSION

The survival periods of 555 postmastectomy patients who underwent various endocrine ablative procedures have been compared with each other and with a similar series treated with sex steroids and an "untreated series."

The survival times of the adrenalectomy and hypophysectomy groups were similar but significantly longer than those of the oophorectomy group. However, the oophorectomy group does not include those cases having had an oophorectomy who later simultaneously underwent further ablative surgery. This, of course, eliminates many cases, which, because of their favorable course, were selected for adrenalectomy or hypophysectomy.

Survival of the endocrine ablative series is similar to the sex steroid-treated series and both have longer survival than the "untreated series."

Sequential oophorectomy-adrenalectomy-treated patients have the same survival as those in whom both procedures were done at the same time.

Comparative survival studies serve a useful purpose in evaluating the efficacy of treatment in disseminated cancer.

### ACKNOWLEDGMENTS

We are indebted to Doctors Howard H. Sky-Peck and Stanley A. Harris for their valuable assistance in the statistical analysis used in this paper.

### REFERENCES

1. Androgens and Estrogens in the Treatment of Disseminated Mammary Carcinoma. Special Report. *J. Am. Med. Assoc.* **172**, 1271-1283 (1960).
2. Cade, Sir Stanford, *Cancer* **10**, 777-788 (1957).
3. Dao, T. L-Y., and Huggins, C. *A.M.A. Arch. Surg.* **71**, 645-657 (1955).
4. Fracchia, A. A., Holleb, A. I., Farrow, J. H., Treves, N. E., Randall, H. T., Finkbeiner, J. A., and Whitmore, W. F., Jr. *Cancer* **12**, 58-68 (1959).
5. Kofman, S., Sky-Peck, H. H., Perlia, C., Economou, S. G., Winzler, R. J., and Taylor, S. G., III. *Cancer* **13**, 425-431 (1960).

6. Lipsett, M. B., Whitmore, W. F., Jr., Treves, N. E., West, C. D., Randall, H. T., and Pearson, O. H. *Cancer* **10**, 111-119 (1957).
7. Luft, R., and Olivecrona, H. *Cancer* **10**, 788-794 (1957).
8. Macdonald, I. *Proc. Natl. Cancer Conf. 3rd Conf. 1956* pp. 87-95 (1957).
9. Pearson, O. H., and Ray, B. R. *Cancer* **12**, 85-92 (1959).
10. Shimkin, M. B., Lucia, E. L., Low-Beer, B. V. A., and Bell, H. G. *Cancer* **7**, 29-46 (1954).
11. Treves, N. E., and Finkbeiner, J. A. *Cancer* **11**, 421-438 (1958).
12. Wade, P. *Brit. J. Radiol.* **19**, 272-280 (1946).
13. Wilson, R. E., Jessiman, A. G., and Moore, F. D. *New Engl. J. Med.* **258**, 312-280 (1958).

## DISCUSSION

**S. J. Melette:** I would like to ask Dr. Taylor what efforts were made, or what criteria used, to determine completeness of operative procedures such as hypophysectomy in this series. For example, if a chart included a laboratory report that showed high follicle-stimulating hormone (FSH) values after the procedure was completed, was this chart excluded?

**S. G. Taylor:** This material is in the process of being collected and has not been included in the paper today. We have excluded cases that have obviously not had hypophysectomy.

**G. S. Gordan:** I agree with Dr. Taylor that a really good procedure should prolong survival. One of the most disturbing features of endocrine therapy has been that it does not affect the survival rate. The survival problem, however, is "loaded," and particularly so with ablative procedures, for fairly obvious statistical reasons. If one plots the number of patients surviving on a logarithmic ordinate against time on a linear abscissa, instead of on a linear plot such as Dr. Taylor used, the rate would appear as a straight line instead of a curve. We can therefore draw parallel lines for any surgical procedure which would obviously be farther to the right simply because of the time required for preoperative preparation and for the operation, plus 30 days of postoperative survival to exclude operative deaths. The survival rate for patients who had castration only is identical with that of what Dr. Taylor calls the Shimkin series (University of California series). This castration survival rate is the one that concerns me most. It necessarily includes two groups—those who responded and those who did not. Whether they responded or not, all of them will eventually have recurrence. In most institutions that do ablative therapy, subsequent adrenalectomy or hypophysectomy will be done only on patients who respond favorably to castration. If I understood correctly, Dr. Taylor threw out cases that had subsequent ablative procedures. In other words, the castration series included only the unfavorable cases.

Finally, one other problem bothers me greatly; i.e., the matter of selecting the patients. In most institutions patients are not selected for hypophysectomy if they have visceral metastases. Therefore one has to show the number of cases in the various subgroups. For example, the data from the Sloan-Kettering Institute show that 50% of the steroid-treated patients had visceral metastases, whereas in the Cooperative Group studies only 37% had visceral involvement. Obviously these series can be tipped either way by the kind of patients selected.

**S. G. Taylor:** I emphasized that we could not compare the oophorectomy series because of just those reasons Dr. Gordan mentioned. That is a very important point and I'm glad it was brought out. The figures on the oophorectomy cannot be included because of that factor. As far as the percentage of patients with a visceral disease is concerned, I did present Fig. 3, demonstrating that the figures of the University of California are similar to those of the adrenalectomy and hypophysectomy groups. The difference comes in the age factor; they have more patients in an older age group. The percentage of patients with long and short free intervals is the same as ours. So they are quite similar groups all the way through except for the age factor.

H. Volk: Dr. Taylor, in Table II, showing the stages of disease, you include pleura in Stage I. When the Breast Cancer Cooperative Group established the various classifications for the protocol, as you are well aware, it included pleura in the visceral disease category, which has a much poorer prognosis. Could you explain why you elected to include pleura in Stage I?

S. G. Taylor: We did that for a particular reason. In the first place, it is so frequently the case that the patient who has pleural effusion and no other evidence of disseminated disease, and who is treated aggressively in that area alone, will frequently have a long survival, compared with patients with other visceral lesions. I am sure you have all had patients who have had a pleural stripping or installation of $HN_2$, following which two or three years elapse before generalized dissemination aside from the pleural occurred. We feel that is a special group. What we are going to do in our final analysis is to have the pleural group in a series of their own where there is just pleural effusion and nothing else.

B. J. Kennedy: When I first heard of this proposed project I was concerned because there was more interest in the ablative procedures themselves than in the problem of utilizing the procedures in a consecutive order for maximum utilization of therapy for patients. The fundamental problem is that too many exclusions have been made, and it is almost impossible to evaluate the statistical results.

S. G. Taylor: These are important points that Dr. Kennedy has brought up, some of which I cannot answer. These cases have been selected by various criteria, varying in different institutions. You know that the A.M.A. patients were all selected. There isn't, as far as I know, any published series of cases of metastatic breast cancer who had had a mastectomy for primary disease completely comparable. The A.M.A. and Shimkin's series had had previous mastectomy. Study of the A.M.A. series shows that patients who had had a mastectomy and then had recurrence behaved differently in regard to survival than patients who entered the series with a primary disease still intact. So we have eliminated the latter cases from all series in order to try to compare similar entities. Most of the survival studies are comparisons of various surgical procedures. I hoped that someone would congratulate me on not using the Darlin-Nathanson series as a comparison.

I know that there are a lot of variables to this survival study, and I have emphasized them in the paper. The thing I am trying to bring out is that survival is a tool for the measurement of end results that should be used together with measurement of objective regression in evaluating the effectiveness of palliative therapy. There is too much disagreement about what a regression is, so let us leave regression out of this. I did peek at regression; I had promised myself not to say anything about it, but it was very interesting to me that the patients with a short "free interval" who had "regression" lived a shorter length of time than did the patients who were classified as not having a regression and who had had a long "free interval," taking the time of survival from recurrence to death.

B. J. Kennedy: There is little difference between the adrenalectomy and the hypophysectomy group. This is of value to know.

# Testosterone Propionate Therapy of Breast Cancer— A Report for the Cooperative Breast Cancer Group

Albert Segaloff

*Alton Ochsner Medical Foundation, and Tulane University School of Medicine, New Orleans, Louisiana*

It has been apparent for some time that it is possible to produce objective regression of advancing metastatic deposits originating from mammary cancer by the administration of adequate amounts of the male sex hormone, testosterone propionate. There have been many publications on this phenomenon as well as the very substantial effort put forth by the American Medical Association's Therapeutics Trials Committee, Subcommittee on Steroids and Cancer (later the Committee on Research of the Council on Pharmacy and Chemistry) (2). Despite this, there has been no study of which we are aware that had an adequate protocol setting up the criteria for entering patients into the study and distributing them into the various experimental groups in a statistically adequate random fashion. The material which constitutes the data for the present report, on the other hand, we believe adequately meets these criteria.

The women studied were treated with testosterone propionate in vegetable oil, 100 mg. intramuscularly three times weekly, or with one of a wide variety of steroidal agents. Only those patients treated with testosterone propionate are the subject of this report. A few additional studies have been made with fluoxymesterone as an oral reference standard which will be briefly discussed subsequently.

All the data herein reported were collected as the reference control data for the study of hormonal therapy for advanced breast cancer being carried out by the Cooperative Breast Cancer Group of the Cancer Chemotherapy National Service Center, National Institutes of Health.

As we have pointed out previously (4), metastatic breast cancer, once it is established, does not grow inexorably, progressing until it brings about the death of the host. On the contrary, it usually goes through alternating periods of rapid growth and of slow growth or quiescence. The quiescent periods may last a substantial length of time and can be of sufficient duration so that the induction of such quiescent periods would indeed be worth while. In view of this, it was thought important that all the patients entered in this study have objective evidence of advancing disease at the time of initiation of therapy, so that there could be no question of the continuation of such a period of inactivity. Conversely, although cognizance will be made of the induction of such a quiescent period in a previously advancing lesion, the protocol's criteria for objective effect on the disease requires regression of all ascertainable lesions before it can be called an objective regression.

A careful protocol[1] was formulated and strictly adhered to, and it is the criteria[2] of this protocol that were applied in the current study.

A body of evidence is also available which indicates that the site of major involvement with metastatic deposits governs the outcome of the disease not only in longevity but in the chance of response to changes of the hormonal environment (1). In order to evaluate this area carefully and to be sure that there would be an equitable distribution of various types of cases prior to randomization, patients were distributed into three categories according to the dominant area of involvement. Where there was major involvement of more than one system, the patient was classified as having the dominant lesion with the least favorable prognosis. These categories, from best to poorest prognosis, are: local breast and skin soft tissue lesions, osseous lesions, and, finally, visceral lesions (including pulmonary and central nervous systems).

Much evidence is available which would indicate that the patient's menopausal age also has an effect on outcome, particularly with respect to response to changes in the hormonal milieu (3). Accordingly, the patients were further subdivided by their menopausal age. The first group covered less than one year following castration. (Patients who had been menopausal less than one year were castrated prior to the use of administrative hormonal therapy because of the frequency of a favorable outcome from castration in such individuals). The other groups were from 1 to 5 years, 5 to 10 years, and more than 10 years postmenopausal. Thus each of the patients was placed into one of the 12 categories depending upon their menopausal age and the site of major involvement with the metastatic deposits.

Since a preliminary review of the accumulated data on testosterone propionate therapy in cases such as these being reported (carried out at the Alton Ochsner Medical Foundation and at the Sloan-Kettering Institute) indicated that previous administrative hormonal therapy may decrease the chance of subsequent response to testosterone propionate, all the patients treated under the present protocol had their therapy as the first administrative hormonal therapy for recurrent or primary inoperable breast cancer.

The necessary randomization schemata, with serially numbered sealed envelopes for each category, and the materials were supplied to the cooperat-

---

[1] The protocol was drawn up by a committee of the Cooperative Breast Cancer Group consisting of: the late Dr. Delbert M. Bergenstal, Dr. George C. Escher, Dr. Robert Huseby, and Dr. Albert Segaloff, Chairman.

[2] Cooperative Breast Cancer Group Protocol I (draft of February 28, 1957 as revised June 3, 1959, p. 9):

ing institutions through the Cancer Chemotherapy National Service Center. Where it was physically possible, the experimental agent and testosterone propionate were "doubly blinded." Thus, when a patient was admitted to the study and assigned to her category, the next numbered envelope covering the appropriate category of dominant lesion and menopausal age was opened and the patient given the material indicated. A report of each patient's entry was sent to the Chairman's office, and at prescribed intervals follow-up reports on her status were also sent. The present study includes those patients who have been on therapy with testosterone propionate and on whom at least one follow-up report is available. Since some patients do not show objective evidence of regression sufficient to satisfy the criteria of the protocol for some time after being started on therapy, the figures given here may be considered as minimum response figures rather than as maximal response figures.

At the conclusion of a study, one or more members of the Cooperative Group visit the institution where the study was carried out and review all the material on the patients to determine whether they agree or disagree with the reports made by the original investigator. The final reports utilized by the Group are those agreed on by the reviewer and the investigator. Wherever feasible, the reviewers are not apprised of the material given to each patient until after the review is completed and the decisions made. In the double-blind studies, wherever possible, this will have been accomplished before the code is broken, so that neither the investigator nor the reviewer is aware of what material the patient received. Serial measurements using a standard caliper, photographs which include a scale, the date, and the patient's name, as well as roentgen films, are the basis on which such decisions are made.

VII. *Evaluation of Response*

D. The following criteria have been established for the evaluation of patient objective remission:

1. Patients in whom all demonstrable tumor masses diminish measurably in size.
   a. Healing of an ulcerated lesion cannot be considered evidence of an objective remission.
2. Patients in whom more than 50% of non-osseous lesions decrease in size although all bone lesions are static.
3. Patients in whom more than 50% of total lesions improve while the remainder are static.

A total of 401 patients have been entered into the testosterone propionate study. Their distribution among the twelve categories is seen in Table I. The patients appear to be about as evenly distributed among the various groups as one could expect. Table II shows the percentage distribution in response of the twelve groups. It should be immediately apparent that we have been fully justified in setting up so many groups in the randomization, since there is a correlation with both the system of major involvement and the menopausal age of the patient. In all major involvement categories there

TABLE I
TESTOSTERONE PROPIONATE: DISTRIBUTION OF PATIENTS

| Dominant lesions | Years postmenopausal | | | | Number of patients |
|---|---|---|---|---|---|
| | < 1 | 1–5 | 5–10 | > 10 | |
| Local | 18 | 18 | 11 | 53 | 100 |
| Osseous | 30 | 28 | 29 | 65 | 152 |
| Visceral | 26 | 28 | 21 | 74 | 149 |
| | 74 | 74 | 61 | 192 | 401 |

TABLE II
TESTOSTERONE PROPIONATE: PERCENTAGE OF OBJECTIVE REGRESSIONS

| Dominant lesions | Years postmenopausal | | | | Per cent of total |
|---|---|---|---|---|---|
| | < 1 | 1–5 | 5–10 | > 10 | |
| Local | 6 | 17 | 27 | 43 | 30 |
| Osseous | 13 | 18 | 21 | 23 | 20 |
| Visceral | 4 | 7 | 14 | 20 | 14 |
| Per cent of total | 8 | 14 | 20 | 28 | 20 |

is a significant increase in response with increase in the menopausal age. Figure 1 shows lines drawn assuming the groups to be placed at equal intervals along the postmenopausal age axis. Although the slopes of these lines are markedly different ($b_L = 2.50$—local; $b_O = 0.61$—osseous; $b_V = 1.13$—visceral), the standard deviations of the estimates of the slopes are so high that these cannot be said at present to show a significant difference. However, as pointed out above, in all the categories of involvement and for the total in each menopausal age group there is a significant increase in the percentage of patients showing objective regressions with increase in menopausal age.

There does not appear to be any significant difference in any of the groups when one relates the time elapsed between the original diagnosis and the start of treatment. For the entire group this averaged 33.3 months. The patients who experienced remission averaged 30.3 months, while the failures averaged a 34.1 month period.

When the investigators started their second study under our protocol, if they used an orally administered agent instead of a parenterally administered one, the patients were then given fluoxymesterone as 20 mg. in three equally divided doses through the day, doubly blinded with the experimental material, in place of the testosterone propionate as the reference standard. The same randomization schema and criteria were applied to these patients as to those considered above. Unfortunately, there are not yet enough patients to justify a full presentation of the data. There are one or more patients in each of the twelve groups, but there is a total of only 54 patients

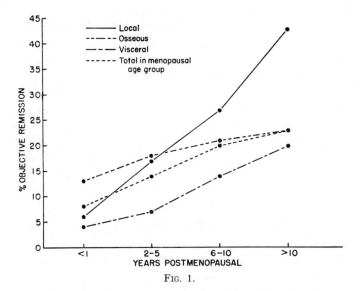

Fig. 1.

entered in this study to date. Of these 54 patients, 5 have been reported as showing objective remission. These remissions are distributed throughout the groups in such a fashion that it is not possible to relate the remission rate adequately to the various groups as yet. However, these 5 remissions constitute only 9 % of the total patients entered into the study, whereas the 81 remissions in the testosterone propionate group constitute 20.2 % of the total number of patients entered.

## DISCUSSION

The present report is a preliminary one since many of the patients are still under therapy. The final report will be very likely to show a greater response rate than that given at present. In addition, in the future it will be possible to give an analysis of duration of responses and some figures on the androgenic effects produced in the patients, as well as the incidence of such non-androgenic effects as the production of hypercalcemia.

It is difficult to equate the presently reported results with those of previous studies for many reasons. We have clearly shown an increasing percentage response with increasing menopausal age, so that studies such as that of the Subcommittee on Steroids and Cancer (5) must be viewed in the light of the bias against testosterone introduced by the use of patients more than 5 years postmenopausal, preferentially for estrogen therapy. In addition to this, our percentage response in the patients who were more than 10 years postmenopausal with local soft tissue disease probably does not differ significantly from that seen, in the American Medical Association study, associated with estrogen therapy in their most comparable group.

It appears to me that, from the data reported, the following is justified: (1) Testosterone propionate in a dose of 100 mg. intramuscularly three times weekly is indeed capable of producing objective regression in women having advancing metastatic deposits from breast cancer. (2) Testosterone propionate therapy is as effective as any well-documented hormonal therapy in any menopausal age group. (3) Testosterone propionate therapy is as effective as any well-documented hormonal therapy in any dominant lesion group. (4) When new hormonal agents are evaluated, due weight must be given to menopausal age and sites of involvement.

## Summary

Four hundred and one patients have been treated with intramuscular testosterone propionate according to a very carefully devised and controlled protocol, under which patients were entered into this study by randomization after being classified into twelve groups according to the dominant lesion and menopausal age of the patient. Eighty-one of these patients have to date sustained an objective remission according to the criteria of the protocol of the Cooperative Breast Cancer Group. The distribution of the objective remissions is such that there is indeed a significant increase in percentage of objective remissions with increase in menopausal age in all three of the dominant lesion categories employed. It would also appear that the percentage objective response is related to the dominant lesion. The highest response rate was seen in those patients more than 10 years postmenopausal having local soft tissue lesions as their major involvement. These patients showed a 43 % objective response rate. The lowest objective response rate was seen in patients with visceral involvement who had been castrated less than one year and only 4 % of these patients showed an objective remission of their advancing breast cancer.

Of 54 patients treated similarly with fluoxymesterone, 5 patients, or 9 %, have shown objective remission.

### ACKNOWLEDGMENTS

This study was made possible by the substantial cooperation of the entire staff of the Cancer Chemotherapy National Service Center, without whose yeoman efforts the study could not have been carried out. Especially important contributions have been made by Dr. Erwin Vollmer, Mr. Morris Graff, Mr. Arthur G. Hilgar, and Dr. T. Philip Waalkes. We should also like particularly to thank the members of the Statistical Section, including Mrs. Nancy B. Engel, Mrs. Opal Rasch, and Dr. David Alling for their invaluable assistance.

\*　　\*　　\*

The data collected here were contributed by all members of the Cooperative Breast Cancer Group. The author is honored to have been designated to present the data for them. The members of the Cooperative Breast Cancer Group are as follows:

†Dr. Paul D. Abramson, Confederate Memorial Hospital, Shreveport, Louisiana

Dr. Fred J. Ansfield, University of Wisconsin, Madison, Wisconsin

Dr. John C. Athans, Boston University, Boston, Massachusetts

Dr. William Baker, Massachusetts General Hospital, Boston, Massachusetts

Dr. Harry Bisel, University of Pittsburgh, Pittsburgh, Pennsylvania

Dr. Charles Blackburn, The Mayo Clinic, Rochester, Minnesota

Dr. Michael Brennan, Henry Ford Hospital, Detroit, Michigan

Dr. Ralph Carabasi, Jefferson Medical College, Philadelphia, Pennsylvania

Dr. Anne Carter, State University of New York, Downstate Medical Center, Brooklyn, New York

Dr. George V. Coleman, Rhode Island Hospital, Providence, Rhode Island

Dr. Thomas Dao, Roswell Park Memorial Institute, Buffalo, New York

Dr. George C. Escher, Sloan-Kettering Institute, New York, New York

Dr. Ira Goldenberg, Yale University, New Haven, Connecticut

Dr. Gilbert Gordan, University of California, San Francisco, California

Dr. Carleton R. Haines, Mary Fletcher Hospital, Burlington, Vermont

Dr. Thomas C. Hall, Lemuel Shattuck Hospital, Boston, Massachusetts

Dr. John Hawk, Jr., Medical College of South Carolina, Charleston, South Carolina

Dr. Mark Hayes, Yale University, New Haven, Connecticut

Dr. Robert Huseby, University of Colorado, Denver, Colorado

Dr. Rita Kelley, Pondville Hospital, Walpole, Massachusetts

Dr. B. J. Kennedy, University of Minnesota, Minneapolis, Minnesota

†Dr. Daniel Laszlo, Montefiore Hospital, New York, New York

Dr. Gerson Lesnick, Mt. Sinai Hospital, New York, New York

Dr. Edward Lewison, Johns Hopkins University, Baltimore, Maryland

Dr. Kenneth F. Olson, Albany Medical College of Union University, Albany, New York

Dr. Robert Ravdin, University of Pennsylvania, Philadelphia, Pennsylvania

Dr. Victor Richards, Stanford University, San Francisco, California

Dr. Chester Rosoff, Beth Israel Hospital, Boston, Massachusetts

Dr. Albert Segaloff, Alton Ochsner Medical Foundation, New Orleans, Louisiana

---

† Deceased.

Dr. Herta Spencer, Montefiore Hospital, New York, New York
Dr. Samuel Taylor, III, University of Illinois, Chicago, Illinois
Dr. Frank Tyler, University of Utah, Salt Lake City, Utah

The following were formerly responsible investigators of the Cooperative Breast Cancer Group:

Dr. Milton Dworin, New York University, New York, New York
Dr. Henry M. Lemon, Boston University, Boston, Massachusetts (now associate responsible investigator)
Dr. H. C. Moss, Roswell Park Memorial Institute, Buffalo, New York
Dr. Herbert Volk, Albert Einstein College of Medicine, New York, New York

### REFERENCES

1. Escher, G. C. "Breast Cancer," p. 199. C. V. Mosby, St. Louis, Missouri, 1958.
2. Nathanson, I. T., Adair, F. E., Allen, W. M., and Engle, E. T. *J. Am. Med. Assoc.* **135**, 987 (1947).
3. Nathanson, I. T. *Radiology* **56**, 535 (1956).
4. Segaloff, A. *Ann. N. Y. Acad. Sci.* **76**, 717 (1958).
5. Subcommittee on Steroids and Cancer of the Committee on Research (a standing committee of the A.M.A. Council on Pharmacy and Chemistry). *J. Am. Med. Assoc.* **146**, 471 (1951).

# Hormonal Therapy of Breast Cancer
## A Summary of Experience with Newer Steroids

CHESTER B. ROSOFF

*Department of Surgery, Beth Israel Hospital, and Harvard Medical School, Boston, Massachusetts*

An evaluation of additive hormonal therapy in advanced breast cancer presents many difficulties for the clinical investigator. In part, this reflects the variation observed in the natural history of the disease as it appears in patients of different physiologic age; and in part, the lack of a uniform approach to patient selection, modes of therapy, and interpretation of results achieved. In an attempt to avoid these difficulties, the Cancer Chemotherapy National Service Center has sponsored an interhospital cooperative study of the therapy of advanced breast cancer. The group of investigators taking part in the study uses a single protocol designed to facilitate the evaluation of presently available and newly created steroids under standard conditions in the treatment of the disseminated stages of the disease. As of May, 1959, over 1000 patients had been entered in the study for treatment with either testosterone propionate, the control material, or with various unproven but apparently promising compounds that have been tested in animals for toxicity, antitumor activity, and general biologic effect. The data from the twelve studies completed prior to September 1, 1959 will be included in this summary of the results of the group effort, results which in most instances are as yet unpublished.

The criteria for admission of patients to the study are as follows: Female patients with recurrent, inoperable, or metastatic carcinoma of the breast, progressive under observation, are eligible providing that they are at least one year postmenopausal. Premenopausal patients or patients less than one year postmenopausal, may be entered only after castration has been carried out. Steroids must not have been administered within 6 months of admission to the study. The initial examination of the patient includes the evaluation of physical condition, an X-ray survey of the bones and chest, measurements of all visible and palpable lesions, blood chemical and vaginal cytological determinations. These tests are repeated at intervals of approximately 4–6 weeks, depending upon the status of the patient.

Once admitted to the study, the patients are randomized and treatment begun in double-blind fashion with either the control material or the new compound to be evaluated. Each study represents a minimum of twenty test patients and twenty simultaneous control patients. Therapy is continued until unequivocal evidence of progression of the disease can be demonstrated or until the life of the patient is endangered by the development of undesirable side effects. The objective response of the tumor to therapy is the sole criterion of the effectiveness of the agent administered. In order for an "objective remission" to be recorded it must be shown that (1) all demonstrable tumor masses diminish in size, or (2) more than half of the nonosseous lesions shrink while the bone lesions remain static, or (3) improvement is noted in more than 50 % of all lesions while the others remain unchanged.

Patients are classified according to the location of the dominant lesion and by the postmenopausal age and are then assigned to a group. Where there is involvement of more than one major area of spread the dominant site with the poorer prognosis is used for classification purposes. The incidence of local or breast recurrence, osseous spread, or visceral involvement is approximately equal, ranging from 27 to 38 % of the total studied (Table I).

TABLE I

CLASSIFICATION (PERCENTAGE) OF 490 STUDY PATIENTS WITH DISSEMINATED
BREAST CARCINOMA

| Dominant Lesions | Years postmenopausal | | | | Total |
| --- | --- | --- | --- | --- | --- |
| | < 1 | 1–5 | 6–10 | > 10 | |
| Local | 4 | 5 | 3 | 15 | 27 |
| Osseous | 8 | 6 | 6 | 18 | 38 |
| Visceral | 6 | 6 | 5 | 17 | 34 |
| | 18 | 17 | 14 | 50 | — |

In the group "less than one year postmenopausal" are included only patients castrated prior to admission to the study, since the protocol requires all other patients to be more than one year postmenopausal. The distribution of patients in the study by menopausal age shows the greatest number of patients—50 % of the entire series—in the "greater than ten years postmenopausal" group. This is not surprising, since in terms of the average age of menopause and life expectancy, the last column covers about as many years as do the first three columns, and a distribution of patients accordingly would be expected.

Many of the test compounds that have been evaluated are androgens, i.e., they are $C_{19}$ steroids with oxygen substituents at C-3 and C-17 and with no side chain at the C-17 position. They are compounds that cause development of the male sex organs or secondary sex characteristics but vary considerably as to their biologic potency. All of the trial group of compounds have been evaluated in the same fashion as have the controls whose therapeutic efficacy has been reported showing a remission rate, over-all, of at least 18 %.

Androsterone (Fig. 1), one of a series of androstane compounds evaluated, was administered by Segaloff (10) in a dosage of 100 mg. intramuscularly three times a week. A remission rate of 4 % was achieved with but one of 22 patients responding to treatment (Table II).

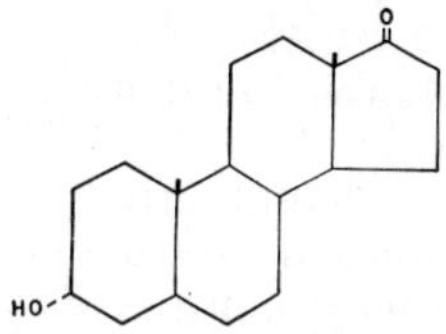

FIG. 1.   Androsterone.

TABLE   II

ANDROSTERONE: SUMMARY OF OBJECTIVE REMISSIONS PER NUMBER OF PATIENTS[a, b]

| | Years postmenopausal | | | | Total | |
|---|---|---|---|---|---|---|
| Dominant Lesions | $< 1$ | 1–5 | 6–10 | $> 10$ | Number | % |
| Local | 0/2 | 0/2 | 0/1 | 0/4 | 0/9 | 0 |
| Osseous | 0/1 | 0/1 | 0/1 | 0/3 | 0/6 | 0 |
| Visceral | 0/1 | 0/1 | — | 1/5 | 1/7 | 14 |
| Total | | | | | | |
| Number | 0/4 | 0/4 | 0/2 | 1/12 | 1/22 | — |
| Per cent | 0 | 0 | 0 | 8 | — | 4 |

[a] Data from Segaloff (10).

[b] Dosage: 100 mg. intramuscularly three times per week.

Androstane-3α,17β-diol, dipropionate (Fig. 2), was also administered by Segaloff (10) in the same dosage of 100 mg. intramuscularly three times a week. This dipropionate form of the compound resulted in a pattern of response quite similar to that found with androsterone. The remission rate was again 4 % (Table III).

Another of the modified androstane molecules is androstane-3β,17β-diol, diacetate (Fig. 3), the assessment of which was carried out by Brennan (3) (Fig. 3). Three of the 21 patients studied, or 14 %, showed objective regression of the disease after treatment with 100 mg. intramuscularly three times weekly (Table IV).

Androstan-3-one, 17β-hydroxy-2α-methyl-, propionate (2-methyldihydro-testosterone) is another (Fig. 4) of this series of modified androstane compounds. The clinical evaluation was carried out by Blackburn (2), who in a series of 27 cases reported 12 objective regressions of disease, a rate of 44 % (Table V). Two-thirds of the regressions reported were in the group of patients whose dominant site of metastatic spread was osseous. There was an even distribution of response observed in each of the age groups except

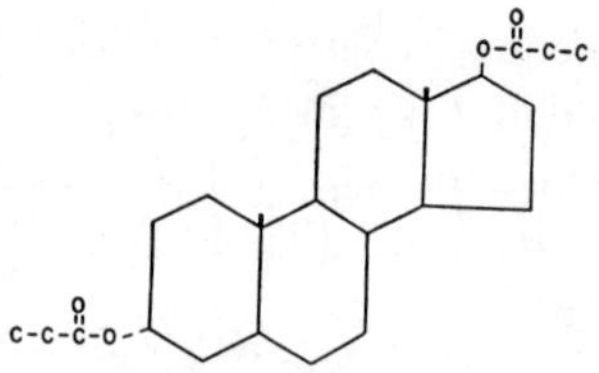

Fig. 2. Androstane-3α,17β-diol, dipropionate.

TABLE III

ANDROSTANE-3α,17β-DIOL, DIPROPIONATE: SUMMARY OF OBJECTIVE REMISSIONS PER NUMBER OF PATIENTS[a, b]

| Dominant Lesions | Years postmenopausal | | | | Total | |
|---|---|---|---|---|---|---|
| | < 1 | 1–5 | 6–10 | > 10 | Number | % |
| Local | 0/1 | — | 0/1 | 0/2 | 0/4 | 0 |
| Osseous | 0/2 | 0/2 | 0/1 | 0/4 | 0/9 | 0 |
| Visceral | 0/2 | 1/2 | 0/1 | 0/5 | 1/10 | 10 |
| Total | | | | | | |
| Number | 0/4 | 1/4 | 0/3 | 0/11 | 1/23 | — |
| Per cent | 0 | 25 | 0 | 0 | — | 4 |

[a] Data from Segaloff (10).

[b] Dosage: 100 mg. intramuscularly three times per week.

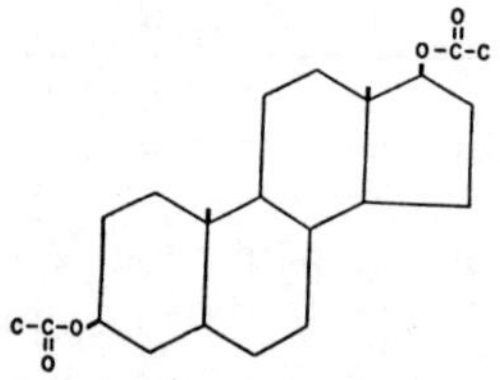

Fig. 3. Androstane-3β,17β-diol, diacetate.

TABLE IV

ANDROSTANE-3β,17β-DIOL, DIACETATE: SUMMARY OF OBJECTIVE REMISSIONS PER NUMBER OF PATIENTS[a, b]

| Dominant Lesions | Years postmenopausal | | | | Total | |
|---|---|---|---|---|---|---|
| | < 1 | 1–5 | 6–10 | > 10 | Number | % |
| Local | — | 0/1 | — | 1/4 | 1/5 | 20 |
| Osseous | 0/3 | 0/2 | — | 0/3 | 0/8 | 0 |
| Visceral | 0/1 | 0/3 | 1/1 | 1/3 | 2/8 | 25 |
| Total | | | | | | |
| Number | 0/4 | 0/6 | 1/1 | 2/10 | 3/21 | — |
| Per cent | 0 | 0 | 100 | 20 | — | 14 |

[a] Data from Brennan (3).

[b] Dosage: 100 mg. intramuscularly three times per week.

for those recently castrated, the "less than one year postmenopausal" group. With the exception of this group of patients, the rate of response approached 50 %, and the over-all figure of 44 % for the series is considerably in excess of that found with testosterone propionate. In all probability, this new

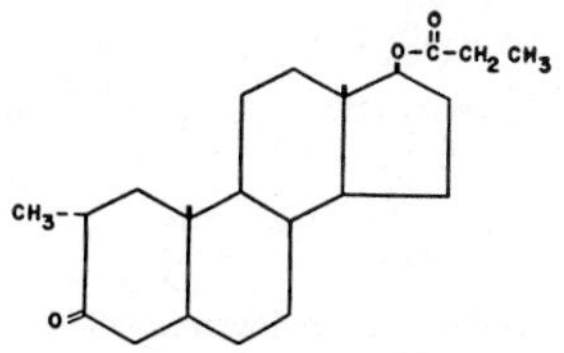

FIG. 4. Androstan-3-one, 17β-hydroxy-2α-methyl-, propionate (2-methyldihydrotestosterone).

### TABLE V
2-METHYLDIHYDROTESTOSTERONE, PROPIONATE:
SUMMARY OF OBJECTIVE REMISSIONS PER NUMBER OF PATIENTS[a, b]

| Dominant Lesions | Years postmenopausal | | | | Total | |
|---|---|---|---|---|---|---|
| | < 1 | 1–5 | 6–10 | > 10 | Number | % |
| Local | 0/1 | 0/2 | 0/2 | 1/1 | 1/6 | 17 |
| Osseous | 1/1 | 3/3 | 2/2 | 2/6 | 8/12 | 67 |
| Visceral | 0/2 | 1/3 | 1/2 | 1/2 | 3/9 | 33 |
| Total | | | | | | |
| Number | 1/4 | 4/8 | 3/6 | 4/9 | 12/27 | — |
| Per cent | 25 | 50 | 50 | 44 | — | 44 |

[a] Data from Blackburn (2).

[b] Dosage: 100 mg. intramuscularly three times per week.

compound offers a therapeutic efficacy significantly better than that of any other compound studied to date.

The 4-androstene form seen in testosterone appears in the 3β,17β-diol diacetate modification (Fig. 5) used by Olson and Ansfield (9). In a group of 23 patients treated, 5, or 22 %, showed satisfactory evidence of regression of disease with the best response observed in the oldest group of patients treated (Table VI).

The next two compounds to be reviewed are closely related and are both 19-nortestosterones. 19-nor-4-androsten-3-one, 17β-hydroxy-17α-methyl- (19-nortestosterone, 17-methyl-) (Fig. 6) was studied by Carter (4), who administered it in a dosage of 30 mg. per day by mouth. Five of 21 patients, or 24 % of those receiving this compound, showed evidence of objective regression of disease (Table VII). It is apparent that the patients in the immediate postmenopausal age group did not do well, but there was a relatively even distribution of responses in other age groups. There was also a suggestion that patients with local recurrence of disease responded more

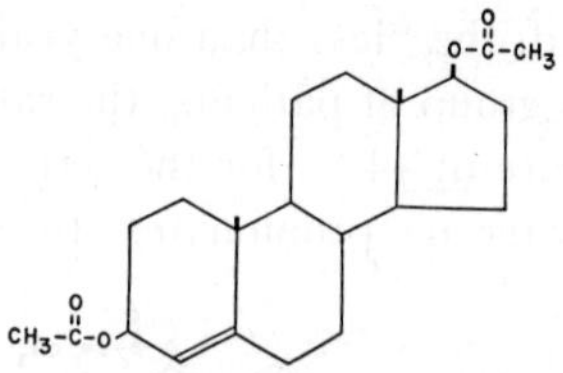

FIG. 5. 4-Androstene-3β,17β-diol, diacetate.

TABLE VI

4-ANDROSTENE-3β,17β-DIOL, DIACETATE: SUMMARY OF OBJECTIVE REMISSIONS PER NUMBER OF PATIENTS[a, b]

| Dominant Lesions | Years postmenopausal | | | | Total | |
|---|---|---|---|---|---|---|
| | < 1 | 1–5 | 6–10 | > 10 | Number | % |
| Local | — | 0/3 | 0/1 | 3/4 | 3/8 | 38 |
| Osseous | 0/3 | 1/3 | 0/1 | 1/4 | 2/11 | 18 |
| Visceral | 0/1 | 0/2 | 0/1 | — | 0/4 | 0 |
| Total | | | | | | |
| Number | 0/4 | 1/8 | 0/3 | 4/8 | 5/23 | — |
| Per cent | 0 | 13 | 0 | 50 | — | 22 |

[a] Data from Olson and Ansfield (9).
[b] Dosage: 100 mg. intramuscularly three times per week.

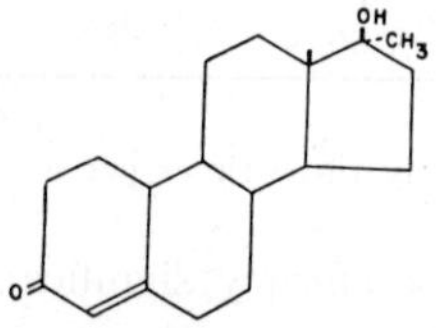

FIG. 6. 19-Nor-4-androsten-3-one,17β-hydroxy-17α-methyl-(19-nortestosterone,17-methyl-).

TABLE VII

19-NORTESTOSTERONE, 17-METHYL-: SUMMARY OF OBJECTIVE REMISSIONS PER NUMBER OF PATIENTS[a, b]

| Dominant Lesions | Years postmenopausal | | | | Total | |
|---|---|---|---|---|---|---|
| | < 1 | 1–5 | 6–10 | > 10 | Number | % |
| Local | 0/1 | 0/1 | 1/1 | 3/7 | 4/10 | 40 |
| Osseous | 0/1 | 1/1 | 0/1 | 0/3 | 1/6 | 17 |
| Visceral | 0/1 | 0/1 | 0/1 | 0/2 | 0/5 | 0 |
| Total | | | | | | |
| Number | 0/3 | 1/3 | 1/3 | 3/12 | 5/21 | — |
| Per cent | 0 | 33 | 33 | 25 | — | 24 |

[a] Data from Carter (4).
[b] Dosage: 30 mg. per day by mouth.

favorably than did those with other areas of involvement. This suggestive pattern of grouping of responses is seen frequently in the compounds investigated.

A closely related compound structurally is 19-nor-4-androsten-3-one, 17α-ethynyl-17β-hydroxy- (19-nortestosterone, 17-ethynyl-). This compound differs from the previous one only in the replacement of the 17α-methyl group by an ethynyl radical (Fig. 7). Lewin (8) used this material in clinical trials in a dosage of 40 mg. by mouth daily and observed a 23 % rate of

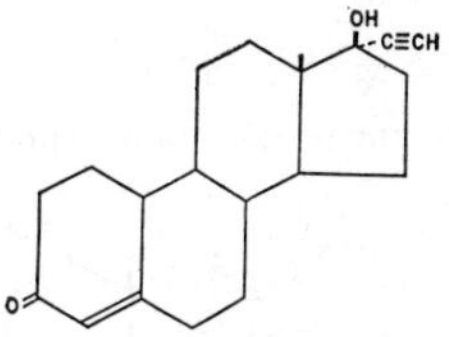

FIG. 7.   19-Nor-4-androsten-3-one,   17α-ethynyl-17β-hydroxy-(19-nortestosterone,   17-ethynyl-).

TABLE VIII

19-Nortestosterone, 17-Ethynyl-: Summary of Objective Remissions per Number of Patients[a, b]

| Dominant Lesions | Years postmenopausal | | | | Total | |
|---|---|---|---|---|---|---|
| | < 1 | 1–5 | 6–10 | > 10 | Number | % |
| Local | 0/2 | 1/2 | — | 0/1 | 1/5 | 20 |
| Osseous | 0/1 | — | 2/2 | 1/5 | 3/8 | 38 |
| Visceral | — | 1/2 | 0/3 | 0/4 | 1/9 | 11 |
| Total | | | | | | |
| Number | 0/3 | 2/4 | 2/5 | 1/10 | 5/22 | — |
| Per cent | 0 | 50 | 40 | 10 | — | 23 |

[a] Data from Lewin (8).
[b] Dosage: 40 mg. per day by mouth.

regression of disease, with 5 of 22 patients studied responding (Table VIII). The most favorable response observed was in those with osseous disease, ½ of whom showed remission of their tumor.

Two representatives of the $C_{21}$ steroid family, progesterone (Fig. 8) and a modified compound, 9α-bromo-11-oxoprogesterone have been studied. Huseby and associates (7) assayed the antitumor effect of progesterone, using a dosage of 2.0 gm. daily by mouth. There was no evidence of tumor response in any of the 26 patients treated despite adequate evidence of absorption from the gastrointestinal tract and a biologic effect on the endometrium. When this parent structure was modified to form 9α-bromo-11-oxoprogesterone (bromoketoprogesterone), a more effective material resulted (Fig. 9). This was evaluated by Hayes and Goldenberg (6) in 25 patients, five of whom, or 20 %, showed objective regression of disease (Table IX). Three hundred milligrams per day was administered orally in the group tested. Half of the regressions observed were in patients with local or breast manifestations of disease, and all of the remissions were in the older groups of patients.

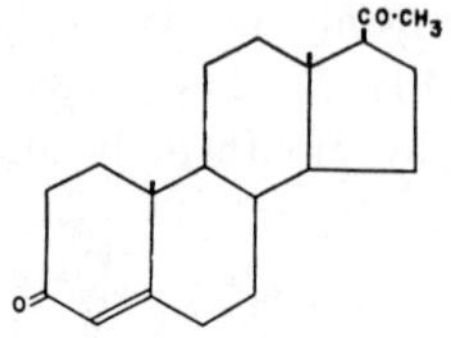

FIG. 8. 4-Pregnene-3,20-dione (progesterone).

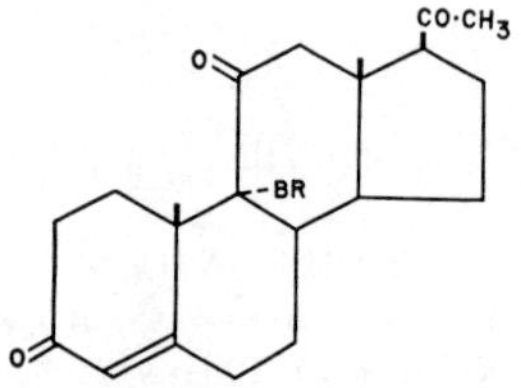

FIG. 9. 9α-Bromo-11-oxoprogesterone.

TABLE IX

9α-BROMO-11-OXOPROGESTERONE: SUMMARY OF OBJECTIVE REMISSIONS PER NUMBER OF PATIENTS[a, b]

| | Years postmenopausal | | | | Total | |
|---|---|---|---|---|---|---|
| Dominant Lesions | < 1 | 1–5 | 6–10 | > 10 | Number | % |
| Local | 0/1 | 0/1 | 1/1 | 2/3 | 3/6 | 50 |
| Osseous | 0/3 | 0/1 | 1/3 | 1/5 | 2/12 | 17 |
| Visceral | 0/2 | 0/1 | 0/1 | 0/3 | 0/7 | 0 |
| Total | | | | | | |
| Number | 0/6 | 0/3 | 2/5 | 3/11 | 5/25 | — |
| Per cent | 0 | 0 | 40 | 27 | — | 20 |

[a] Data from Hayes and Goldenberg (6).
[b] Dosage: 300 mg. per day by mouth.

Two of the compounds studied demonstrated estrogenic effects. The first, 5(10)-estren-3-one, 17α-ethynyl-17β-hydroxy-, or Norethynodrel (Fig. 10) was tested in 20 patients by Baker and Kelley (1). Four patients of the 20 receiving 40 mg. daily by mouth showed regression of the disease (Table X). All the patients who responded were in the oldest age group and showed various evidences of estrogen effects.

The second of the estrogenic compounds studied was estriol, 16α-methyl-, 3-methyl ether (Fig. 11). This material, also known as Manvene, was

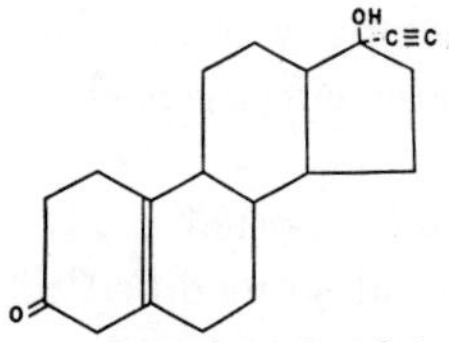

Fig. 10.   5(10)-Estren-3-one,   17α-ethynyl-17β-hydroxy-   (Norethynodrel).

TABLE X

Norethynodrel: Summary of Objective Remissions per Number of Patients[a, b]

| Dominant Lesions | Years postmenopausal | | | | Total | |
|---|---|---|---|---|---|---|
| | < 1 | 1–5 | 6–10 | > 10 | Number | % |
| Local | — | 0/1 | — | 2/6 | 2/7 | 29 |
| Osseous | 0/1 | 0/2 | — | 0/3 | 0/6 | 0 |
| Visceral | 0/1 | 0/1 | 0/1 | 2/4 | 2/7 | 0 |
| Total | | | | | | |
|   Number | 0/2 | 0/4 | 0/1 | 4/13 | 4/20 | — |
|   Per cent | 0 | 0 | 0 | 31 | — | 20 |

[a] Data from Baker and Kelley (1).

[b] Dosage: 40 mg. per day by mouth.

studied by Dao (5), who used 50 mg. of this material orally each day. Four of 25 patients treated responded favorably to the medication, a regression rate of 16 % (Table XI). As was noted for the previous compound, all the

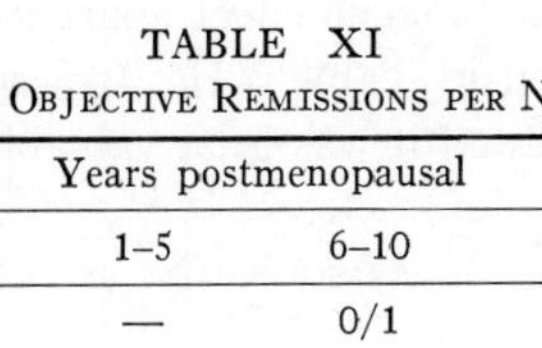

Fig. 11.   Estriol, 16α-methyl-, 3-methyl ether (Manvene).

TABLE XI

Manvene: Summary of Objective Remissions per Number of Patients[a, b]

| Dominant Lesions | Years postmenopausal | | | | Total | |
|---|---|---|---|---|---|---|
| | < 1 | 1–5 | 6–10 | > 10 | Number | % |
| Local | 0/1 | — | 0/1 | 0/4 | 0/6 | 0 |
| Osseous | — | — | 0/3 | 0/5 | 0/8 | 0 |
| Visceral | 0/1 | 0/1 | — | 4/9 | 4/11 | 36 |
| Total | | | | | | |
|   Number | 0/2 | 0/1 | 0/4 | 4/18 | 4/25 | — |
|   Per cent | 0 | 0 | 0 | 22 | — | 16 |

[a] Data from Dao (5).

[b] Dosage: 50 mg. per day by mouth.

patients who responded to therapy were over ten years postmenopausal. This was the only compound whose effectiveness was demonstrated in patients with visceral involvement.

The last of the compounds reported deals with $\Delta^1$-testololactone. The insertion of a C-1,2 double bond so modified the activity of this material as compared with the parent compound testololactone, that it resulted in the second most effective antitumor drug studied (Fig. 12). As pointed out by Segaloff (10), who used the compound in a dosage of 100 mg. intramuscularly three times a week, one of the most interesting aspects of its use was the

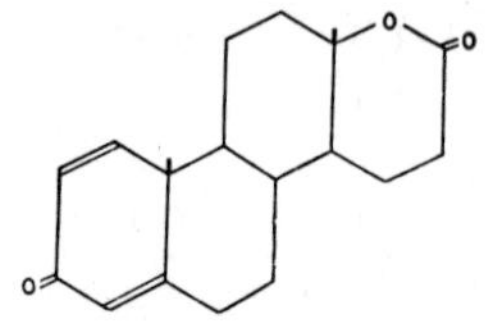

FIG. 12. 13,17-Seco-1,4-androstadien-17-oic acid, 13α-hydroxy-3-keto-, lactone ($\Delta^1$-testololactone).

TABLE XII

$\Delta^1$-TESTOLOLACTONE: SUMMARY OF OBJECTIVE REMISSIONS PER NUMBER OF PATIENTS[a, b]

| Dominant Lesions | Years postmenopausal | | | | Total | |
|---|---|---|---|---|---|---|
| | < 1 | 1–5 | 6–10 | > 10 | Number | % |
| Local | — | 1/2 | — | 2/3 | 3/5 | 60 |
| Osseous | 1/2 | — | 1/1 | 1/5 | 3/8 | 38 |
| Visceral | 0/1 | 0/2 | 0/1 | 1/6 | 1/10 | 10 |
| Total | | | | | | |
| Number | 1/3 | 1/4 | 1/2 | 4/14 | 7/23 | — |
| Per cent | 33 | 25 | 50 | 29 | — | 30 |

[a] Data from Segaloff (10).
[b] Dosage: 100 mg. intramuscularly three times per week.

total lack of any observable biologic effect apart from its antitumor activity. The results are summarized in Table XII. Its greatest effect was noted in patients with local disease, and it was least valuable in patients with visceral involvement.

## DISCUSSION

This brief summary of results represents the experience gained with 282 patients who have received these new compounds. The over-all rate of regression of disease in this entire group was 19 %, a figure quite comparable to that obtained with testosterone propionate, and reassuring to the investigator that experimental therapy on the whole has been at least as good as standard therapy. The relationship of molecular structure and biologic effect is slowly becoming more clear, and it is apparent that definite hints for effective substitution can be found in the evaluation of data such as those presented here. It is expected that it will be progressively more feasible to make use of such information in the preparation of more effective antitumor compounds which have side effects less distressing than was observed in many of those studied in this effort to date.

The 92 regressions achieved in the entire group of the 490 patients making up both the experimental and the control series are classified in table XIII.

TABLE XIII

RESULTS OF THERAPY: CLASSIFICATION (PERCENTAGE) OF 92 REMISSIONS[a]

| Dominant Lesions | Years postmenopausal | | | | Total |
|---|---|---|---|---|---|
| | < 1 | 1–5 | 6–10 | > 10 | |
| Local | 0 | 8 | 29 | 29 | 23 |
| Osseous | 15 | 24 | 26 | 18 | 20 |
| Visceral | 0 | 15 | 4 | 20 | 14 |
| Total | 7 | 16 | 20 | 23 | 19 |

[a] Total number of patients: 208 in control group; 282 in group treated with twelve new steroids.

Only 7 % of the patients treated in the group "less than one year post-menopausal," that is those with progressive disease in the first year after castration, had regression of their disease. As the postmenopausal interval increased, the rate of response improved from this low figure of 7 % to a high of 23 %. This same trend holds for the experimental or the control series considered separately. If the results obtained are divided according to site of dominant lesions, it is apparent that those patients with visceral disease did less well than the others, with a remission rate of 14 % compared to 23 % for local (skin or breast) recurrence and 20 % for bone disease. It is also apparent that in the individual reports are suggestions that one or another compound would seem to have more promise in treating certain manifestations of the advanced disease than others. For example, 19-nor-testosterone, 17-methyl-, produced regression of disease in 40 % of local recurrences, bromoketoprogesterone a 50 % rate, and $\Delta^1$-testololactone, a 60 % rate. In osseous disease, 2-methyldihydrotestosterone was effective in two-thirds of the patients treated, while the use of Manvene (estriol, 16α-methyl-, 3-methyl ether) resulted in a remission in one-third of patients with visceral disease.

The course and activity of breast cancer in women is so variable and protean in nature as to suggest that this is not one disease, but several. It is certainly premature to indicate a specific drug for treatment of each age group and dominant lesion, but it is reasonable to expect that these studies, when extended, will eventually point the way toward this goal.

## SUMMARY AND CONCLUSIONS

A study of the use of twelve new steroids in 282 patients with advanced breast cancer has been reported. The remission rate of 18 % achieved in the control group of 208 patients treated with testosterone propionate was approximated in the over-all by the new compounds, the use of which resulted in 19 % remission. Individually, there were two very promising materials studied. One of these, $\Delta^1$-testololactone, resulted in a remission rate of 30 % and apparently demonstrated no other biological action. The most effective drug was $2\alpha$-methyldihydrotestosterone, which caused objective regression of disease in 44 % of patients treated.

### ACKNOWLEDGMENTS

The assistance of the statistical section of the Cancer Chemotherapy National Service Center in the compilation of data for this report is gratefully acknowledged.

### REFERENCES

1. Baker, W., and Kelley, R. Personal communication.
2. Blackburn, C., and Childs, D.S. *Proc. Staff Meetings Mayo Clinic* **34**, 113 (1959).
3. Brennan, M. Personal communication.
4. Carter, A. C. Personal communication.
5. Dao, T. Personal communication.
6. Hayes, M., and Goldenberg, I. Personal communication.
7. Huseby, R., Tyler, F., and Volk, H. Personal communication.
8. Lewin, I. Personal communication.
9. Olson, K., and Ansfield, F. Personal communication.
10. Segaloff, A. Personal communication.

### DISCUSSION*

**B. J. Kennedy:** I would like to compliment both Dr. Rosoff and Dr. Segaloff on their very nice presentation of this material. Dr. Segaloff made reference to the A.M.A. study. This was the first study of the cooperative type. Much of the present study was the result of those earlier efforts. There is a good deal of similarity between the two studies, and I do hope that at some point Dr. Segaloff might request that the A.M.A. study be presented at one of its meetings. That testosterone has produced an increasing regression rate in the postmenopausal patient is comparable to results shown in the A.M.A. study. One difference between the two groups is that the Public Health study does include local disease and in the A.M.A. study, primary breast lesions or local recurrence groups were not included. Testosterone appears to have produced a very high regression rate among the local lesions, as you demonstrated from your chart.

One thing that is lacking in the present study is a comparison of estrogenic compounds and androgens. The importance of this is obvious, and I think that this has still to be done under the same conditions as those of the testosterone study. Am I right in understanding that the two estrogenic compounds that were studied were compared to testosterone and not to stilbestrol as a standard?

---

\* This discussion followed the reports by Drs. Segaloff and Rosoff.

**A. Segaloff:** The two compounds were compared with testosterone propionate. I think you all ought to remember that the studies presented here include only the completed ones. There are additional studies of estrogen being done.

**S. J. Taylor, III:** I went into this group study with a lot of trepidation and have become more enthusiastic as time has gone on; but I feel there is one point that Dr. Kennedy has brought up, which is very obviously missing here, that I have been trying to put across since the first meeting. We could have used diethylstilbestrol as our control, along with some of the groups that are using testosterone propionate, and, having that as a control, a comparison between testosterone and diethylstibestrol would now have been available.

**R. Hertz:** What I need to know, in order to be able to evaluate the significance of these groups of 20 patients on each substance, is how much variation there would be from group to group if you were simply to take serially, in groups of 20 each, the patients that you pooled on testosterone propionate. What would the variation be around your 20% figure in such groups? I think it is a basic requirement that we have some idea of intrinsic variability of the control data.

**A. Segaloff:** I don't remember all the figures; also, not all the groups have completed their first study. As I recall, the study with the smallest number of regressions had 3 of their 22 or 23 patients with regression. The one with the largest had, I think, 7. This is well within the random distribution for the groups. We have had none that have differed significantly from what one would expect.

**H. M. Lemon:** Following up Dr. Kennedy's remarks, I would like to point out that there is a second area in the studies which we are trying to help fill out, and that is with reference to adrenal corticoid therapy in breast cancer. During the last five years there are a number of encouraging and documented remissions reported in reputable journals in this country and abroad concerning the usefulness of cortisol or prednisone against breast cancer. I would like to point out that Dr. Lieberman, the other night, showed in one of his charts that the average daily output of adrenal cortisol was in the range of 20–25 mg. per day and most patients that have survived adrenalectomy and hypophysectomy usually receive somewhat larger maintenance doses of cortisol; so that I think we have to consider in interpreting any ablative type of treatment the simultaneous administration of an agent which also has direct antiestrogenic activity. There is a lot of very nice work in the literature, such as published studies by Szego and Roberts, Hisaw and his collaborators from Harvard, and Huggins and Jensen, on this topic. These studies all show that cortisol acts on the rat uterus as an effective local estrogen antagonist. I think this is a very real possibility.

The other thing that struck me yesterday was the large number of adrenal cortical compounds that showed antitumor activity against human and animal cancers, including mammary tumors; they were more numerous than the available estrogens and androgens tested. I would like to emphasize that one of the problems that faces anyone who tries to evaluate adrenal corticoid therapy in breast cancer, is that the postmenopausal ovary which is not inhibited continues to secrete estrogens. Dr. Herbert Wotiz in our laboratory, has ample proof now that human postmenopause ovaries will synthesize estrone and estradiol from radioactive acetate in the presence of human chorionic gonadotropin. Dr. Marrian has been skeptical of our technique, but two of his co-workers have recently reduplicated our procedure and have confirmed our findings, studying polycystic ovaries from patients who are in a younger age group. At present I wonder if the low rate of regressions, noted in the last two papers in the years immediately following the menopause is due to continued estrogenic activity in some patients. We all know, and Dr. Pincus has emphasized, the very high ratio of androgen that is necessary to block estrogen stimulation, if indeed estrogens have anything to do with mammary cancer.

Finally, I would just like to emphasize that in our present thinking the best sequential therapy for the control or palliation of most patients with mammary cancer is (1) oophorectomy, not prophylactically but oophorectomy at the time there is progressive distant metastatic disease, (2) some form of sex hormone therapy, when these patients relapse from oophorectomy, and finally, (3) adrenal corticoid therapy which we and some other people believe is as effective as adrenalectomy plus oophorectomy or hypophysectomy, either in survival or objective remission rate.

**A. Segaloff:** This gives me an opportunity to point out again that all our reports to date are in the form of progress reports. We are a long way from having final answers, indeed as Dr. Lemon knows, since his group is the one that is studying prednisolone. In this regard we also have under way a study which maybe we can report on at another meeting; in this, adrenal corticoids, estrogens, and androgens are being compared in patients previously treated with hormones.

**O. Mühlbock:** I was much impressed by the very good results you get in the group of local recurrences as compared with recurrences in the bones. In a recent analysis Dr. Gerbranoy made of 200 cases at our institute, it was found that response to hormone treatment in cases with local recurrences was very poor as compared with the group with recurrences in bones. After mastectomy all patients are irradiated, and we thought that maybe this was the reason for poor response to hormonal treatment. I would like to have your comment on this.

**C. B. Rosoff:** It should be made clear that recurrences termed "local" in the slides shown were so labeled for the sake of brevity. This classification includes instances of skin or breast involvement at any site, not just the operative area. I have no explanation for Dr. Mühlbock's observation of a poor response to hormonal therapy of skin recurrences in previously irradiated skin, but our data do show that there is a considerable variation of response depending on the steroid employed.

**W. H. Fishman:** The purpose of the conference, as Dr. Pincus has mentioned several times, is to relate the biological activity of steroids to cancer. The data that were presented today provide the information which has been missing from the picture visible to people studying biological activities of steroids with a view to making correlations with cancer. I am stimulated to present briefly some of our work, as a result of seeing these data of Drs. Segaloff and Rosoff for the first time.

The biological activity with which we are concerned is the kidney β-glucuronidase response [Fishman, W. H., *Ann. N.Y. Acad. Sci.* **54**, 548 (1951) ; Fishman, W. H., and Farmelant, M. H., *Endocrinology* **52**, 536 (1953)]. The kidney is an end organ for the action of androgen, i.e., the so-called adrenotropic activity described years ago by Kochakian and others. The enzyme β-glucuronidase increases very strikingly in the kidney in inbred strains of mice in response to the administration of androgens. If the average activity of the Ajax mouse is 3000 plus or minus 300 Fishman units per gram, responses up to 50,000 units per gram can be obtained depending upon the experimental conditions [Fishman, W. H., Artenstein, M., and Green, S., *Endocrinology* **57**, 646 (1955)]. The kidney β-glucuronidase is a specific protein whose amount actually does increase as a result of androgen administration, on the basis of $C^{14}$-glycine experiments which are in progress in the laboratory. When we first encountered this phenomenon we were interested in its specificity and studied some 85 steroids including a great many pregnane derivatives. Briefly, estrogens were inactive, progesterone was inactive, and a few of the corticoids were weakly active. The greatest activity was seen with testosterone, methyltestosterone, and particularly the esterified testosterones. The correlation of structure and biological activity was very striking—to us at any rate. First of all, epitestosterone was negative, the 17-keto androgens were less active than testosterone, and the introduction of the methyl group at position 17 enhanced activity. Ring A hydroxyls didn't seem to be too important with regard to enhancing activity. Elimination of the angular 19-methyl group gave more potency. The conclusion we drew in 1955 was that the kidney $\beta$-glucuronidase response was definitely not correlated with the virilizing property of androgen, and we implied that it might be associated with the protein anabolic property of these steroids.

In the intervening years a number of compounds have become available, which are characterized by a higher ratio of protein anabolic to virilizing activity. I refer to the various nortestosterones, substituted position 17. We determined [Fishman, W. H., and Lipkind, J., *J. Biol. Chem.* **232**, 729 (1958)] that these were more potent than testosterone by the kidney glucuronidase response, with eight- to elevenfold increases in response to the nortestosterone compared to threefold increase of the kidney in response to testosterone under standard conditions. More recently several compounds were made available to the laboratory which were reputed to be progestins. On assay we found that all these were very potent (Table A). Protein anabolic activity was reported in a publication of Dr. Bartter for the 17α-vinylnortestosterone, and 17α-ethynylnortestoster-

TABLE A

| No. Compound | Renal $\beta$-glucuronidase factor | Response units[b] | Protein in | Anabolism in the Rat | Therapeutic value[c] (TP = +) |
|---|---|---|---|---|---|
| 1 Control (no steroid) | 1.0[a] | — | Yes | Yes | |
| 2 Testosterone | 3.0 | 3.0 | Yes | Yes | |
| 3 19-Nortestosterone | 4.1 | | Yes | Yes | |
| 4 Methyltestosterone | 6.3 | 24.0 | Yes | Yes | |
| 5 17α-Ethynyl-19-nortestosterone | 7.6 | 15.16 | Yes | Little | + |
| 6 17α-Vinyl-19-nortestosterone | 10.8 | Q.N.S. | Yes | Little | + |
| 7 9α-Fluoro-11β-hydroxy-17α-methyl-testosterone | 10.9 | Q.N.S. | Yes | Yes | + |
| 8 2α-Methyldihydro-testosterone | 10.4 | 40.3 | Yes | Yes | + + |
| 9 2α,17α-Dimethyldi-hydrotestosterone | 15.0 | 127.5 | Yes | Yes | |

[a] Mean kidney $\beta$-glucuronidase activity, 3100 ± 300 units per gram.

[b] The reciprocal of the dosage in milligrams required to produce a kidney assaying 10,000 units per gram, multiplied by 24.

[c] Rosoff's data.

one in man but not in the rat (levator ani test). Both of these gave us very good kidney β-glucuronidase responses. In our view, at the present time the response is correlated much more closely with the protein anabolic activity of steroids in man than with any other property of these steroids. What correlation existed between kidney β-glucuronidase response and effectiveness of steroids in cancer of the breast, I could only guess at since the information wasn't available until today. The compounds which we have assayed and which show potencies greater than testosterone tend to be those which are, as a rule as effective as testosterone propionate in cancer of the breast. Particular note should be taken of 2α-methyldihydrotestosterone which gave us a very good result. In this regard, the most potent compound we have assayed is the 2α,17α-dimethyldihydrotestosterone. I don't know what the clinical result is with this compound, but on the basis of what we know we would predict that it would be at least as active as testosterone propionate in cancer of the breast. Consequently, I feel that this kidney enzyme response offers new information that is not ordinarily forthcoming from presently available bioassay methods.

**G. S. Gordan:** Before reporting the thirteenth protocol series, I would like to reply to Dr. Fishman that if you use the original Eisenberg and Gordan levator ani test instead of the Hershberg modification, 19-nortestosterone is a potent androgen and stimulates the growth of levator ani muscle extremely well.

The test compound used by the University of California group was fluoxymesterone (9α-fluoro-11β-hydroxy-17α-methyltestosterone), also known as Halotestin (Upjohn), Oratestryl (Squibb), or Ultandren (Ciba). This compound was given in a dose of 40 mg. per day and was compared with testosterone propionate, 100 mg. intramuscularly three times a week. In 21 patients it produced 3 regressions, a rate of 14 %; testosterone propionate produced 5 regressions in 24 patients (21 %). These rates are, of course, not significantly different.

I would like to ask Dr. Segaloff, as chairman of the cooperative group, whether his data indicating only 7 % regressions in patients less than one year after castration indicate that we should abandon administrative hormonal therapy for young women.

**A. Segaloff:** Actually, Dr. Gordan, I don't know of anything in this group that is this good. I think this would indicate that you should continue to use such patients. In our experience this group, subsequently treated with promising nonhormonal forms of chemotherapy, fare equally poorly in comparison with others.

**G. Pincus:** One of the familiar biological phenomena that we observe with steroids is dosage-response curves. Now all these data are at a single dosage. I presume from what I hear that the groups cannot report on dosage variations in this study, but I wonder if any of you have data with testosterone propionate that would indicate some dosage response. I am particularly struck by this because in the case of progesterone the regression rate was zero with 2 gm. by mouth per day. On the basis of some studies that we undertook on the biological activity of oral progesterone in women it has 1/50 to 1/200 the activity of injectible progesterone upon the endometrium, so that you would be giving roughly the equivalent of 10 mg. by injection three times a week. This is a rather low dose. Results with higher dosage levels would be most interesting.

**A. Segaloff:** I would disagree with the idea that 2 gm. of progesterone orally is no more effective than 10 mg. injected. We have been able to produce in a rather high percentage of patients decidual casts of the endometrium on 2 gm. of oral progesterone a day. I have never seen this with 10 mg. intramuscularly. We have ourselves, before these present studies were initiated, given progesterone in larger doses intramuscularly and have seen an occasional remission. I might point out that one of the problems one encounters here, and this is why oral progesterone was used, is that it is exceedingly difficult to get women to take parenteral progesterone, in doses of any size, very long. It just can't be done. If you will find some way of doing it, we will be glad to try.

The dosage-response problem I agree is a real one, and one which should be investigated. One is in a very difficult situation where he is torn between the problem of virilization and that of decreased response. Since the dosage employed here seems to be an optimal one that neither excessively virilized nor gave away too much in terms of response, it was employed. Actually in our newer compounds, for which we are starting with more extensive studies, we are investigating dosage-response relationships.

**P. C. Merker:** Dr. Mühlbock has presented the very interesting observation that prior radiation therapy seems to block the efficacy of steroid treatment of breast cancer. Has this observation been made by other investigators here?

**G. C. Escher:** This particular question was raised by Ted Nathanson years ago, and several of us in the old cooperative group attempted to answer it. We could never satisfy ourselves that there was any difference in response to areas that had been irradiated as opposed to those that had not been irradiated.

I would like briefly to raise a few other points. I think, from the discussion we have had today, we can see that it will be possible in the not too distant future to compare adequately the relative efficacy of additive androgen therapy and the more extensive ablative procedures. In doing this, I think if one is going to estimate survival one must include every patient subjected to the therapeutic procedure.

**R. Hertz:** I still need a little more statistical help, Dr. Segaloff. I understood you to say that if you divide the control series into separate groups of 20, you would have a variation of 3 positives to 7 positives within the separate groups of 20. That is a difference of 4 out of 20 cases within your control reporting groups. Your progesterone is zero, your over-all average is 5 out of 20; you tell me on one hand you can't tell the difference between zero and 5 out of 20. I think I need a little statistical help to differentiate these considerations.

**A. Segaloff:** I must say that the problem is a very simple one. We haven't been presenting either the statistical background or what was wanted in these studies. We have presented our results to date for you to look at. I will try to explain the statistical basis on which this study was built. This study was not designed to compare androgens or other agents with the reference standard in any way other than to reject those less active than testosterone and to offer a valid preliminary basis for selecting others for more definitive study. The objective upon which this protocol was based was an attempt to find compounds that are better than the presently available compounds. Therefore, the study was designed to do two things. First, to get for the first time an adequately controlled comparable group of reference data. Secondly, to reject those compounds which either because of their toxicity or because of their low rate of response are significantly poorer than the reference compound, so that a decision can then be made that compounds which look promising can be studied on a large enough sample to show whether a given compound is better than the reference material. The data presented today, for example, would show in the size sample and the way it was done for progesterone, in the dose given with a zero response, that it was rejected because it was significantly less effective than our reference standard. There are some agents that look as good as testosterone, and among these 19-nor-17α-methyltestosterone is very interesting. This type of compound is being discarded from further study because of obvious toxicity that has showed up in the studies. Two compounds have been selected for further study. One is 2α-methyldihydrotestosterone propionate, which seems in the preliminary trial to be better than the control substance. The other is the $\Delta^1$-testololactone, which does not seem to be significantly better, but does have a very interesting absence of other biological activity. I think that, in terms of our objective, this study gives a suitable answer.

**R. Huseby:** I think that the analysis of the data need not be strictly according to the statistician. In the progesterone study a number of the failures were treated with another hormone as secondary therapy and eight regressions were obtained. This would indicate that in this group of 29 patients there were at least 8 patients with hormone responsive tumors which had not responded to progesterone. To our way of thinking this increases the probability that the first compound that we were giving was inactive.

**S. J. Taylor, III:** I would like to answer the criticism about not including the operative deaths in the survival figure. The survival figures were done for one purpose: to compare the relative effectiveness of the two procedures, that is, adrenalectomy versus hypophysectomy and sex steroid therapy. You cannot compare the relative effectiveness in a patient who does not live long enough to have the effectiveness of the ablative procedure or steroid therapy show up. Now, from the point of view of survival alone, of course, operative deaths would have to be included.

**M. J. Brennan:** Dr. Taylor's indication that hypophysectomy and adrenalectomy produce essentially comparable results would appear to be borne out by figures that I saw at Dr. Adkins' clinic in which the response and survival curves on these patients were very closely parallel, with the hypophysectomy perhaps a little better. I am sure Dr. Pearson may have some comments on them himself. Secondly, I think one of the things bothering Dr. Hertz and myself about these figures is that Dr. Blackburn has a regression rate with his androgen that is better than we get with adrenalectomy and hypophysectomy. This is something that is hard to accept. The problem that this poses for interpretation becomes apparent when we consider that there appeared to be a smaller frequency of responses in the testosterone group than would have been expected and a higher frequency of responses in the test compound. If by some accident the higher frequency of responses in the test compound was due to hormonally sensitive cases having been concentrated in that group, we can see that it would have a marked effect on these figures on a small sample. We think that the thing that counts is that we see 2 or 3 regressions in 20 patients. When we see that, we are satisfied that we have an active compound. We never think that on the basis of 40 patients we can make any valid prediction of the ultimate usefulness of the compound as compared in a large series against testosterone propionate.

I would like to ask the Chairman or others to comment on one problem. Wee have done 45 hypophysectomies in the past five years. Initially, we started it as a heroic procedure which was indicated more by sympathetic considerations than by scientific decisions. We were fortunate to get two very good remissions on the first two patients. Later the odds caught up with us and we haven't done a great many hypophysectomies in the past two years. The greater part of the series was in that early group. Initially we were operating on very sick people, very far advanced disease. We now select these subjects much more restrictively. I don't know if our criteria are right and would like to hear some comment about other people's ideas about the proper sequence of therapeutic management in this disease.

**A. Segaloff:** Rather than being surprised, I will be delighted if we find compounds that are better than hypophysectomy; I would say that this means that although we have had a nice hypothesis, which some agree with and some don't, of hormonal dependency as the reason why hormones work, it may have to be replaced. This is why I like to talk about hormonal *responsiveness;* this is actually what we are measuring. The small sample is not designed to give you a definitive answer but does give you enough of an indication to extend the study, and that is why several of your colleagues are extending Dr. Blackburn's study.

**O. Pearson:** I believe that it is difficult to outline the optimum endocrine therapy for patients with metastatic breast cancer at the present time. The reports by Drs. Taylor, Segaloff, and Rosoff constitute very preliminary and incomplete results and are not suitable for comparison at the present time. I believe that there is fairly general agreement that oophorectomy is superior to hormone administration in the premenopausal patient with metastatic breast cancer because this procedure yields a higher incidence and longer duration of remissions. In the previously castrated patient or in the postmenopausal patient, it is my opinion that removal of endocrine glands (i.e., ovaries and adrenals or the pituitary) yields better results than hormone administration. However, further evaluation of the results of both additive and ablative therapy in this setting is needed before general agreement can be reached. In the treatment of the patient, other factors must be considered and weighed, such as the undesirable virilizing effects of androgen administration, the risks of surgery, and the requirement for hormonal replacement therapy. Further evaluation of the preliminary results reported here should provide an answer to this problem. It is also to be hoped that these studies will lead to new approaches to the treatment of these patients. If optimum results can be obtained without resort to surgery, I am sure that everyone concerned will be most pleased.

**H. M. Lemon:** I was unable to determine from Dr. Leiter's slides just how many of the steroids Dr. Rosoff has reported showed any activity in the animal tumor screening program. It seems to me that here is a very important consideration, i.e., whether this human program is detecting anticancer activity that has not shown up in the animal screening program.

**J. Leiter:** I didn't intend to present any specific data, merely illustrative data; and I didn't gear my talk to this because I presented a thesis that the screening we were doing probably had very little to do with the endocrinological properties of material; we were just screening for an effective chemical. I still believe this, and I don't think this would demonstrate anything that could be considered an endocrine response.

**U. Kim:** In order to obtain some base line, we have done comparative studies of various ablative therapies simultaneously on a given hormone-responsive mammary carcinoma. We grafted a given tumor to many isologous rats of same age and sex, divided them into five groups, and performed hypophysectomy, oophorectomy, adrenalectomy and/or gave them androgen therapy. From this experiment we have observed that hypophysectomy was the most beneficial ablative measure in mammary tumor inhibition, oophorectomy or androgen therapy next, and adrenalectomy last.

**E. Jensen:** In regard to the relative merits of ablative therapy versus hormonal chemotherapy, I would like to express a thought, which may reflect my own bias as a chemist rather than a surgeon:

> "A lady, with growth neoplastic,
> Thought castration to be a bit drastic.
> She would fain cure her ill
> Just by taking a pill,
> Which isn't completely fantastic."

**S. Werner:** I had hoped Dr. Lemon would repeat his question since I didn't quite get the answer as to what the animal screen showed for these compounds.

**A. Segaloff:** As I remember it, none of these compounds was positive in the standard screen.

**A. P. Harris:** I thought Dr. Taylor made an important point about the latent period between surgery for the initial lesion and the recurrence, showing that therapy was more effective in groups in which the latent period was longest. The curve Dr. Segaloff showed implied that in his series he had long latent periods. I wonder if this is so; and if not, has the question of latent period been analyzed with respect to therapy?

**A. Segaloff:** We unfortunately do not have data on the interval between the mastectomy and the first recurrence. The data on the interval between the original diagnosis and the time they have a sufficient recurrence for us to be treating them, do not show a significant difference between the responders and the nonresponders.

**D. J. Taylor:** Actually I have to come to our defense on the results on the clinical steroids. Dr. Leiter did have a slide for this program which he did not get to show. We had some 33 steroids that are represented in the clinical compounds. Of those 33, as I recall, there were 6 or 8, all corticoids, that were active in one or more of the test systems. There were several, I know, that were positive in both S-180 and in Ca-755.

**G. W. Woolley:** In consideration of $\Delta^1$-testololactone, we do have a few preliminary experimental observations that might be worth recording. Dr. Merker made an observation that $\Delta^1$-testololactone when used in the cortisone-conditioned mouse appeared to increase liver pathology. We tested this against our experimental breast tumor in the mouse ($C_3HBA$). $\Delta^1$-Testololactone at 500 mg./kg. was almost without effect as an inhibitor of this tumor. Cortisone acetate at 25 mg./kg. per day was a good inhibitor over the 10-day test period. When combined at the above two dosages, tumor inhibition was increased over that expected for cortisone alone. This additive effect was obtained in two successive tests. The respective inhibitions were $\Delta^1$-testololactone 17 % or negative, cortisone 60 %, and the two combined 79 %.

**L. J. Lerner:** The interesting observations just reported by Dr. Woolley, together with those reported by Dr. Rosoff, prompt me to make a few remarks about our laboratory findings with $\Delta^1$-testololactone. Biologic tests have shown that this compound is not androgenic, antiandrogenic, estrogenic, antiestrogenic, progestational, antiprogestational, glucocorticoid, mineralocorticoid, antimineralocorticoid, gonadotropin inhibitory, or hypocholesterolemic. In fact we have found no biological activity for this compound when it is administered by itself to the test animal. However, when $\Delta^1$-testololactone is administered to castrated immature male rats together with testosterone, the resultant accessory sex organ weights are augmented above that obtained with testosterone alone. This augmentation of an androgen, and, as Dr. Woolley has reported, the augmentation of a corticoid by this otherwise "inactive" compound is unusual and should be explored further.

**K. B. Olson:** Drs. Rosoff and Segaloff have presented a large amount of important material. Dr. Rosoff recognized the pitfalls of this as well as I, when he emphasized that local lesions responded well. It should be borne in mind that many of the patients with osseous and visceral lesions also had skin lesions with local recurrences which did not necessarily respond. In discussing this with Dr. Anne Carter we have wondered if, sometime in this study, it might not be possible to tabulate the ancillary lesions as well as the dominant lesions. The local lesions were the dominant lesion in the cases presented by Dr. Rosoff and the only lesion really in those patients. This does not indicate the results noted in all local lesions.

Finally, I should like to disagree with Dr. Kennedy. I think the figures on testosterone are quite significant and different from results that I know of in the A.M.A. study. At the outset of this study group, there were a number of investigators who felt it was criminal to give androgen to people in the older age group, and this was on the basis of the A.M.A. study. They felt that estrogens were so much superior that we were actually doing a real disservice. I think the study of Dr. Segaloff on testosterone has demonstrated that it is as good although it may not be any better.

**B. J. Kennedy:** I disagree with Dr. Olson. Testosterone was not contraindicated in the older age group, but estrogens were contraindicated in the young group. As a result more patients in the older group received estrogen. There are comparative data for both compounds in the postmenopausal group. The data show that the older patient responds more freqeuntly to an androgen than does the younger patient.

I would like to ask one last question. In comparing an unknown to testosterone propionate there is a 6-week cut-off period, at the end of which time, if the patient hasn't responded, the investigator can stop the agent. Is it possible that some of the very good compounds act faster, so that within the first 6-week period an improvement would appear, while the same investigator at the end of 6 weeks may be discouraged with testosterone and drop it? If he had treated the same patient for longer period of time an improvement might have occurred. This was an arbitrary figure of 6 weeks.

**A. Segaloff:** There doesn't appear to be any difference in the time at which you get your first regression. Of the now about 1150 patients that we have had, there have been two patients who initially were thought to be progressing but were kept on therapy longer, and who subsequently went on to good objective remission. I don't think this is a big danger because they represent only two out of the over 200 patients with objective remissions.

If I may, I would like to close by commenting that I personally am unable to bring a meeting like this to a close without paying homage to the late Dr. Nathanson to whom we are all tremendously indebted. He really started us off on this type of clinical investigation, and I hope and believe that he would be proud of what we have presented here.

**C. B. Rosoff:** In closing, it is pertinent to point out that this effort has demonstrated that it is quite feasible for a group of cooperating investigators to work together on this type of problem. Their unified efforts and common protocol does speed the accumulation of data and need not affect their scientific integrity.

If this approach to patient selection and evaluation of therapy were applied to ablative treatment, we would all be able to view these efforts in a clearer light and reach some valid conclusions as to the best means of coping with the advanced stages of breast cancer.

# Evaluation of 4-Androstene-3β,17β-diol Diacetate in the Treatment of Advanced Breast Cancer

KENNETH B. OLSON, AND FRED J. ANSFIELD

*Albany Medical College, Albany, New York, and University of Wisconsin Medical School, Madison, Wisconsin*

As a study initiated by the cooperative group studying breast cancer with the assistance of the Cancer Chemotherapy Section of the United States Public Health Service, the compound, 4-androstene-3β,17β-diol diacetate, hereinafter referred to as the "test" compound, was selected for trial on patients with advanced breast cancer. Endocrinological assays of the test compound furnished by the Service Center indicated that it produced a marked increase in androgenic and myogenic activity in castrate rats as compared to testosterone propionate. This effect was profound with subcutaneous injection and hardly apparent with oral administration. The inhibition of androgenic and myogenic effects as measured by the inhibiting effect of the test material on androgen--stimulated secondary sex structures and muscle in castrate rats was slight and the same with oral and subcutaneous administration. There was no uterotropic effect as measured by the uterine weight changes of immature mice. The antiuterotropic effect noted on the estrogen-stimulated secondary sex structures in immature mice was appreciably less than that of testosterone propionate. There was no alteration of glycogen deposition in the liver of adrenalectomized rats and the thymolytic and anti-inflammatory stimulating and inhibiting effects were negligible. In summary, this material appeared to have a significant effect in increasing the weight of the ventral prostate, seminal vesicle, and levator ani muscle of castrate rats when administered subcutaneously, but otherwise had minimal or no endocrinological activity.

## METHODS

Methods of evaluation were those outlined in a protocol agreed upon by the cooperative study group. Patients were admitted to the study if they demonstrated progressive disease in the previous 6 months with measurable lesions that could be tabulated or recorded by means of photographs or radiographs. Cases having had previous hormone or ablative procedures (except castration) were excluded. No menstruating women were accepted, but could be admitted to the study if they demonstrated progressive disease 6 weeks or more after surgical or adequate radiation castration. All cases eligible for the study and under the control of the investigator were admitted to the study regardless of their condition. Previous X-ray therapy, chemotherapy, or surgical treatment did not exclude patients providing that

385

measurable, untreated, progressive lesions existed. In several cases with multiple osseous lesions, radiation therapy was given concurrently with hormone therapy to involved weight-bearing skeletal areas when other measurable lesions beyond the zone of radiation were present for evaluation. Histological evidence of the original disease and of recurrent lesions when possible was obtained in all cases. Radiographic skeletal surveys, photographs, and measurements were obtained prior to therapy and at 6-week intervals thereafter in all cases. Serial serum protein-bound iodine studies were obtained on 6 patients before and after drug treatment, and serum calcium, phosphorus, alkaline phosphatase, albumin and globulin determinations, and hemograms were obtained before and after treatment in most patients.

Cases were randomized according to menstrual age and dominant lesion (i.e., osseous, soft tissue, or visceral) prior to the start of therapy, and a code number indicated the compound to be used so that the investigator did not know whether the patient was receiving the test compound or testosterone propionate, both of which were administered intramuscularly in a dose of 100 mg. (2 ml.) three times per week. In the event that a patient died before receiving at least 2 weeks of therapy, another case was admitted so that a minimum of 20 patients receiving the test compound and 20 receiving testosterone propionate for more than 2 weeks were admitted to the study. A patient was considered to be in remission only when there was diminution in size of at least 50 % of measurable lesions or recalcification of lytic osseous lesions and the absence of any new lesions. This state had to be evident for at least two observations separated by at least a month.

## RESULTS

A summary of the results (Table I) indicates that 4 of 23 patients obtained a remission with testosterone and 5 of 23 with the test compound. Four remissions in 24 cases treated were observed at Madison, Wisconsin, and 5 remissions were observed at Albany, New York, where 22 cases were treated, indicating astonishing agreement between findings in the two institutions. Four cases received treatment for less than 2 weeks; the longest period of treatment was 68 weeks.

The average interval from the original diagnosis to start of treatment was 34.7 months in the testosterone-treated group, and 29.3 months in the test compound-treated group. The median periods were 16 and 18 months, respectively. Of the 23 patients who received testosterone propionate, 4 (17.4 %) experienced a remission of disease (the 95 % confidence interval for this percentage is 5 %–38 %). On the other hand, of the 23 patients who were treated with the test compound, 5 (21.7 %) had a remission (the 95 %

confidence interval for this percentage is 7 %–44 %). There was no significant statistical difference in the response of patients to the test compound
as compared to testosterone propionate. Five of the nine remissions occurred
in patients with osseous lesions, but this is of no significance because the
largest number of patients admitted were in the osseous group. The length

TABLE I

COMPARISON OF 4-ANDROSTENE-3β,17β-DIOL DIACETATE AND TESTOSTERONE PROPIONATE
IN ADVANCED BREAST CANCER[a]

| Site | Menopausal age | | | | Total | % Remission |
|---|---|---|---|---|---|---|
| | $< 1$ | 1–5 | 6–10 | $> 10$ | | |
| Testosterone propionate | | | | | | |
| Breast, skin, lymph nodes | 0/2 | 0/1 | 0/1 | 0/1 | 0/5 | 0.0 |
| Osseous | 1/3 | 1/2 | 0/2 | 1/3 | 3/10 | 30.0 |
| Visceral | 0/2 | 0/2 | 0/2 | 1/2 | 1/8 | 12.5 |
| | 1/7 | 1/5 | 0/5 | 2/6 | 4/23 | (17.4%) |
| 4-Androstene-3β,17β-diol Diacetate | | | | | | |
| Breast, skin, lymph nodes | 0/0 | 0/3 | 0/1 | 3/4 | 3/8 | 37.5 |
| Osseous | 0/3 | 1/3 | 0/1 | 1/4 | 2/11 | 18.2 |
| Visceral | 0/1 | 0/2[b] | 0/1 | 0/0 | 0/4 | 0.0 |
| | 0/4 | 1/8 | 0/3 | 4/8 | 5/23 | (21.7%) |

[a] Remissions per total cases.
[b] One patient remained unchanged for 68 weeks of therapy.

of hormone treatment for those cases receiving more than 2 weeks of
therapy is indicated in Table II. The length of remission in cases treated
with the test compound appears to be slightly longer than in those cases
treated with testosterone propionate, but the small number of cases involved
and the wide range does not allow a statistical conclusion.

In all patients receiving treatment for 4 weeks or more, there was some
degree of virilization and the impression was gained that the test compound
might be more androgenic than testosterone. In 20 cases, hirsutism, acne,
hoarseness, and libido were tabulated crudely on a one to four plus basis.
The pluses were added and divided by the weeks of treatment before the
code was broken. The ratio 0.3 divided the cases into two groups, and it was
assumed that those patients with a ratio of less than 0.3 received testosterone and those with a higher ratio, the test compound. The guesses were
right in 10 cases and wrong in an equal number, indicating that the test

compound was no more or less virilizing than testosterone as judged by this crude measure.

TABLE II

LENGTH OF TREATMENT

| Statistics | Testosterone propionate | 4-Androstene-3β,17β-diol diacetate |
|---|---|---|
| Remissions | | |
| Total cases | 4 | 5 |
| Range | 18–60 wk. | 17–81 wk. |
| Median | 20 wk. | 30 wk. |
| Mean | 31.2 wk. | 40.6 wk. |
| Progressions | | |
| Total cases | 16 | 17[a] |
| Range | 4–23 wk. | 4–68 wk. |
| Median | 6.0 wk. | 6.0 wk. |
| Mean | 9.1 wk. | 10.0 wk. |

[a] Includes 1 case classed as unchanged after 68 weeks of therapy.

Fluid retention of some degree occurred in about half the cases, but was severe in only 4 cases and was divided between the two groups. Hypercalcemia was not observed.

## SUMMARY

4-Androstene-3β,17β-diol diacetate was found to produce approximately the same rate of remission in advanced breast cancer as testosterone propionate in 46 patients divided into two equal groups and treated in a double-blind study. The remission rate for testosterone was 17.4 % and for the test compound 21.7 %. Duration of remission was slightly longer in the group treated with the test compound. Virilism and fluid retention had about the same incidence and severity in both groups of patients treated.

### ACKNOWLEDGMENTS

This investigation was supported by research grants Cyp-4594 and Cyp-3365, from the National Institutes of Health, United States Public Health Service.

We wish to acknowledge, with thanks, statistical advice and assistance given by Nancy Engel and Opal Rasch of the Cancer Chemotherapy National Service Center.

# $\Delta^1$-Testololactone, Androsterone, and 5α-Androstane-3α, 17β-diol Dipropionate in the Treatment of Advanced Breast Cancer[1]

ALBERT SEGALOFF, J. B. WEETH, P. J. MURISON, AND E. L. RONGONE

*Alton Ochsner Medical Foundation, and Tulane University School of Medicine,
New Orleans, Louisiana*

As members of the Cooperative Breast Cancer Group, we made our first study on Protocol I a comparison between androsterone, 5α-androstane-3α,17β-diol dipropionate, and $\Delta^1$-testololactone. The androsterone and the $\Delta^1$-testololactone were prepared as 50 mg./ml. aqueous suspensions and the androstanediol as a 50 mg./ml. solution in sesame oil. All three steroids were given intramuscularly, 100 mg. three times weekly, except during periods of urine collections for study of hormonal excretion, when 50 mg. were given daily.

The randomization and evaluation procedures of the Cooperative Breast Cancer Group were followed.

Studies of hormonal excretion were done following the standard procedures of our laboratory (1).

## RESULTS

Table I shows the distribution of the patients and their responses among the three compounds and the twelve randomization categories. As has fre-

TABLE I

DISTRIBUTION AND RESPONSE OF PATIENTS IN STUDY[a]

| Years postmenopausal | < 1 | | | 1–5 | | | 5–10 | | | > 10 | | | Totals |
|---|---|---|---|---|---|---|---|---|---|---|---|---|---|
| Dominant lesions[b] | L | O | V | L | O | V | L | O | V | L | O | V | |
| $\Delta^1$-Testololactone | — | 1/2 | 0/1 | 1/2 | — | 0/2 | — | 1/1 | 0/1 | 2/3 | 1/5 | 1/6 | 7/23 |
| 5α-Androstane-3α, 17β-diol-dipropionate | 0/1 | 0/2 | 0/2 | — | 0/2 | 1/2 | 0/1 | 0/1 | 0/1 | 0/3 | 0/4 | 0/5 | 1/24 |
| Androsterone | 0/2 | 0/1 | 0/1 | 0/2 | 0/1 | 0/1 | 0/1 | 0/1 | — | 0/4 | 0/3 | 1/5 | 1/22 |

[a] Objective remissions/number of patients.

[b] Lesions: L = local; O = osseous; V = visceral.

quently been the case at our institution, half of the patients fell into the more-than-10-year postmenopausal group.

There is a significantly greater objective response rate for the $\Delta^1$-testololactone than for the other two compounds. Seven of 23 patients showed

---

[1] This study was aided in part by a grant from the American Cancer Society, Inc., New York; and in part by a research grant (CY-3364) from the National Cancer Institute of the National Institutes of Health, United States Public Health Service.

TABLE II

| Drug | Creatinine (gm./24 hr.) | | Creatine (gm./24 hr.) | | Urine calcium (mg./24 hr.) | | Pregnanediol (mg./24 hr.) | |
|---|---|---|---|---|---|---|---|---|
| | Before | During | Before | During | Before | During | Before | During |
| Δ¹-Testololactone objective remissions | 0.81(7) | 0.91(7) | 0.09(7) | 0.08(7) | 157(3) | 244(3) | 0.40(7) | 0.35(7) |
| Δ¹-Testololactone failures | 0.83(5) | 0.63(5) | 0.18(5) | 0.21(5) | 222(5) | 140(5) | 0.35(5) | 1.14(5) |
| 5α-Androstane-3α, 17β-diol dipropionate | 0.81(13) | 0.86(13) | 0.12(13) | 0.21(13) | 183(10) | 109(10) | 0.27(13) | 0.52(13) |
| Androsterone | 0.76(16) | 0.79(16) | 0.18(16) | 0.13(16) | 112(9) | 152(9) | 0.32(16) | 0.68(16) |

TABLE III

| Drug | 17 Ketosteroids (mg./24 hr.) | | Formaldehydogenic corticoids (mg. DOC/24 hr.)[a] | | Porter-Silber (mg./24 hr.) | | Fluorometric phenols (μg./24 hr.) | |
|---|---|---|---|---|---|---|---|---|
| | Before | During | Before | During | Before | During | Before | During |
| Δ¹-Testololactone, objective remissions | 6.6(7) | 8.2(7) | 0.47(7) | 0.66(7) | 0.63(7) | 0.43(7) | 62(7) | 130(7) |
| Δ¹-Testololactone, failures | 11.0(5) | 11.1(5) | 0.96(5) | 0.63(5) | 1.18(5) | 0.47(5) | 76(5) | 68(5) |
| 5α-Androstane-3α, 17β-diol dipropionate | 5.9(13) | 9.8(13) | 0.74(13) | 0.85(13) | 0.46(13) | 0.47(13) | 109(13) | 129(13) |
| Androsterone | 5.5(16) | 15.5(16) | 0.46(16) | 0.54(16) | 0.50(16) | 0.61(16) | 51(16) | 40(16) |

[a] DOC, Deoxycorticosterone.

objective remission on the $\Delta^1$-testololactone. In sharp contrast, androsterone produced only 1 objective remission out of 22 patients; and androstanediol produced only one objective remission out of 24 patients treated.

TABLE IV

| Drug | Gonad-stimulating hormones (M.U./24 hr.) | | Prolactin (I.U./24 hr.) | | Luteinizing hormones (µg./24 hr.) | |
|---|---|---|---|---|---|---|
| | Before | During | Before | During | Before | During |
| $\Delta^1$-Testololactone, objective remissions | 146(7) | 160(7) | 36(4) | 37(4) | 381(7) | 193(7) |
| $\Delta^1$-Testololactone, failures | 31(3) | 134(3) | 21(3) | 25(3) | 117(3) | 92(3) |
| 5α-Androstane-3α, 17β-diol dipropionate | 154(13) | 165(13) | 35(12) | 51(12) | 273(10) | 139(10) |
| Androsterone | 64(16) | 89(16) | 40(14) | 37(14) | 168(14) | 103(14) |

Tables II–IV show that there was no substantial effect of the therapies on creatine, creatinine, calcium, pregnanediol, corticoids (by either the formaldehydogenic or the Porter-Silber method), fluorometric phenols, gonad-stimulating hormone (as mouse units or as hypophysectomized male rat ventral prostate stimulating material), or prolactin. The only substantial effect on urinary excretion patterns was seen in the 17-ketosteroids, where $\Delta^1$-testololactone had no effect, androstanediol produced a modest increase, and androsterone produced a threefold increase.

$\Delta^1$-Testololactone showed no evidence of virilizing the patients whereas the other two agents showed a mild virilizing propensity.

## Summary

$\Delta^1$-Testololactone seemed remarkably free of biologic activity other than the production of objective remission of advancing breast cancer in 7 of 23 patients treated.

Androsterone and 5α-androstane-3α,17β-diol dipropionate produced significantly smaller remission rates—only 1 each of 22 and 24 patients treated, respectively. The latter two compounds were mildly virilizing and increased the 17-ketosteroid excretion but produced no other significant change in the urinary hormonal pattern.

### Acknowledgments

We would like to thank E. R. Squibb and Company, through the courtesy of Dr. Josef Fried, for their gift of the $\Delta^1$-testololactone; Syntex, S.A., through Dr. Carl Djerassi and Dr. Howard Ringold, for their gift of the androsterone and the 5α-androstane-3α,17β-diol dipropionate. We are appreciative of Dr. George C. Escher's effort in reviewing our clinical material. We should also like to thank the staff of the Cancer Chemotherapy National Service Center for their assistance in many matters concerned with the prosecution of this study.

REFERENCE

1. Segaloff, A., Bowers, C. Y., Rongone, E. L., and Murison, P. J. *Cancer* **12**, 735 (1959).

# An Evaluation of 9α-Bromo-11-ketoprogesterone in the Treatment of Metastatic Breast Carcinoma[1]

Ira S. Goldenberg and Mark A. Hayes

*Department of Surgery, Yale University School of Medicine, New Haven, Connecticut*

Progesterone has had limited application in the therapy of metastatic breast carcinoma because potent, easily administered forms have not been developed. While halogenating steroids to enhance their action, Fried *et al.* (2) synthesized 9α-bromo-11-ketoprogesterone (Fig. 1), which was found to have powerful progestational qualities (4). Because of the apparent regression of metastatic breast carcinoma which followed early use of this preparation by Jonsson *et al.* (3), it was felt that further controlled evalua-

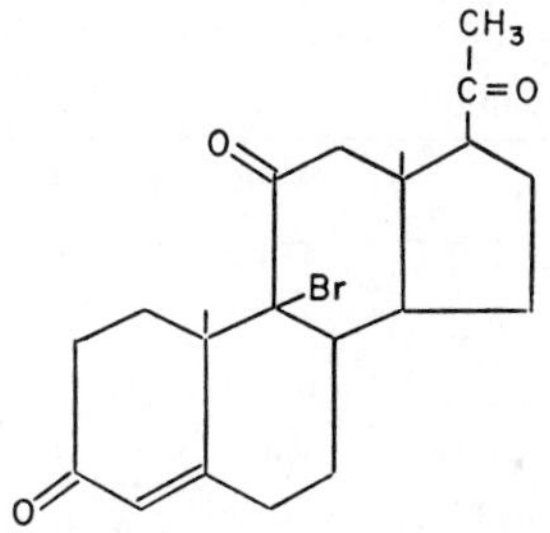

FIG. 1.   9α-Bromo-11-ketoprogesterone.

tion of its efficacy was indicated. As a result the drug was included in the Cooperative Study sponsored by the Cancer Chemotherapy National Service Center.

Testosterone propionate was chosen as the standard against which the halogenated progesterone was compared. Patients received either testosterone propionate or the new preparation according to statistical randomization schedules based on menopausal age and dominant metastatic lesion.

An arbitrary daily dosage schedule of 300 mg. of the progesterone administered orally was utilized to be compared to 100 mg. of testosterone propionate administered three times weekly intramuscularly. Only patients demonstrating objective evidence of improvement of metastatic foci were included as remissions.

It has been suggested in the past that hormone therapy of breast cancer is effective only when functional pituitary suppression occurs. To test this

---

[1] This investigation was supported by a research grant (CY-3360) from the National Cancer Institute, of the National Institutes of Health, United States Public Health Service, and was made possible by the cooperation of the physicians of Connecticut.

hypothesis 24-hour urine excretion of pituitary gonadotropin was determined prior to starting therapy and at varying periods during therapy in 10 patients. The method of Albert (1) was utilized for these determinations.

## RESULTS

A total of 49 patients were studied—24 received testosterone propionate and 25, the halogenated progesterone. Objective remission was present in 25 % of the patients receiving testosterone propionate (6 of 24), and 20 % of those receiving progesterone had remissions (5 of 25). This difference of one greater could be expected to occur by chance in 20 to 50 % of similar experiments and hence the difference is not statistically significant.

Of the 10 patients in whom serial determinations of urinary gonadotropins were completed, a definite decrease was noted in 9 (Table I). This group

TABLE I
POSITIVE DILUTION—MOUSE UTERINE WEIGHT

| Name | Age | Menopausal status[a] | Weeks of therapy | | | | | HPG[b] |
| | | | 0 | 1–4 | 5–8 | 9–12 | 13+ | |
|---|---|---|---|---|---|---|---|---|
| B.O.P.[c] Failures | | | | | | | | |
| M.B. | 55 | 10+ | 276 | 0 | — | — | — | Decrease |
| O.B. | 77 | 10+ | 138 | 69 | 17 | — | — | Decrease |
| E.C. | 57 | 5–10 | 138 | — | — | — | 9 | Decrease |
| A.G. | 65 | 10+ | 17 | 9 | — | — | — | Decrease |
| A.M. | 57 | 10+ | 69 | 17 | 276 | — | — | Decrease |
| R.S. | 43 | R.C. | 69 | — | — | — | 17 | Decrease |
| B.O.P. Remissions | | | | | | | | |
| L.B. | 58 | 5–10 | 17 | 276 | 17 | 69 | 17 | Increase |
| T.B. | 72 | 10+ | 52 | 13 | — | — | — | Decrease |
| M.G. | 50 | 5–10 | 138 | 0 | — | — | — | Decrease |
| J.H. | 64 | S.C. | 138 | 69 | — | — | — | Decrease |

[a] Figures indicate years postmenopausal; R.C.—radiation castration, S.C.—surgical castration.

[b] Human pituitary gonadotropin.

[c] B.O.P.—9α-Bromo-11-ketoprogesterone.

included 3 patients in whom an objective remission of the metastases occurred and 6 patients who had no remission.

Side effects including hypokalemia, sodium retention with edema formation, and gastrointestinal disturbances reported in the early use of the progesterone occurred here in only 6 women. One patient developed anasarca which remained to the time of death. Nausea and vomiting forced discontinuation of the medication in 2 patients.

## COMMENTS

Although the progesterone proved to be less effective than testosterone propionate in this study, it offers some value in treating metastatic breast cancer. Its virtue may be its use in those patients who have failed to respond to other forms of hormone therapy. It is possible that the remission rate could be increased if a higher dosage schedule were utilized.

## SUMMARY

A halogenated progesterone, 9α-bromo-11-ketoprogesterone was evaluated for its efficacy in the therapy of metastatic breast cancer. It was found to be about as effective as testosterone propionate in causing remissions.

### REFERENCES

1. Albert, A. *Recent Progr. in Hormone Research* **12**, 227 (1956).
2. Fried, J., Kessler, W. B., and Borman, A. *Ann. N. Y. Acad. Sci.* **71**, 494 (1958).
3. Jonsson, U., Colsky, J., Lessner, H. E., Roath, O. S., Alper, R. G., and Jones, R., Jr. *Cancer* **12**, 509 (1959).
4. Wied, G. L., and Davis, M. E. *Obstet. Gynecol. Survey* **10**, 411 (1957).

# Comparison of the Antitumor Effects of 17α-Methyl-19-Nortestosterone and Testosterone Propionate in Advanced Mammary Carcinoma[1,2]

ANNE C. CARTER, ELAINE BOSSAK FELDMAN, AND GEORGE C. ESCHER

*The State University of New York, College of Medicine at New York City, and The Medical Service (Division II) Kings County Hospital, Brooklyn, New York*

Studies of the antitumor effects of 17α-methyl-19-nortestosterone (17-MNT) the experimental compound, and testosterone propionate (TP), the reference standard, were carried out in 43 women with advanced progressive metastatic carcinoma of the breast placed on one or the other steroid according to a randomized scheme (2). Patients were admitted to the study in accordance with the criteria listed in the protocol for a Cooperative Study to Evaluate Experimental Steroids in the Therapy of Advanced Breast Carcinoma. Base-line studies, measurements, and evaluation of response were made also in accordance with the requirements of the protocol. The records and roentgenograms of the patients were reviewed by one other investigator.[3]

The 21 subjects receiving 17-MNT ranged in age from 39 to 79 years, with a mean age of 61 years. The 22 subjects on therapy with TP ranged in age from 35 to 82 years with a mean age of 59 years. Dosage of 17-MNT was 10 mg. thrice daily by mouth. Patients were treated for from 2 to 30 weeks with a mean treatment period of 13 weeks. The total dose administered ranged from 300 to 6610 mg. TP was administered intramuscularly in doses of 100 mg. thrice weekly. The treatment period ranged from 2 days to 65 weeks with a mean duration of 22 weeks. The total dose ranged from 300 mg. to 19,600 mg. Two patients of the original group are still under therapy.

In terms of menopausal age and dominant lesion of the two groups of patients, the comparability is presented in Tables I and II.

Of the group treated with 17-MNT, progression of disease occurred in 12 patients; 1 patient died during the first 2 weeks of therapy and 3 died 4,

[1] This work was supported in part by Grant CY3601 from The National Cancer Institute, The National Institutes of Health, United States Public Health Service.

[2] These studies were part of a Cooperative Study to Evaluate Experimental Steroids in the Therapy of Advanced Breast Carcinoma, sponsored by the Cancer Chemotherapy National Service Center, which supplied the 17α-methyl-19-nortestosterone (Parke Davis & Co.) and testosterone propionate.

[3] We should like to thank Dr. Kenneth Olson, The Albany Medical College of Union University, Albany, New York, for reviewing the records and roentgenograms of all of the patients.

6, and 10 weeks after therapy was instituted. No change occurred in 3 patients. In 1 subject there was a mixed response. Objective regression occurred in 5 patients. Of these, 3 subjects were classified more than 10 years menopausal, dominant breast, and 1 each in the category 6–10 years menopausal, dominant breast, and 1 to 5 years menopausal, dominant osseous (Table I). Regressions lasted for from 10 to 30 weeks with an average duration of 21 weeks. In two instances, therapy was terminated because jaundice developed while the patients were still in regression.

TABLE I

INCIDENCE OF OBJECTIVE REGRESSION IN 21 SUBJECTS RECEIVING 17α-METHYL-19-NORTESTOSTERONE[a] CLASSIFIED ACCORDING TO MENOPAUSAL AGE AND DOMINANT METASTATIC LESION

| Dominant lesion | Menopausal age in years | | | | Total |
| | < 1 | 1–5 | 6–10 | > 10 | |
| --- | --- | --- | --- | --- | --- |
| Breast | 0/1 | 0/1 | 1/1 | 3/7 | 4/10 |
| Osseous | 0/1 | 1/1 | 0/1 | 0/3 | 1/6 |
| Visceral | 0/1 | 0/1 | 0/1 | 0/2 | 0/5 |
| | 0/3 | 1/3 | 1/3 | 3/12 | 5/21 |

[a] Dosage: 30 mg. daily per os.

Of the group treated with TP, progression of disease occurred in 13 patients, of whom 2 died during the first 2 weeks of therapy and 4 died 3, 4, 4, and 8 weeks after therapy was instituted. No change occurred in 3 patients, and in 1 subject there was a mixed response. Regression occurred in 5 patients. Four subjects were more than 10 years menopausal, 2 dominant visceral and 2 dominant osseous. One subject was castrated less than 1 year, dominant osseous (Table II). Regressions lasted for from 19 to 49 weeks with an average duration of 36 weeks. Two patients, still on therapy, show continuing regression for 37 and 49 weeks.

TABLE II

INCIDENCE OF OBJECTIVE REGRESSION IN 22 SUBJECTS RECEIVING TESTOSTERONE PROPIONATE[a] CLASSIFIED ACCORDING TO MENOPAUSAL AGE AND DOMINANT METASTATIC LESION

| Dominant lesion | Menopausal age in years | | | | Total |
| | < 1 | 1–5 | 6–10 | > 10 | |
| --- | --- | --- | --- | --- | --- |
| Breast | 0/1 | 0/0 | 0/0 | 0/2 | 0/3 |
| Osseous | 1/2 | 0/2 | 0/1 | 2/4 | 3/9 |
| Visceral | 0/2 | 0/1 | 0/1 | 2/6 | 2/10 |
| | 1/5 | 0/3 | 0/2 | 4/12 | 5/22 |

[a] Dosage: 300 mg. weekly, intramuscularly.

Adverse effects observed in patients receiving 17-MNT included retention of fluid in 11 subjects, elevation of bilirubin above 1 mg. % in 10 women, and signs of virilization in 7 subjects. Retention of fluid occurred in 8 subjects given TP, and signs of virilization were noted in 10 women. One subject developed hypercalcemia while receiving TP.

The endocrinologic and metabolic effects of 17-MNT and TP in these subjects are reported elsewhere (1).

## SUMMARY

Objective regression of disease lasting an average of 21 weeks occurred in 5 of 21 women with advanced metastatic breast carcinoma treated with 17α-methyl-19-nortestosterone. Jaundice in 2 of these women necessitated cessation of therapy. Retention of fluid and virilization were prominent adverse effects of the drug. In comparison, testosterone propionate induced regression of an average duration of 36 weeks in 5 of 22 women. Somewhat less retention of fluid and more virilization accompanied the use of this hormone.

## REFERENCES

1. Feldman, E. B., and Carter, A. C. *J. Clin. Endocrinol. and Metab.* **20**, 842 (1960).
2. Segaloff, A. *Ann. N.Y. Acad. Sci.* **76**, 717 (1958).

# The Cooperative Study Program in Therapy of Advanced Prostatic Cancer

HERBERT BRENDLER

*New York University School of Medicine, Bellevue Medical Center, New York, New York*

## INTRODUCTION

Prostatic cancer constitutes a problem of increasing magnitude. The annual mortality from this disease in the United States is about 11,000, or 12 % of the number of men over 50 dying each year of all causes (650,000) whose prostates contain histological evidence of cancer (90,000). Although only 1 in 8 men with clinical or occult cancer of the prostate presently succumbs to the disease, it is important to recognize that the total number of deaths attributable to this condition has risen steadily with the years. Perhaps the chief reason for this has been the fact that, as life expectancy has increased, hitherto quiescent cases have had time to become clinically active. Clinical prostatic cancer is recognized as one of the most common forms of malignancy in men over 50, if not the most common. This is true, not only in this country, but in those Western European countries possessing reliable tumor registries, such as Denmark, where prostatic cancer incidence is almost identical with our own (4, 5).

Since 1940, the initial therapy of advanced prostatic cancer has been characterized by the use of methods designed to nullify the effects of endogenous androgens, i.e., castration and estrogen administration. A favorable response has been observed in the majority of patients so treated, perhaps 60–80 %. Nevertheless, after varying periods of remission, the disease has become reactivated. The subsequent treatment of relapse need not be recited in detail, except to point out that it has largely been directed at the elimination of extragonadal androgen production and utilization by the use of such measures as intensified estrogen therapy, cortisone administration, adrenalectomy, and hypophysectomy. The treatment of such reactivated cases has generally proved disappointing owing, perhaps, not so much to the failure to counteract persistent androgenic stimulation, as to mutational changes favoring the survival of cancer cells which have achieved a considerable degree of "androgen independence." Satisfactory responses have occurred following the use of the methods described, but not with regularity or for an appreciable time. Some patients in relapse have actually benefited from such unorthodox therapy as testosterone (1), progesterone (10), or certain of the newer testosterone derivatives (2). Abrupt cessation of all administrative therapy has even on occasion been followed by general clinical improvement.

Observations such as those just described have prompted sporadic therapeutic trials; most of these studies, unfortunately, have suffered from lack of
sufficient case material, unsatisfactory experimental design, and inadequate
financial support. It is paradoxical, indeed, that there exist no accurate
therapeutic evaluations based on the application of accepted principles of
medical statistics in the very field, i.e., prostatic cancer, where, in 1941, there
occurred the first conclusive demonstration of the value of endocrine therapy
in human cancer (8). It is also sobering to reflect that a number of otherwise promising leads in the treatment of reactivated prostatic cancer may
have been discredited and discarded in the past without fair and thorough
evaluation.

## Organization of the Study

In 1956, plans were begun for a nation-wide, cooperative study program
in prostatic cancer, the first such effort in this country, to be conducted
under the auspices of the Cancer Chemotherapy National Service Center
(CCNSC). During 1957, a preliminary study protocol was drafted and the
membership of the study group completed. In May, 1958, the final protocol
was approved by the Experimental Design Committee of the Clinical Studies
Panel, and, in September of that year, the first clinical trial was begun.

The Prostate Cancer Study has the following aims:

1. To conduct studies in the therapy of advanced prostatic cancer, using
patients who have either relapsed following previous therapy, or who have
proved refractory to such measures from the outset. Previously untreated
cases are not included, inasmuch as most of these (60–80 %) respond satisfactorily to castration, with or without estrogen supplementation; to uncover
an agent which might conceivably improve on this regime would require an
exorbitant case load and many years of study.

Determinations, as quantitative as possible, are to be made of: (a) The
short-term response to promising agents, according to appropriate objective
and subjective criteria. (b) The duration of response in those patients in
whom such therapy may prove effective.

2. To discover, during the course of the study, improvements in study
methods which may be useful in similar cooperative programs.

The twelve research centers listed in the tabulation on the following page
are presently participating in the Cooperative Study.

Since the earliest planning stages of the Study, the Statistical Center,
which is located at New York University, has participated closely in all
phases of the cooperative program, including protocol design, drafting and
supplying standard record forms, random allocation of patients at all participating institutions, constant surveillance of data, processing of study

records and analysis of data, statistical evaluation of results, and rendering periodic reports to cooperating investigators and the Cancer Chemotherapy National Service Center. Dr. Donald Mainland is Consultant Biometrician and Miss Elisabeth Street, Executive Biometrician.

| Research center | Principal investigator |
| --- | --- |
| New York University | Dr. Herbert Brendler |
| University of Iowa | Dr. Rubin Flocks |
| University of California | Dr. Willard Goodwin |
| (Los Angeles) | |
| Northwestern University | Dr. John Grayhack |
| Vanderbilt University | Dr. A. Page Harris |
| University of Oregon | Dr. Clarence Hodges |
| Columbia University | Dr. Perry Hudson |
| University of Rochester | Dr. Donald McDonald |
| University of Miami | Dr. George Prout |
| Johns Hopkins University | Dr. William W. Scott |
| University of Kansas | Dr. William Valk |
| Memorial Center (New York) | Dr. Willet F. Whitmore, Jr. |

The Pathology Center, which is located at Columbia University (Francis Delafield Hospital), reviews histological slides on all potential study patients to confirm the tissue diagnosis. No patient may be admitted to the Study without such confirmation. Dr. Arthur Purdy Stout and Dr. Edith Sproul are Consultant Pathologists.

## CLINICAL TRIALS

The selection of patients for the Study is rigidly controlled. All patients with a presumptive diagnosis of advanced, (i.e., surgically incurable), disseminated (osseous or soft-parts) cancer of the prostate, are considered potential candidates for the Study and must be registered. Acceptance of such patients into the Study is determined from the criteria for admission enumerated in the protocol. If a patient is found acceptable, but is not admitted to the Study, the Statistical Center must be so notified, and a summary of the case submitted, together with the reason(s) for rejection.

The principal criteria for admission to the Study include:

1. Evidence of advanced, disseminated prostatic cancer, with histological confirmation.

2. A history of surgical castration, at least 6 weeks prior to admission to the Study.

3. Evidence of active progression of the disease, as determined from selected criteria enumerated in the protocol, such as increasing size of primary growth, increasing size or number of metastases, elevated serum acid phosphatase, etc. Quiescent cases do not qualify for the Study because

failure of an experimental compound to induce a beneficial response may be attributable to the latent state of the cancer, rather than to a lack of carcinostatic potency of the agent under investigation. As expected, this criterion has resulted in a temporary loss of about 75–90 % of the total prostatic cancer population to the formal clinical trials. Eventually, however, most of these patients will become reactivated and thereby qualify for admission.

4. A period of at least 2 weeks prior to admission into the Study, during which time no anticancer therapy, e.g., estrogens, shall have been administered.

All potential patients for the Study must first receive a careful preliminary evaluation, in order to determine whether they exhibit the necessary criteria for admission to the clinical trials. A record is made of dates of onset and initial diagnosis. The nature of prior therapy is determined as accurately as possible. The degree of pain is classified according to sedation requirements. The physical examination stresses such items as mental attitude, ambulatory status, weight (and height), soft-part metastases, rectal findings, neurological signs, and amount of residual urine. The laboratory studies include a hemogram, urea nitrogen determination, serum acid and alkaline phosphatase assays, skeletal survey, chest X-ray, and intravenous urogram. The foregoing items represent only minimal procedure; all members are encouraged to make whatever supplementary studies they desire, provided that such studies do not bias, or interfere with, those required by the protocol.

At present, no attempt is made to stratify patients according to such factors as age, duration of disease, morphological characteristics of the primary, original extent of metastases, prior serum acid phosphatase levels, and quality of response to previous therapy. One reason for the decision not to stratify patients has been the unreliability of histories elicited from these elderly men and their families, and the difficulty experienced in obtaining accurate information uniformly from the original physician. Another reason has been the wish to preserve as large a number of patients as possible for statistical purposes. Most important of all is the lack of valid data supporting stratification along the lines indicated above. Subsequent experience may prompt changes in the present arrangement.

Each clinical trial has been designed as a double-blind comparison of the effectiveness of two different therapies. Each trial is planned so that it may be carried out simultaneously at all participating institutions. This method of simultaneous testing has been adopted by the Study Group, at least for the present, in order to assure ample case material for statistical analysis. The first and second clinical trials, for example, will each require a total of 200 patients, in order to provide a 97.3 % chance of showing a significant (14 %) difference between compounds (9). This number of patients will also facilitate early testing of the protocol. Although this requirement may seem somewhat stringent, it must be pointed out that the Study Group not only is interested in discovering an effective compound, but also is concerned lest one, perhaps only slightly better than stilbestrol, be missed. This is a most important consideration in reactivated prostatic cancer, where no form of therapy, however dubious, seems available at the moment.

It is recognized that simultaneous testing may temporarily hamper individual investigators interested in special compounds; however, none of the participants, but one, possesses large enough individual case loads to warrant separate trials. Moreover, the comparatively short duration of each trial (4 weeks, if no improvement is noted) should permit inclusion of any one patient in five to six trials annually. Eventually, as the registries build up at the participating institutions, it is hoped that an ample number of patients will be available for separate drug testing, or at least testing by groups of two to four institutions. Finally, it must be pointed out that, apart from the formal trials, the individual participants are free to carry out ancillary pilot studies on compounds of their own choosing, in as confidential a manner as they may desire. Such individual pilot studies are encouraged by the Group, for only by unrestricted inquiries of this nature can promising compounds be brought to light. The Study Program, while being conducted as a collaborative venture, nevertheless seeks to preserve the autonomy of individual participants insofar as is compatible with the joint effort.

The first three trials, which are currently in progress, consist of evaluations of the following:

I.   stilbestrol 5 mg./day vs. placebo (oral)

II.  stilbestrol 5 mg./day vs. stilbestrol 500 mg./day (oral)

III. testosterone propionate 300 mg./week vs. stilbestrol 30 mg./week (parenteral)

Subsequent trials now being planned involve the use of potent corticoid and progestational agents, as well as newer steroids manifesting a variety of biological properties in experimental animal studies.

Each study patient is re-evaluated 4 weeks after starting therapy, as specified in the protocol. If a patient has improved on study therapy, he is kept on that compound until the investigator decides it is no longer beneficial. During this period, the patient is evaluated again at 8 weeks, 12 weeks, and 16 weeks, then every 2 months as long as he stays on the compound.

## Method of Evaluation

There exists at this time no single criterion, or group of criteria, according to which the progress of the disease may be accurately determined. It was necessary in the beginning, therefore, to draft a scheme for evaluation of therapeutic effect, which would permit patients to be classified at the Statistical Center not only for purposes of statistical analysis, but also to facilitate selection of appropriate standard compounds for succeeding trials. Despite its somewhat arbitrary nature, every effort was made to conform to the spirit of the protocol, so that it was accordingly based on the criteria of active progression which qualify patients for admission to the Study.

It was realized soon after the first and second trials had begun, that collection of the necessary 200 patients would require 18 months or more. In order to save time in subsequent trials, as well as the effort and expense involved (especially should the compounds being evaluated appear to be ineffective early in the trial), it was determined to employ sequential testing in the third and succeeding trials. The details of this method, which is now in use in the Prostate Cancer Study, lie outside the scope of this paper. Briefly, however, sequential testing offers a good chance that fewer patients will be needed to reach a conclusion as to the relative effectiveness of two modes of therapy, than when a fixed sample size is employed, as is presently the case in Trials I and II. The disadvantages of sequential testing are first, that it occasionally requires *more* patients than the more conventional method; second, that it determines only the relative effectiveness of the two compounds and is complicated, sometimes unreliable, for analysis of other variables; third, that it may reach the verdict that a particular trial should be terminated and thus interfere with ancillary studies being run concurrently, which may require additional patients.

## Results

The Cooperative Study in prostatic cancer has completed its first year.

Of 122 patients admitted to Trial I, 99 have completed the trial. Of 66 patients admitted to Trial II, 58 have completed the trial. (Each of the foregoing trials requires a fixed sample size of 200 patients: 100 tests and 100 controls.)

Of 23 patients admitted to Trial III, 18 have completed the trial. (This trial is being evaluated by the sequential procedure, so that the number of patients required is not fixed.)

In view of the double-blind nature of the trials, the results will not be made known by the Statistical Center until the respective trials have been completed. Nevertheless, it is possible to record at this time a number of clinical impressions which have developed as the Study has progressed.

In Trial I (stilbestrol vs. placebo), which is well past the half-way mark, experiences with patients in whom the code has been broken for one reason or another, convey the distinct impression that stilbestrol is slightly, but definitely, more effective than placebo in the treatment of relapse. It is only fair, however, to point out that a few objective remissions have actually been observed in patients receiving placebo.

According to several of the participating institutions, estrogen withdrawal, which is required for at least 2 weeks prior to admission to the Study, has been followed promptly by serious relapses, even death in a few instances, raising the question of a causal relationship. Others in the Study Group, however, feel that such evidence is largely circumstantial. Whether a direct relationship exists between the two is a moot point at present, and more data are needed to resolve it. Patients who deteriorate when taken off prior estrogens, are now being removed from the Study and placed on appropriate therapy.

Testosterone, which is being evaluated in Trial III against stilbestrol, has been reported to cause adverse reactions in a number of patients, who have consequently had to be removed from the Study. Here again, opinion is divided. Studies in the past have shown that, although testosterone does, indeed, cause exacerbations in a few, it has little, if any, effect in most patients, and it may even be responsible for temporary subjective remissions in a small number, probably because of its anabolic properties (1). One patient, not included in the present study, experienced definite regression of skin metastases following testosterone administration; when treatment was discontinued, the metastases recurred, only to disappear again on resumption of testosterone (7).

As required by the protocol, a minimum of 6 weeks must elapse after castration before the disease may be considered to be progressing actively, and thereby qualify the patient for admission to the Study. This stipulation is based on clinical experiences in the past, which have seemed to indicate that a beneficial response to castration, including return of acid phosphatase values to normal levels, occurs quite promptly, usually within the first week or so. The present study has produced some doubts on this score. A number of patients have been observed in whom initially elevated serum acid phosphatase levels fell so slowly after castration, that the values were still abnormal by the end of the 6-week waiting period. One case, who was admitted to the Study on the basis of a still-elevated serum acid phosphatase level after castration, demonstrated what seemed to be an objective remission of bone metastases at the end of 4 weeks of placebo therapy; it was soon realized that this unquestionably represented a delayed castration response, acid phosphatase values also having receded to normal by the end of the 4-week treatment period. The 6-week waiting period after castration may have to be revised upward for subsequent trials.

Difficulties in interpretations of extent and density of bone metastases from X-rays have been experienced by all member institutions. Variations in X-ray technique from one patient to the next constitute a major factor; lack of definition caused by coalescence of individual tumor deposits, another. This problem is a serious one and demands further study. If unresolved, it may lead to the abandonment of this criterion as a measure of therapeutic effect.

## New Compounds

The Compound Evaluation Subcommittee of the Prostate Cancer Study Group meets five or six times annually, to consider available data on new steroids. Approximately 125 of these compounds have been carefully reviewed during the past 15 months. It is the practice of this Subcommittee to select those compounds which appear promising on the basis of chemical configuration and of available bioassay, experimental tumor, and toxicity data. The four members of the Study Group who are serving on the Subcommittee together with members of the CCNSC, carry out their own bioassays and clinical pilot studies of selected compounds and render reports at the meetings of the Subcommittee. Compounds which are deemed of special value are eventually recommended for consideration by the entire Study Group for inclusion in the program of clinical trials.

Difficulty has been experienced in making use of information derived from animal studies. Bioassay data may prove misleading because potent hormonal agents often exert little or no antitumor effect; in fact, the two are not necessarily correlated. Antitumor screening itself may be hard to assess unless one can be certain that the tumor being used represents a suitable yardstick, that is, resembles its human counterpart biologically or biochemically. More often than not the data derived from such studies ultimately cannot be transferred to the clinical level, leaving one with nothing more than an endocrine profile, as it were, of a particular animal tumor. The possibility exists that we may well become quite proficient at treating mouse and rat cancers, but not those found in man. This is not to say that animal bioassay and antitumor data are valueless. They simply must be used with care when selecting compounds for clinical trial. Although pilot studies of a clinical nature have thus far provided more useful information in the Prostate Cancer Study, this method has obvious limitations and must be supplemented by animal work. Heterologous transplantation of human tumors offers promise in the screening of steroidal agents; so far, however, human prostatic cancer has not proved amenable to this technique.

At present, no new compounds have been found in the clinical pilot trials which are consistently effective in the treatment of reactivated prostatic cancer. Objective remissions occur occasionally, subjective ones somewhat more often and probably on an anabolic basis. For example, the 17α-ethylated derivative of 19-nortestosterone (Norethandrolone) has been found to exert a favorable anabolic response in about 50 % of the patients in whom it has been used, and without the androgenic effects sometimes noted following testosterone (2). In one very sick patient treated by us recently with this compound, however, a severe exacerbation occurred 48 hours after starting therapy; this may have been caused by the compound, which is slightly androgenic, or it may have been coincidental. Objective remissions have not been observed in our series with Norethandrolone; very recently, however, an otherwise resistant patient treated elsewhere, experienced not only complete cessation of pain, but a drop in chronically elevated serum acid phosphatase values to normal (6). Norethandrolone effectively reduces the daily excretion of urinary 17-ketosteroids in all patients we have studied (2), a finding also reported by Brooks and Prunty (3). Animal bioassays show, moreover, that it partially inhibits testosterone in intact and castrated rats (2). These two observations may mean that Norethandrolone interferes with androgen utilization in the body, suggesting promise in the treatment of relapse.

It is rather difficult to reconcile the observed reductions in urinary 17-ketosteroids following Norethandrolone, with the view held by some that 17-ketosteroid levels constitute an index of prostatic cancer activity. The fact that the disease apparently continues unabated in the presence of such reductions may mean that reactivation is due to factors other than extragonadal androgens, perhaps mutational changes favoring androgen independence. This possibility is of practical importance in the search for new compounds, for it means that endocrine properties apart from antiandrogenicity have to be considered.

Various alkylating agents, antimetabolites, and antibiotics have been used sporadically in the last few years in prostatic cancer patients. Although the Study Group is presently concentrating its efforts on steroid evaluations, a number of its members are carrying out pilot trials of certain antitumor agents which do not fall into the steroid category. Should a promising agent be discovered as the result of the pilot studies now in progress, a formal trial of such a compound would be included in the Cooperative Program.

Apart from the manifest advantages of conducting clinical studies on a cooperative basis, there is one, perhaps not so apparent, which deserves special mention at this time. A group effort, such as the one described in this paper, provides the individual investigator with direct access to experimental information concerning new compounds, which would otherwise require years of wasteful and disorganized research effort. A group study thus facilitates the selection of compounds for clinical trial on a more reasoned basis than would otherwise be possible. The enormous number of new agents currently available—one is tempted at this point to say, after King Louis XV, *"après* Huggins, *le déluge"*—makes it important that compounds be selected with care, and for reasons based on sound experimental evidence. In a disease such as prostatic cancer where little, if any, real therapeutic progress has occurred in almost the last twenty years, compounds with strange names and even stranger formulas may prove too much to resist, unless one bears in mind the comparatively limited number of patients currently available for study.

REFERENCES

1. Brendler, H., Chase, W. E., and Scott, W. W. *A. M. A. Arch. Surg.* **61**, 433 (1950).
2. Brendler, H., and Winkler, B. S. *J. Clin. Endocrinol. and Metabolism* **19**, 183 (1959).
3. Brooks, R. B., and Prunty, F. T. G. *J. Endocrinol.* **15**, 385 (1957).
4. Clemmesen, J., and Nielsen, A. *Danish Med. Bull.* **3**, 36 (1956).
5. Dorn, H. F., and Cutler, S. J. Morbidity from Cancer in the U.S. *U. S. Public Health Monograph No.* **56** (1959).
6. Gordan, G. Personal communication.
7. Hudson, P. B. Personal communication.
8. Huggins, C., and Hodges, C. V. *Cancer Research* **1**, 293 (1941).
9. Mainland, F., Herrera, L., and Sutcliffe, M. I. Tables for Use with Binomial Samples. Dept. Med. Statis., New York Univ., New York, 1956.
10. Trunnell, J. B., and Duffy, B. J., Jr. *Trans. N. Y. Acad. Sci.* [2] **12**, 238 (1950).

DISCUSSION

**A. Segaloff:** I'd like to compliment Dr. Brendler on all that the prostate group has accomplished and to ask one question about the very elegant method of sequential analysis. Suppose you have had the misfortune of picking two compounds of approximately the same degree of activity, with sequential analysis you may then end up with a very large sample of patients, even larger than the one that you are trying to get away from. Have you set up some arbitrary cut-off point to try to allow for this?

**H. Brendler:** I have discussed this problem with Dr. Mainland and Miss Street, and it is my understanding that an arbitrary cut-off point has been established. Although I did not go into it tonight for reasons of time, there are a number of disadvantages to the sequential procedure, not the least of which is the fact that on occasion it requires more patients than the more conventional method involving fixed sample size. There are other disadvantages as well. For example, on occasion the sequential may interfere with ancillary studies which are in progress, by reaching the verdict that a particular trial should be terminated, before the ancillary studies have been completed. Also, it determines only the relative effectiveness of the two compounds being compared and is complicated, often unreliable, for analysis of other variables.

**G. E. Block:** Dr. Brendler, there seem to be three schools of thought on the treatment of advanced prostatic carcinoma: those who feel that orchiectomy alone is preferable, those who feel that stilbestrol alone is preferable, and those who combine the two. Our institution combines the two and feels that there is a slight increase in survival. I wonder what you are using as your base line and if it would not be advisable to investigate which method is preferable? If a combination of methods is preferable, which of the drug therapies that you have outlined should be used? Are you investigating any of those possibilities at this time?

**H. Brendler:** The problem which you have posed is certainly an important one, and one concerning which there is a great difference of opinion among urologists. It is extremely difficult to conduct a study of this particular problem because it would involve previously untreated patients, or rather those who have not yet been castrated. As I said before, probably 65–80% of these patients respond so well to castration, with or without estrogen supplementation, that it would be impractical to conduct a good statistical evaluation because of the exorbitant amount of clinical material and many years of effort that would be required. Even then, I do not know whether we would turn up with something significantly better than castration. I wish I could answer this question, but our study does not concern previously untreated cases, for the reason I have given.

**P. B. Hudson:** I would like to ask Dr. Brendler how it would influence his committee in selecting drugs if our group (Drs. Viscelli, Lombardo, and Fox) are successful in defining castration biochemically. This hasn't been done yet. There is no definition either from the point of view of the changes in the target tissue (prostatic cells) or from the point of view of just what is being removed by castration. If this is elucidated would it influence the committee which selects drugs? We have been intrigued to learn how they select compounds for clinical trial.

**H. Brendler:** If castration can be defined in the biochemical sense, this information would provide the key to a great many doors. It would enable us to characterize relapse biochemically, something we have been trying to do for years, for example, by means of 17-ketosteroid excretion studies. If such knowledge were available, compounds could be selected more rationally than by the essentially empirical approach which we have been compelled to use. Perhaps I could be more specific if I knew what biochemical test you have discovered.

**R. Hertz:** Dr. Brendler, I think one of the most significant things you mentioned this evening was the occurrence of objective regression in the placebo group in your Trial I. Could you tell us how many of those were observed and could you qualify what was observed in terms of the degree of response and just what was seen clinically? Would you give us your own appraisal of the probability that such phenomena are confusing us in the evaluation of such therapeutic efforts?

**H. Brendler:** The observations I reported in my paper were based on a very few patients, in whom the code was broken for one reason or another. I believe, therefore, it would be premature to discuss these in detail until a more suitable time. However, as I recall, we have seen three or four such cases, one of whom I remember quite clearly. This was a man in whom there occurred definite regression of bilateral hydronephrosis and hydroureter, while he was on placebo therapy. This may have been a delayed castration response, of course, and might signify that our protocol is at fault in requiring only a 6-week waiting period after castration.

The reason I mentioned this phenomenon tonight was because it demonstrates, perhaps, the inadequacy of the somewhat arbitrary criteria for measurement of effect which we have been forced to select. Results such as these will enable us to evaluate our own criteria. In other words, we are not only finding out about the relative efficacy of our test compounds from our clinical trials, but we are also testing our protocol. In time we shall undoubtedly eliminate some of these criteria for measurement of effect which we have found wanting, but which have been accepted in the past without question. I cannot answer your question more precisely, until such time as I can be more certain of the validity of our criteria of therapeutic effect.

**E. E. Sproul:** One thing that has interested me very much, not just in this study but in study of cancer of the prostate in general as it appears at autopsy, is that so often patients have shown a very striking effect on the prostate gland itself and yet the metastases have looked as if the drug had no effect at all. I think this is going to make it quite difficult to evaluate drug effects in general. I wonder if Dr. Brendler has had this experience in clinical observations—that there seems to be atrophy of the prostate yet the bone lesions are apparently progressing.

**H. Brendler:** I quite agree with Dr. Sproul's observation. One frequently sees patients in whom the prostatic tumor has melted away after castration, yet in whom the metastases are progressing steadily. One also sees patients with huge primary tumors, but without metastases. I do not know how to explain those phenomena, unless they indicate that prostatic cancer actually is a generic term for a variety of malignant states. I would agree heartily with Dr. Sproul that it certainly makes evaluation of therapeutic effect a difficult problem.

**S. Werner:** Would you like to characterize the acid phosphatase as a criterion for effectiveness of these agents?

**H. Brendler:** Unfortunately, the serum acid phosphatase is elevated in only about two-thirds of previously untreated patients with metastases, so that a normal value does not rule out the disease. Again, in castrated patients relapse is not correlated with acid phosphatase levels in the blood. When these are elevated, of course, one can assume that the disease is progressing actively; but many patients die of the disease without acid phosphatase increases. Furthermore, the actual serum value, in units of enzyme activity, is not related to the degree of activity of the cancer. In our study, we simply require any elevation above normal in order to catalogue a patient as active. Wide fluctuations are quite normal in an already elevated serum acid phosphatase, so that the actual values are difficult to interpret.

# The Sex Hormones and Cortisone in the Treatment of Inoperable Bronchogenic Carcinoma[1]

JULIUS WOLF, PAUL SPEAR, RAYMOND YESNER, AND MARY ELLEN PATNO

Except in patients with acute leukemia or possibly with one of the lymphomas (4, 19, 20, 31), the steroid hormones have not proved to be of much value in the treatment of non-hormonal-dependent tumors. However many analogs of the basic hormones are now available, some without endocrine activity, which deserve a trial in the various clinical cancer chemotherapy programs because of their interesting and favorable effects observed in the animal screening studies (3, 6, 27, 32). Before these newer compounds can be effectively evaluated, it seemed to us essential that a careful study be done of the effects of the four basic steroid hormones to serve as a guide line for selection of drugs in future studies.

A cooperative study group involving fourteen of the larger Veterans Administration Hospitals was organized to insure a sufficient number of patients so that statistically reliable conclusions could be reached relatively quickly. Bronchogenic carcinoma was chosen as the tumor to be studied because of the large number of patients available.

Since it was estimated that more than half the patients admitted to Veterans Administration Hospitals with inoperable bronchogenic carcinoma die within three months (12) prolongation of life should be satisfactory as a measure of drug effectiveness, thus avoiding difficulties inherent in subjective evaluation. Four drugs were selected for this first study[2]—diethylstilbestrol, testosterone propionate, progesterone, and cortisone—to be

[1] This study was conducted by members of the Veterans Administrative Cooperative Study of Lung Cancer Group through the auspices of the Cancer Chemotherapy National Service Center, National Cancer Institute, National Institutes of Health, Public Health Service, U. S. Department of Health, Education and Welfare. The following investigators participated:

Amatruda, Thomas, M.D. (West Haven, Connecticut); Close, Henry P., M.D., (Philadelphia, Pennsylvania); Ferguson, Donald J., M.D. (Minneapolis, Minnesota); Finegold, Sydney, M.D. (Los Angeles, California); Gillesby, William J., M.D. (Hines, Illinois); Hyde, Leroy, M.D. (Long Beach, California); Lobe, Samuel, M.D. (Cleveland, Ohio); Spear, Paul W., M.D. (Brooklyn, New York); Wade, Frank A., M.D. (Richmond, Virginia); Walkup, H. E., M.D. (Oteen, North Carolina); Weiner, H. A., M.D. (East Orange, New Jersey); Wilson, Russell, M.D. (Dallas, Tex.); Wolf, Julius, M.D. (Bronx, New York); Yee, James, M.D. (Oakland, California); Auerbach, Oscar, M.D. (East Orange, New Jersey); Gerstl, Bruno, M.D. (Oakland, California); Yesner, Raymond, M.D. (West Haven, Connecticut); Lee, Lyndon E., Jr., M.D. (Washington, D.C.); Patno, Mary Ellen, Ph.D. (University of Pittsburgh, Pennsylvania).

[2] Drugs supplied through the courtesy of The Upjohn Company, Merck Sharp & Dohme, and Syntex Chemical Company, Inc.

compared with a regimen in which the patient received the same intensive supportive care but without any additional specific agent. Except for testosterone propionate, the drugs were given orally as coded agents in a double-blind manner with the patients on the nonspecific regimen receiving lactose.

Since the occurrence of lung cancer is at least four to five times higher in males than in females, it had occurred to some earlier investigators that either diethylstilbestrol or perhaps even an orchiectomy might halt the progression of disease (17). In very small groups of patients these treatments had no effect. But testosterone propionate used to test the hypothesis, instead of making the patients worse, seemed to relieve bone pain in some (22, 37). One investigator reported exceptionally good results in a series of five patients with testosterone combined with cortisone (23).

Progesterone was included since this too had been thought to be of beneficial effect in carcinomas ordinarily responsive to the sex hormones (cervix, breast, and prostate) (33) and would complete our study of sex hormone prototypes.

Cortisone has appealed to many investigators interested in the treatment of bronchogenic carcinoma not only for its nonspecific effects, but also because experiments had indicated that the growth of many animal tumors could be inhibited by the use of the adrenal corticosteroids (21). However, in animals there is a divergence of effect since cortisone appears to facilitate heterologous transplantation of tumors and even when the primary tumor is inhibited metastases develop in much greater numbers than in the controls (2, 5, 7, 8, 10, 11, 13, 14, 18, 24, 29, 30, 35, 36, 38). Clinically the corticosteroids do appear to have some effect on leukemias and lymphomas (4, 19, 20, 31), but little or no effect has been noted in bronchogenic carcinoma except for the suggestion of subjective improvement in very few patients (1, 9, 16, 25, 26, 28, 34).

The principal investigators from the fourteen Veterans Administration Hospitals agreed to participate under the chairmanship of Dr. James W. Hollingsworth and accepted patients into the study between February 17, 1958 and February 16, 1959. All patients with primary carcinoma of the lung who could not benefit from surgery or irradiation were included if there was either biopsy proof of the diagnosis of carcinoma of the lung or satisfactory cytologic evidence. All morphologic types of carcinoma were included.

Patients who had received either irradiation or antineoplastic drugs were accepted provided there was no residual toxicity from the prior treatment and the patient either had not responded or had relapsed after some temporary improvement. Patients who had had "curative" surgery but had evidence of recurrence or in whom only a palliative resection had been done were also included.

A complete history and physical examination were performed on each patient in addition to indicated X-ray examinations and other laboratory studies. When it was determined that a patient met the criteria for inclusion in the study, treatment was begun. During the period of treatment the patients were examined twice weekly and sufficient laboratory studies were done to guard against development of corticosteroid toxicity as well as to follow the course of the illness.

In addition to the specific therapeutic regimen, the patient was given the best possible supportive treatment. Antibiotics, transfusions, and other measures were given when necessary. Palliative irradiation to extrathoracic sites for relief of pain or irradiation to the superior mediastinum because of superior vena caval obstruction was given without dropping the patient from the study. However, if it became necessary to deliver radiotherapy to the primary lesion, subsequent observations on the patient were not included in the analysis.

Testosterone propionate was given intramuscularly in 100-mg. dosages three times a week for a period of 12 weeks. The three other drugs and the inert compound (lactose) were identical in physical form and were given orally, two tablets four times a day after meals for 12 weeks and then reduced by one tablet weekly thereafter. This gradual reduction was done since one of the drugs was cortisone and it was felt desirable to decrease its dosage gradually to prevent acute adrenal insufficiency. Cortisone was given thus in a dose of 100 mg. a day; progesterone, 2 gm. a day; and diethylstilbestrol 10 mg. daily. Code names were assigned to the oral drugs. The code was held by the Clinical Pharmacology and Therapeutics Section of the National Cancer Institute.

Randomization of treatments was carried out for each hospital separately and in three basic groups of patients: (1) those who had received irradiation previously, (2) those who had had surgical resection, and (3) those who were termed "without previous therapy" (including patients who had received antineoplastic drugs). Within each group, treatments were assigned by unrestricted randomization. After the randomization was done, each investigator was supplied with three series of sealed envelopes, numbered consecutively and designating treatments. Pooled results of the randomization are given in Table I and show the fairly even distribution among the five treatment groups.

Thirty-four patients were removed from the study; in most instances this was either because the diagnosis was not confirmed by the participating pathologists or because subsequent autopsy proved the primary site to be other than the lung. A few inadvertently received other forms of treatment or died before treatment could be started.

TABLE I
TOTAL NUMBER OF PATIENTS ADMITTED TO STUDY

| | Accepted | | | | |
| Drug | No previous therapy | With resection | With irradiation | Removed | Total |
|---|---|---|---|---|---|
| Diethylstilbestrol | 64 | 12 | 6 | 7 | 89 |
| Inert compound | 62 | 16 | 6 | 4 | 88 |
| Testosterone propionate | 74 | 18 | 7 | 7 | 106 |
| Cortisone | 55 | 17 | 6 | 8 | 86 |
| Progesterone | 67 | 10 | 6 | 8 | 91 |
| | 322 | 73 | 31 | 34 | 460 |

Three pathologists independently examined the original slides upon which the diagnosis was made. Since the pathologist in the originating hospital had first examined the slide(s), in most cases four opinions were available. Each pathologist classified the material as squamous cell carcinoma, adenocarcinoma, or undifferentiated carcinoma which was subdivided into the small and large cell types. Smears of sputa, bronchial secretions, or pleural fluid were read as positive or negative for carcinoma cells. Where doubtful, they were classified as negative. The final diagnosis rested upon the agreement of at least two of the three pathologists. Where there was no agreement as to type, the tumor was classified as undifferentiated large-cell carcinoma.

## RESULTS

Analysis of the patients' survival times after start of treatment was made as of August 1, 1959. On this date 366 patients were deceased, 48 were still living, and 12 were termed "limited observations." Among those who were alive, the shortest observation time was 171 days; the longest, 514 days. The 12 "limited observations" came about through the patient's receiving added therapy or being lost to follow-up. In either case, observations prior to the happening were used in the analysis.

The four drugs and the inert compound have been compared by considering the proportion of patients who survived to the 30th, 60th, 90th, 120th, 150th, and 180th days after treatment was begun. The estimated average survival time after treatment is also presented. All estimates were made by what Kaplan and Meier have termed the "Product Limit" method (15).

The experience of patients who had been treated previously either by surgery or irradiation was analyzed and found to be no different from that of persons without previous therapy. Therefore presentation of data has been limited to that for the entire group.

The distribution of the four principal tumor types did not differ statistically among the various drug groups, so that the end result could not have been influenced by any possible difference in responsiveness. No attempt was made to analyze the survival rates of patients with different tumor types. Those with squamous cell carcinoma constituted the largest group (56 %) and adenocarcinoma, the smallest (4 %). Twenty-seven per cent of the patients had what was termed undifferentiated small-cell carcinoma and 13 % were diagnosed as having undifferentiated large-cell carcinoma.

The proportion of patients who survived to a given time has been presented in two ways: (1) the point estimate and (2) the 90 % confidence interval estimate (Table II; Fig. 1). In most instances, the point estimate was simply the actual proportion of patients surviving to the indicated time, since, with the exception of the twelve limited observations, all persons were observed for at least 171 days or until death. The confidence interval estimates were obtained by merely computing the 90 % confidence limits for each point estimate (the probability that the "true" proportion lies somewhere within the range of the interval is 90 %).

With prolongation of life as the measurement, the least favorable experience was among those patients who received cortisone; the most favorable, among those who were treated with the inert compound. For example, only 37 % of the cortisone-treated patients survived to the 90th day compared to 51 % of those who received the inert compound. The survival rates at the 90th day for diethylstilbestrol, testosterone propionate, and progesterone fell between those for cortisone and inert compound.

The possible deleterious effects of cortisone were noted in the second month (Table III; Fig. 2). At the end of the 29th day, the survival rate for the cortisone group equaled that for the control group. Among the patients who lived to the second month, however, the survival rate of those on cortisone was 62 %; of those in the control group, 83 %. The probability that this difference was the result of sampling variation is less than 2 %.

In view of the previous reports of the beneficial effects of cortisone, it was surprising to find the increased mortality among those patients receiving it during their second month of treatment. A careful analysis of the major contributory causes of death (Table IV) failed to disclose any increased incidence of heart failure or pulmonary infection which we first thought might be the explanation. We are unable to account for this increased mortality among the cortisone-treated patients. While one patient did die of a perforated ulcer, there was one such death in the inert compound group.

It is noteworthy that few if any of the usually observed adrenal cortico steroid side effects were found in our patients receiving 100 mg. of cortisone daily for three months. Actually no appreciable number of side effects was observed with any of the drugs. During the study gynecomastia developed in a few patients. Some of these, when the code was broken, were found to have received the inert compound rather than the expected diethylstilbestrol.

Also of considerable interest are the 11 patients who died of pulmonary hemorrhage. Six had received diethylstilbestrol. Four had keratinizing squamous carcinoma (defined as well differentiated), and two had moderately well-differentiated squamous carcinoma. In this small series almost two-thirds of the cases having severe hemorrhage had squamous carcinoma, but more strikingly, 4 out of 11 had keratinizing squamous carcinoma (in contrast to the general figure of 6 % of all biopsies). Since the distribution of the 28 cases of this highly differentiated form of squamous carcinoma was approximately the same throughout the five treatment groups, the use of diethylstilbestrol in keratinizing squamous carcinoma may have led to more rapid necrosis with subsequent hemorrhage.

TABLE II

PROPORTION SURVIVING TO INDICATED DAY

| Day | Diethyl-stilbestrol | Inert compound | Testosterone propionate | Cortisone | Progesterone |
|---|---|---|---|---|---|
| | | | Point estimate | | |
| 30 | 0.80 | 0.75 | 0.75 | 0.74 | 0.73 |
| 60 | .58 | .62 | .62 | .46 | .51 |
| 90 | .44 | .51 | .44 | .37 | .41 |
| 120 | .33 | .46 | .37 | .26 | .33 |
| 150 | .26 | .38 | .28 | .21 | .27 |
| 180 | .25 | .30 | .22 | .18 | .23 |
| | | | 90% Confidence interval estimate | | |
| 30 | 0.72–.87 | 0.66–.82 | 0.66–.82 | 0.65–.82 | 0.64–.81 |
| 60 | .48–.67 | .52.–71 | .53–.70 | .37–.56 | .41–.60 |
| 90 | .35–.54 | .42–.61 | .36–.53 | .28–.47 | .32–.51 |
| 120 | .24–.42 | .37–.56 | .29–.46 | .18–.35 | .25–.43 |
| 150 | .19–.36 | .29.–48 | .20–.36 | .14–.30 | .19–.36 |
| 180 | .18–.34 | .22–.39 | .16–.30 | .11–.27 | .16–.32 |

Except for this possible influence of hemorrhage in patients with keratinizing squamous carcinoma the sex hormones had no effect on the life span of the patients that could be distinguished from that of the inert compound. There is the suggestion that progesterone may have exerted almost as deleterious an effect as cortisone, but its difference from that of the inert compound is not sufficiently great to enable us to make such a statement with 90 % confidence as we can for cortisone.

Observed median survival and the estimated survival times are presented in Table V. These data give added evidence to the apparent unfavorable results among patients who received cortisone (56 and 106 days as compared to 93 and 138 days for the inert compound group) and to the suggestion that the three sex hormones are of no value in prolonging life.

Although the therapeutic implications that can be drawn from this first study by our group are all on the negative side, we have demonstrated that bronchogenic carcinoma can be well studied by the large-scale cooperative technique using the proportion of patients surviving to a given day as the index of drug comparison. The advantages of such an end point are obvious

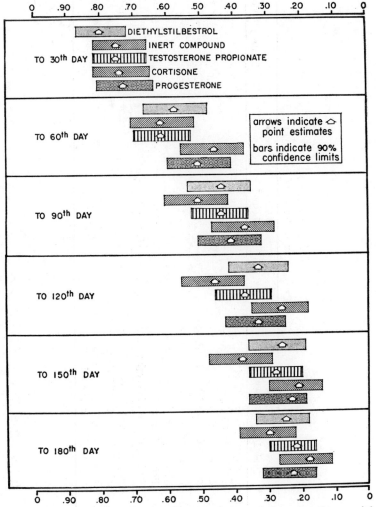

Fig. 1. Ninety per cent confidence interval estimates of the proportion surviving to indicated day.

TABLE III

PROBABILITY OF SURVIVING TO A GIVEN DAY

| Probability of survival | Diethyl-stilbestrol | Inert compound | Testosterone propionate | Cortisone | Progesterone |
|---|---|---|---|---|---|
| Probability (proportion) of surviving to 30 days | | | | | |
| Point estimate | 0.80 | 0.75 | 0.75 | 0.74 | 0.73 |
| 90% Confidence interval estimate | .72–.87 | .66–.82 | .66–.82 | .65–.82 | .64–.81 |
| Probability of surviving to 60th day having survived to 30th day | | | | | |
| Point estimate | 0.72 | 0.83 | 0.82 | 0.62 | 0.69 |
| 90% Confidence interval estimate | .61–.81 | .71–.90 | .73–.89 | .50–.73 | .58–.79 |
| Probability of surviving to 90th day having survived to 60th day | | | | | |
| Point estimate | 0.76 | 0.83 | 0.72 | 0.81 | 0.80 |
| 90% Confidence interval estimate | .63–.86 | .71–.90 | .61–.81 | .66–.90 | .67–.90 |

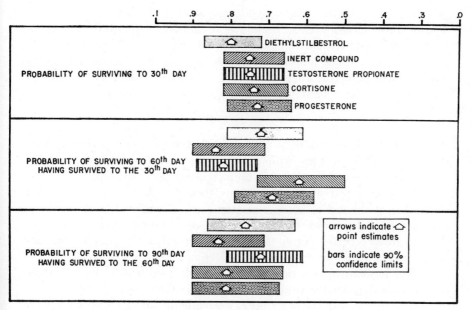

FIG. 2. Conditional probabilities of survival.

TABLE IV
PRINCIPAL CONTRIBUTORY CAUSES OF DEATH

| Drug | Total | None | Pulmonary infection | Hemorrhage | Heart failure | Perforated ulcer | Other |
|---|---|---|---|---|---|---|---|
| Diethylstilbestrol | 65 | 38 | 16 | 6 | 2 | 0 | 3 |
| Inert compound | 72 | 47 | 14 | 1 | 4 | 1 | 5 |
| Testosterone propionate | 87 | 66 | 17 | 0 | 2 | 1 | 1 |
| Cortisone | 72 | 49 | 15 | 1 | 2 | 1 | 4 |
| Progesterone | 70 | 46 | 16 | 3 | 2 | 0 | 3 |
| | 366 | 246 | 78 | 11 | 12 | 3 | 16 |

TABLE V
MEDIAN SURVIVAL TIMES AND ESTIMATED AVERAGE SURVIVAL TIMES

| Survival time | Diethylstilbestrol | Inert compound | Testosterone propionate | Cortisone | Progesterone |
|---|---|---|---|---|---|
| Median survival (days) | 75 | 93 | 78 | 56 | 60 |
| Estimated mean survival (days) | 138 | 138 | 117 | 106 | 122 |

when compared to the other commonly used ones of subjective evaluation and/or tumor measurements. Both present many difficulties involving agreement between different investigators and the elimination of many patients whose tumors are not measurable. Long-range survival studies are always difficult because of the large number of patients who have to be dropped because they receive additional treatment or are lost to follow-up.

## SUMMARY

1. Four hundred and sixty patients with bronchogenic carcinoma were treated for three months with either diethylstilbestrol, testosterone propionate, progesterone, cortisone, or an inert compound (lactose).

2. Fifty-one per cent of the patients treated with the inert compound were alive at the end of 90 days of treatment as compared to 37 % of the patients treated with cortisone. Most of the fatalities in the cortisone-treated group occurred during the second month of treatment. No explanation could be found for the apparent deleterious effects of cortisone.

3. The median survival time for the control group was 93 days as compared to 56 days for the group receiving cortisone.

4. The results with the other drugs were intermediate between those with the inert compound and those with cortisone, with the experience in the progesterone group almost as bad.

5. There were 11 patients who died of exsanguinating hemorrhage; 6 had received diethylstilbestrol; 4 had keratinizing squamous carcinoma as compared to an over-all incidence of 6 % of this type of bronchogenic carcinoma in our series.

6. We have demonstrated the feasibility of studying the therapy of bronchogenic carcinoma in a large-scale cooperative project, with the proportion of patients surviving to a given day as the index of drug comparison.

## REFERENCES

1. Alpert, L. K., Zimmerman, H. S., and Scherr, E. H. *Proc. Clin. ACTH Conf. 2nd Conf. 1951* p. 235 (1951).
2. Bollag, W., and Meyer, C. *Oncologia* **7**, 66 (1954).
3. Clarke, D. A. *Cancer Research* **3**, 14 (1955).
4. Fessas, P., Wintrobe, M. M., Thompson, R. B., and Cartwright, G. E. *A. M. A. Arch. Internal Med.* **94**, 384 (1954).
5. Foley, E. J., and Silverstein, R. *Proc. Soc. Exptl. Biol. Med.* **77**, 713 (1951).
6. Gellhorn, A., Kells, A., and Golino, M. *Cancer Research* Suppl. No. 3, 38 (1955).
7. Ghose, T. *Indian J. Med. Sci.* **12**, 629 (1958).
8. Green, H. N., and Whiteley, H. J. *Brit. Med. J.* **II**, 538 (1952).
9. Griboff, S. I. *A. M. A. Arch. Internal Med.* **89**, 812 (1952).
10. Herbut, P. A., and Kraemer, W. H. *Cancer Research* **16**, 408 (1956).
11. Hoch-Ligeti, C., and Hsu, Y. T. *Science* **117**, 360 (1953).

12. Hollingsworth, J. W. Unpublished data.
13. Howes, E. L. *Yale J. Biol. and Med.* **23**, 454 (1951).
14. Iversen, H. G. *Acta Pathol. Microbiol. Scand.* **41**, 273 (1957).
15. Kaplan, E. L., and Meier, P. *J. Am. Statist. Assoc.* **53**, 282 (1958).
16. Karnofsky, D. A., Meyers, W. P. L., and Phillips, R. *Am. J. Surgery* **89**, 526 (1955).
17. Kembler, R. L., and Graham, E. A. *Cancer* **3**, 735 (1950).
18. Lapis, K., and Sagi, T. *Acta Morphol. Acad. Sci. Hung.* **7**, 91 (1956).
19. Lewis, S. M. *Post Grad. Med. J. London* **34**, 340 (1958).
20. Louis, J., Sanford, H. N., and Limarzi, L. R. *J. Am. Med. Assoc.* **167**, 1913 (1958).
21. Noble, R. L. *Pharmacol. Revs.* **9**, 367 (1957).
22. Olson, K. B. *Am. J. Med. Sci.* **230**, 157 (1955).
23. Ornstein, G., Lercher, L., and Robitzek, E. *Quart. Bull. Sea View Hosp.* **12**, 125 (1951).
24. Patterson, W. B., Chute, R. N., and Sommers, S. C. *Cancer Research* **14**, 656 (1954).
25. Pearson, O. H., and Eliel, L. P. *J. Am. Med. Assoc.* **144**, 1349 (1950).
26. Raab, A. P., and Gerber, A. *N.Y. State J. Med.* **53**, 1333 (1953).
27. Skipper, H. E., and Thomson, J. R. *Cancer Research* Suppl. No. 3, 44 (1955).
28. Spies, T. D., Stone, R. E., Lopez, G. G., Milanes, F., Toca, R. L., and Reboredo, A. *Lancet* **2**, 241 (1950).
29. Stock, C. C. *Ciba Foundation Colloq. Endocrinol.* **1**, 135 (1952).
30. Stock, C. C. *Recent. Progr. Hormone Research* **11**, 425 (1954).
31. Straus, B., Jacobson, A. S., Berson, S. A., Bernstein, T. C., Fadem, R. S., and Yalow, R. S. *Am. J. Med.* **12**, 170 (1952).
32. Sugiura, K. *Cancer Research* Suppl. No. 3, 19 (1955).
33. Taylor, S. G., III, Ayer, J. P., and Morris, R. S., Jr. *J. Am. Med. Assoc.* **144**, 1058 (1950).
34. Taylor, S. T. *Proc. Clin. ACTH Conf. 2nd Conf. 1951* **2**, 230 (1951).
35. Toolan, H. W. *Cancer Research* **13**, 389 (1953).
36. Toolan, H. W. *Cancer Research* **14**, 660 (1954).
37. Truhaut, R. *Semaine hôp.* **33**, 366 (1957).
38. Watson, B. E. *J. Natl. Cancer Inst.* **20**, 219 (1958).

## DISCUSSION

**G. W. Woolley:** It may be of interest to state that many of us in experimental animal study find that we get into serious trouble if we use cortisone on a steady regime. We have learned that it is often better, if we wish to continue treatment over a long period of time, to alternate heavy with low dosage or periods of treatment with periods of nontreatment.

**J. Wolf:** Clinically, 100 mg. of cortisone a day for 3 months has been fairly well tolerated. Although we would get into some trouble when we treated rheumatoid patients with this dose, we didn't see any complication in our bronchogenic patients. Now most of the hospitals gave the cortisone after meals and at bed time. A few gave the cortisone four times a day running from 7 o'clock in the morning to 5 o'clock in the evening so there was some difference in the range of cortisone therapy. I'm not sure that a change of administration of cortisone might prove deleterious, but I hardly expect that it would prove beneficial.

**G. C. Escher:** When this program was originally set up the 3-month treatment was based on the experience in breast cancer, where we have found that if a case was going to respond it would probably do this within a 3-month period. We felt that since we were running a blinded study as much as possible, we would avoid altering dose schedules. This would confound the picture even more.

**J. Lampkin-Hibbard:** In reference to Dr. Woolley's discussion I would like to mention a few things about cortisone treatment in mice. Dr. Potter and I found that the best treatment in mice for a long period with cortisone was, first, to give the maximal tolerated dose for mice, which is 25 mg./kg., for 1 week. Then we reduced it to 15 mg./kg. for 61 days without losing any mice. If we treated them any longer than seven days with 25 mg./kg., many mice died with infections and other mani- festations. So I think one might study the possibility of having a large dose at first, and then reducing it.

**H. M. Lemon:** It just occurred to me in hearing this that there is maybe some- thing rather important here, because Dr. S. Sommers has published some very careful studies of the endocrine pathology in patients with lung cancer. I know the general picture which he obtained in study of a good many tens of thousands of cells counted in the anterior hypophysis indicated a hyperactivity of the pituitary adrenal-cortical axis. His interpretation of these cell counts was that these individuals were pretty much extroverted and possibly prone to certain types of violent lives, with excessive drive and often excessive habits of smoking and drinking. I notice there was mention that some of them died of accidents during the course of this study. In view of the fact that 100 mg. daily of cortisone appeared to have rather small end organ effects, if I understood the speaker correctly, maybe this was just adding a further push in the same direction that they were already apt to follow on the basis of their endocrine and personality make-up.

**J. Wolf:** These people were watched very carefully. At the beginning the electrolytes were done weekly, blood sugars, blood pressures, and weights twice a week, but toward the end of the study all of us became less concerned. I don't know the answer; a good many of these people at autopsy had most of their adrenals replaced by tumor, as is common for people with bronchogenic carcinoma with adrenals so completely replaced that he is an Addisonian for all intents and purposes.

**K. B. Olson:** This is a subject that I've been quite interested in, but I am not sure if what I have to say is relevant. Dr. Skiff who worked in our Albany Medical College laboratory, transplanted about 70 human tumors—and I believe 10 of these were bron- chogenic cancers—to cortisone-conditioned hamsters. His greatest success was with lung cancer. He developed the tumor, A-42, reported last night by Dr. Woolley, and in addition to that had three other tumors that grew for several generations and several others that survived. I think 8 out of the 10 tumors survived for one or two transplants. Only 2 survived for any long period of transplantation. I have wondered if this finding has any relevance to the apparent bad clinical effect of cortisone on these patients.

The second question I would like to ask is the importance of the sex difference in bronchogenic squamous and undifferentiated carcinoma. No such difference is found in adenocarcinoma. Clinically, one finds a number of observations that are not statistical and not subject to analysis. Feminization of some degree with loss of chest hair, loss of axillary hair, and testicular atrophy has been commented on for a number of years by many thoracic surgeons. Maybe thoracic surgeons are not competent to comment on these findings in patients with lung cancer, but they do. This is an observation that is handed down from older surgeons. I wonder if anyone here has studied urinary steroid excretion patterns or gonadotropins in these patients. We studied urinary 17- ketosteroid excretion in a small number of cases, but found no alteration from normal. I wonder if more extensive studies ever have been carried out in this group of cancer patients, because the sex differential favoring the male is striking in squamous and undifferentiated types of cancer. This differential is usually attributed to environment, but it seems to me that some other factor might be present in this type of cancer that we may be missing.

J. Wolf: I can't answer the first question. There are animal experiments of cortisone-treated tumors where the primary tumor may be inhibited but it seems there are more pulmonary metastases than in the controls. As for the second question, I didn't state, but I assumed that everyone would take for granted, that in fourteen Veterans Administration Hospitals all the patients would be males. As far as gynecomastia is concerned even nonthoracic surgeons do see it. We have done a few studies but have not been able to detect any change in the endocrine pattern. Particularly intriguing is the unilateral gynecomastia on the same side of the tumor.

W. H. Baker: I wanted to ask whether in this series of cases you have had any cases of overt Cushing's syndrome associated with bronchogenic carcinoma. This finding was first reported in England and had since been corroborated in other areas. In a large series of cases like this, I wondered also if you had found any cases in which a high blood calcium and low serum phosphorus like hyperparathyroidism-type syndrome existed.

J. Wolf: In this first study there were really about 550 cases. There was a sixth drug group—nitrogen mustard—the results will be reported later. In the 560 patients we did not see a case of Cushing's, but in our second study with 400 additional cases, we have seen one man with Cushing's disease and one man with a syndrome of salt loss simulating Addison's disease. There has been a number of cases of hypercalcemia, but I don't know the precise number.

S. Werner: Do the patients with Cushing's disease have a more fulminating course than the other patients?

J. Wolf: No.

B. J. Kennedy: Am I correct in interpreting the figures, that only 31 of your 460 patients with lung cancer received irradiation therapy? If this is so, the lung cancer must be initially advanced and irradiation therapy is very seldom considered.

J. Wolf: You are right. There were 31 patients who had received irradiation before being admitted to the V.A. Hospital. A good many of these people would have received irradiation if they had not been on the study. They were all advanced patients. Most of our patients came to us with the first symptom of their disease and were not referred after having gone through extensive courses of treatment elsewhere. I think our mortality figures would indicate these were severely ill patients.

R. Grinberg: We have had some experience with patients affected with malignant lung tumors. We treated some of them with TEM and prednisone, and the results showed improvement in 3 out of 10 patients. I want to ask Dr. Wolf if he did electrolyte balance studies in his patients treated with cortisone. Second, if he has seen some signs in the lungs that could explain the rapid downhill course of his patients.

J. Wolf: We did not do balance studies in any of our patients. We simply did occasional electrolytes. We cannot see any difference in the rate of progression of the lesions, either in X-ray or at the time of autopsy, in the cortisone-treated group as compared to the placebo group.

R. W. Talley: I would like to compliment Dr. Wolf for compiling these statistics. I think it brings forth one point very clearly, at least to me, that even though animal work has shown that the corticoids probably are an effective group of agents this hasn't been the case in nonendocrine, nonlymphoid human disease, again emphasizing the species difference problem. It also suggests that caution should be employed in treating patients with terminal cancer with corticoids as a supportive measure. I think a study of this type should be considered in other disseminated cancers to determine if corticoids might accelerate the progress of the patient.

**J. Wolf:** Thanks for the last comment. I thought somebody was going to ask me whether these patients may have died sooner but perhaps they died happier. Actually we did set up a system of trying to evaluate the clinical status of the patient using the performance status of the Memorial group of several years ago, and we found this not very useful. First of all it was hard to attribute what part the cancer played in the performance status and what part the pneumonia or other complications did. But using what we had, we found in no group any evidence of an improvement in the performance status. On the other hand if we asked each investigator to vote for which drug was making his people feel better, they all said it was testosterone propionate, and this was so clear to everyone that halfway through the study we thought that testosterone was going to be a favorable drug and began a new study using other anabolic agents. I think the reason for this was first, that this was the one drug that was not given blinded, and secondly, that the patients were getting injections. But the testosterone group performance status was no different from the performance status of the cortisone group, and the people did not die any happier.

# Clinical Observations on the Effect of Progesterone in the Treatment of Metastatic Endometrial Carcinoma[1,2]

RITA M. KELLEY AND WILLIAM H. BAKER

*Department of Medicine, Massachusetts General Hospital, Boston, Massachusetts, and Department of Medicine, Pondville Hospital, Walpole, Massachusetts; The John Collins Warren Laboratories of the Huntington Memorial Hospital of Harvard University at the Tumor Clinic of the Massachusetts General Hospital, Boston, Massachusetts*

The successful treatment of cancer of the uterus is usually accomplished by total hysterectomy, irradiation, or a combination of both procedures (2).

Data from 27 clinics, in 8366 cases, are surveyed in the 10th Annual Report of the Results in Treatment of Carcinoma of the Uterus (5). The over-all five-year cure rate was 54.3 %. When the tumor was confined to the uterus (Stage I, Group I), the five-year cure rate was 60 %, but only 19.6 % for those patients in whom the growth had spread outside of the uterus (Stage II) (5).

Metastatic inoperable carcinoma of the uterus is usually treated by irradiation, and much symptomatic benefit can be achieved by this form of therapy. Recurrent local disease after radiotherapy has been a problem in management. Also, the treatment of lung metastases is less successfully managed by radiotherapy, since adequate radiation to metastatic lung lesions carries with it the hazard of producing pulmonary fibrosis.

The beneficial effects of changes in the hormonal environment of certain metastatic tumors from the prostate and breast prompted us to investigate the use of sex hormones in the treatment of endometrial cancer. The relationship of sex hormones to human endometrial cancer is not well defined at present. The coexistence of endometrial hyperplasia and endometrial carcinoma in humans has given rise to the concept that endometrial cancer may be related to overstimulation with estrogens (4). Endometrial cancer has been induced with long-term estrogen administration in guinea pigs and rabbits (1). Long-term administration of progesterone in rabbits has not as yet produced endometrial cancer (7, 8).

Progesterone has a profound effect upon the endometrium and synergistically with estrogen produces the secretory endometrial phase of the menstrual cycle (3). If progesterone is continued alone over a prolonged

[1] This is publication No. 1010 of the Cancer Commission of Harvard University and publication No. 216 of Pondville Hospital.

[2] This investigation was supported by a National Cancer Institute Research Grant, No. C2421.

time, disappearance of acini will occur with marked decidual reaction of the endometrium (3, 6). This latter effect is usually obtained without any consistent measurable effect upon the urinary gonadotropins (3). Because of the known effects of progesterone on the uterine endometrium, we felt that this steroid was worthy of trial in the treatment of metastatic endometrial carcinoma, which could not be effectively treated by radiotherapy.

In 1951, we began treating patients with metastatic recurrent endometrial carcinoma with progesterone or progesterone-like compounds. At the present time, we have treated 15 such cases, and it is the purpose of this report to depict the results obtained in these patients. All 15 patients had a previous pathologic diagnosis of adenocarcinoma of the endometrium. Most of the cases had been previously treated by panhysterectomy, local radiotherapy, or both treatments in conjunction. Only those patients are included who have been treated for longer than $3\frac{1}{2}$ weeks with progesterone. Five of these 15 cases have shown objective regression of metastatic disease, lasting from 6 months to $4\frac{1}{2}$ years. In 4 of the 5 patients, the metastatic disease was evidenced by lung metastases, and thus no biopsy material was available. In the fifth patient, local disease was present, but biopsy material was not obtained. In all the cases that have responded, gratifying symptomatic relief was obtained with objective remission of the metastatic chest lesions or local disease. At the present time, 2 of the 5 responders have died of recurrent disease and the 3 living patients all now have evidence of recurrent disease, either locally or within the chest.

Early in our studies, we administered progesterone intramuscularly in the form of Proluton[3] at a dose level of 50–200 mg. daily. More recently, we have been using Delalutin[4] in a dose schedule of 250–500 mg. twice a week. The structural formulas are shown in Fig. 1. The 5 cases that responded are reported next in detail and the 10 patients not responding are summarized in Table I.

*Case 1.* A. G., MGH 572590, age 61. In 1945 a panhystectomy was performed for adenocarcinoma of the endometrium. In 1947, a recurrence in the vagina was treated with 4200 r with a good response. In October 1950, the patient developed cough, anorexia, and complained of weight loss of 24 pounds over the preceding three months. She was seen by us in November 1950, at which time a chest X-ray (Fig. 2a) was taken. On November 14, 1950, the patient was begun on 200 mg. of Proluton intramuscularly daily (4 cc.). Follicle-stimulating hormone (FSH) titer taken prior to therapy was positive for 52 mouse units and negative for 104 mouse units. Two weeks after beginning Proluton therapy, she felt symptomatically much improved. Repeat chest X-ray at that time showed no change. One month after beginning therapy, she continued to improve with a gain in weight of 5 pounds; again no change was seen in

---

[3] Progesterone in oil, Schering Corp., Bloomfield, New Jersey.

[4] 17α-Hydroxyprogesterone 17-*n*-caproate, E. R. Squibb & Sons, New York.

her X-rays. On January 14, 1951, improvement was maximal with no cough and X-rays showed definite diminution of all lung metastases. On March 22, 1951, further X-rays showed more regression in the right upper lobe lesion (Figure 2b). The patient was continued on Proluton, 200 mg. daily, and no further regression of the metastatic tumor nodules in the chest occured. In June 1951, since her condition was static, she was put on Proluton 100 mg. three times a week; in September 1951, definite increase in the

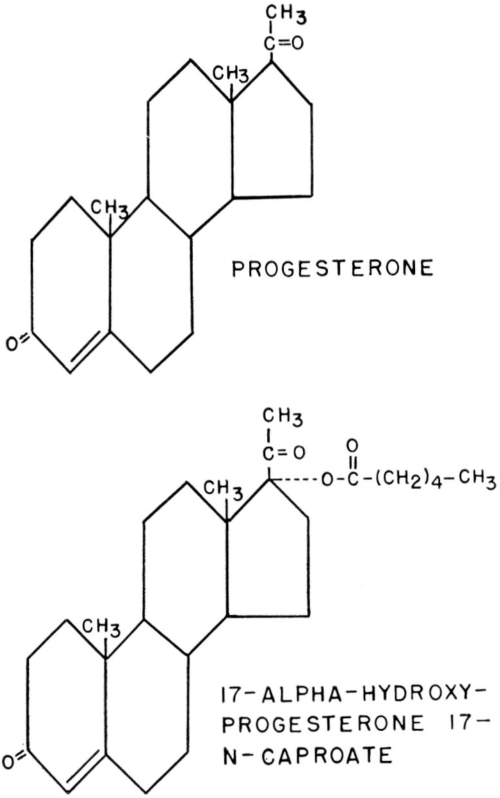

FIG. 1. Structural formula of progesterone and 17α-hydroxyprogesterone 17-*n*-caproate (Delalutin).

size of the right upper lobe lesion and left upper lobe lesion occurred. In October 1951, there was further increase in the size of the lesions and in November 1951, X-ray therapy was given to the right and left upper lobes, 1800 r to each area. X-ray therapy was completed on November 23, 1951. The patient became progressively worse and died in December 1951. Permission for autopsy was refused. Total dose of Proluton was 38,400 mg.

*Case 2.* R. W., MGH 845077, age 61. In March 1951, a panhysterectomy was done for adenocarcinoma of the uterus with metastasis to one ovary. Local vaginal recurrence in April 1954 was treated by 3300 r. One month after completion of X-ray therapy,

TABLE I

BRIEF SUMMARY OF PATIENTS WHO DID NOT RESPOND TO PROGESTERONE

| Patient Unit, No. Age | Prior therapy[a] | Extent of disease | Duration of therapy and total dose[b] | Response |
|---|---|---|---|---|
| E. R. PH 40789 59 | 8/56: H + 5000 r 6/57: 1800 r | 8/57: Huge mass in vagina, invasion of bladder, multiple nodules in chest | Proluton 100 mg. tiw. 36 weeks 12,000 mg. | No change in pulmonary disease. Pelvic exenteration 8/58 because of progression of symptoms. Died 12/58 at home; no postmortem |
| R. H. MGH 736216 55 | 4/51: R 4400 mg.-hr. 6/51: 5000 r | 11/51: Supraclavicular; Horner's on left. Pulmonary and pelvic wall metastases | Proluton 200 mg. 6 d./week, 4 weeks 200 mg. tiw. 1 week, 5400 mg. | Progression to death 1/6/52. Massive peripheral edema |
| B. K. MGH 1041561 51 | 5/58: H + 4000 r | 1/59: Mass in lf. supraclavicular area. Mass in pelvis. Bilateral leg edema | Delalutin 500 mg. biw. 5 weeks 5000 mg. | 2 weeks: regression of neck and abdominal masses; then progression to death in 5 weeks. |
| C. P. MGH 795784 33 | 1/52: H 1/53: 1800 r | 1/53: Local recurrence extensive pulmonary metastases | Proluton 200 mg. biw. 4 weeks 100 mg. biw. 7200 mg. 8 weeks | No response. Steady downhill course. Developed acne. Died 5/53 at home. |
| N. S. MGH 668882 47 | 6/49: H 3/50: 5000 r | 2/51: Massive rt. pleural effusion positive for tumor cells; multiple pulmonary metastases | Proluton 200 mg. qd. 6 weeks 100 mg. qd. 8000 mg. 1 week | No response. Repeated thoracenteses required. Died 5/3/51 (buttock abscess) |

TABLE I (*continued*)

| | | | | |
|---|---|---|---|---|
| F. E.<br>MGH 729814<br>73 | 3/51: H + 1800 r (no chest film) | 5/51: Local recurrence, multiple pulmonary metastases and metastases in pelvic bones | Proluton<br>200 mg. qd.<br>4 weeks<br>5600 mg. | No response. Died at home 7/7/51 |
| M. H.<br>MGH 360451<br>63 | 1949: H + X-ray (? amount)<br>2/55: 4000 r | 3/57: Mass in left pelvis. Partial intestinal obstruction | Delalutin<br>250 mg. biw.<br>8 weeks<br>4000 mg. | No response. Died in terminal care hospital |
| I. P.<br>MGH 336647<br>62 | 6/52: H<br>10/53: 9600 r (skin dose) | 2/54: Vaginal recurrence rt. lower abdomen and pelvic wall; involvement of iliac vessels with lymph obst, rt. leg. | Proluton<br>200 mg. qd.<br>2 weeks<br>100 mg. qd.<br>5600 mg. 4 weeks | No response. Developed pleural effusion on Rx. Died shortly after discharge |
| S. A.<br>PH 39634<br>64 | 1947: H<br>1954: colostomy<br>11/56: large bowel obstruction | 12/56: Huge RLQ mass and many smaller tumor masses. Bilateral leg edema. Terminal state | Delalutin<br>100 mg. qd.<br>2 weeks<br>250 mg. biw.<br>12 weeks<br>8900 mg. | Marked subjective improvement for 3 months. Appetite stimulation, loss of edema, resumption of activity. 4/57: partial obst. 8/58: died at home |
| R. W.<br>P.H. 41152<br>58 | 4/57: R 300 mg.-hr. (ext. radiation ? amount) | 11/57: Recurrence, metastases to vagina, vulva, perineum, skin. Phlebitis and edema rt. leg. Terminal state | Delalutin<br>250 mg. biw.<br>3 weeks<br>1500 mg. | No response. Died 12/19/57 |

[a] H = Panhysterectomy; R = local radiation or radium.

[b] tiw. = Three times a week; biw. = twice a week; qd. = per day.

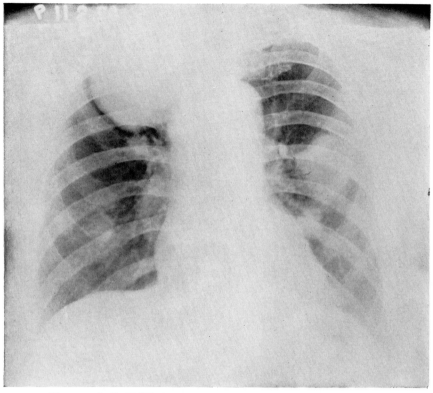

FIG. 2a.   A. G., MGH 572590 11/2/50.   Multiple pulmonary metastases.

multiple nodular densities in both lungs were present and she was referred to our clinic. At that time, metastatic series was negative. Serum calcium was 12.5 mg. %, phosphorus was 2.3 mg. %, and alkaline phosphatase was 3.3 Bodansky units. In June 1954, a repeat X-ray of her lung indicated increase in the nodular densities in both lung fields (Fig. 3a). She was placed on Proluton, 50 mg. three times a week, intramuscularly. In September 1954, repeat X-rays (Fig. 3b) showed definite regression of her chest metastatic lesions, and in one year, the nodular densities had all disappeared (Fig. 3c). Because of this dramatic response, she was continued on Proluton, 50 mg. three times a week for the next four years; no change in chest X-rays occurred during periodic examinations. She tolerated the medication well. In March 1958, a small increase in the right hilum of the chest was seen and over the next six months gradually it increased in size. In September 1958, because of increase in size of the hilar mass (Fig. 3d), Proluton was discontinued, to see whether a withdrawal response could be obtained. No change occurred following discontinuance and over the next ten months no therapy was given. In July 1959, further increase in hilar disease was seen in her chest and Delalutin therapy, 500 mg. twice a week, was begun. X-Rays taken in December 1959 showed definite but slight decrease in size of the hilar metastatic disease and a peripheral nodular lesion of the right lower lung and left upper lung fields had disappeared. She

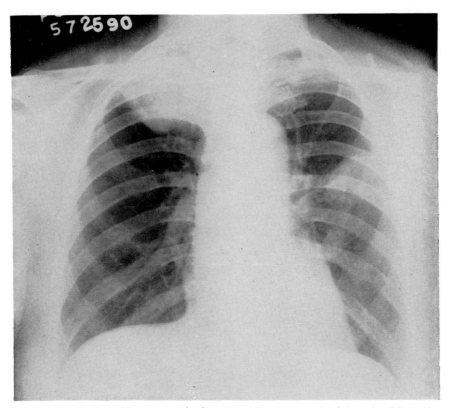

FIG. 2b.  A. G., MGH 572590, 3/22/51. Note disappearance of lesions in right mid-lung field and marked shrinkage of lesions in right upper lobe and left mid-lung.

is at present, alive, well, and being continued on Delalutin 500 mg. twice a week. Hypercalcemia and hypophosphatemia have persisted throughout this entire period. Metastatic series including bone biopsy is negative for metastatic disease. She has refused parathyroid exploration. Total dose, 26,000 mg. first course and 20,000 mg. second course to date.

Case 3. R. H., MGH 961541, age 64. In February 1957, dilatation and curettage were performed because of intermittent vaginal spotting. A diagnosis of adenocarcinoma of the fundus was made. Ether examination revealed implants in the vulva and enlargement of the uterus to three times normal with penetration of posterior uterine wall. X-Rays of her chest revealed bilateral nodular densities with increased linear markings in both lung fields, interpreted as lymphatic spread of carcinoma. Primary disease in the uterus was treated with 5400 mg.-hours of radium. Because of the metastatic disease in her chest Delalutin therapy, 250 mg. three times a week, was begun. She was treated with this compound from March 1957 to May 1957. In one month her chest X-ray had begun to clear and in two months, it was completely negative. All palpable local disease disappeared, but vaginal smears were positive intermittently. Chest X-rays have remained free of disease but in August 1959, retroperitoneal recurrence appeared. At

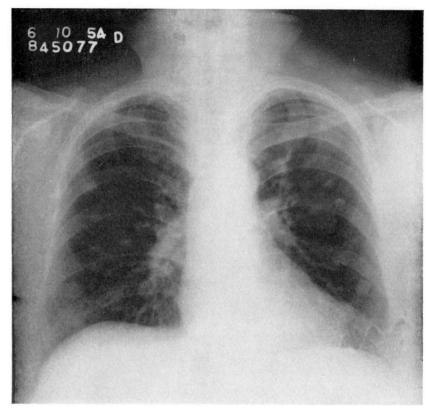

Fig. 3a.  R. W., MGH 845077, 6/10/54. Multiple nodular densities.

the present time, she is on her second course of Delalutin therapy 250 mg. three times a week but is getting no response to this second course and is gradually going downhill. X-Rays of her chest were lost and are not available for reproduction.

*Case 4.* V. C., PH 39432, age 55. In March 1951, a panhysterectomy was performed for adenocarcinoma of the endometrium. Postoperative irradiation of unknown amount was given to the operative site. In March 1956, because of loss of weight, lymphedema of the left leg, recurrent partial intestinal obstruction, and a mass felt on physical examination, abdominal exploration was done and a mass was found fixed to the left pelvic wall extending up into the left upper quadrant. The left kidney was not functioning by IVP examination. Multiple pulmonary metastases were seen, 1–3 cm. in diameter, and in November, 1956, because of metastatic pulmonary disease, Delalutin 250 mg. three times a week was begun (Fig. 4a). This was continued until March, 1957, when dose was reduced to 250 mg. twice weekly until December 1958. In March 1957, there was definite decrease in metastatic pulmonary disease, disappearance of lymphedema and marked improvement in bowel function. The left lower quadrant mass was no longer palpable and the left kidney was still nonfunctioning. In February (Fig. 4b) and November 1958, X-rays revealed continued decrease in pulmonary

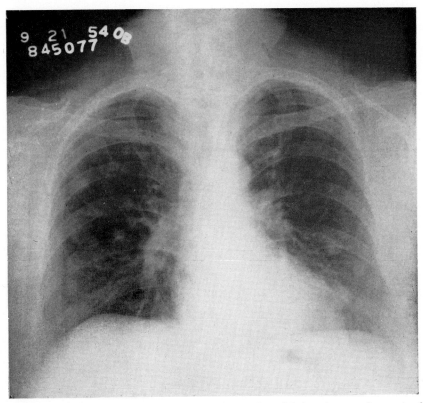

FIG. 3b.  R. W., MGH 845077, 9/21/54.  Slight, but definite, decrease in most of the metastatic lesions.

metastases.  In December 1958, she developed intestinal obstruction treated at an outside hospital.  She died at home in February 1959.  No autopsy was obtained.

*Case 5.*  M. J., MGH 1009968, age 67.  In March 1957, a vaginal hysterectomy was performed for adenocarcinoma of the endometrium.  This was followed by 3000 r of X-ray therapy.  One year later, in March 1958, there was local recurrence in the vagina with multiple ulcerating nodules in the anterior and posterior walls of the vagina. The local disease disappeared with 2000 mg.-hours of radium.  In December 1958, new nodules appeared in the vagina, multiple in number, measuring from 1 to 4 cm.  They were ulcerated and bleeding and Delalutin therapy was begun, 500 mg. twice a week, and continued until March 1959.  In March 1959 the nodules showed definite evidence of decrease in size and 250 mg. of Delalutin were given twice a week.  In June 1959, all evidence of ulcerating nodules had disappeared and she was begun on 375 mg. of Delalutin weekly.  In September 1959, she developed steady pain in the left lower quadrant, palpable disease in the vaginal apex, and an extrinsic mass elevating the rectosigmoid junction on barium enema.  Delalutin was discontinued and she received 2000 r of X-ray of the left lower quadrant with relief of pain.  She now (November 1959) has advancing disease throughout the pelvis and is going slowly downhill.

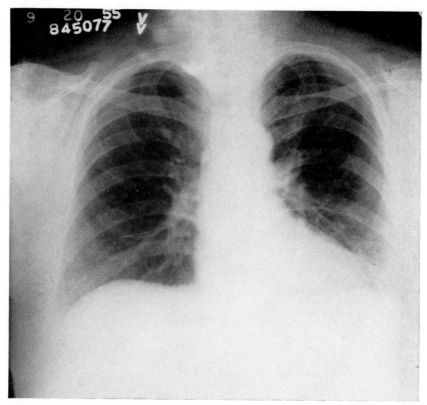

FIG. 3c. R. W., MGH 845077, 9/20/55. Regression and disappearance of all nodular densities.

## DISCUSSION

We feel that these five cases represent definite objective regression of metastatic endometrial adenocarcinoma following progesterone therapy. How progesterone affects metastatic endometrial carcinoma is unknown. The major action is probably one of direct local effect upon the endometrial carcinoma in much the same way that progesterone affects normal endo-metrial tissue. It is of interest that approximately one-third of the patients treated responded objectively to administration of progesterone. This is approximately the same percentage of patients that respond to other forms of hormonal management in carcinoma of the breast. It is felt that these tumors probably represent slowly growing tumors, which might be deemed hormonally dependent carcinomas. In none of the cases have we found any indirect evidence of estrogen activity as measured by changes in vaginal smears or by a measurable increase in estrogen excretion performed in one

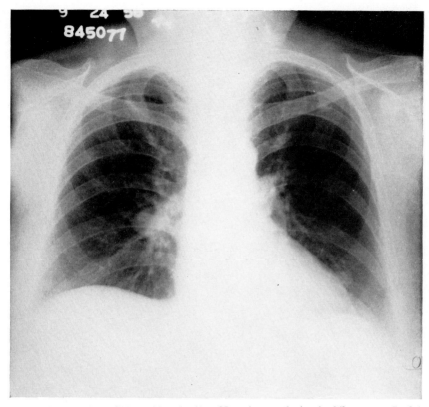

FIG. 3d. R. W., MGH 845077, 9/24/58. Note increased size in hilar area. In left lower lung field, adjacent to the cardiac silhouette, note reappearance of nodular density.

patient. There also has been no evidence of androgenic activity, as measured by hirsutism, acne, increased libido, or increased clitoral size. Because of the large doses of Delalutin which were used, we have done repeated measurements of pH and $CO_2$ on two of the five patients, and in neither has there been a lowering of the $CO_2$ or change of the pH to the alkaline side. An FSH titer done on one patient, R. W., during therapy was 80 rat units, indicating no suppression of FSH. No LH measurements have been performed. Two patients showed evidence of peripheral edema with weight gain and ankle edema, beginning approximately 2 weeks after institution of therapy. In one patient who did not respond, massive edema developed which was thought to be due to the salt-retaining effect of progesterone. In no case, following discontinuance of progesterone, have we noted a change in the vaginal smear or withdrawal bleeding. Since progesterone occupies a key role in steroid metabolism, it seemed possible that progesterone could

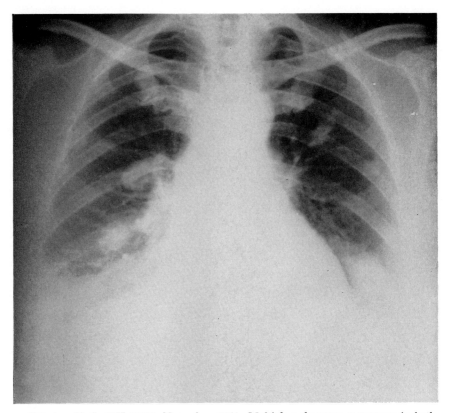

FIG. 4a.  V. C., P.H. 39432, November, 1956.  Multiple pulmonary metastases in both lung fields.

be acting through one of its many metabolic end products, estrogens, androgens, or corticoids.  As stated before, there was no evidence that appreciable conversion to estrogen or biologically active androgen has occurred.  Aldosterone and corticosterone levels were not obtained.

## SUMMARY AND CONCLUSIONS

Fifteen patients with metastatic adenocarcinoma originating in the endometrium have been treated from 3½ weeks to 4½ years with progesterone in varying quantities, from 50 mg. three times a week in the form of Proluton to as much as 1 gm. of Delalutin weekly.  Five out of 15 cases showed definite objective regression lasting from 6 months to 4½ years.  In none of the patients do we have available pathological material to document the objective benefit obtained with the administration of the drug.  In no cases have we noted any evidence of estrogen effect as measured by vaginal smear

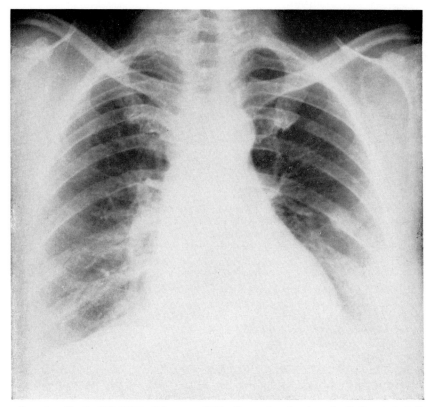

Fɪɢ. 4b. V. C., PH 39432, February, 1958. Regression in size of all the metastatic pulmonary nodules. Lesions remained the same size up to November 1958.

change or pigmentation of nipples or withdrawal bleeding. Progesterone seems to be an effective compound in the treatment of some cases of metastatic endometrial adenocarcinoma and should be given a clinical trial in all cases of metastatic endometrial carcinoma which are not amenable to other forms of therapy. Because of the small number of patients treated in this series, the exact percentage of patients responding to progesterone is unknown. It is of interest that the percentage obtained in this small series corresponds to the approximate percentage of patients who usually respond to hormone therapy in breast carcinoma. The exact mode of action of progesterone in endometrial carcinoma is unknown, but the major effect is undoubtedly related to its direct local effect, which occurs on the endometrium in the absence of endometrial carcinoma. We believe this is another example of a target organ cancer which retains its hormonal identity and responsiveness in spite of neoplastic transformation.

ACKNOWLEDGMENTS

We are indebted to Dr. Howard Ulfelder, Chief of Vincent Memorial Hospital (Gynecology Service of the Massachusetts General Hospital), whose assistance made this study possible. Schering Corp., Bloomfield, New Jersey, and E. R. Squibb and Sons, New Brunswick, New Jersey, generously supplied the Proluton and Delalutin, respectively.

REFERENCES

1. Burrows, H., and Horning, E. "Oestrogens and Neoplasia." C. C Thomas, Springfield, Illinois, 1952.
2. Graham, J. B. *New Engl. J. Med.* **254**, 1112-1119 (1956).
3. Greenblatt, R. B., and Clark, S. L. "The Medical Clinics of North America." Saunders, Philadelphia, Pennsylvania, 1957.
4. Hertig, A. T., and Sommers, S. C. *Cancer* **2**, 946-956 (1949).
5. Heyman, J., ed. "Tenth Annual Report on the Results of Treatment in Carcinoma of the Uterus," 345 pp. P. A. Norstedt, Stockholm, 1955.
6. Kistner, R. W. *Cancer* **12**, 1106-1110 (1959).
7. Meissner, W. A. Personal communication.
8. Meissner, W. A., Sommers, S. C., and Sherman, G. *Cancer* **10**, 500-509 (1957).

DISCUSSION

**R. Hertz:** Dr. Baker, could you tell us the course of events in the ten patients not responding? How rapidly could you detect progression by X-ray on those so-called nonresponding patients? How short a term would it take before you knew the difference between a responding and nonresponding case?

**W. H. Baker:** In about 4–8 weeks. Most of the patients have been treated with progesterone for periods longer than 2 months before evaluation. If you are interested in the natural duration of this neoplasia, it varied from patient to patient as you might expect. I would like to show an X-ray of an unusual patient who demonstrated a slow but definite advance of disease without regression over four years. This patient was followed by Dr. Langdon Parsons and was not treated with progesterone. She does demonstrate what Dr. Hertz, I think, is trying to bring out; namely that endometrial neoplasia has an unpredictable course, with some patients surviving long periods without therapy. This patient has metastatic disease in the chest which slowly progressed over four years, as you can see by these serial X-rays taken about every 6 months. This patient is under Dr. Lemon's care at present and is receiving cortisone.

**H. M. Lemon:** The patient referred to by Dr. Baker has been under treatment with cortisone and prednisone during the last five years. About five years ago she came into the Massachusetts Memorial Hospital, quite dyspneic, with approximately 50% of her visible lung area filled up with these large shadows. She went back to work within a week after starting cortisone, with her vital capacity improved somewhat and her exercise tolerance improved a great deal. She has been working since. She has had two episodes of bronchial penumonia; I can't really say there has been any major regression of these pulmonary metatases. She certainly has had a tremendous subjective response, but in view of her very slow previous course that is all you can say. I think this is a major problem in interpreting one's results in this field.

**E. C. Reifenstein, Jr.:** We have been following the observations of Drs. Baker and Kelley on the effect of Delalutin (17α-hydroxyprogesterone caproate) in patients with advanced metastatic endometrial cancer, with great interest. We wish to express our appreciation to them for initiating this exciting study. Considerable data on the use of Delalutin in various clinical conditions have been reported to us at The Squibb Institute for Medical Research during the past four years in which this unusual steroid ester has been available for investigation and therapeutic administration. This background of information prompts me to make several comments concerning these studies of Delalutin in endometrial cancer.

First, some remarks concerning the dosage of Delalutin that is being used. As pioneers in the use of this long-acting progestational agent in endometrial cancer, Drs. Baker and Kelley were understandably cautious in utilizing this new steroid ester. The dosage originally employed in their study ranged from 250 mg. per injection, two or three times a week, to 500 mg. per injection once or twice a week. The complete absence of undesirable effects of any kind has encouraged them to use larger doses, so that now they are giving 1 gm. or more per week. During the past year, we have supplied Delalutin to several other groups of investigators who had suitable cases for treatment. Some of these workers are using as much as 5000 mg. per week by injection without any untoward effects. Currently, it is our impression that the malignant process responds more promptly and to a greater degree to the larger doses. We believe that it will be necessary to treat a considerable number of suitable cases with large doses of Delalutin beginning when the steroid ester is first administered in order to determine whether the incidence of remission and other aspects of the course of the malignant disease will be influenced favorably by this massive therapy. Treatment to date has been limited to patients who are not amenable to established therapy or who are given surgery and radiation in addition. It will take much study to determine whether we can use Delalutin in early cases instead of surgery and radiation. We would be pleased to supply Delalutin on an investigative basis to the investigators attending this conference and to other qualified workers who have suitable cases of advanced endometrial cancer for study.

**J. Brener:** I would like to mention some observations that have been published in the British literature. The investigators concluded that this disease occurs more frequently in women who have delayed menopause. They also observed diabetes in many, and they go so far as to advise prophylactic hysterectomy in women with this background. I wonder if Dr. Baker in his group of patients has observed anything like that.

**W. H. Baker:** One of the 15 patients had diabetes. This subject was reviewed at Pondville by Dr. Vander, who was unable to find any increased evidence of diabetes in patients with endometrial carcinoma. In regard to their being fat women, I think they were about average size for women beyond the menopause.

**G. E. Block:** I have two patients with endometrial carcinoma in whom we did adrenalectomy and had complete failure. We had no difficulty in seeing progression, as the patients soon died of their disease. I would like to ask Dr. Baker if any of the 15 patients in his series had either benign or malignant breast tumors. We have seen the last five cases that are in our hospital and two of them had mammary cancers.

**W. H. Baker:** In this small series we have not seen any patient with mammary carcinoma.

**R. M. Kelley:** Dr. Segaloff said this morning he hadn't seen a patient with breast cancer who was able to tolerate progestational agents for very long. Most of the patients whom I have treated tolerated the preparations well for as long as two years. In addition to the objective regressions shown here, there has been marked subjective improvement in some of the patients, both the ones who had objective remission and some who did not. One of these patients, who had the best response with pulmonary metastases, was a nurse and a very intelligent person. She used to try herself off the preparation and found that after a month or 6 weeks symptoms of subacute intestinal obstruction would recur, and when she went back on the compound her bowel movements would come back to normal within a couple of weeks. She felt much better on than off therapy, and this went on for two and one-half years during the period when her chest became clear. This happened also in two or three of the other patients, so the preparation is well tolerated. I think it would compete with Dr. Lemon's cortisone in making the patients feel better, and in addition possibly cause a regression of pulmonary metastases.

None of these patients had diabetes except the one Dr. Baker mentioned. Most of them were fat women. They were all, I think, over weight for their age except the premenopausal girl, who was 33. We reviewed all our endometrium cancer at Pondville for diabetes, and there is no increased incidence of diabetes in our series of patients.

**A. Segaloff:** I didn't say progestational agents, I said progesterone. I agree that Delalutin is well tolerated in large amounts, but it is difficult to get people to take 200 mg. of progesterone intramuscularly a day for any length of time. I believe endometrial carcinoma is a responsive tumor. We have not treated any of them with progesterone. However, we treated several patients with testosterone and have one quite striking regression of pulmonary lesions, and several failures. One of the problems of getting patients with this disease for hormonal therapy is that the other therapies do exceedingly well. I wonder whether this really is better than other therapies.

**W. H. Baker:** The favorable thing about progesterone is the singular lack of serious complications. Alkylating agents and radiation have serious effects on the bone marrow and gastrointestinal tract, and this does not occur with progesterone. As far as administration of progesterone is concerned, one of our patients has been treated for four and one-half years with weekly injections. In general, Delalutin is very well tolerated.

**M. J. Brennan:** As many of us remember, this is the first tumor in which the Sommers group of abnormalities of nodular pituitary hyperplasia, nodular adrenal hypoplasia, ovarian stromal hyperplasia, and nodular thyroid hyperlasia as a configuration in endocrine pathology was described. For this reason, we have always hoped that by disturbing the hormonal status of the patients we might be able to upset the tumor. We have a patient with a good long-term result of 9 months on corticoids. I wanted to ask whether anyone has experience with hypophysectomy in this tumor.

**W. H. Baker:** Is Dr. Pearson in the audience? I am fairly sure that they have not done hypophysectomies in endometrial carcinoma. We have not, but if you can obtain this kind of remission with administered hormones, I maintain this would probably be the best way to treat them. In the tumors that are not hormone dependent some other form of therapy, such as alkylating agents and antibiotics, might well be useful.

**H. Volk:** In regard to Dr. Kelley's statement on the symptomatic improvement and well-being of patients who received parental progesterone, I would like to mention that in our series, in which we gave oral progesterone—2 gm. a day to 29 women—we failed to observe subjective improvement. We had evidence that the oral progesterone was absorbed from the gastrointestinal tract and was metabolically active, since we demonstrated a catabolic effect; and Dr. Tyler's group showed that in patients primed with estrogen there was a definite progestational effect on the endometrium.

I would like to add that this stimulating and provocative report of Dr. Baker raises again the point made this morning by Dr. Pincus concerning the daily oral dose of 2 gm. of progesterone. Originally, it was believed this represented an exceedingly large amount, but now one wonders whether this is necessarily so in terms of systemically absorbed agent.

**B. J. Kennedy:** I think it is encouraging to find that uterine carcinomas do respond so nicely to hormones. We have employed arterial nitrogen mustard, using a brachial artery catheter inserted into the descending aorta. Striking regressions lasting more than a year occurred in two patients.

# Steroid Metabolism in Endocrine Tumors[1]

RALPH I. DORFMAN

*Worcester Foundation for Experimental Biology,
Shrewsbury, Massachusetts*

## INTRODUCTION

Advances in our knowledge of steroid metabolism coupled with the availability of precise methods have made possible the study of functional tumors of steroid-producing tissues. These studies are contributing significantly to our understanding of the type of biochemical abnormality involved, frequently indicating how the abnormal state is maintained, and may eventually lead to a more rational system for the classification of functional tumors. The precise methods include quantitative and qualitative studies of blood and urinary steroids, *in vivo* biosynthetic studies using singly or doubly labeled precursors, incubation of tumor tissues obtained at surgery with non-labeled and labeled precursors, and finally direct analysis of tumors obtained at operation or autopsy.

In this communication representative steroid-producing tumors in man will be discussed in the light of newer biochemical findings.

## BIOSYNTHESIS OF STEROID HORMONES

Briefly stated, steroid hormones in the main appear to be derived from acetate and cholesterol. Cholesterol is converted into pregnenolone, which on oxidation to progesterone yields the basic versatile intermediate for the formation of androgens and in turn estrogens as well as corticoids such as cortisol, corticosterone, and aldosterone (reviewed in 12–16, 24, 25).

Specifically, in the gonad, adrenal, and placenta the bulk of the androgens are biosynthesized by the following reaction sequence: cholesterol → pregnenolone → progesterone → 17α-hydroxyprogesterone → $\Delta^4$-androstene-3,17-dione → testosterone. In the adrenal 11β-hydroxylation of $\Delta^4$-androstene-3,17-dione leads to a unique series of androgens. Dehydroepiandrosterone may be formed from pregnenolone through 17α-hydroxypregnenolone in the adrenal. The bulk of the estrogens are produced from androgens by a mechanism involving a 19-hydroxy intermediate and this reaction takes place in all steroid-producing tissue and perhaps in liver tissue as well.

Corticoids are produced in the adrenal by a sequence involving cholesterol → pregnenolone → progesterone. Progesterone on hydroxylation at

[1] Some of the work discussed here has been supported by The Jane Coffin Childs Memorial Fund for Medical Research, American Cancer Society, and the Atomic Energy Commission.

positions 11β, 17α, and 21 yields cortisol, on hydroxylation at positions 11β and 21 yields corticosterone, and on hydroxylation at positions 11β, 18, and 21 (plus further oxidation of the 18-hydroxy group to the aldehyde) yields aldosterone.

These biosynthetic reactions form the basis for our study of steroid metabolism in endocrine tumors.

## TUMORS OF THE GONADS

### Ovarian Tumors

*Masculinizing Tumors. Virilizing malignant lipoid cell tumor of the ovary.* This tumor, found in both the benign and malignant form in females of all ages, has also been termed hypernephroma, hypernephroid tumor of the ovary, luteinoma, interstitioma, luteoma, adrenal tumor of the ovary, and masculinovoblastoma. Only limited biochemical studies have been done, one quite recently and another over fifteen years ago.

Recently, through the cooperation of Doctors R. M. Clark and A. Ross, of the Oshawa General Hospital, Oshawa, Ontario, Canada, we have studied the urine of a patient with the diagnosis of a malignant lipoid cell tumor, established by clinical observations, surgical removal and histological examination of the tumor, and the finding of a high 17-ketosteroid excretion of 220 mg. per day. The individual 17-ketosteroids were analyzed by the method of Rubin *et al.* (36) as indicated in Table I.

TABLE I

INDIVIDUAL 17-KETOSTEROID EXCRETION IN THE URINE OF A PATIENT WITH
A LIPOID CELL TUMOR OF THE OVARY

| 17-Ketosteroid | Mg./24 hr. | % Increase over normal |
|---|---|---|
| Androsterone | 66.0 | 1600 |
| Etiocholanolone | 48.9 | 1200 |
| 11-Ketoandrosterone | 5.3 | 5000 |
| 11β-Hydroxyandrosterone | 29.8 | 4000 |
| 11-Ketoetiocholanolone | 6.3 | 1200 |
| 11β-Hydroxyetiocholanolone | 7.5 | 1500 |

Although the tumor was located in the ovary, the biochemical evidence agreed with histological evidence indicating an adrenal origin of this tissue. This statement is made on the basis of the enormous increase in 11-keto-androsterone and 11β-hydroxyandrosterone (fifty times and forty times, respectively), which indicated the production by the tumor of the adrenal androgens 11β-hydroxy-$\Delta^4$-androstene-3,17-dione and adrenosterone (6, 38).

Steroid studies on the urine of a second patient with the diagnosis of non-malignant luteoma of the ovary was reported in some detail (18), but unfortunately at the time the isolations were done (almost twenty years ago), methods were relatively crude and 11-oxygenated $C_{19}$ steroids in urine were still to be discovered. Androsterone in concentrations up to 16 mg. per liter was isolated from the urine of the 21-year-old virilized female bearing the ovarian tumor. Of interest was the isolation of 0.5 mg. per liter of $\Delta^{16}$-androsten-3$\alpha$-ol (18). This steroid has been isolated in increased amounts from the urine of patients with adrenocortical tumors (30), from the urine of a patient with adrenal hyperplasia (31), and from normal men's urine (8).

Although both tumors, the lipoid cell tumor and the luteoma, may have had the same steroid biosynthetic potentials and in fact similar urinary steroid patterns on the basis of the available evidence, the only similarity that is known with certainty is the high androsterone excretion. The urine of the patient bearing the luteoma may also have had a high content of 11-oxygenated $C_{19}$ steroids, but this would not have been detected. At the present time, pending additional studies of this type of tumor, the following tentative conclusions may be drawn: (a) the tumor is derived from adrenal tissue, and (b) the steroid biosynthetic capacity of the tumor includes the formation of 11-deoxy-$C_{19}$ steroids and 11-oxygenated-$C_{19}$ steroids, but that the formation of corticoids in significant concentrations does not take place. Both patients were considerably virilized, and this can be explained on the basis of the excessive production of $\Delta^4$-androstene-3,17-dione and testosterone by the tumor tissue.

*Arrhenoblastoma tumor.* This tumor, also known as androblastoma and masculinoma, occurs in patients from 15 to 60 years of age. The tumor is almost always unilateral and most often causes atrophy of the contralateral ovary. In size it may vary from almost a pin-point nodule to a mass 5 inches in diameter. The origin of the tumor has not been established with certainty, but it is generally believed that the tumor arises from certain male-directed cells in the ovary persisting from an early ambivalent stage of gonadogenesis. The original description of this tumor was by Pick (33), who found the tumor in an ovotestis of a hermaphrodite, but this has been the only published case of this type.

Hormonally, the tumor produces excessive androgens and, rarely, excessive estrogens as well (23). Determination of urinary 17-ketosteroids has in the main indicated a tendency toward an increase in some patients, normal values in others, and in a few, increases up to 300 % above normal (15).

Recently direct analyses have been done on the tumor tissue. These important studies are those of Anliker et al. (1), who isolated progesterone, testosterone, $\Delta^4$-androstene-3,17-dione, and androsterone from an arrhenoblastoma. The fact that testosterone was isolated was indeed important, since this gave a possible explanation for the observed virilism or even masculinization in the face of an insignificant or slight increase in urinary 17-ketosteroids in the urine. The finding of testosterone in arrhenoblastoma tissue has been confirmed by Savard *et al.* (41), who showed that progesterone-4-$C^{14}$ was converted into 17α-hydroxyprogesterone, Δ⁴-androstene-3,17-dione, and testosterone. The former two steroids were also found by Wiest *et al.* (45) to be biosynthetic products of progesterone in arrhenoblastoma tissue.

On the basis of existing evidence, the modification of steroid biosynthesis seems to involve the increased production of testosterone without necessarily modifying other aspects of the biosynthetic pathway. This may be illustrated as follows:

$$\text{Cholesterol} \rightarrow \text{Pregnenolone} \rightarrow \text{Progesterone}$$
$$\text{Primary Defect}$$
$$\downarrow$$
$$\text{Testosterone} \rightleftharpoons \Delta^4\text{-Androstene-3,17-dione} \leftarrow 17\alpha\text{-Hydroxyprogesterone}$$

*Feminizing Tumor: Granulosa cell tumor.* The granulosa cell tumor usually shows a low-grade malignancy and occurs most frequently during active sex life and less frequently after the menopause or in the childhood. It is believed that the tumor is derived from remnants of the early mesenchymal core of the ovary. These tumors are capable of producing excessive amounts of estrogens.

A typical example is a tumor detected by clinical observations in a postmenopausal woman. The bioassay, using an immature mouse uterus method, of the phenolic fraction of urine, indicated a titer of 100 μg. of estrone equivalent, which for a subject in this age range is about fifty times normal by the methods employed. This high titer of estrogenic material was confirmed by chemical analysis by the Brown Method (7). The chemical assay indicated an excretion of more than 200 μg. per day for the combined estrone, estradiol-17β, and estriol fractions (unpublished observation).

Since $C_{19}$ steroids appeared to be excreted in normal amounts and since the estrogen was assumed to be produced in the tumor, the biosynthetic abnormality was placed somewhere between the androgens and the estrogens. This statement assumes that the principal pathway for estrogen biosynthesis is from androgens. On this basis one may suggest an excessive concentration of 19-hydroxylase and the enzyme system which aromatizes the 19-hydroxy $C_{19}$ steroid to estrogens.

## TUMORS OF THE TESTIS

*Chorionepithelioma.* At least some tumors of this type in men produce androgens. This is deduced from the fact that urinary 17-ketosteroids may be increased (15, 29). Also striking, at least in one case that was studied some years ago (29), was the fact that the urine of a 20-year-old male with metastases yielded pregnanediol at the elevated rate of 4 mg. per day and 75 µg. of estrone equivalent per day. Actually this case illustrated the basic biosynthetic pattern from progesterone to androgens to estrogens, but it was not recognized at the time. In addition to progesterone, androgen, and estrogens, this chorionepithelioma tumor also produced gonadotropins.

*Interstitial Cell Tumor (Masculinizing).* This tumor is an androgen-producing tumor and has as its clinical feature in young boys precocious puberty. Up to recently it was considered to be simply a condition of over-production of testosterone. This hypothesis was consistent with the steroid studies on a patient who excreted 1000 mg. of 17-ketosteroids per day. From this urine, excessive amounts of androsterone and etiocholanolone were isolated, although the titer of dehydroepiandrosterone was not increased (44). Recent studies, however, have reopened the question of steroid biosynthesis by such a tumor, since 11β-hydroxylase activity was detected in the tissue and a corresponding excessive concentration of 11-oxygenated $C_{19}$ catabolites in the urine (Table II) (39, 40, 42).

TABLE II

17-KETOSTEROID EXCRETION IN THE URINE OF A PATIENT WITH AN INTERSTITIAL CELL TUMOR (42)

| 17-Ketosteroid | Preoperative (mg./day) | Postoperative (mg./day) |
|---|---|---|
| Androsterone | 2.4 | 0 |
| Etiocholanolone | 2.0 | 0.1 |
| Dehydroepiandrosterone | 1.4 | 0 |
| 11β-Hydroxy- and 11-ketoandrosterone | 1.8 | 0.1 |
| 11β-Hydroxy- and 11-ketoetiocholanolone | 0.4 | 0 |

The urinary studies revealed an elevated excretion of pregnanetriol which decreased to one-tenth the value 2 days after surgery. This component is an indication of the increased production of 17α-hydroxyprogesterone, the intermediate in androgen production. Corticoids were normal and remained unchanged as a result of the operation. The 17-ketosteroids were 13.6 mg. for the 5½-year-old boy and dropped to 1.4 mg. per day after surgery. When the 17-ketosteroids were fractionated a significant increase in all components was found, including dehydroepiandrosterone. The increase in this component which is corroborated by the conversion of acetate to dehydroepiandrosterone (Table II) in the incubation experiments with tumor tissue strongly suggests the presence of adrenal tissue. Dehydroepiandrosterone is not considered to be a product of testicular tissue. The finding of increased amounts of the 11-oxygenated derivatives of androsterone and etiocholanolone and in a ratio of 5α:5β of 4.5:1 (6, 38) indicates that the precursor in the tumor was 11β-hydroxy-$\Delta^4$-androstene-3,17-dione (or testosterone derivative), a fact which is in accord with the incubation experiments demonstrating 11β-hydroxylase in the tumor tissue (Table III).

TABLE III

BIOSYNTHESIS OF STEROIDS IN AN INTERSTITIAL CELL TUMOR
BY SELECTED SUBSTRATES (42)

| Substrate | Product |
|---|---|
| Acetate | Testosterone; $\Delta^4$-androstene-3,17-dione; 11β-hydroxy-$\Delta^4$-androstene-3,17-dione; adrenosterone; dehydroepiandrosterone; 17α-hydroxyprogesterone |
| Progesterone | Testosterone; $\Delta^4$-androstene-3,17-dione; 11β-hydroxy-$\Delta^4$-androstene-3,17-dione; 17α-hydroxyprogesterone |
| Testosterone | $\Delta^4$-Androstene-3,17-dione; 11β-hydroxy-$\Delta^4$-androstene-3,17-dione; 11β-hydroxy-testosterone, adrenosterone |

*Interstitial Cell Tumor (Feminizing)*. This type of interstitial cell tumor is rarer than that which produces excessive androgens, but about 7 cases are now reported. In a typical case reported recently by Herrmann *et al.* (26) the patient had an elevated urinary excretion of estriol and estradiol-17β while the estrone level was normal. Although the estrogen levels were not determined postoperatively, the gynecomastia receded slowly and the depressed sperm count increased to normal. The 17-ketosteroid excretion was not especially changed from normal in the 20-year-old male patient. The 11-oxy-17-ketosteroids showed no significant increase from normal, nor was there a decrease after removal of the tumor. It appears that, quite unlike the masculinizing interstitial tumor here described, no 11β-hydroxylase could be demonstrated.

The primary defect in this type of tumor seems to depend upon the efficiency with which a normal amount of androgens is converted to estrogens. As with the granulosa cell tumor where the same conditions obtain, a possible cause could be relative increases in the specific enzyme content concerned with the conversion of androgens to estrogens.

*An Undifferentiated Testicular Tumor*. In one extensive study on the urine and tumor tissue the biochemical facts indicate that the tumor possessed properties usually attributable to adrenal tissue. The urine of a 3-year-old boy, who was virilized as a result of this type of tumor, contained increased quantities of urocortisol and urocortisone, which indicated the strong possibility that cortisol was produced by the tumor tissue. Increased amounts of 11-oxygenated derivatives of androsterone without a proportionately larger amount of 11-oxygenated derivatives of etiocholanolone indicated an elevated production of 11β-hydroxy-$\Delta^4$-androstene-3,17-dione, usually considered to be an adrenal androgen. Finally, the urine contained increased amounts of dehydroepiandrosterone, an androgen as yet undetected in testicular tissue but known to be produced by the adrenal (5, 34).

Incubation of the tumor tissue with acetate-$1$-$C^{14}$ afforded a means of testing the biosynthetic capacities of the tissue directly. When this was done all the suspicions generated by the urinary studies were confirmed. Labeled cortisol was isolated and presumptive evidence was found for the formation of the characteristic adrenocortical steroids dehydroepiandrosterone and 11β-hydroxy-$\Delta^4$-androstene-3,17-dione (3).

## Adrenal Tumors

### Adrenal Cancer with Virilism

This type of adrenal hyperactivity is characterized usually by an excessive excretion of dehydroepiandrosterone and related steroids having the $\Delta^5$-3β-hydroxy configuration in ring A. Dehydroepiandrosterone has been isolated from adrenal cancer tissue (34). It is possible that even the high levels of dehydroepiandrosterone are not sufficiently androgenic to account for the severe masculinization seen in these patients. It is likely that the responsible virilizing agent is actually testosterone, which is present probably in excessive amounts in these adrenal tumors. Precise determinations of the circulating testosterone to establish this point cannot be done at the present time owing to lack of adequate methods.

A striking biosynthetic peculiarity in this syndrome appears to be a relative deficiency in the enzyme 3β-ol-dehydrogenase which oxidizes the $\Delta^5$-3β-hydroxy steroid group to the $\Delta^4$-3-ketone. The enzyme deficiency results in a high concentration of dehydroepiandrosterone, the related $C_{19}$ steroids, $\Delta^5$-androstene-3β,17β-diol, and $\Delta^5$-androstene-3β,16α,17β-triol, and the $C_{21}$ compounds $\Delta^5$-pregnene-3β,20α-diol, $\Delta^5$-pregnene-3β,16α,20α-triol, and others (15). On the other hand, cortisol and corticosterone may be produced in normal or only slightly elevated amounts.

Steroid production by adrenal tumors of the virilizing variety may or may not be sensitive to ACTH control. In general, these tissues appear to have a high degree of autonomy (27).

Finkelstein and Shoenberger (20) have demonstrated that patients with adrenal cancer and virilism do not have measurable (less than 0.2 mg. per day) amounts of pregnanetriolone (3α,11β,17α-trihydroxypregnan-20-one) although the pregnanetriol and 17-ketosteroids may be greatly increased. Actually, as Finkelstein and Shoenberger (20) have indicated, the test for the triolone is an aid to differential diagnosis. If 17-ketosteroids and/or pregnanetriol are increased and triolone cannot be detected, then an adrenal tumor of the virilizing type, either benign or malignant, is possible.

## Adrenal Cancer—Feminizing Tumor

Some patients with adrenal cancer with masculinization and no cortisol disease have an increased titer of estrogens in their urine. The physiological effects may be obscured by an enormously increased amount of androgens. In other instances, however, the quantity of estrogens may reach such high levels that distinct feminization results. The biochemical defects in these patients seem to involve an excessive production of estrogens by a mechanism in the adrenal involving $\Delta^4$-androstene-3,17-dione aromatization to estrone or testosterone to estradiol-17$\beta$. In a typical case, an adrenal cortical carcinoma removed from a 66-year-old man with gynecomastia was incubated with testosterone-3-$C^{14}$, and $C^{14}$-labeled estrone and estradiol-17$\beta$ were formed. This corroborated the preoperative high daily excretion of estrogens: estrone, 187 µg.; estradiol-17$\beta$, 47 µg.; and estriol, 170 µg. (4). An important report by Salhanick and Berliner (37) described the isolation of equilenin from an adrenal carcinoma which produced excessive amounts of estrogens. This ring B unsaturated estrogen has been isolated heretofore only from the urine of the pregnant mare and may indicate a second pathway for the biosynthesis of estrogens (13).

## Cushing's Syndrome—Cancer

This condition, caused by excessive secretion of cortisol, is characterized primarily by protein loss, diabetes mellitus, hypertension, obesity, weakness, and osteoporosis. One adrenal bears the tumor while the contralateral adrenal is atrophied. This is due to the fact that the high concentration of cortisol causes a decreased production and/or release of ACTH. 17-Ketosteroids may be low to excessive. No pregnanetriolone can be detected (20). The tumor tissue has established an autonomous steroid production and is usually not receptive to ACTH stimulation. The important changes in biosynthesis involve an excessive production of $C_{21}$ steroids, which means an increase in pregnenolone from cholesterol, an increase in progesterone, and that the hydroxylation reactions leading from progesterone to cortisol and corticosterone are also operating maximally. Under certain conditions, however, partial blocks in corticoid synthesis have been observed. In a study on a woman with Cushing's syndrome due to a metastasizing adrenal cancer, in the terminal stage of the disease evidence for a relatively low level of 11$\beta$-hydroxylation was found. The urine contained a major amount of 3$\alpha$,17$\alpha$-dihydroxypregnan-20-one, indicating a high tumor production of deoxycortisol. Similar findings have been reported by other workers (17, 35, 43).

## Cushing's Syndrome—Adenoma

This condition also results in excessive cortisol secretion, atrophy of the contralateral adrenal, usual minimum virilism, and normal or relatively decreased titers of 17-ketosteroids; only rarely are increased 17-ketosteroids observed. No pregnanetriolone can be detected in the urine (20). The adenoma seems to possess some autonomous qualities, and it is this feature in face of a decreased ACTH (as seen by an atrophied contralateral adrenal) that keeps the cortisol production at a high level. About one-half of the patients respond to ACTH stimulation.

The biosynthetic capacities of two adrenal adenomas in association with Cushing's syndrome have been studied in our laboratory. In one experiment slices of tissue were incubated with acetate-$1$-$C^{14}$, and it was possible to show that a variety of corticoids including cortisol, cortisone, corticosterone, 11-dehydrocorticosterone, and 11-deoxycortisol were formed. Corticosterone and 11-dehydrocorticosterone were formed in greater quantities than cortisol and cortisone. The $C_{19}$ steroids dehydroepiandrosterone, $\Delta^4$-androstene-3,17-dione, and 11$\beta$-hydroxy-$\Delta^4$-androstene-3,17-dione were also biosynthesized from the acetate (21).

In a second experiment (22) a homogenate of adenomatous adrenal tumor from a patient with Cushing's syndrome was incubated with cholesterol-$C^{14}$ and pregnenolone-$H^3$ and yielded $C^{14}$- and $H^3$-labeled cortisol, cortisone, 11-deoxycortisol, deoxycorticosterone, dehydroepiandrosterone, and 11$\beta$- hydroxy-$\Delta^4$-androstene-3,17-dione. The ratio of $H^3$ to $C^{14}$ for the $C_{21}$ corticoids varied from 1:10 to 1:16, while the ratios for the two $C_{19}$ steroids were 1:7 for dehydroepiandrosterone and 1:9 for 11$\beta$-hydroxy-$\Delta^4$-androstene-3,17-dione.

These results demonstrated that pregnenolone, probably by way of 17$\alpha$-hydroxypregnenolone, was converted to dehydroepiandrosterone and that possibly a portion of the dehydroepiandrosterone was formed from cholesterol without going through a $C_{21}$ intermediate such as pregnenolone.

## Virilizing Benign Adenoma—without Cushing's Syndrome

This is a nonmalignant, partially autonomous tumor showing a highly elevated production of androgens, of which dehydroepiandrosterone appears to be the principal one. In some patients estrogens may also be elevated. The fact that pregnanediol and pregnanetriol seem to be deficient indicates that both progesterone and 17$\alpha$-hydroxyprogesterone are secreted in normal, and certainly not abnormal, quantities. Pregnanetriolone could not be detected at the 50 μg./24 hour level (19). The ACTH stimulation test caused little increase in 17-ketosteroid excretion, a minimum corticoid increase, and a minimum increase in estrogens. The corticoid inhibition test indicated a slight decrease in 17-ketosteroids, but corticoid and estrogens may not be altered.

From a biochemical viewpoint there seems to be a relative deficiency of 3β-ol-dehydrogenase similar to that described under adrenal cancer with virilism.

### Prepuberal Virilism—Benign Adenoma

This condition is characterized by a high concentration of circulating androgens as reflected by high urinary 17-ketosteroids with a corresponding normal corticoid production. The contralateral adrenal is normal or at least not atrophied. ACTH tests indicate a normal increase in corticoid production but an increased responsiveness with respect to androgen output. Normal responsiveness to cortisol therapy has been found and no data are available on pregnanetriol excretion or effects of irradiation.

### Primary Aldosteronism—Adenoma and Cancer

A syndrome described by Conn (10, 11) for the first time involves a variety of symptoms including intermittent tetany, periodic severe muscular weakness and paralysis, paresthesia, polyuria, polydipsia, hypertension, impairment of renal function, but no edema. Conn (10, 11) was able to demonstrate that the urine of these patients contained excessive concentrations of sodium-retaining material, presumably aldosterone, and that removal of the tumor resulted in a dramatic reversal of the symptoms, in fact a cure. These observations have been amply confirmed [collected cases cited (2)].

In many of the reported cases both 17-ketosteroid and corticoid excretion were normal; the increase in steroid production was essentially limited to aldosterone. Increased amounts of aldosterone have been detected by direct analysis of tumors from patients with primary aldosteronism (32) and by tumor incubation studies (2).

### Summary and Conclusions

The metabolism of steroids in certain endocrine tumors has been briefly reviewed and compared with that in normal tissues. Although the data concerning the various tumors are fragmentary, certain patterns are emerging. The biosynthetic pathways in tumor tissue appear to be similar to those of the normal tissues from which they are derived. The differences in steroid production between normal and tumor tissue appear to be quantitative rather than qualitative. The single observation that goes contrary to this last statement, that is, isolation of equilenin from an adrenal carcinoma causing feminization, still awaits confirmation; if it can be confirmed it will be necessary to show that this estrogen does not occur in normal adrenal tissue.

More detailed information on the biosynthesis of steroids in tumor tissue supplements existing clinical and pathological findings in various states of hyperactivity and may be expected to aid in the establishment of a more precise classification of the tumors. The detailed study of these tumors may be expected to continue to be a convenient method for the elucidation of normal steroid biosynthesis.

### REFERENCES

1. Anliker, R., Rohr, O., and Ruzicka, L. *Ann. Chem. Liebig's* **603**, 109 (1957).
2. Ayres, P. J., Garrod, O., Tait, S. A. S., and Tait, J. F. *In* "Aldosterone" (A. F. Muller and C. M. O'Connor, eds.), p. 143. Little, Brown, Boston, Massachusetts, 1958.
3. Baggett, B., Engel, L. L., Savard, K., and Dorfman, R. I. *Federation Proc.* **16**, 149 (1957).
4. Baggett, B., Engel, L. L., Balderas, L., Lanman, G., Savard, K., and Dorfman, R. I. *Endocrinology* **64**, 600 (1959).
5. Bloch, E., Dorfman, R. I., and Pincus, G. *Arch. Biochem. Biophys.* **61**, 245 (1956).
6. Bradlow, H. L., and Gallagher, T. F. *J. Biol. Chem.* **229**, 505 (1957).
7. Brown, J. B. *Biochem. J.* **60**, 185 (1955).
8. Brooksbank, B. W. L., and Haslewood, G. A. D. *Biochem. J.* **44**, iii (1949).
9. Brown, J. B. *Biochem. J.* **60**, 185 (1955).
10. Conn, J. W. *J. Lab Clin. Med.* **45**, 6 (1955).
11. Conn, J. W. *J. Lab. Clin. Med.* **45**, 661 (1955).
12. Dorfman, R. I. *Proc. Intern. Congr. Biochem., 4th Congr., Vienna, 1958* p. 175 (1959).
13. Dorfman, R. I. *Am. J. Med.* **21**, 679 (1956).
14. Dorfman, R. I. *Ann. Rev. Biochem.* **26**, 523 (1957).
15. Dorfman, R. I., and Shipley, R. A. "Androgens." Wiley, New York, 1956.
16. Dorfman, R. I., and Ungar, F. "Metabolism of Steroid Hormones." Burgess, Minneapolis, Minnesota, 1954.
17. Eberlein, W. R., and Bongiovanni, A. M. *Helv. Paediat. Acta* **2**, 105 (1956).
18. Engel, L. L., Dorfman, R. I., and Abarbanel, A. R. *J. Clin. Endocrinol. and Metabolism,* **13**, 903 (1953).
19. Finkelstein, M. *Acta Endocrinol.* **30**, 489 (1959).
20. Finkelstein, M., and Shoenberger, J. *J. Clin. Endocrinol. and Metabolism,* **19**, 609 (1959).
21. Goldstein, M., Gut, M., and Dorfman, R. I. Unpublished.
22. Goldstein, M., Gut, M., Dorfman, R. I., Soffer, L. J., and Gabrilove, J. L. Unpublished.
23. Greene, R. R. *In* "Progress in Clinical Endocrinology" (S. Soskins, ed.), p. 323. Grune and Stratton, New York, 1950.
24. Hechter, O. "Cholesterol" (R. P. Cook, ed.), p. 309. Academic Press, New York, 1958.

25. Hechter, O., and Pincus, G. *Physiol. Revs.* **34**, 459 (1954).
26. Herrman, W. L., Buckner, F., and Baskin, A. *J. Clin. Endocrinol. and Metabolism* **18**, 834 (1958).
27. Jailer, J. W., Gold, J. J., and Wallace, E. Z. *Am. J. Med.* **16**, 340 (1954).
28. Jones, G. S., and Everett, H. S. *Am. J. Obstet. Gynecol.* **52**, 614 (1946).
29. Laipply, T. C., and Shipley, R. A. *Am. J. Pathol.* **21**, 921 (1945).
30. Mason, H. L., and Schneider, J. J. *J. Biol. Chem.* **184**, 593 (1950).
31. Miller, A. M., Rosenkrantz, H., and Dorfman, R. I. *Endocrinology* **53**, 238 (1953).
32. Neher, R. *In* "Aldosterone" (A. F. Muller and C. M. O'Connor, eds.), p. 21. Little, Brown, Boston, Massachusetts (1958).
33. Pick, L. *Arch. Gynäkol.* **76**, 191 (1905).
34. Plantin, L. O., Diczfalusy, E., and Birke, G. *Nature* **179**, 421 (1957).
35. Rosselet, J. P., Overland, L., Jailer, J. W., and Lieberman, S. *Helv. Chim. Acta* **37**, 1933 (1954).
36. Rubin, B. L., Dorfman, R. I., and Pincus, G. *J. Biol Chem.* **203**, 629 (1953).
37. Salhanick, H., and Berliner, D. L. *J. Biol. Chem.* **227**, 583 (1957).
38. Savard, K., Burstein, S., Rosenkrantz, H., and Dorfman, R. I. *J. Biol. Chem.* **202**, 717 (1953).
39. Savard, K., Dorfman, R. I., Baggett, B., and Engel, L. L. *Federation Proc.* **15**, 346 (1956).
40. Savard, K., Dorfman, R. I., Baggett, B., and Engel, L. L. *J. Clin. Endocrinol. and Metabolism* **16**, 1629 (1956).
41. Savard, K., Dorfman, R. I., Gabrilove, J. L., and Soffer, L. J. *J. Clin. Endocrinol. and Metabolism* (in press).
42. Savard, K., Dorfman, R. I., Baggett, B., Fielding, L. L., Engel, L. L., McPherson, H. T., Lester, L. M., Johnson, D. S., Hamblen, G. C., and Engel, F. L. *J. Clin. Invest.* **39**, 534 (1960).
43. Touchstone, J. C., Richardson, E. M., Bubaschenko, H., Landolt, I., and Dohan, F. C. *J. Clin. Endocrinol. and Metabolism* **14**, 676 (1954).
44. Venning, E. H., Hoffman, M. M., and Brown, J. S. L. *J. Biol. Chem.* **146**, 369 (1942).
45. Wiest, W. G., Zander, J., and Holmstrom, E. G. *J. Clin. Endocrinol. and Metabolism* **19**, 297 (1959).

### DISCUSSION

**R. Huseby:** We are all grateful to Dr. Dorfman for bringing this large amount of material together and presenting it in such a straightforward manner. There is, however, some possible variation in interpretation. Over the past several years working with Drs. Oscar Dominguez and Leo Samuels, we have been investigating the biosynthetic pathways in the induced interstitial cell testicular tumors of the mouse. Here we do have a good idea of the tissue of origin: we are fairly certain from histological and from developmental studies of the tumors, that they did, in fact, arise from interstitial cells. We can more easily get normal tissue of origin with which to work, since we can easily obtain normal testicular tissue from the mouse. From the start it became very evident that quantitation was the big problem, and I agree with Dr. Dorfman whole-heatedly that quantitation in the *in vitro* systems is still the biggest problem. However, one of these tumors very early was found to have appreciable 21-hydroxylase activity and yet was typically an interstitial cell tumor. We had never seen 21-hydroxylase in normal testicular tissue up to that time and the observation worried us. In subsequent studies this tumor actually was producing adrenal corticoidlike substances, in all probability deoxycorticosterone (DOC), for we isolated and identified DOC in the blood of animals carrying the tumor, and the tumor was able to protect adrenalectomized animals against a potassium load. We then went back to normal rodent testes and with improved methods could show that a small amount of 21-hydroxylase was present.

Our thesis is that all the steroid-producing tissues probably have at least a majority of the enzymes that are present in the others. The testis, for instance, produces primarily androgens because in this tissue the conditions, enzyme concentrations, etc., are such that the androgenic biosynthetic pathways take precedence over the others, that is, over the corticoid- or estrogen-producing pathways. But when a neoplasm develops, certain enzyme systems may drop out, and again we feel that this may happen in a rather random fashion, so that tumors can develop in which the corticoid pathways, for example, can express themselves as one of the dominant pathways of steroidogenesis. We do not have to assume that we have adrenal rest tissue in the ovaries or in the testis as a necessary alternative, but rather that in certain tumors developing from these tissues the enzymatic situation has been altered so that the production of adrenal corticoids can now take precedence over the originally dominant type of hormone production.

**R. Dorfman:** I have followed the work of Dr. Huseby's group with great interest and there is little doubt that they have demonstrated 21-hydroxylase in normal mouse testis tissue. This is something that still remains to be demonstrated in normal human testis.

**M. E. Lombardo:** Dr. Viscelli, Dr. Hudson, and I have been interested in studying the biosynthesis of androgens in the normal human testis. We have done a number of *in vitro* experiments along these lines in which we found that the substrate most readily metabolized was progesterone. When progesterone was incubated with normal human testicular tissue, the main transformation product was 17α-hydroxyprogesterone. The second product formed is $\Delta^4$-androstene-3,17-dione. Once or twice we got traces of a substance that looked like testosterone, but we were never able to confirm this with certainty. We proceeded from this type of experiment to an *in situ* perfusion of the human testis with 4-$C^{14}$-progesterone. The main transformation product was again 17α-hydroxyprogesterone and the second product isolated was $\Delta^4$-androstene-3,17-dione. We were never able to detect any C-21 hydroxylated substances and as yet we have been unable to pick up testosterone in radioactive form. It appears to me that the scheme for the biosynthesis of androgens by the normal human testis agrees very well with the scheme proposed by Dr. Dorfman.

**R. Dorfman:** I am delighted to hear of Dr. Lombardo's experiment. Work of this type will give us the proper background against which to interpret studies on various testicular tumors.

**C. J. Migeon:** Most pathologists would be willing to admit that it is very difficult to differentiate the various types of testicular tumors. This is why incubation work is very important, since it gives us some idea of the nature of the steroids produced by these tumors and, therefore, permits a better classification. However, in this incubation technique one adds all sorts of cofactors and consequently I believe that the end results indicate a potential synthesis of steroids rather than a true *in vivo* production by the tumor.

We have tried to avoid the possible pitfalls inherent in incubation methods. In collaboration with Dr. Howard Jones of the Department of Gynecology at the Johns Hopkins Hospital, we have been able to collect some ovarian vein blood in several cases with ovarian pathology. In a case with the pathological diagnosis of adrenal rest tumor of the ovary we have detected in the ovarian blood $\Delta^4$-androstene-3,17-dione (45 μg. per 100 ml. of plasma) and, strangely enough, etiocholanolone (30 μg. per 100 ml.). In a case of Stein-Leventhal syndrome we have detected $\Delta^4$-androstene-3,17-dione (29 μg./100 ml.) and androsterone (36 μg./100 ml.), but in two other cases no free 17-ketosteroids were found. In a single case of arrhenoblastoma we have observed the presence of $\Delta^4$-androstene-3,17-dione (20 μg./100 ml.), androsterone (about 10 μg./100 ml.), and etiocholanolone (about 8 μg./100 ml.). It must be emphasized that these androgens were found as unconjugated steroids and were not detectable in the antecubital vein blood of these patients. In our present experience, extracts of ovarian vein blood from normal females have not yielded any 17-ketosteroids. Finally, I must add that very large pools of antecubital vein plasma from normal males and females usually contain less than 1.0 μg. per 100 ml. of any individual free 17-ketosteroids (Migeon, C. J., Androgens in human plasma. *In* "A Symposium on Hormones in Human Plasma" (H. Antoniades, ed.), Part 4, Chapter 10. Little, Brown, Boston. In press.

**R. Dorfman:** You are right, Dr. Migeon—our studies are really more concerned with the biosynthetic capability of the gland. In many studies we add cofactors to assess the biosynthetic enzymes that are present. It is said that crystalloids of Reinecke in a tissue from the testis indicate an interstitial cell tumor. It so happens that these were present in both of the glands that produced adrenal steroids and appeared to be absent in the one that did not produce these steroids.

**E. E. Sproul:** May I ask you, Dr. Dorfman, whether you have had occasion to study more than one sample from isolated portions of one tumor, especially whether you have studied the primary tumor and a metastasis in the same patient? Being, I hope, an honest pathologist, I have to admit that we are very often confronted with a metastasis first and find it very difficult to suggest the source of origin of this tumor. It often varies tremendously in histological appearance in different areas, and I wonder if this is reflected in its function.

**R. Dorfman:** We really have not had an occasion to study metastasis, nor has any special effort been made to study different parts of any single tumor.

**M. Ehrenstein:** I should like to make a brief statement concerning organic chemical transformations. Dr. Dorfman has referred to the biochemical conversion of androgens to estrogens and to the role of steroids oxygenated in the 19-position as possible metabolic intermediates. A few years ago, we published the synthesis of 19-hydroxy-$\Delta^4$-androstene-3,17-dione. Recently we selectively reduced this compound and obtained 19-hydroxytestosterone, which by acetylation gave the 17,19-diacetate. By subsequent treatment with selenium dioxide, an additional double bond was introduced in the A ring leading to 19-hydroxy-1-dehydrotestosterone diacetate. When this compound was treated with potassium hydroxide, instantaneous aromatization took place resulting in the isolation of estradiol-17β. On choosing milder conditions, e.g., on using potassium carbonate or potassium bicarbonate, conversion occurred into the 17-monoacetate of estradiol-17β. This demonstrates that, with the $\Delta^1$-double bond present in such a 19-hydroxylated $\Delta^4$-3-ketone, aromatization proceeds with the greatest of ease. If one considers that this conversion occurs in the presence of bicarbonate, we are really approaching biological conditions. I might emphasize that the end products of these aromatization reactions, i.e., estradiol-17β and the corresponding 17-monoacetate, were obtained in excellent yields. In conclusion, on the basis of our observations, 19-hydroxy-$\Delta^{1,4}$-dien-3-ones may well be intermediates in the metabolic conversion of androgens into estrogens.

**G. Pincus:** I'd like to ask Dr. Dorfman to comment on the possibility that if one can get steroid-producing tumors in animal tissue, either adrenal or interstitial cell tumors of the type of Dr. Huseby's, might we be able to supply one of Dr. Huggins' requirements. In other words if you wish to test an anti-tumor agent, it may be that the effect on the steroidogenic process might be so rapid that within a matter of days one could see an effect instead of having to measure tumor sizes over a longer period of time.

**R. Dorfman:** This would assume that there is a correlation between the growth of the tumor and the enzymes that produce the steroids. As yet we have no proof that this is so.

**G. Gordan:** It's been done, Dr. Pincus. You recall that amphenone stops the production of steroids without affecting the growth of the tumor.

**K. Paschkis:** Is there any information, either in your preparations, Dr. Dorfman, or in the experiments of those who studied the ovarian and testicular effluents, whether chorionic gonadotropin or ACTH would shift the synthesis to nonhydroxylated or to hydroxylated compounds?

**R. Dorfman:** No information is available on this point.

**S. Kushinsky:** I'd like to return, if I may, to a topic that was discussed earlier in the conference, namely, possible differences in the metabolism of estrogens in responsive and nonresponsive women with mammary carcinoma. The work I shall describe is in progress at the University of Southern California Medical School and the Los Angeles County Hospital in collaboration with Drs. James Demetriou, Ian Macdonald, Oliver Kuzma, and Lawrence Crowley. You will recall that earlier it was said by Dr. Greenwood and others that no correlation has been found between estrogen metabolism and responsiveness. It was mentioned also that a slight correlation has been found by Dr. Brown (Brown, J. B. *In* "Endocrine Aspects of Breast Cancer" (A. R. Currie, ed.), p. 206. Livingstone, Edinburgh and London, 1958) between normal women and women with mammary carcinoma, wherein the ratio of estriol to estrone in urine is higher on the average in the cancer group following an administered dose of estradiol.

We became interested in this problem several years ago and have been studying the metabolism of an administered dose of estradiol-4-$C^{14}$ in postmenopausal women with mammary carcinoma, to see if we could distinguish between patients who respond favorably to estrogen therapy and those who do not. Figures A and B summarize some of the results we found. The methodology has been published in part [Kushinsky, S., Demetriou, J., Nasutavicus, W., and Wu, J. *Nature* **182**, 874 (1958)] and will be published in greater detail in the near future. The compounds which we have been able to analyze for, and assign tentative designations to, include estrone, estradiol, estriol, 2-methoxyestrone, 16-ketoestrone, 16-epiestriol, and possibly 17-epiestriol. Many others have been detected. In Fig. A is shown the excretion of estriol. The data have been expressed in terms of several parameters. These are: (1) percentage of injected dose; (2) cumulative percentage of injected dose; (3) percentage of daily excretion; and (4) percentage of neutral and phenolic fraction.

Note that depending on how the data are expressed, owing to variability in hydrolysis, there can be a fall or rise in estriol excretion as seen on day 3. In Fig. B are shown some additonal data. The data have been expressed in terms of the ratio of estrone to estriol excreted on day 1. Note that on top there is a normal control—a woman with no mammary carcinoma. Below this is a woman who was responsive to estradiol benzoate therapy. Below this is a patient who was not responsive to therapy, but who was studied while she was under estrogen therapy. Lower down is shown the same

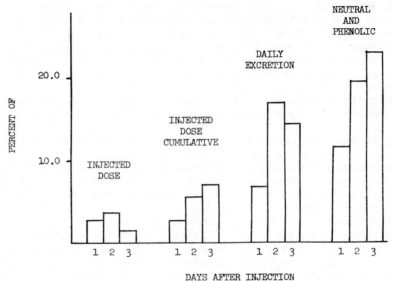

FIG. A.  Excretion of estriol.

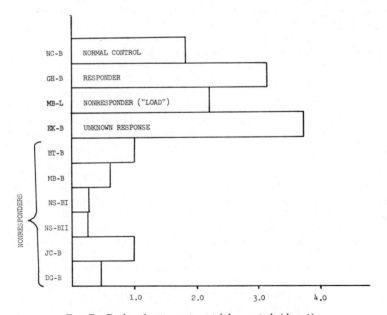

FIG. B.  Ratio of estrone to estriol excreted (day 1).

patient prior to therapy. A large difference in ratio is apparent which may be due to the effect of estrogen therapy. Next is one patient who died shortly after hypophysectomy and is of unknown response. The remaining subjects did not respond favorably to therapy. In each case the ratio is considerably lower than those described above. Since the time this figure was prepared we have been able to obtain data on another responsive patient and on several additional nonresponsive patients, and this difference still is maintained. It is certainly of interest to continue with this approach to see if it will stand up. One additional point is that another woman was studied who had cystic disease. Curiously enough, when expressed in this manner, the ratio fell between those of patients with mammary carcinoma and the normal control. However, when the data were expressed in terms of the sum of estrone, 2-methoxyestrone, and 16-keto-estrone divided by estriol, the difference between the two responders, the normal woman and the nonresponder under therapy, on one hand, and the nonresponsive patients on the other hand was maintained. But in the latter case the patient with cystic disease looked more like a normal. These data possibly may account for the lack of clear-cut distinction between normal women and women with breast cancer reported by Brown in that those women with breast cancer who respond to therapy have excretion patterns similar to those of normal women. Much more work will have to be done before we can clarify these points.

# Regression of Adrenal Cancer and Suppression of Adrenal Function in Man by o,p'-DDD[1]

D. M. BERGENSTAL, M. B. LIPSETT, R. H. MOY, AND ROY HERTZ

*Endocrinology Branch, National Cancer Institute, National Institutes of Health, Bethesda, Maryland*

During an investigation into the toxicologic effects of certain insecticides, Nelson and Woodward (5) noted that DDD [2,2-bis(p-chlorophenyl)-1,1-dichloroethane] caused necrosis of the zona fasciculata and reticularis of the canine adrenal cortex. Subsequently, Nichols and Gardner (6) demonstrated increased insulin sensitivity in the DDD-treated dog and inferred decreased production of glucocorticoids. Attempts were made to utilize this effect of DDD clinically to produce a chemical adrenalectomy (8, 9, 11) but these proved unsuccessful. A major break-through in the field was reported by two groups (2, 3, 7) who showed that the active constituent in the DDD was an isomer, 2-o-chlorophenyl-2-p-chlorophenyl-1,1-dichloroethane (o,p'-DDD). Hence, studies of the treatment of metastatic adrenal carcinoma with o,p'-DDD in man were undertaken.

Our approach to the problem of dosage has been largely empirical. In general, we have tried to give 10 gm. of the drug daily to adults and proportionally smaller doses to children, with individual adjustment of the dose up to the point of tolerance. When an effective level of therapy was attained, the dose of the drug was reduced by about two-thirds and the patients then received this as a maintenance dose. This regimen was adopted on the premise that it is necessary to maintain high levels of o,p'-DDD in the body fat depots for considerable periods of time in order to continue to suppress the disease process. The experimental evidence for this is discussed subsequently. The dosage figures listed in the tables and figures should not be interpreted as reflecting the amount of drug absorbed since a nonpolar aromatic hydrocarbon such as o,p'-DDD might be expected to be absorbed only with difficulty. Our preliminary results with the measurement of o,p'-DDD in plasma and in the stool suggest that absorption is variable and this may account for the high doses of o,p'-DDD that are apparently needed in some patients.

Fourteen patients with histologically proved adrenal carcinoma have received o,p'-DDD since April 1958. The case material is listed in Table I. The patients ranged from 1½ years to 59 years of age and included 4 children. Twelve of the 14 patients had measurable metastatic disease before treatment and in 13 of the patients there was evidence of excessive steroid

---

[1] Read on behalf of Dr. D. M. Bergenstal, who died on September 12, 1959.

TABLE I
RESULTS OF TREATMENT

| Patient | Effect of treatment | | Total dose o,p'-DDD (gm.) | Current therapy | Duration of remission (months) | Current status |
| | Tumor | Urinary steroids | | | | |
|---|---|---|---|---|---|---|
| F. Fox | Decrease | Normal | 1100 | None | 8 | Progressing |
| L. Str | Progression | Normal | 312 | — | — | Died |
| P. Vei | No lesions measurable | Normal | 1200 + | o,p'-DDD 3 gm. | 8 + | Remission |
| R. Sher | Unchanged | 50% | 316 | — | — | Died |
| M. Nir | Progression | Unchanged | 940 | Prednisone | — | Progressing |
| M. Cher | Unchanged | 70% | 212 | — | — | Died |
| M. Mal | Decrease | Normal | 600 + | o,p'-DDD 3.5 gm. | 3 + | Remission |
| P. Ioz | Progression | 50% | 1300 + | o,p'-DDD 9 gm. | — | Progressing |
| G. Hop | Decrease | Normal | 450 | Prednisone | 18 + | Remission |
| S. Sch | Decrease | Normal | 200 + | o,p'-DDD 1 gm. | 5 + | Remission |
| D. Ale | Unchanged | Normal | 311 | Dexamethasone | — | Died |
| H. Hom | Decrease | Normal | 302 | — | 3 | Died |
| A. Vic | Unchanged | Normal | 500 + | Prednisone | — | No Change |
| A. Smi | Unchanged | Normal | 1100 | Prednisone | — | Died |

production. Hirsutism was noted in all the females and Cushing's syndrome was apparent in 7 of the 8 females. The excretion of 17-ketosteroids and 17-hydroxycorticoids tended to fluctuate during the initial periods of observation and the values listed are the average daily excretion of each class of steroid. Our method for these determinations has been previously cited (4).

### TABLE II
#### PATIENTS AND CLINICAL SYNDROMES

| Patient | Age (years) | Sex | Average initial 17-KS (mg./ 24 hr.) | 17-OHCS (mg./ 24 hr.) | Viriliza- tion | Cushing's Syndrome | Sites of metas- tases[a] |
|---|---|---|---|---|---|---|---|
| F. Fox | 56 | F | 250 | 25 | + | + | L |
| L. Str | 57 | F | 50 | 15 | + | + | L |
| P. Vei | 33 | F | 60 | 30 | + | + | A |
| R. Sher | 36 | F | 60 | 70 | + | + | A |
| M. Nir | 55 | F | 30 | 10 | + | | L |
| M. Cher | 38 | F | 600 | 170 | + | + | A |
| M. Mal | 38 | F | 50 | 12 | + | + | L |
| P. Ioz | 11 | F | 40 | 170 | + | + | A |
| G. Hop | 1½ | M | 150 | 1 | + | | A |
| S. Sch | 7 | M | 30 | 5 | + | | L |
| D. Ale | 9 | M | 80 | 3 | + | | A |
| H. Hom | 52 | M | 25 | 8 | | | L A |
| A. Vic | 59 | M | 14 | 6 | | | A |
| A. Smi | 56 | M | 110 | 20 | | | A |

[a] L = lung; A = abdomen.

In Table II, the over-all results of therapy have been presented. In no instance has there been progression of measurable disease with a concurrent sustained decrease in urinary steroids to normal levels.

There is one patient (Vei) who did not have clinically demonstrable metastatic disease but whose clinical manifestations of cancer, namely, Cushing's syndrome and virilization, have been completely suppressed for 9 months.

Five patients exhibited measurable decrease in tumor size. One of these (Fox) has refused further therapy with $o,p'$-DDD because of gastric intolerance and now has progressive disease. Hom died of septicemia although there had been marked regression of pulmonary and abdominal metastases. The other three patients remain in remission.

There are three patients currently under treatment who demonstrate relative resistance to the drug. It seems probable, from the plasma levels of $o,p'$-DDD, that the progression of disease in one of these patients despite large amounts of $o,p'$-DDD cannot be attributed to poor absorption of the drug.

There have been six deaths in this series. Two of the patients (Str and Cher), died of progression of disease early in the course of therapy. There was suppression of steroid excretion in both patients at the time of death. The cause of death in Ale was a cerebellar astrocytoma. Hom died of septicemia associated with severe inanition.

In two patients, the cause of death is not apparent. Smi, a patient with hepatic metastases, had been treated with $o,p'$-DDD resulting in normal urinary steroids. He died suddenly at home while receiving 7 gm. of $o,p'$-DDD daily. Autopsy permission was not granted. A patient (Sher) with advanced Cushing's syndrome died during the early phase of treatment after 4 days of somnolence and increasing respiratory paralysis. There was no apparent cause of death at autopsy. Thus, we have observed 3 patients in whom drug toxicity may have contributed to the fatal outcome. Careful examination of the brain in the 5 patients on whom a postmortem examination was performed has not revealed any unusual histological changes that could be attributed to $o,p'$-DDD.

In order to illustrate some of the problems encountered, several case histories are pertinent. In Fig. 1, we have plotted the effect of $o,p'$-DDD on steroid levels in Smi. The first course of therapy was interrupted because of a generalized red, pruritic, macular rash. Before we could resume treatment, the excretion of urinary steroids had returned to pretreatment levels. The subsequent course of therapy was accomplished without toxic skin manifestations and the urinary steroids fell and subsequently remained at normal levels. We have observed a similar response in other patients in whom drug therapy was interrupted after an initial decrease in the urinary steroids.

After receiving 900 gm. of $o,p'$-DDD over a period of 5 months, Fox demonstrated regression of pulmonary metastases (Fig. 2) and a drop in steroids to below normal levels which persisted for 4 months without further therapy. Following this period, the 17-ketosteroids began to rise and a second short course of 132 gm. again reduced the steroid excretion. When further therapy was refused by the patient, the steroid excretion promptly rose and metastases subsequently increased.

It is likely that the sensitivity of the cancer cells to $o,p'$-DDD varies widely among patients. We have mentioned one patient who has received over 1400 gm. of $o,p'$-DDD with little effect in spite of the fact that high blood levels reflect adequate absorption of the drug. The other end of the spectrum of responsiveness is illustrated in Fig. 3. This 7-year-old boy had progressive enlargement of his pulmonary metastasis during the initial 2 weeks of observation (Fig. 4). However, there was a marked decrease in the excretion of 17-KS after less than 25 gm. of $o,p'$-DDD (Fig. 3), and a decrease in the pulmonary lesion was noted after 5 weeks of therapy.

Very substantial regression of tumor size can be obtained. We have previously reported (1) regression of a large inoperable adrenal carcinoma in a 1½-year-old boy. This child has now been followed for 19 months and the abdominal mass has continued to regress and has become calcified (Fig. 5). Because of increasing anorexia recently, $o,p'$-DDD was discon-

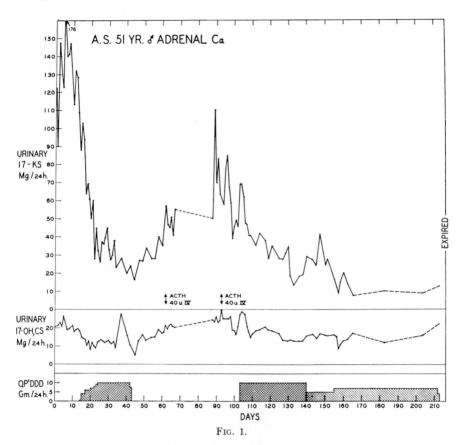

Fig. 1.

tinued and improvement was noted. We plan to observe the child and examine his 17-KS excretion at frequent intervals.

Detailed studies of the urinary steroids in the patients will be reported elsewhere, but certain generalizations can be made. $o,p'$-DDD does not exert a selective effect on the biosynthesis of specific steroids. The excretion of 17-OHCS, 17-KS, and dehydroepiandrosterone has always either decreased or increased proportionately. In 3 patients, there was a return of menses during therapy, suggesting that estrogen secretion by the ovary continued.

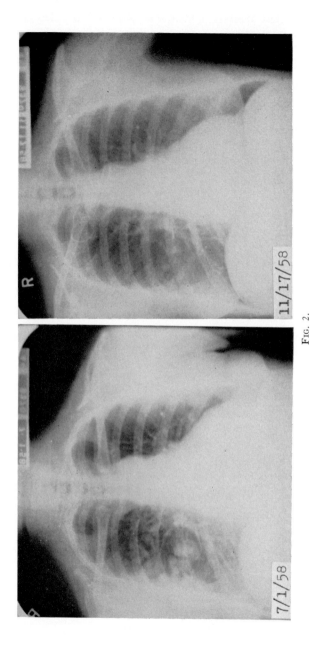

Fig. 2.

It was generally necessary to place the patients on some type of gluco-corticoid replacement, since the secretion of hydrocortisone by the remaining normal adrenal gland was suppressed by the *o,p'*-DDD. In these instances, prolonged stimulation with adrenocorticotropin failed to stimulate the normal adrenal gland. This was noted even in those patients whose endogenous adrenal function had not been suppressed by the secretions of the cancer. Although we have not measured aldosterone secretion after prolonged treat-

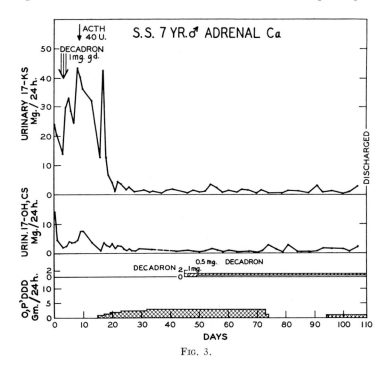

FIG. 3.

ment with *o,p'*-DDD, 3 patients have responded to a low sodium intake by a normal decrease in urinary sodium excretion, probably denoting adequate secretion of aldosterone. Thus the glomerulosa of the human adrenal gland, like that of the dog, appears to be relatively more resistant to the action of *o,p'*-DDD than are the other zones of the adrenal cortex.

## DISCUSSION

The reported effects of *o,p'*-DDD on the dog adrenal gland (10) permit an explanation of the temporary suppression of steroid excretion seen with the drug in man. After 2 days of therapy with *o,p'*-DDD in the dog, adrenal vein 17-OHCS have greatly decreased although there are only minimal his-

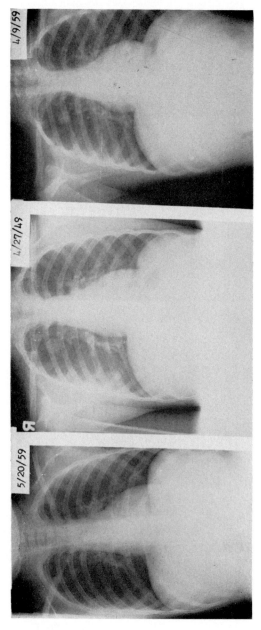

FIG. 4.

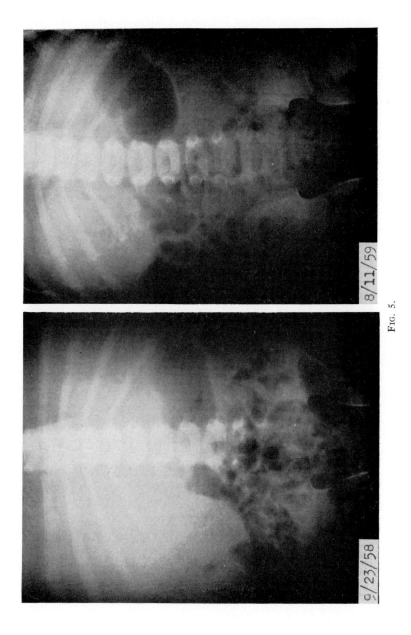

FIG. 5.

tological changes. If $o,p'$-DDD is a selective cell poison, it is a reasonable hypothesis that at some dose of the drug, cellular metabolic processes may be sufficiently suppressed so that steroid biosynthesis is halted but cellular death does not occur. Only when $o,p'$-DDD is given for longer periods of time is there obvious necrosis of cells in the dog adrenal cortex and regression of metastases in man. Our experience with $o,p'$-DDD administration in two breast cancer patients with normal adrenal glands (1) supports the experimental findings that function is impaired before significant histological damage can be demonstrated.

A decrease in steroid excretion after the administration of $o,p'$-DDD has been almost uniformly noted. Although these changes were significant in each case, some patients did not survive long enough for appreciable tumor regression. From these data it does not seem possible to differentiate sharply between responsive and resistant types of adrenal cancer. Rather, there appear to be varying degrees of susceptibility to the cytotoxic effect of $o,p'$-DDD among the adrenal carcinomas so far observed.

We have mentioned some of the possible toxic effects of $o,p'$-DDD. Somnolence was encountered in several patients but was generally quickly reversible when the drug was stopped or caffeine was given. Electroencephalographic changes have not been observed during therapy. Psychometric examinations have been unchanged. There is thus little evidence for irreversible central nervous system toxicity.

There have not been any changes suggestive of hepatic, renal, or bone marrow damage after prolonged courses of therapy. This is in accord with the initial observations of Nelson and Woodard (5), who found only fatty infiltration of the liver in dogs that had received $o,p'$-DDD[2] for long periods of time and had been anorectic for many days. Nausea and anorexia have been frequently observed. A drug rash has been encountered several times.

With respect to the treatment of cancer, the unique properties of $o,p'$-DDD open new areas of investigation, for here is an agent which is selectively toxic to a specific organ. The mechanism of this selectivity and the possibility of finding other chemicals similarly unique in their effects upon other organs should be vigorously explored.

## Summary

Objective regression of metastatic adrenal cortical carcinoma has been obtained in 5 of 14 patients given $o,p'$-DDD (2-$o$-chlorophenyl-2-$p$-chlorophenyl-1,1-dichloroethane). An almost uniform suppression of steroid output by the tumors of all treated patients has been noted. Prolonged oral therapy

---

[2] Commercial product Rothane (Rohm and Haas) of which $o,p'$-DDD is a contaminant in varying percentages.

with this drug has been found necessary to obtain significant tumor regression.

There has been no evidence of toxic damage to liver, kidneys, or bone marrow. The somnolence encountered in some patients suggests a reversible effect on the central nervous system.

## REFERENCES

1. Bergenstal, D. M., Lipsett, M. B., Moy, R., and Hertz, R. *Trans. Assoc. Am. Physicians* (in press).
2. Cueto, C., and Brown, J. H. U. *Endocrinology* **62**, 226 (1958).
3. Cueto, C., and Brown, J. H. U. *Endocrinology* **62**, 334 (1958).
4. Hertz, R., Bergenstal, D. M., Lubs, H. A., and Jackson, S. J. *Cancer* **10**, 765 (1957).
5. Nelson, A., and Woodard, G. *A.M.A. Arch. Pathol.* **48**, 387 (1949).
6. Nichols, J., and Gardner, L. I. *J. Lab. Clin. Med.* **37**, 229 (1951).
7. Nichols, J., and Hennigar, G. R. *Exptl. Med. Surg.* **15**, 310 (1957).
8. Sheehan, H. L., Summers, V. K., and Nichols, J. *Lancet* **1**, 312 (1953).
9. Tornblom, N. *Acta Med. Scand.* **154**, 83 (1956).
10. Vilar, O., and Tullner, W. W. *Endocrinology* **65**, 80 (1959).
11. Zimmerman, B., Block, H. W., Williams, W. L., Hitchcock, C. R., and Hoelocher, B. *Cancer* **9**, 940 (1956).

## DISCUSSION

**S. C. Werner:** For the sake of the record I think the fourteenth case should be presented. This patient was treated through the kindness of Dr. Bergenstal and Dr. Hertz. Functional depression of the tumor was obtained, but unfortunately, despite adequate dosage given throughout her course, the tumor progressed and the patient died of cancer of the adrenal. She was a woman in her early forties, and presented a fairly clear-cut syndrome of Cushing's disease. There was a large palpable mass in the right upper quadrant. At operation, the decision was made to try to excise the tumor. This had already compressed liver and it was problematical whether it had invaded enough to defeat excision or not. Excision was undertaken. The surgeon however, was not sure whether a thin shell of surviving tumor tissue remained. It proved, unfortunately, that there was residual tissue, and at that point we heard about Dr. Bergenstal's work. Dr. Hertz was kind enough in the absence of $o,p'$-DDD to provide some DDD, which was tried for about 3 weeks, when Dr. Bergenstal provided the $o,p'$-DDD. Thus there was a 3-week period in which the tumor presumably had ample chance to grow, although inhibited to some degree, I presume, by the DDD. Then for the next 2 months this woman tolerated and took 10 gm. of the $o,p'$-DDD. For the first few weeks, there was really quite an improvement in the Cushing's aspect of the disease. There was no change in sedimentation rate, and, of course, at that time there was no mass that one could follow by examination. Despite the encouraging early start, she began rapidly to go downhill, not from Cushing's disease but from being ill. Ultimately, she succumbed at the end of about 10 weeks of therapy, on 10 gm. per day with perhaps a few days off every now and then. At autopsy, the tumor showed necrosis which was consistent with the size of the recurrence just as well as with an effect of the drug upon the tumor. The steroid excretion had fallen to normal by the time of her later decline.

**R. Hertz:** Dr. Werner has brought out a significant point which I had meant to make. All our patients who have come to autopsy had unequivocal evidence of residual tumor. There has been, in fact, very extensive necrosis, but this is one of the predominant natural characteristics of adrenocortical carcinoma, so that the pathologists cannot really give us any good evaluation of the effects of the drug on previously existing lesions.

I had meant to mention that, owing to the limitations of oral administration, Dr. Tullner and I have been exploring other methods of the administration of $o,p'$DDD and would like to ask the chairman's indulgence to have Dr. Tullner present in a word some of his more recent observations on this point.

**W. W. Tullner:** We would like to present a tabulation of results obtained in studies on dog adrenal vein plasma 17-hydroxycorticoids following the intravenous administration of $o,p'$-DDD. Because of the problem of overcoming the incomplete absorption that is frequently found after oral administration of this drug to patients and also because we do have several related drugs in short supply which we would like to test, but do not have enough to test by the oral route, we have been interested in developing an intravenous method of administering this type of fat-soluble compound.

In Table A, the first two dogs represent controls which received vehicle only. The vehicle found to be suitable for intravenous administration of $o,p'$-DDD was Lipomul, an emulsion, in combination with propylene glycol (in which the drug was initially dissolved) and absolute ethanol in the proportions of 90:5:5 as you see in the footnote of Table A. The vehicle alone was given at a rate of 4–5 ml. per minute over a period of approximately 30–40 minutes while the dog was under Nembutal anesthesia. Vehicle alone had no effect on the adrenocortical secretion of Porter-Silber chromogens. These levels are quite within the normal range for our laboratory. In the series below this, in which the drug had been administered at doses of 50–54 mg. per kilogram daily for a period of 3-days, one finds a marked decrease in 17-hydroxycorticoid output based on the adrenal vein plasma content. This marked decrease approximates that found in the hypophysectomized dog. Thus it is apparent that it is possible to use the drug intravenously to obtain effects similar to those obtained by the oral route. In addition, we have been able to use smaller doses than we have been able to use previously to produce a similar inhibitory effect.

TABLE A

INHIBITION OF 17-HYDROXYCORTICOID OUTPUT AFTER INTRAVENOUS ADMINISTRATION OF $o,p'$-DDD

| Dog. No. | Sex | Weight (kg.) | Daily dose $o,p'$-DDD[a] (mg./kg.) | Infusion rate (ml./min.) | 17-OH Corticoids (plasma) (μg./min.) |
|---|---|---|---|---|---|
| 576 | ♀ | 19.5 | None | 4–5 | 5.4,  5.6,  7.2 |
| 581 | ♂ | 13.4 | None | 4–5 | 10.1, 10.5, 11.0 |
| 571 | ♀ | 10.0 | 50 | 4–5 | 0.3,  0.3,  0.2 |
| 580 | ♂ | 16.2 | 54 | 4–5 | 0.5,  0.6 |
| 575 | ♀ | 13.3 | 50 | 4–5 | 0.5,  0.5,  0.5 |

[a] Given intravenously at a concentration of 5 mg. $o,p'$-DDD per milliliter Lipomul (Upjohn), propylene glycol, and absolute ethanol in the proportions of 90:5:5, respectively.

**A. C. Carter:** Dr. Masterson and I have treated the fifteenth patient with $o,p'$-DDD. This patient has adrenal carcinoma with abodominal metastases, and no pulmonary metastasis. The patient has improved subjectively on therapy. Prior to therapy she required large amounts of analgesics and now requires none. Her 17-ketosteroid excretion at the time therapy was instituted was in the range of 450 mg. per 24 hours, and on the $o,p'$-DDD regimen it is on the order of 150–200 mg. per 24 hours. The therapeutic regimen that we have employed is 7 gm. of the $o,p'$-DDD for 10 days, no therapy for 10 days, and so on for 9 months.

**R. Hertz:** Dr. Masterson told me about that case, Dr. Carter. I understand she was completely amenorrhoeic for several years, during the course of development of her tumor, and has since resumed menstruation; is that correct? This would indicate that there is sufficient suppression of whatever it is that causes ovarian atrophy in the presence of high endogenous adrenal steroid, presumably the ketosteroid phase, to allow the ovary to escape from inhibition. We have seen this in the one patient I showed you also, and I think its one of the most interesting phases of the response. Your patient has also been a very favorable one in tolerating the medication as well as she has. I understand, that, like three or four of our patients, she has had no subjective reaction to the drug.

**D. West:** We recently administered $o,p'$-DDD to a patient with feminizing adrenal carcinoma. This patient is excreting very high levels of estrogens, levels that are only seen in late pregnancy. The study is incomplete, but at this time the patient has received DDD for 10 days and already the excretion of estrone and estradiol has decreased to approximately a third of the control levels. Strangely enough estriol has not decreased. It may be that the estriol levels will decrease with further treatment. We also saw the decrease in the 17-hydroxycorticoids measured by the Porter-Silber reaction, and 17-ketosteroids which Dr. Hertz describes so beautifully. One of the impressive things, at least to us, was the lack of toxicity in this patient. We went to some trouble to obtain a rather pure preparation of $o,p'$-DDD as determined by melting point, mixed melting points, and infrared spectra. I know you can't draw any conclusions from one patient, but I'm wondering what the degree of purity of $o,p'$-DDD was that Dr. Hertz and the others have used, and whether or not the toxic symptoms might still be due to contamination with $p,p$-DDD.

**R. Hertz:** I think considerations of possible trace contaminations such as Dr. West raises are very tenable. In the early phase of any such therapeutic attempts this frequently arises. I give you the case of stilbestrol, which for its first two years of use was regarded as an extremely toxic agent but has subsequently through better methods of preparation proved not to be. I think this may occur in this case, but we can't say at this time.

# Serum Proteins in Breast Carcinoma: Effects of Androgen Therapy

M. J. BRENNAN AND W. L. SIMPSON

*Oncology Division, Henry Ford Hospital, Detroit Institute of Cancer Research, and Wayne State University College of Medicine, Detroit, Michigan*

The search for objective indices of response to therapy in cancer patients has led to a re-examination of the systemic manifestations of cancer. Immunochemical methods developed in this laboratory have been employed for the determination of several serum proteins and the effects of changes in disease state on these proteins in several hundred cancer patients during the past five years.

Previous reports describing the immunochemical techniques employed for albumin (3), gamma globulin (3), and orosomucoid (4) have been published. For the past year serial paper electrophoretic analyses have also been done as a part of the study, using a Spinco cell, bromophenol blue staining, and an automatized scanner (Spinco Analytrol).

Mean values for protein fractions of normal serum as determined by paper electrophoresis, moving boundary electrophoresis, and the immunochemical method, are shown in Table I. Values obtained in our laboratory by use of either paper electrophoresis or immunochemical precipitation closely approximate those reported by other workers.

Albumin falls as disseminated cancer progresses, whereas orosomucoid tends to rise (10, 6). Orosomucoid is a glycoprotein, and a fraction of seromucoid that moves in the α-1 electrophoretic fraction. In our series, γ-globulin showed no major shift away from an initial mean of 1.2 gm. % as measured immunochemically.

These changes do not depend on the presence of metastases in any specific organ system (10), nor are they specific to breast cancer. They represent the general trends encountered in over 300 patients with various kinds of malignant disease.

When an objective regression of any disseminated neoplastic process develops, the albumin curve generally turns back upward and the orosomucoid levels recede toward normal (10). The restoration of initially abnormal levels of these two proteins to the normal range does not occur as promptly as does the cessation of hypercalcuria under similar circumstances (10). A fall in orosomucoid is noted earlier than a rise in albumin, but several weeks are usually required for the former to reach a normal level.

Infection may prevent these trends from becoming apparent. Severe liver impairment may be associated with an abrupt and paradoxical decline in

TABLE I
SERUM PROTEIN FRACTIONS[a]

| Study | Method | Number of subjects | Total serum protein[b] | Albumin | α-1-Globulin | α-2-Globulin | β-Globulin | γ-Globulin | Orosomucoid |
|---|---|---|---|---|---|---|---|---|---|
| Present | Paper electrophoresis | 42 | 7.40 ± 0.46 | 4.84 ± 0.39 | 0.27 ± 0.05 | 0.55 ± 0.11 | 0.76 ± 0.12 | 1.00 ± 0.20 | — |
| Faulkner (2) | Paper electrophoresis | 61 | 7.05 ± 0.42 | 4.73 ± 0.41 | 0.23 ± 0.07 | 0.48 ± 0.10 | 0.64 ± 0.14 | 0.95 ± 0.20 | — |
| Reiner et al. (9) | Moving boundary electrophoresis | 60 | 7.22 ± 0.48 | 4.10 ± 0.32 | — | — | — | 1.00 ± 0.20 | |
| Goodman et al. (3, 4) | Immuno-chemical | 45 | 7.63 ± 0.44 | 4.59 ± 0.35 | — | — | — | 1.20 ± 0.18 | 76.0 ± 3.0 |

[a] Normal values with standard errors are expressed as grams per 100 ml. serum except orosomucoid, which is given as milligrams per cent.

[b] Total serum proteins were determined by Kjeldahl or biuret methods.

orosomucoid values in the presence of a rapidly advancing tumor. Under these circumstances the concentration of albumin also falls and thus minimizes confusion.

We have divided our androgen-treated breast cancer patients into three groups. Group I consists of those who experienced objective regressions. Group II are those in whom, during the period of observation recorded, we were unable to make out any notable change of clinical state. Group III are those who manifested progression of disease as objectively measured. Mean values for three serum protein fractions in each group are recorded in Table II.

TABLE II

SERUM PROTEIN CHANGES VERSUS DISEASE STATUS

|  | Orosomucoid (mg.%) | Albumin (gm.%) | γ-Globulin (gm.%) |
|---|---|---|---|
| Group I (regressions—10 patients) | | | |
| Prior to androgen treatment | 135 | 4.1 | 1.4 |
| 1 month | 124 | 4.0 | 1.2 |
| 2 months | 113 | 4.0 | 1.3 |
| 3 months | 120 | 4.3 | 1.3 |
| Group II (no change—8 patients) | | | |
| Prior to androgen treatment | 109 | 4.3 | 1.2 |
| 1 month | 110 | 4.1 | 1.2 |
| 2 months | 114 | 3.6 | 0.9 |
| 3 months | 111 | 4.3 | 1.1 |
| Group III (progressions—15 patients) | | | |
| Prior to androgen treatment | 121 | 4.0 | 1.3 |
| 1 month | 159 | 4.0 | 1.3 |
| 2 months | 163 | 4.0 | 1.3 |
| 3 months | — | — | — |

A prompt move in orosomucoid toward clearly elevated levels, or a failure to come down from such levels if initially present, occurred in Group III. Mean orosomucoid values for this group were significantly elevated at 1 and 2 months. By this time obvious progression of disease required a change in therapy. An opposite trend was seen in Group I. Group II remained unchanged. Mean values of albumin did not change significantly in any of the groups during these studies.

The down trend of serum albumin in the later stages of progressive neoplastic disease is well known (3, 11). Our experience has confirmed this finding and, heretofore, demonstrated a consistent rise in albumin with regression (10) in such far-advanced disease. In the present series, certain patients failed to exhibit an improvement of their serum albumin levels at a time when they showed objective evidences of remission. In part this may be attributed to the fact that we were dealing with patients whose initial albumin levels were but slightly below normal. In addition data will be presented later suggesting that factors other than those related simply to progression-regression are operative with respect to protein metabolism in this group of androgen-treated breast cancer patients.

A review of the literature concerning the influence of gonadal steroids on plasma proteins revealed a paucity of information on changes induced in serum albumin and globulin concentrations by the androgens. Pincus (8) cites Nava and Zilli (7) as demonstrating a "decrease in all blood proteins in men." In their study twelve well subjects were given 40–100 mg. testosterone propionate intramuscularly for 5 days. In rats treated with gonadotropin, paper electrophoresis showed a definite and sustained increase in total serum protein and all individual fractions in the female, but no change in proteins in the male (1). Increases in β-lipoproteins have been noted after methyl testosterone administration in man (5).

When the serial electrophoretic data in a group of 6 patients classified as equivalent in state of disease to those of Group II were examined, an effect was noted which seemed related to the agent employed.

These patients were selected because it was felt that they were in an essentially steady state with regard to tumor-host interaction. Hence, changes developed in the serum proteins on therapy could probably be attributed primarily to metabolic influences not directly concerned with a change in the disease state as such. Two patients had been treated with 17-nonmethylated androgens and 4 with 17-methylated androgens. The 4 given 17-methylated androgens showed a significant fall in albumin of 0.75–1 gm. in the first month of treatment and a rise in α-2- and β-globulin. Two patients treated with nonmethylated androgens showed no change in albumin or in α-1-, a suggestive drop in α-2, and a fall in β- and γ-globulin. In two of the methylated series, bromosulfaphthalein retention was measured and found increased. The methylated steroids used were 9α-fluoro-11β-hydroxy-17α-methyltestosterone 20 mg. per day orally (2 patients); 2,17-dimethyltestosterone 50 mg. per day orally (1 patient); and 2-hydroxymethylene-17α-methyldihydrotestosterone (RS 992) 125 mg. per day orally (1 patient). The nonmethylated steroids were testosterone propionate 100 mg. in sesame oil intramuscularly three times a week (1 patient) and 3β,17β-androstanediol same dose as testosterone (1 patient).

Although the number of observations is limited, it appears that a very early effect on protein synthesis compatible with altered hepatocellular function may be produced by 17-methylated steroids and that 17-nonmethylated steroids may differ from them in this regard.

## TABLE III
### RELATIONSHIP OF ANDROGEN THERAPY TO SERUM PROTEIN VALUES IN BREAST CANCER PATIENTS[a,b]

#### 17-Methylated androgens

| Patient | Total serum protein[c] | | | | Albumin | | | | α-1-Globulin | | | |
|---|---|---|---|---|---|---|---|---|---|---|---|---|
| | A | B | C | D | A | B | C | D | A | B | C | D |
| Before treatment | 5.8 | 7.0 | 7.3 | 6.9 | 3.3 | 4.6 | 4.6 | 2.7 | 0.38 | 0.28 | 0.17 | 0.76 |
| 1 month on therapy | 5.6 | 7.3 | 7.3 | 5.9 | 2.3 | 3.6 | 4.0 | 2.0 | 0.56 | 0.40 | 0.33 | 0.40 |

| Patient | α-2-Globulin | | | | β-Globulin | | | | γ-Globulin | | | |
|---|---|---|---|---|---|---|---|---|---|---|---|---|
| | A | B | C | D | A | B | C | D | A | B | C | D |
| Before treatment | 0.65 | 0.50 | 0.50 | 1.58 | 0.55 | 0.65 | 1.18 | 0.85 | 0.94 | 0.96 | 1.50 | 1.12 |
| 1 month on therapy | 0.83 | 1.00 | 1.05 | 1.65 | 0.78 | 1.00 | 1.78 | 0.90 | 1.14 | 1.28 | 1.20 | 0.98 |

#### 17-Nonmethylated androgens

| Patient | Total serum protein[c] | | Albumin | | α-1-Globulin | | α-2-Globulin | |
|---|---|---|---|---|---|---|---|---|
| | E | F | E | F | E | F | E | F |
| Before treatment | 7.25 | 7.0 | 3.15 | 2.60 | 0.52 | .56 | 1.04 | 0.92 |
| 1 month on therapy | 6.75 | 6.6 | 3.25 | 2.75 | 0.43 | .48 | 0.90 | 0.77 |
| Normal and std. error | 7.40 ± 0.46 | | 4.84 ± 0.39 | | 0.23 ± 0.07 | | 0.48 ± 0.10 | |

| Patient | β-Globulin | | γ-Globulin | |
|---|---|---|---|---|
| | E | F | E | F |
| Before treatment | 1.30 | 1.62 | 1.30 | 1.40 |
| 1 month on therapy | 1.10 | 1.30 | 1.10 | 1.34 |
| Normal and std. error | 0.64 ± 0.14 | | 0.95 ± 0.20 | |

[a] Paper electrophoresis.
[b] All values in grams per cent.
[c] Biuret.

## Summary

Elevated orosomucoid concentrations tend to return toward normal levels in breast carcinoma patients when a regression is induced by androgen (or any other effective therapy).

In patients with progressive disease, a poor response to therapy was associated with a prompt change from near normal to more severely displaced levels of this protein or maintenance of initially abnormal levels.

17-methylated androgens appeared to have an early effect on serum protein levels in 4 patients. This effect, which may be attributable to decreased hepatocellular function, was not observed in 2 patients treated with 17-nonmethylated androgens.

## Acknowledgments

Supported in part by grant No. CY-2903 USPHS, NCI, NIH; grant No. CY-3357; Institutional grants to the Detroit Institute of Cancer Research from United Foundation of Greater Detroit through American Cancer Society, Southeastern Michigan Division.

We are indebted to D. Remp, Ph.D., for assistance with electrophoretic studies and to Monica Cichon and Bernice Bond who carried out the immunochemical determinations.

## References

1. Bernasconi, C. *Acta Endocrinol.* **24**, 50 (1957).
2. Faulkner, W. R. *Clin. Chem.* **5**, 375 (1959).
3. Goodman, M., Ramsey, D. S., Simpson, W. L., Remp, D. G., Basinski, D. H., and Brennan, M. J. *J. Lab. Clin. Med.* **49**, 151 (1957).
4. Goodman, M., Ramsey, D. S., Simpson, W. L., and Brennan, M. J. *J. Lab. Clin. Med.* **50**, 758 (1957).
5. Higano, N., Cohen, W. D., and Robinson, R. W. *Ann. N. Y. Acad. Sci.* **72**, 970 (1959).
6. Mider, G. B., Alling, E. J., and Morton, J. J. *Cancer* **3**, 56 (1950).
7. Nava, G., and Zilli, E. *Arch. "E Maragliano" patol. e clin.* **5**, 637 (1950).
8. Pincus, G. *In* "The Hormones" (G. Pincus and K. V. Thimann, eds.), Vol. 3, p. 665. Academic Press, New York, 1955.
9. Reiner, M., Fenichel, R. W., and Stern, K. G. *Acta Haematol.* **3**, 202 (1950).
10. Simpson, W. L., Brennan, M. J., and Goodman, M. *Proc. 2nd Internat. Symposium on Mammary Cancer, Perugia, Italy, 1957* pp. 399-412 (1958).
11. Winzler, R. J. *Advances in Cancer Research* **1**, 503 (1953).

# Cellular Prognostic Factors in Breast Cancer Hormone Therapy

Thomas C. Hall, Margarida M. Dederick, Hans B. Nevinny, and Rita M. Kelley

*Division of Oncology, Medical Services, Lemuel Shattuck Hospital, Boston, Massachusetts; Harvard Medical School, Boston, Massachusetts; Department of Medicine, Massachusetts General Hospital, Boston, Massachusetts, and Department of Medicine, Pondville Hospital, Walpole, Massachusetts*

## Introduction

The present report attempts to examine some of the factors operating in the host-tumor biologic relationship which may condition responses to therapy, as well as some of the early changes in tumor isotope uptake which may presage ultimate response to therapy. The encouraging reports of Drs. Segaloff and Rosoff still leave us faced with the unpleasant fact that between three and four of every five patients treated with hormones will *not* respond, and Dr. Kennedy reminded us yesterday of Dr. Nathanson's classic observation that many patients do not begin to show beneficial responses to hormone therapy until after more than 6 or 8 weeks of therapy. One is left with the discouraging prospect of having to treat patients over long periods of time with drugs that may have unpleasant and even life-endangering side effects (as with induced hypercalcemia) before being sure that they are going to be among the failing majority. Any information leading to intelligent pre-selection of patients for therapy would be helpful.

## Results

The cases were first examined from the point of view of prevailing clinical impressions that age in relation to menopause, type of dominant lesion, estrogen production by ovaries, adrenals, or other source, and previous responses to therapy were important factors in predicting patient response to hormonal therapy.

### Age

Table I shows the response rate, according to Cooperative Breast Group criteria of patients first treated with hormones, as related to their age. The data on androgen treatment are similar to those reported by the Cooperative Group and indicate unexpected effectiveness in the older age groups. Of interest is the fact that the estrogen data show the same trend toward increasing effectiveness with age and a significantly higher rate of objective responses. No such trends are seen in the castrated or corticoid-treated patients, although the figures are probably too incomplete to be very definite about this aspect.

## Lesion

Another clinical impression regarding prognostic factors in therapy deserving of critical examination concerns the importance of dominant type of lesion. Because of difficulties in classifying disease of the opposite breast or of the skin of the thigh as "local," as well as the anomalous position of pleural disease in classification, in addition to the fact that patients oophorectomized for "local" recurrences were often found to have intra-abdominal metastases at the time of surgery, it was decided to put patients with pre-

TABLE I

BREAST CANCER: EFFECT OF AGE OF PATIENT ON PERCENTAGE OF OBJECTIVE RESPONSES ACHIEVED WITH THERAPY

| Age | Castration | Androgens | Estrogens | Corticoids |
|---|---|---|---|---|
| To 40 yr. | 25% | 11% | 0% | 0% |
| 40 to 50 yr. | 24% | 12% | 7% | 18% |
| 50 to 60 yr. | 26% | 22% | 19% | 6% |
| 60 to 70 yr. | 0/4 | 20% | 20% | 12% |
| 70 to 80 yr. | — | 29% | 48% | — |
| Over 80 yr. | — | 0/2 | 46% | 1/2 |
| No. of patients | 113 | 102 | 269 | 58 |

TABLE II

BREAST CANCER: EFFECT OF DOMINANT LESION ON PERCENTAGE OF RESPONSES ACHIEVED WITH THERAPY

| | Castration | | Androgens | Estrogens | | Corticoids | |
|---|---|---|---|---|---|---|---|
| | | | | Years postmenopausal | | | |
| Group | Radiation | Surgical | | $< 5$ | $> 5$ | $< 5$ | $> 5$ |
| Subjective responses | 17% | 31% | 80% | 15% | 11% | 48% | 41% |
| Objective responses | | | | | | | |
| Soft tissues | 39% | 23% | 23% | 3% | 28% | 7% | 7% |
| Bones | 22% | 16% | 24% | — | 1% | 7% | 0% |
| No. of patients | 25 | 88 | 102 | 34 | 235 | 29 | 29 |

dominantly osseous disease in one group, and consider together all those with soft-tissue disease not treatable by local X-ray or surgery. The results are shown on Table II in which (1) there is a suggestion that castration by whatever route causes more regressions in soft-tissue disease than in bone disease; and (2) there is no suggestion that testosterone is superior for osseous disease, and the effect of estrogen is largely on the soft-tissue disease. The objective response rate of cortisone in these patients is low in both groups.

## Ovary

Next examined was the controversial problem of the ovary. One of the impressions that has long underlain our approach to therapy is that certain tumors are not so much "estrogen dependent" as "hormonally manipulable," and if a patient responds to castration, this may be less related to tumor cell dependence upon estrogen from whatever source than to tumor cell sensitivity to alterations of many sorts in the hormonal environment. The responses to subsequent therapy on the part of patients undergoing castration and relapsing are summarized in Table III. Patients who respond

TABLE III

BREAST CANCER: PREDICTIVE VALUE OF RESPONSES TO CASTRATION

| Group | Number of patients | Number of responses | % Responses |
|---|---|---|---|
| I. Castration primary therapy | 113 | 20 | 17 |
| II. Secondarily treated | 87 | 11 | 13 |
| 1. Primary castration responders | | | |
| a. Secondary estrogen therapy | 3 | 1 | 33 |
| b. Secondary androgen therapy | 10 | 3 | 30 |
| c. Secondary corticoid therapy | 4 | 3 | 75 |
| 2. Primary castration failures | | | |
| a. Secondary estrogen therapy | 9 | 0 | 0 |
| b. Secondary androgen therapy | 38 | 2 | 5 |
| c. Secondary corticoid therapy | 23 | 2 | 9 |

initially to castration appear to have a better likelihood of responding to subsequent therapy of any sort, and there is a suggestion that in such patients corticoid therapy may be especially suitable. This may be in the nature of "medical hypophysectomy" since others have suggested that such patients may respond well to subsequent hypophysectomy.

Two comments may answer the query as to why not try to achieve synergism between corticoids and castration at the start: (1) The incidence of responses to castration in the older age groups is low so that such an approach might best be confined to women less than ten years postmenopausal. And (2) there may be a serious hazard in the use of corticoids in patients with liver disease. Nine such patients developed rapidly progressive and fatal liver involvement shortly after being started on corticoids. A similar situation seems to obtain with secondary hormonal therapy after initial estrogen therapy (Table IV) and after initial androgen therapy (Table V). In each of these instances, patients who respond well to primary therapy tend to respond well to secondary therapy whereas those who respond poorly initially rarely respond well later.

## Cortical Stromal Hyperplasia (CSH)

In addition to the type of response after removal of the ovaries, the cellular status of the organ itself at the time of surgery has come under suspicion as indicating something about the biologic propensities of the breast tumor in the host. Specifically, Sommers (5) and others have described a higher than normal incidence of cortical stromal hyperplasia in breast cancer patients. However, the data are not impressive regarding the

TABLE IV

BREAST CANCER: PREDICTIVE VALUE OF RESPONSES TO PRIMARY THERAPY WITH ESTROGENS

| Group | Number of patients | Number of responses | % Responses |
|---|---|---|---|
| I.  Estrogen primary therapy | 162 | 58 | 36 |
| II.  Secondarily treated | 29 | 4 | 14 |
| 1.  Primary estrogen responses | | | |
| a. Secondary estrogen therapy | 15 | 4 | 25 |
| 2.  Primary estrogen failures | | | |
| a. Secondary estrogen therapy | 10 | 0 | 0 |
| b. Secondary androgen therapy | 3 | 0 | 0 |
| c. Secondary castration therapy | 1 | 0 | 0 |

TABLE V

BREAST CANCER: PREDICTIVE VALUE OF RESPONSES TO PRIMARY THERAPY WITH ANDROGENS

| Group | Number of patients | Number of responses | % Responses |
|---|---|---|---|
| I.  Androgen primary therapy | 58 | 14 | 24 |
| II.  Secondarily treated | 14 | 3 | 21 |
| 1.  Primary androgen responses | | | |
| a. Secondary estrogen therapy | 2 | 1 | "50" |
| b. Secondary androgen therapy | 7 | 2 | 30 |
| 2.  Primary androgen failures | | | |
| a. Secondary estrogen therapy | 4 | 0 | 0 |
| b. Secondary androgen therapy | 3 | 0 | 0 |

incidence of CSH in oophorectomized patients, nor is the relationship between CSH at operation and subsequent good responses to antiestrogenic therapy, including oophorectomy. In order to evaluate the incidence of this condition objectively, two pathologists were asked to examine the slides on all patients having ovarian tissue sufficient for adequate diagnosis. Although each pathologist chose 26 % of these as showing significant cortical stromal hyperplasia, the cases they chose were often different ones, so that they were able to agree on only 13 % of the specimens. These figures are not significantly different from those given by Morris and Scully (3) for nontumor patients by age groups and do not confirm the higher reported cortical stromal hyperplasia incidence.

The prognostic value of cortical stromal hyperplasia for future therapy was not so easily dismissed. However, Table VI shows that patients who had CSH subsequently developed a 43 % objective response to castration as compared with a 19 % rate for the group as a whole. However, other data do not show that similarly high response rates were achieved on secondary administrative therapy with androgens (17 % response). To enable a more comparative view of the prognostic significance of cortical stromal hyperplasia, the prognostic significance of another, usually overlooked, ovarian cellular factor is shown in the same table. In this series, 22 % of patients were found to have ovarian metastases at operation—the pathologists had no difficulty in

TABLE VI

BREAST CANCER: CORTICAL STROMAL HYPERPLASIA AND METASTASES TO OVARIES FOUND AT CASTRATION AS PREDICTIVE FACTORS IN RESPONSE OF PATIENTS TO OOPHORECTOMY[a]

| | |
|---|---|
| Patients with cortical stromal hyperplasia | 13% |
| Responses with cortical stromal hyperplasia | 43% |
| Patients with ovarian metastases | 22% |
| Response with ovarian metastases | 43% |
| Over-all castration response | 19% |

[a] Total number of patients: 116.

agreeing on this figure—and these patients were found to have a higher response rate than patients with uninvolved ovaries. There was no higher rate of metastases to ovaries showing CSH than to others. Since ovarian metastases were found twice as commonly as CSH they may be a prognostic factor of much greater practical importance.

### Estrogenic Stimulation Test (EST)

There has been considerable interest in the estrogen stimulation test (2) as a prognostic factor in response to estrogenic therapy. Dr. B. J. Kennedy (1) long ago proved conclusively that untoward responses to estrogen, including hypercalcemia, malaise, and bone pain, did not necessarily preclude an ultimate clinical remission. We undertook to push estrogen therapy in a group of patients having such "positive" tests. Among nine such patients, in five therapy had to be stopped because of uncontrollable hypercalcemia, but in the four remaining patients three objective remissions were achieved. One wonders whether the positive estrogen test may merely be comparable to the "androgenic flare" which has come almost to be expected during the first two weeks of androgen therapy. At any rate, the over-all response rate of one-third is comparable to the series as a whole for estrogen responses in this age group. In our opinion a positive test is not necessarily a sign of poor prognosis.

### $P^{32}$ *Incorporation*

An attempt has been made (4) to relate the incorporation of $P^{32}$ by super-ficial nodules of breast tumor before and after therapy to the objective changes in tumor size induced by therapy, with a view to using these $P^{32}$ responses as an index of predictability in choice of patients for therapy. This technique is simpler than that of Drs. Taylor, Winzler, Perlia, Sky-Peck,

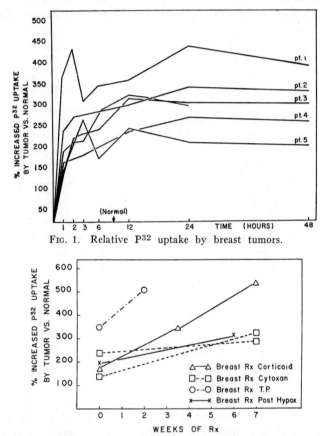

Fig. 1.  Relative $P^{32}$ uptake by breast tumors.

Fig. 2.  $P^{32}$ uptake during tumor progression.

and Kofman, and less biochemically informative but quite practical clini-cally in patients who are unwilling to undergo repeated biopsies. Figure 1 shows that breast tumor nodules when actively growing have uptakes which are significantly higher than the normal breast at periods from 24 hours on. Figure 2 shows that the 24-hour uptake tends to increase as tumor progres-sion occurs. Figure 3 shows that tumor regression is relatable to falls in

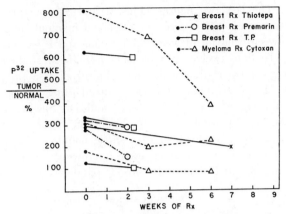

FIG. 3.   P³² uptake during tumor regression.

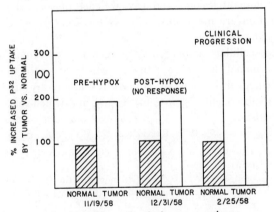

FIG. 4.   P³² uptake during progression.

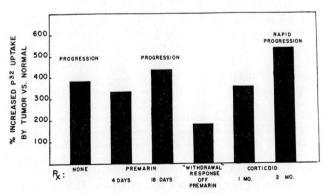

FIG. 5.   Predictive value of P³² uptake.

P³² uptakes. The last two figures (Figs. 4 and 5) chart the changes in single patients treated with a series of hormonal manipulations. The goodness of fit between behavior of measurable tumor and P³² uptake changes is encouraging. To date twelve such patients have been studied repeatedly; nine show a good correlation with their clinical disease progression, and three do not. There are many drawbacks in adapting the procedure to a test giving information of predictive value, and Dr. Nevinny is struggling with these. Among the problems are the limitation of the test to superficial tumors, nonrepresentative character of a single nodule (falls in P³² uptake may occur in one area while another lesion is growing), and the cumulative danger of giving repeated doses of P³² to one patient.

## CONCLUSIONS

Among cellular host factors that might predict the outcome of therapy, (1) age, (2) dominant lesion, and (3) presence of cortical stromal hyperplasia at castration are important, but (4) estrogen stimulation tests seem of doubtful prognostic value.

Among tumor cellular factors, (1) the tendency of tumor to respond to castration or hormonal therapy, (2) the propensity of tumor to go to ovaries, and (3) the changes in P³² uptake induced by therapy are often factors well correlated with subsequent response to therapy and which may be helpful in predicting responses.

### REFERENCES

1. Kennedy, B. J., Tibbetts, D. M., Nathanson, I. T., and Aub, J. C. *Cancer Research* **13**, 445-459 (1953).
2. Jessiman, A. G., and Moore, F. D. *In* "Carcinoma of the Breast," Medical Progress Series (*New Engl. J. Med.*) pp. 33-36. Little, Brown, Boston, Massachusetts, 1956.
3. Morris, J. McL., and Scully, R. E. "Endocrine Pathology of the Ovary," p. 151. Mosby, St. Louis, Missouri, 1958.
4. Nevinny, H. B., and Hall, T. C. *Proc. Am. Assoc. Cancer Research* **3**, 1, 47 (1959).
5. Sommers, S. C., and Teloh, H. A. *A.M.A. Arch. Pathol.* **53**, 160-166 (1952).

### DISCUSSION

**H. M. Lemon:** Dr. Bradford Patterson of Boston some years ago obtained an undifferentiated carcinoma of the testis which has now been carried through more than forty serial transplants in the hamster. Dr. Herbert Wotiz and I have studied this tumor and have found that it is synthesizing *in vivo* very large quantities of testosterone. Indeed, it was possible to obtain free testosterone from the transplant in considerable amounts, and this may be a research tool of interest to some individuals.

First, with reference to ovarian cortical stroma hyperplasia our impression is quite similar to yours—we do not find a clear-cut correlation between endocrine responsiveness to therapy and presence of this lesion. We also have found that the presence of metastatic carcinoma in the ovary seems to be, if there is any significance to these ovarian changes, as significant for prognosis as nodular cortical stroma hyperplasia. We do think, however, and this is important in relation to the age group of the patients whom you have oophorectomized, that ovarian stromal hyperplasia indicates estrogen secretion. This lesion is noteworthy as occurring in the postmenopausal patient over 60, and I notice a small portion of your oophorectomies in that age group, so I think you might find a higher incidence if you were practicing oophorectomy, as we do, up to the age of 70. Now this is pertinent also to your responses in cortisone-treated breast cancer cases. We have seldom seen—I personally have never seen—a remission on cortisone or prednisone in a patient below the age of 65 who has intact or irradiated ovaries. A single exception occurred in a woman who had had ovarian irradiation some ten years before. We think that this is due to the fact that cortisone and perhaps prednisone have some influence on the hypophysis which augments pituitary gonadotropin secretion. This has been the subject of a number of reports in the literature, including one by Dr. Segaloff, in which an increase in gonadotropin excretion following cortisone administration occurred. Dr. Agnes Burt Russell of Boston for several years has been assaying human pituitaries at autopsy and finds routinely in the cortisone-treated patients an extremely high content of gonadotropic hormone which would tend to bear this out. Everyone has encountered numerous failures in treating postmenopause breast cancer patients with intact ovaries with cortisone or prednisone. We think that what you are accomplishing with prednisone therapy is possibly some direct anti-estrogenic action on the tumor, but of course a very profound adrenal cortical atrophy also may result. This does result in disappearance of androsterone and etiocholanolone from the urine of treated patients, but not in a very regular or impressive or durable reduction in estrogen excretion (either bioassay or Brown method). Although adrenal estrogen stimulus to the tumor or possibly an adrenal androgen stimulus is reduced, it seems to me that the postmenopausal ovary and particularly these nodular hyperplastic ovaries which may retain capacities for steroid biogenesis, may be stimulated by the hypergonadotropic pituitary response, resulting in persistent estrogen secretion. I am encouraged very much to see that you have had some objective remissions in some of your oophorectomized patients.

T. Hall: The data that we have are really largely tangential to your data as regards cortical stromal hyperplasia and oophorectomy in the older age groups; it certainly does go up both in normals and patients with breast cancer. We wouldn't know very much about the older folk, although the data that we do have seem to suggest that there actually may be an augmentation of the effect of castration when cortisone is subsequently used in treatment.

E. E. Sproul: I should like to give some practical advice to Dr. Hall. I don't think it's necessary to have two pathologists look at these sections. One pathologist looking at the sections at different times would give you an equal difference of opinion. At the risk of singing the same tune too often I would like to point out that it is extremely important to study a large portion of any organ like the ovary for stromal hyperplasia. We cut sections at several levels through the block; this is extremely important in making any estimate of anything one is studying. The pathologist, I think, realizes this very strongly, but I find that very many chemists and clinicians will take a small biopsy and then extrapolate the findings to apply to the entire tumor and entire tissue.

# Glossary

NOTE: The glossary is for the convenience of the reader who encounters unfamiliar terms in this book and wants at least a helpful synonym. Self-explanatory terms, which are well defined in context or which have no common synonym, are not included. Synonyms for steroids are given principally in the IUPAC System to show interrelationships.

| Term | Synonym or definition |
|------|----------------------|

## A

| Term | Synonym or definition |
|------|----------------------|
| 2-AAF | 2-Acetylaminofluorene |
| ACTH | Adrenocorticotropic hormone; Corticotropin |
| Adrenosterone | 4-Androstene-3,11,17-trione |
| Aldosterone | 4-Pregnene-3,20-dione, 18-al-11β,21-dihydroxy- |
| 3β,17β-Androstanediol | Androstane-3β,17β-diol |
| Androstanedione | Androstane-3,17-dione |
| Androstan-3α-ol-17-one | Androstan-17-one, 3α-hydroxy-; Androsterone |
| Androstan-3β-ol-17-one | Androstan-17-one, 3β-hydroxy-; Epiandrosterone; Isoandrosterone |
| Androstan-17β-ol-3-one | Androstan-3-one, 17β-hydroxy-; Dihydrotestosterone |
| Androstan-3-one, 17β-hydroxy-2α-methyl-, propionate | 2α-Methyldihydrotestosterone propionate; Testosterone, 4,5α-Dihydro-2α-methyl-, propionate |
| Androstenediol | 5-Androstene-3β,17β-diol |
| 4-Androsten-17α-ol-3-one | 4-Androsten-3-one, 17α-hydroxy-; Epitestosterone; Cis-testosterone |
| 4-Androsten-17β-ol-3-one | 4-Androsten-3-one, 17β-hydroxy-; Testosterone |
| 5-Androsten-3β-ol-17-one | 5-Androsten-17-one, 3β-hydroxy-; Dehydroisoandrosterone; Dehydroepiandrosterone |
| Androsterone | Androstan-17-one, 3α-hydroxy-; Androstan-3α-ol-17-one |

## B

| Term | Synonym or definition |
|------|----------------------|
| BOP | 4-Pregnene-3,11,20-trione, 9α-bromo-; 9α-Bromo-11-ketoprogesterone |
| 9α-Bromo-11-ketoprogesterone | 4-Pregnene-3,11,20-trione, 9α-bromo-; 9α-Bromoxoprogesterone (BOP) |
| n-Butyl-19-nortestosterone | 19-Nor-4-androsten-3-one, 17α-n-butyl-17-hydroxy- |

## C

| Term | Synonym or definition |
|------|----------------------|
| CBG | Corticosteroid binding globulin; Transcortin |
| 4-Chloro-17α-methyl-testosterone | 4-Androsten-3-one, 4-chloro-17β-hydroxy-17-methyl- |
| Cholesterol | 5-Cholesten-3β-ol |
| Compound S (Reichstein) | 4-Pregnene-3,20-dione, 17α,21-dihydroxy- |
| Corticosterone | 4-Pregnene-3,20-dione, 11β,21-dihydroxy |
| Cortisol | 4-Pregnene-3,20-dione, 11β,17α,21-trihydroxy-; Hydrocortisone |
| Cortisone | 4-Pregnene-3,11,20-trione, 17α,21-dihydroxy- |
| Cortisone acetate | 4-Pregnene-3,11,20-trione, 17α,21-dihydroxy-, 21-acetate |

493

| Term | Synonym or definition |
|------|----------------------|
| | **D** |
| DDD | Ethane, 1,1-dichloro-2,2-bis(*p*-chlorophenyl)- |
| *o,p'*-DDD | Ethane, 1,1-dichloro-2-(*o*-chlorophenyl)-2-(*p*-chlorophenyl)-; 2-*o*-Chlorophenyl-2-*p*-chlorophenyl-1,1-dichloroethane |
| Decadron | 1,4-Pregnadiene-3,20-dione, 9α-fluoro-11β,17α,21-trihydroxy-16α-methyl-; 9α-Fluoro-16α-methylprednisolone; Dexamethasone; Hexadecadrol |
| Dehydrocorticosterone | 4-Pregnene-3,11,20-trione, 21-hydroxy- |
| Dehydroepiandrosterone | 5-Androsten-17-one, 3β-hydroxy-; 5-Androsten-3β-ol-17-one; Dehydroisoandrosterone |
| 6-Dehydroestradiol | 1,3,5(10),6-Estratetraene-3,17β-diol |
| 6-Dehydroestrone | 1,3,5(10),6-Estratetraen-17-one, 3-hydroxy- |
| 9(11)-Dehydroestrone | 1,3,5(10),9(11)-Estratetraen-17-one, 3-hydroxy- |
| 1-Dehydrohydrocortisone | 1,4-Pregnadiene-3,20-dione, 11β,17α,21-trihydroxy-; Prednisolone |
| Dehydroisoandrosterone | See Dehydroepiandrosterone |
| 1-Dehydrotestololactone | 13,17-Seco-1,4-androstadien-17-oic acid, 13α-hydroxy-3-keto-, lactone; Δ¹-Testololactone |
| Delalutin | 4-Pregnene-3,20-dione, 17α-hydroxy-, hexanoate; 17α-Hydroxyprogesterone 17-*n*-caproate; Progesterone, 17α-hydroxy-, hexanoate |
| Deoxycorticosterone | 4-Pregnene-3,20-dione, 21-hydroxy-; DOC |
| 11-Deoxycortisol | 4-Pregnene-3,20-dione, 17α-21-dihydroxy- |
| 3-Deoxyestradiol-17α | 1,3,5(10)-Estratrien-17α-ol |
| 17-Deoxyestradiol | 1,3,5(10)-Estratrien-3-ol |
| Dexamethasone | See Decadron |
| Dienestrol | Phenol, 4,4'-(1,2-diethylideneethylene)di- |
| Diethylstilbestrol | 4,4'-Stilbenediol, α,α'-diethyl-; Stilbestrol |
| 6α,9α-Difluoro-16α-hydroxy-prednisolone acetonide | 1,4-Pregnadiene-3,20-dione, 6α,9α-difluoro-11β,16α,17α,21-tetrahydroxy-, acetonide |
| 6α,9α-Difluoro-16α-methyl-prednisolone | 1,4-Pregnadiene-3,20-dione, 6α,9α-difluoro-11β,17α,21-trihydroxy-16α-methyl- |
| 6α,9α-Difluoroprednisolone acetate | 1,4-Pregnadiene-3,20-dione, 6α,9α-difluoro-11β,17α,21-trihydroxy-, 17-acetate |
| Dihydrotestosterone | Androstan-3-one, 17β-hydroxy-; Androstan-17β-ol-3-one |
| 17β,19-Dihydroxy-1,4-androstadien-3-one | 1,4-Androstadien-3-one, 17β,19-dihydroxy- |
| 3α,17α-Dihydroxypregnan-20-one | Pregnan-20-one, 3α,17α-dihydroxy- |
| 2,2-Dimethyldihydro-testosterone | Androstan-3-one, 17β-hydroxy-2,2-dimethyl-; Testosterone, 4,5α-dihydro-2,2-dimethyl- |
| 2α,17α-Dimethyldihydro-testosterone | Androstan-3-one, 17β-hydroxy-2α,17-dimethyl-; Testosterone, 4,5α-dihydro-2α,17-dimethyl- |
| 4,4-Dimethyldihydro-testosterone | Androstan-3-one, 17β-hydroxy-4,4-dimethyl-; Testosterone, 4,5α-dihydro-4,4-dimethyl- |

| Term | Synonym or definition |
|------|----------------------|
| 2α,17-Dimethyltestosterone | 4-Androsten-3-one, 17β-hydroxy-2α,17-dimethyl- |
| 6α,17-Dimethyltestosterone | 4-Androsten-3-one, 17β-hydroxy-6α,17-dimethyl- |
| DOC | See Deoxycorticosterone |

### E

| Term | Synonym or definition |
|------|----------------------|
| Epiandrosterone | Androstan-17-one, 3β-hydroxy-; Androstan-3β-ol-17-one; Isoandrosterone |
| 16-Epiestriol | 1,3,5(10)-Estratrien-3,16β,17β-triol |
| Epitestosterone | 4-Androsten-3-one, 17α-hydroxy-; 4-Androsten-17α-ol-3-one; Cistestosterone |
| 9β,11β-Epoxy-17-methyl-testosterone | 4-Androsten-3-one, 9β,11β-epoxy-17β-hydroxy-17-methyl- |
| Equilenin | 1,3,5(10),6,8-Estrapentaen-17-one, 3-hydroxy-; D-Equilenin |
| α-Estradiol | 1,3,5(10)-Estratriene-3,17α-diol |
| Estradiol-17β | 1,3,5(10)-Estratriene-3,17β-diol |
| Estradiolbenzoate | 1,3,5(10)-Estratriene-3,17β-diol, 3-benzoate; Estradiol-17β, 3-benzoate |
| Estriol | 1,3,5(10)-Estratriene-3,16α,17β-triol |
| Estrololactone | 13,17-Seco-1,3,5(10)-estratrien-17-oic acid, 3,13α-dihydroxy-, lactone |
| Estrone | 1,3,5(10)-Estratrien-17-one, 3-hydroxy- |
| 17-Ethyl-5(10)-estrenolone | 5(10)-Estren-3-one, 17α-ethyl-17-hydroxy- |
| 17α-Ethyl-19-nortestosterone | 19-Nor-4-androsten-3-one, 17α-ethyl-17-hydroxy-; Norethandrolone; Nilevar |
| Ethynyl estradiol | 1,3,5(10)-Estratriene-3,17β-diol, 17-ethynyl- |
| Ethynyl estradiol, 3-methyl ether | 1,3,5(10)-Estratriene-3,17β-diol, 17-ethynyl-, 3-methyl ether |
| 17-Ethynyl-5(10)-estrenolone | 5(10)-Estren-3-one, 17α-ethynyl-17-hydroxy- |
| Ethynyltestosterone | 4-Androsten-3-one, 17α-ethynyl-17-hydroxy-; 17-Ethynyltestosterone |
| Etiocholanolone | Etiocholan-17-one, 3α-hydroxy-; 5β-Androstan-17-one, 3α-hydroxy- |
| Etiocholan-17β-ol-3-one | Etiocholan-3-one, 17β-hydroxy-; 5β-Androstan-3-one, 17β-hydroxy- |

### F

| Term | Synonym or definition |
|------|----------------------|
| 6α-Fluoro-17α-acetoxy-progesterone | 4-Pregnene-3,20-dione, 6α-fluoro-17α-hydroxy-, 17-acetate |
| 10β-Fluoro-$\Delta^{1,4}$-androstadien-17β-ol-3-one | 1,4-Androstadien-3-one, 10β-fluoro-17β-hydroxy- |
| 9α-Fluorocorticosterone | 4-Pregnene-3,20-dione, 9α-fluoro-11β,21-dihydroxy- |
| 9α Fluorocortisol | 4-Pregnene-3,20-dione, 9α-fluoro-11β,17α,21-trihydroxy-; 9α-Fluorohydrocortisone |
| 9α-Fluorocortisone | 4-Pregnene-3,11,20-trione, 9α-fluoro-17α,21-dihydroxy- |
| 9α-Fluorocortisone bisethylene ketal | 4-Pregnene-3,11,20-trione, 9α-fluoro-17α,21-dihydroxy-, bisethylene ketal |

| Term | Synonym or definition |
|------|----------------------|
| 6-Fluoro-6-dehydro-17α-acetoxyprogesterone | 4,6-Pregnadiene-3,20-dione, 6-fluoro-17α-hydroxy-, 17-acetate |
| 2α-Fluoro-4,5α-dihydro-testosterone | Androstan-3-one, 2α-fluoro-17β-hydroxy- |
| 10β-Fluoro-4,5-dihydro-testosterone | Androstan-3-one, 10β-fluoro-17β-hydroxy- |
| 9α-Fluorohydrocortisone | 4-Pregnene-3,20-dione, 9α-fluoro-11β,17α,21-tri-hydroxy-; 9α-Fluorocortisol |
| 6α-Fluoro-17β-hydroxy-5α-androstan-3-one | Androstan-3-one, 6α-fluoro-17β-hydroxy- |
| 9α-Fluoro-11β-hydroxy-androstenedione | 4-Androstene-3,17-dione, 9α-fluoro-11β-hydroxy- |
| 9α-Fluoro-11β-hydroxy-17-methyltestosterone | 4-Androsten-3-one, 9α-fluoro-11β,17β-dihydroxy-17-methyl-; Halotestin; Fluoxymesterone |
| 9α-Fluoro-16α-hydroxy-prednisolone | 1,4-Pregnadiene-3,20-dione, 9α-fluoro-11β,16α,17α,21-tetrahydroxy- |
| 9α-Fluoro-11β-hydroxy-progesterone (FHP) | 4-Pregnene-3,20-dione, 9α-fluoro-11β-hydroxy- |
| 9α-Fluoro-11-keto-17-acetoxyprogesterone | 4-Pregnene-3,11,20-trione, 9α-fluoro-17-hydroxy-, acetate |
| 9α-Fluoro-11-keto-17-methyltestosterone | 4-Androstene-3,11-dione, 9α-fluoro-17β-hydroxy-17-methyl- |
| 9α-Fluoroprednisolone | 1,4-Pregnadiene-3,20-dione, 9α-fluoro-11β,17α,21-tri-hydroxy- |
| 9α-Fluoro-11β,16α,17α-trihydroxyprogesterone | 4-Pregnene-3,20-dione, 9α-fluoro-11β,16α,17α-trihydroxy- |
| 12α-Fluoro-11β,16α,17α-trihydroxyprogesterone | 4-Pregnene-3,20-dione, 12α-fluoro-11β,16α,17α-tri-hydroxy- |
| Fluoxymesterone | 4-Androsten-3-one, 9α-fluoro-11β,17β-dihydroxy-17-methyl-; Testosterone, 9α-fluoro-11β-hydroxy-17-methyl-; Halotestin; Oratestryl; Ultrandren |
| Fraction III-0 (Cohn) | A β-lipoprotein |
| FSH | Follicle-stimulating hormone |

**G**

| | |
|------|----------------------|
| GH | Growth hormone; Somatotropin |
| Globulin, corticosteroid binding | CBG; Transcortin |
| Glycoprotein, in α-1 fraction of seromucoid | Orosomucoid |

**H**

| | |
|------|----------------------|
| Halotestin | 4-Androsten-3-one, 9α-fluoro-11β,17β-dihydroxy-17-methyl-; 9α-Fluoro-11β-hydroxy-17-methyltestosterone; Fluoxymesterone |
| HCG | Human chorionic gonadotropin |
| Hexestrol | Phenol, 4,4'-(1,2-diethylethylene)di- |
| Hydrocortisone | See Cortisol |

| Term | Synonym or definition |
|------|----------------------|
| Hydrocortisone acetate | 4-Pregnene-3,20-dione, 11β,17α,21-trihydroxy-, 21-acetate |
| 11β-Hydroxy-Δ⁴-androstene-3,17-dione | 4-Androstene-3,17-dione, 11β-hydroxy- |
| 11β-Hydroxyandrosterone | Androstan-17-one, 3α,11β-dihydroxy- |
| 2-Hydroxyestradiol-17β | 1,3,5(10)-Estratriene-2,3,17β-triol |
| 4-Hydroxyestradiol-17β | 1,3,5(10)-Estratriene-3,4,17β-triol |
| 16α-Hydroxyestrone | 1,3,5(10)-Estratrien-17-one, 3,16α-dihydroxy- |
| 16β-Hydroxyestrone | 1,3,5(10)-Estratrien-17-one, 3,16β-dihydroxy- |
| 18-Hydroxyestrone | 1,3,5(10)-Estratrien-17-one, 3,18-dihydroxy- |
| 16α-Hydroxy-9α-fluoro-prednisolone | 1,4-Pregnadiene-3,20-dione, 9α-fluoro-11β,16α,17α,21-tetrahydroxy- |
| 17β-Hydroxy-17α-methyl-4,9(11)-androstadien-3-one | 4,9(11)-Androstadien-3-one, 17β-hydroxy-17-methyl-; Testosterone, 9(11)-dehydro-17-methyl- |
| 17β-Hydroxy-17-methyl-androstane-3,11-dione | Androstane-3,11-dione, 17β-hydroxy-17-methyl- |
| 2-Hydroxymethylene-17α-methyldihydrotestosterone | Androstan-3-one, 2-hydroxymethylene-17β-hydroxy-17-methyl- |
| 11α-Hydroxy-17-methyl-testosterone | 4-Androsten-3-one, 11α,17β-dihydroxy-17-methyl- |
| 17α-Hydroxypregnenolone | 5-Pregnen-20-one, 3β,17α-dihydroxy- |
| 17α-Hydroxypregnenolone-3-monoacetate | 5-Pregnen-20-one, 3β,17α-dihydroxy-, 3-acetate |
| 11α-Hydroxyprogesterone | 4-Pregnene-3,20-dione, 11α-hydroxy- |
| 11β-Hydroxyprogesterone | 4-Pregnene-3,20-dione, 11β-hydroxy- |
| 17α-Hydroxyprogesterone | 4-Pregnene-3,20-dione, 17α-hydroxy- |
| 17α-Hydroxyprogesterone-17-n-caproate | See Delalutin |
| 19-Hydroxytestosterone | 4-Androsten-3-one, 17β,19-dihydroxy- |

## I

| | |
|------|----------------------|
| ICSH | Interstitial cell-stimulating hormone |
| Isodienestrol | Phenol, 4,4′-(1,2-diethylideneethylene)di- |
| Isopropyl-19-nortestosterone | 19-Nor-4-androsten-3-one, 17β-hydroxy-17-isopropyl- |

## K

| | |
|------|----------------------|
| 11-Ketoandrosterone | Androstane-11,17-dione, 3α-hydroxy- |
| 7-Ketodehydroisoandrosterone | 5-Androstene-7,17-dione, 3β-hydroxy- |
| 16-Ketoestradiol | 1,3,5(10)-Estratrien-16-one, 3,17β-dihydroxy- |
| 16-Ketoestrone | 1,3,5(10)-Estratriene-16,17-dione, 3-hydroxy- |
| 11-Keto-17-methyltestosterone | 4-Androstene-3,11-dione, 17β-hydroxy-17-methyl- |
| 11-Ketoprogesterone | 4-Pregnene-3,11,20-trione |

## L

| | |
|------|----------------------|
| LH | Luteinizing hormone |
| β-Lipoprotein | Fraction III-0 (Cohn) |

| Term | Synonym or definition |
|------|----------------------|

**M**

Manvene — 1,3,5(10)-Estratriene-3,16β,17β-triol, 16-methyl-3-methyl ether; Mytatrienediol; Estradiol-17β,16β-hydroxy-16-methyl-, 3-methyl ether; 16α-Methyl-epiestriol-3-methyl ether

6-MAP — 4-Pregnene-3,20-dione, 17α-hydroxy-6α-methyl-, acetate; 6α-Methyl-17α-acetoxyprogesterone; Provera

Methallenestril — 2-Naphthalenepropionic acid, β-ethyl-6-methoxy-α,α-dimethyl-; Vallestril

17-(2-Methallyl)-19-nortestosterone — 19-Nor-4-androsten-3-one, 17β-hydroxy-17-(2-methallyl)-

2-Methoxyestradiol — 1,3,5(10)-Estratriene-3,17β-diol, 2-methyl ether

2-Methoxyestriol — 1,3,5(10)-Estratriene-3,16α,17β-triol, 2-methyl ether

2-Methoxyestrone — 1,3,5(10)-Estratrien-17-one, 3-hydroxy-, 2-methyl ether

6α-Methyl-17α-acetoxyprogesterone — 4-Pregnene-3,20-dione, 17α-hydroxy-6α-methyl-, acetate; Provera; 6-MAP

17-Methylandrostenediol — 5-Androstene-3β,17β-diol, 17-methyl-; Methylandrostenediol

16α-Methylandrosterone — Androstan-17-one, 3α-hydroxy-16α-methyl-

11α-Methyl-9α-chlorocortisol — 4-Pregnene-3,20-dione, 9α-chloro-11,17α,21-trihydroxy-11α-methyl-

Methylcholanthrene — 3-Methylcholanthrene; 20-Methylcholanthrene

9α-Methylcortisol — 4-Pregnene-3,20-dione, 11β,17α,21-trihydroxy-9α-methyl-; 9α-Methylhydrocortisone

6α-Methyl-21-deoxy-9α-fluoroprednisolone — 1,4-Pregnadiene-3,20-dione, 9α-fluoro-11β,17α-dihydroxy-6α-methyl-

2α-Methyldihydrotestosterone — Androstan-3-one, 17β-hydroxy-2α-methyl; Testosterone, 4,5α-dihydro-2α-methyl-

16-Methyleneandrosterone — Androstan-17-one, 3α-hydroxy-16-methylene-

1-Methylestradiol-17β — 1,3,5(10)-Estratriene-3,17β-diol, 1-methyl-

6α-Methyl-9α-fluoro-17-acetoxy-21-deoxyprednisolone — 1,4-Pregnadiene-3,20-dione, 9α-fluoro-11β,17α-dihydroxy-6α-methyl-, 17-acetate; U-17323

6α-Methyl-9α-fluoroprednisolone — 1,4-Pregnadiene-3,20-dione, 9α-fluoro-11β,17α,21-trihydroxy-6α-methyl-

9α-Methyl-11-ketoprogesterone bisethylene ketal — 4-Pregnene-3,11,20-trione, 9α-methyl-, bisethylene ketal

12α-Methyl-11-ketoprogesterone bisethylene ketal — 4-Pregnene-3,11,20-trione, 12α-methyl, bisethylene ketal

Methyl-19-nortestosterone — 19-Nor-4-androsten-3-one, 17β-hydroxy-17-methyl-; 17-MNT

2-Methyl-19-nortestosterone — 19-Nor-4-androsten-3-one, 17β-hydroxy-2-methyl-

6α-Methylprednisolone — 1,4-Pregnadiene-3,20-dione, 11β,17α,21-trihydroxy-6α-methyl-

17α-Methyltestosterone — 4-Androsten-3-one, 17β-hydroxy-17-methyl-

Mytatrienediol — See Manvene

| Term | Synonym or definition |
|------|----------------------|

## N

| | |
|------|----------------------|
| Nilevar | 19-Nor-4-androsten-3-one, 17α-ethyl-17-hydroxy-; 17α-Ethyl-19-nortestosterone; Norethandrolone |
| 2-Nitroestrone | 1,3,5(10)-Estratrien-17-one, 3-hydroxy-2-nitro- |
| 4-Nitroestrone | 1,3,5(10)-Estratrien-17-one, 3-hydroxy-4-nitro- |
| A-Norcortisol | A-Nor-3(5)-pregnene-2,20-dione, 11β,17α,21-trihydroxy- |
| Norethandrolone | See Nilevar |
| Norethyndrone | 19-Nor-4-androsten-3-one, 17α-ethynyl-17-hydroxy-; 19-Norethynyltestosterone; Norlutin; 17-Ethynyl-19-nortestosterone |
| Norethynodrel | 5(10)-Estren-3-one, 17α-ethynyl-17-hydroxy-; Enovid |
| 19-Norethynyltestosterone | See Norethyndrone |
| Norlutin | See Norethyndrone |
| A-Norprogesterone | A-Nor-3(5)-pregnene-2,20-dione |
| 19-Norprogesterone | 19-Nor-4-pregnene-3,20-dione |
| B-Nortestosterone | 16-Nor-4-androsten-3-one, 17β-hydroxy- |
| 19-Nortestosterone | 19-Nor-4-androsten-3-one, 17β-hydroxy- |

## O

| | |
|------|----------------------|
| Orosomucoid | A glycoprotein, in α-1 fraction of seromucoid |

## P

| | |
|------|----------------------|
| PBI | Protein-bound iodine |
| Prednisolone | 1,4-Pregnadiene-3,20-dione, 11β,17α,21-trihydroxy-; 1-Dehydrohydrocortisone |
| Prednisone | 1,4-Pregnadiene-3,11,20-trione, 17α,21-dihydroxy- |
| Pregnanediol | Pregnane-3α,20α-diol |
| Pregnanetriol | Pregnane-3α,17α,20α-triol |
| Δ⁵-Pregnene-3α,20α-diol | 5-Pregnene-3α,20α-diol |
| Δ⁵-Pregnene-3β,16α,20α-triol | 5-Pregnene-3β,16α,20α-triol |
| Pregnenolone | 5-Pregnen-20-one, 3β-hydroxy- |
| Premarin | Conjugated equine estrogen (estrone sulfate) |
| Progesterone | 4-Pregnene-3,20-dione |
| Progesterone, 17α-hydroxy-hexanoate | 4-Pregnene-3,20-dione, 17α-hydroxy-, hexanoate; 17α-Hydroxyprogesterone 17-n-caproate; Delalutin |
| Prolactin | A protein of anterior pituitary origin, with luteotropic and lactogenic properties |
| Proluton (progesterone in oil) | See Progesterone |
| 17β-Propionoxy-2α-methyl-androstan-3-one | Androstan-3-one, 17β-hydroxy-2α-methyl-, propionate; Testosterone, 1,5α dihydro 2α methyl-, propionate |
| 17-Propyl-19-nortestosterone | 19-Nor-4-androsten-3-one, 17β-hydroxy-17-propyl- |
| Propynyl-19-nortestosterone | 19-Nor-4-androsten-3-one, 17β-hydroxy-17-propynyl- |
| Provera | 4-Pregnene-3,20-dione, 17α-hydroxy-6α-methyl-, acetate; 6-MAP; 6α-Methyl-17α-acetoxyprogesterone |

| Term | Synonym or definition |
| --- | --- |
| | **S** |
| Somatotropin | Pituitary growth hormone |
| SPF-17874 | A suspending vehicle containing an aqueous solution of sodium chloride, polysorbate 80, carboxymethylcellulose, and benzyl alcohol |
| Stilbestrol | 4,4'-Stilbenediol, α,α'-diethyl-; Diethylstilbestrol |
| | **T** |
| TBP | Thyroxine-binding protein |
| Testololactone | 13,17-Seco-4-androsten-17-oic acid, 13α-hydroxy-3-keto-, lactone |
| Δ¹-Testololactone | 13,17-Seco-1,4-androstadien-17-oic acid, 13α-hydroxy-3-keto-, lactone; 1-Dehydrotestololactone |
| Testosterone | 4-Androsten-3-one, 17β-hydroxy-; 4-Androsten-17β-ol-3-one |
| Testosterone enanthate | 4-Androsten-3-one, 17β-hydroxy-, heptanoate; Testosterone heptanoate |
| Tetrahydrocortisone | Pregnane-11,20-dione, 3α,17α,21-trihydroxy- |
| Tetrahydro S | Pregnane-20-one, 3α,17,21-trihydroxy- |
| Thyroxine | 3,5,3',5'-Tetraiodothyronine |
| Transcortin | A specific cortisol-binding protein |
| Triamcinolone | 1,4-Pregnadiene-3,20-dione, 9α-fluoro-11β,16α,17α,21-tetrahydroxy- |
| 2,2,17α-Trimethyldihydro-testosterone | Androstan-3-one, 17β-hydroxy-2,2,17-trimethyl-; Testosterone, 4,5α-dihydro-2,2,17-trimethyl- |
| 7-Tritiated dehydroiso-androsterone | 5-Androsten-17-one, 3β-hydroxy-, 7-tritiated |
| 6,7-Tritiated estradiol | 6,7-Tritiated-1,3,5(10)-Estratriene-3,17β-diol |
| 6,7-Tritiated estrone | 6,7-Tritiated-1,3,5(10)-Estratrien-17-one, 3-hydroxy- |
| 9,11-Tritiated estrone | 9,11-Tritiated-1,3,5(10)-Estratrien-17-one, 3-hydroxy- |
| | **V** |
| Vallestril | See Methallenestril |
| 17α-Vinylnortestosterone | 19-Nor-4-androsten-3-one, 17β-hydroxy-17-vinyl- |
| 17α-Vinyltestosterone | 4-Androsten-3-one, 17β-hydroxy-17-vinyl- |

# Author Index

Numbers in parentheses are reference numbers and are included to assist in locating the reference where the authors' names are not mentioned in the text. Numbers in italics refer to the page on which the reference is listed.

## A

Abarbanel, A. R., 446 (18), 447 (18), *455*

Adair, F. E., 40 (88), *56,* 199 (1), *207,* 355 (2), *362*

Adams, J. A., 149 (29), *155*

Adams, R. A., 307 (7), *327*

Aegerter, E. A., 3 (18), 4 (18), *6*

Aitken, E. H., 118, *122*

Aizawa, Y., 131 (1), 133 (1), *141*

Akazawa, T., 153, *155*

Albert, A., 33, *54,* 393, *395*

Albert, S., 45, *54*

Albright, F., 93, *105,* 189, *195, 196*

Allen, W. M., 40 (88), *56,* 355 (2), *362*

Alling, E. J., 477 (6), *482*

Alper, R. G., 393 (3), *395*

Alpert, L. K., 414 (1), *422*

Andervont, H. B., 211 (1), *220*

Andrec, K., 115 (51), *123*

Anliker, R., 447, *455*

Ansfield, F., 367, 368, *374*

Antoniades, H. N., 61 (11), 62 (11), 71 (11), *73*

Applegate, H. E., 21, *23*

Arhelger, S. W., 46, *54*

Armaghan, V., 323 (1), *327*

Armstrong, E. C., 3, *5*

Artenstein, M., *376*

Astwood, E. B., 130 (2), *141*

Aub, J. C., 189 (26), *196,* 487 (1), *490*

Avery, R. C., 308 (23), *328*

Awapara, J., 180 (1, 18), *186*

Axelrod, J., 114 (2), *122*

Ayer, J. P., 414 (33), *423*

Ayres, P. J., 99, *105,* 454 (2), *455*

## B

Babcock, J. C., 16 (17), *22*

Baggett, B., 113 (19), 114 (20a, 21), 116 (3), *122,* 449 (39, 40, 42), 450 (42), 451 (3), 452 (4), *455, 456*

Bailey, G. A., 20 (14), *22*

Baker, W., 370, 371, *374*

Balderas, L., 116 (3), *122,* 452 (4), *455*

Barnes, L. E., 269 (9), *300*

Barron, E. S. G., 180 (2), *186*

Bartter, F. C., 66 (8), 69, *73*

Basinski, D. H., 477 (3), 478 (3), 479 (3), *482*

Baskin, A., 450 (26), *456*

Batres, E., 16 (25), 18 (26), *22*

Bauer, G. C. H., 189 (4, 6), 192, *196*

Bauld, W. S., 112 (42), 118, *122, 123*

Beckett, V. L., 26 (3), 34 (3), *54*

Bell, H. G., 345 (10), 346 (10), 351, (10), *353*

Bellin, J., 189 (7), 191 (7), *196*

Benda, C. E., 189 (8), *196*

Benua, R. S., 77 (1), *89*

Bergenstal, D. M., 465 (4), 467 (1), 472 (1), *473*

Berger, E., 191 (24), *196*

Bergstresser, D., 323 (1), *327*

Bergstrom, S., 151, *155*

Berliner, D. L., *76,* 113 (49), *123,* 452, *456*

Bern, H. A., 319 (20), *327*

Bernasconi, C., 480 (1), *482*

Bernstein, T. C., 413 (31), 414 (31), *423*

Berson, S. A., 413 (31), 414 (31), *423*

Bertrand, J., 66 (7), *73, 75*

Beyler, R. E., 19 (15), *22*

Bianchi, A., 11 (19), 22 (18), *22*

Bielschowsky, F., 3, *5,* 332 (1), *338*

Birke, G., 96 (19), *105,* 451 (34), *456*

Black, F., 96 (4), 99 (4), *105*

Blackburn, C. M., 30, 31, 33, 34 (5), 36 (5), *54,* 365, 367, *374*

Blair, S., 258 (7), 287 (7), *300*

Bleisch, V. R., 39 (31), *54*

Bloch, E., 104 (18), *105,* 451 (5), *455*

Block, H. W., 463 (11), *473*

Bloom, B. M., 16, *22*

Bloomberg, E., 189 (2), *195*

Bodansky, O., 77 (1), *89*

# Subject Index

## A

Ablation therapy
effect of timing in breast cancer, 350
effects on mammary tumors
in Sprague-Dawley rats, 5
various species, 2
evaluation by joint project, 343
evaluation of survival statistics, 351
use in mammary carcinoma, 343, 352
Acetate, as precursor of steroid hormones, 445
Acetate-1-C$^{14}$, incubation with tumor tissue, 451, 453
2-Acetylaminofluorene, used to induce tumors, 3
3-Acetylpyridine, as hydrogen receptor, 149
ACTH
action with testosterone on rat prostate, 180
effect on C3H mammary tumor, 286
responsiveness of adrenal tumors, 451, 453, 454
Adenocarcinoma
endometrial, 427
mammary, in C3H mice
affected by gonadotropin, 286
effect of luteotropin and growth hormone, 286
growth retarded by ACTH, 286
growth retarded by corticoids, 287
not affected by deoxycorticosterone, 287
not affected by sex steroids, 286
prednisolone effects related to host hormone, 287-290
Adrenal
site of hormone-producing tumors, 452-454
Adrenal androgen
evidence for existence, 93
source of precursors, 96
Adrenal cancer, regression induced by o,p'-DDD, 463
Adrenalectomy
inhibition of rat mammary fibroadenoma, 266
use in mammary carcinoma, 344

Adrenal function, suppression by o,p'-DDD, 463
Adrenocortical steroids, see also Individual compounds
effect on mammary adenocarcinoma in rats, 241, 247
Adrenocorticotropic hormone, see ACTH
Adrenosterone, produced by ovarian tumor, 446
Albumin
relationship to regression and progression, 477, 479
in serum of breast cancer patients, 477
and steroid binding, 61, 62
Aldosterone, from adrenal tumors, in vitro and in vivo, 454
Aldosteronism, relieved by removal of tumor, 454
American College of Physicians, study of endocrine ablative surgery, 343
American College of Surgeons, study of endocrine ablative surgery, 343
American Medical Association, statistics on survival in breast cancer, 346, 351
Anabolicity
of 17-ethyl-19-nortestosterone, 34
of 2-methyldihydrotestosterone, 34
of testosterone in cancer patients, 34
Anabolism, see also Metabolism
effects of estrogen in rat uterus, 130, 134, 136
protein synthesis induced by estrogen, 132, 134
Androgen, effects on calcium pool, 191, 192
Androgenicity
as a factor in prostatic cancer, 37
preputial gland as test object, 31
as related to antitumor effect, 31, 34
related to effect on mammary fibroadenoma, 271-275, 279, 285
virilizing effects in cancer drugs, 26, 31
Androgens
in adrenal cancer, 451
in benign adrenal tumor, 453
effect on biochemistry of the prostate, 179

11α-Hydroxyprogesterone, effects on human tumor implants in hamsters, 322

11β-Hydroxyprogesterone, as starting material for glucocorticoids, 12

17α-Hydroxyprogesterone, produced by ovarian tumor, 448

17α-Hydroxyprogesterone, 17-acetate
effects on human tumor implants in hamsters, 322

17β-Hydroxysteroid dehydrogenase, 148

16α-Hydroxytestosterone, conversion to 16α-hydroxyestrone, 117

Hyperplasia
benign nodular, of the prostate, 181

Hypokalemia, during treatment with steroids, 394

Hypophysectomy
effect on dependent tumors in mice, 216
effect on mouse mammary tumor, 340
use in mammary carcinoma, 343-344

## I

Incorporation, see Uptake

Incorporation pattern
of radioactive estrogens
in rat tissues, 164
in target and non-target organs, 166-167
in uteri and liver of rats, 171-172
related to hormone antagonism, 172

Inhibition
of estrogen responses by progestins, 172
of pituitary
other than gonadotropin, 32, 33
related to antitumor effect, 32
by steroids, 38, 48

Isocitrate, in hydrogen transfer, 147

Isoflavones, in hydrogen transfer, 150

## J

Jaundice, in patients treated with 17-MNT, 399

## K

11-Ketoandrosterone, excreted by patient with ovarian tumor, 446

16-Ketoestradiol
in vivo from estradiol, 114
in normal urine, 112
use in treatment of breast cancer, 40

16-Ketoestrone
in normal urine, 112
use in treatment of breast cancer, 40

α-Ketoglutarate, in hydrogen transfer, 147

$\Delta^4$-3-Ketone, introduction of 6-fluorine atom, 16

17-Ketosteroid
contribution by the testes, 103
11-deoxy and 11-oxygenated compounds, 94
excretion, relation to clinical effectiveness, 35

17-Ketosteroids
in Cushing's syndrome, 453
effect of o,p'-DDD on excretion, 467
increased in chorionepithelioma, 448
as index of prostatic cancer activity, 409
and interstitial cell tumor, 449-450
and masculinizing adrenal cancer, 451
originating in arrhenoblastoma, 447
originating in lipoid cell tumor, 446
and undifferentiated testicular tumor, 450

17-KS, see 17-Ketosteroids

## L

Liver, and 3α-hydroxysteroid, 149

Lung cancer, see Bronchogenic carcinoma

Luteinizing hormone (LH), effect on dependent tumors in mice, 215-216

Luteotropin, effect on C3H mammary tumor, 286

## M

Malignancy, criteria in experimental tumors, 301

Mechanism of action
meaning in biological studies, 161
method used in uptake studies, 130
objectives of estrogen studies, 129, 132
résumé of estrogen studies, 140-141
uptake hypothesis of antagonism, 173

Menopausal age, as factor in response of breast cancer to treatment, 356

Metabolism, see also Biosynthesis
of acetate-1-$C^{14}$ in tumors, 451
of calcium
affected by steroids, 189, 196
compared with strontium, 197

globulin, 63

α-glycoprotein, 65

progesterone binding, 62

steroid binding, 61, 73

testosterone binding, 62

transcortin, 67

Protocol study

criteria for admission, breast cancer, 363

of standard reference steroids, 356

of steroids used in breast cancer, 363, 386, 389, 397

*Pseudomonas testosteroni,* dehydrogenases, 149

3-Pyridine aldehyde, as hydrogen receptor, 149

Pyridine nucleotide

reduction inhibited by steroids, 159

reduction by placental enzyme, 148

reduction by uterine cytoplasmic particles, 154

Pyrogenicity

of etiocholanolone, 115

### R

Resistance, *see* Hormone resistance

Responsiveness, to dihydrotestosterone, loss by rat tumor, 258

Ribonucleic acid, changes in rat uterus after estrogen, 131, 144

RNA, and incorporation of formate-C-14, 206

### S

Screening, use of denervated muscle for implants, 303

Sequential testing, use in prostatic cancer trials, 406

Serine, protein-bound

and incorporation of formate-$C^{14}$, 205

Serine aldolase activity, estrogen-induced alterations, 139

Shimkin's series, statistics on survival in breast cancer, 349, 350, 351

17-Spirolactones, as competitive antagonists to aldosterone, 44

Steroids, *see also* individual compounds

affecting morphology and biochemistry, 160

effect on methylcholanthrene-induced tumors, 30

effects on heterologously transplanted tumors, 307

and *in vitro* uptake of formate-$C^{14}$, 199

reasons for association with cancer, 307

as substrates in hydrogen transfer, 149

toxicity associated with tumor effects, 314

$C_{18}$ Steroids, antitumor effects in Swiss mice, 316-318

$C_{19}$ Steroids, antitumor effects in Swiss mice, 316

$C_{21}$ Steroids, antitumor effects in Swiss mice, 314

Steroid structure

cleavage between 17 and 20, 13 and 17, 10

contraction of ring structure, 20

dehydrogenation at the 1,2-position, 10

9α-halogenation, 11, 14

16α-halogenation, 19

hydroxylation

at the 18-position, 10

at 11β,17α- and 21-positions, 9

introduction of 6-fluorine atom, 16

methylation in 2- and 6-position, 11

microbial transformations, 9

related to effects on rat tumors, 279, 295

scission between carbon atoms, 10

structure-activity relationships, 12

synthesis of A-norcortisol, 20

Stilbenes, *see also* Estrogens, Diethylstilbestrol, Hexestrol

Stilbestrol, *see also* Diethylstilbestrol

in treatment of prostatic cancer, 405

### T

TACE [Ethylene, 1-chloro-1,2,2-tris(*p*-methoxyphenyl)-], effect on induced mammary tumor, 6

Target tissue, contrasted with non-target tissue, 174, 176

Testis, site of hormone-producing tumors, 448-452

Testololactone, oxidation to ring-D lactones, 11

Δ¹-Testololactone

derived from progesterone, 10

in treatment of breast cancer, 372, 389